This book is dedicated to all of our curr
former residents at the Ventura County Med

a LANGE medical book

CURRENT
Practice Guidelines in
Primary Care
2023

Jacob A. David, MD, FAAFP
Associate Program Director
Family Medicine Residency Program
Ventura County Medical Center
Clinical Instructor
UCLA School of Medicine
Ventura, California

New York   Chicago   San Francisco   Athens   London   Madrid
Mexico City   Milan   New Delhi   Singapore   Sydney   Toronto

CURRENT Practice Guidelines in Primary Care, 2023

1 2 3 4 5 6 7 8 9   LCR   27 26 25 24 23 22

ISBN 978-1-264-89222-8
MHID 1-264-89222-5
ISSN 1528-1612

This book was set in Minion Pro by MPS Limited.
The editor was Kay Conerly.
The production supervisor was Catherine Saggese.
Project management was provided by Poonam Bisht, MPS Limited.

This book is printed on acid-free paper.

Contents

*= updated guideline for 2023 edition
**=new topic for the 2023 edition

Contributors

Jemma Alarcón, MD MPH

Resident Physician, Family Medicine Residency Program, Ventura County Medical Center
Ventura, California
[Chapters 4, 7]

Ryan Arams, MD MS

Resident Physician, Family Medicine Residency Program, Ventura County Medical Center
Ventura, California
[Chapters 19, 28]

David Araujo, MD FAAFP

Program Director and DIO, Family Medicine Residency Program, Ventura County Medical Center
Associate Clinical Professor, David Geffen School of Medicine at UCLA
Ventura, California
[Chapters 6, 10, 15, 16, 24, 31]

Mariam Asper, DO

Resident Physician, Family Medicine Residency Program, Ventura County Medical Center
Ventura, California
[Chapters 17, 20, 27, 32]

Wallace Baker, MD FAAFP

Director Global Health Fellowships, Family Medicine Residency Program, Ventura County Medical Center
Ventura, California
[Chapters 9, 22, 30]

Sarah Manon Begert, DO

Resident Physician, Family Medicine Residency Program, Ventura County Medical Center
Ventura, California
[Chapters 25, 26]

Nastassja Bell, MD

Resident Physician, Family Medicine Residency Program, Ventura County Medical Center
Ventura, California
[Chapters 1, 14, 18, 29]

Allyson Brome, DO
Resident Physician, Family Medicine Residency Program, Ventura County Medical Center
Ventura, California
[Chapters 2, 3, 5, 8, 11, 15]

Margaret Clark, MD
Resident Physician, Family Medicine Residency Program, Ventura County Medical Center
Ventura, California
[Chapters 6, 10, 15, 16, 24, 31]

Jacob David, MD FAAFP
Associate Program Director, Family Medicine Residency Program, Ventura County Medical Center
Clinical Instructor, David Geffen School of Medicine at UCLA
Ventura, California
[Chapters 21, 23]

Dorothy DeGuzman, MD MPH FAAFP
Associate Program Director, Family Medicine Residency Program, Ventura County Medical Center
Ventura, California
[Chapters 12, 13]

Daniel Farnsworth, DO
Resident Physician, Family Medicine Residency Program, Ventura County Medical Center
Ventura, California
[Chapters 9, 22, 30]

Micah Gamble, MD
Resident Physician, Family Medicine Residency Program, Ventura County Medical Center
Ventura, California
[Chapters 21, 23]

Neil Jorgensen, MD
Core Faculty, Family Medicine Residency Program, Ventura County Medical Center
Ventura, California
[Chapters 2, 3, 5, 8, 11, 15]

Tipu Khan, MD FAAFP FASAM
Fellowship Director, Primary Care Addiction Medicine Fellowship
Core Faculty, Family Medicine Residency Program, Ventura County Medical Center
Adjunct Associate Clinical Professor, USC Keck SOM
Ventura, California
[Chapters 1, 14, 18, 29]

Cheryl Lambing, MD

Core Faculty, Family Medicine Residency Program, Ventura County Medical Center
Ventura, California
[Chapters 17, 20, 27, 32]

Rachel Mueller, DO

Resident Physician, Family Medicine Residency Program, Ventura County Medical Center
Ventura, California
[Chapters 6, 10, 15, 16, 24, 31]

John Nuhn, MD

Faculty Development Fellow, Family Medicine Residency Program, Ventura County Medical Center
Ventura, California
[Chapters 19, 28]

Michael Paglia, DO

Resident Physician, Family Medicine Residency Program, Ventura County Medical Center
Ventura, California
[Chapters 1, 14, 18, 29]

Kristi Schoeld, MD

Core Faculty, Family Medicine Residency Program, Ventura County Medical Center
Clinical Instructor, David Geffen School of Medicine at UCLA
Ventura, California
[Chapters 4, 7]

Zachary Zwolak, DO FAAFP FASAM

Associate Program Director, Family Medicine Residency Program, Ventura County Medical Center
Core Faculty, Primary Care Addiction Medicine Fellowship, Ventura County Medical Center
Ventura, California
[Chapters 25, 26]

Preface

Current Practice Guidelines in Primary Care 2023 is intended for all clinicians interested in updated evidence-based guidelines for primary care topics in ambulatory and hospital settings. This handy reference consolidates information from national medical associations and government agencies into concise recommendations and guidelines covering virtually all primary care topics. This book is organized into topics related to disease screening and prevention for the general population, for specific population groups, and disease management, and further subdivided into organ systems for quick reference to the evaluation and treatment of the most common primary care disorders.

The 2023 edition of *Current Practice Guidelines in Primary Care* contains updates reflecting more than 140 new guidelines. There are significant updates to several guidelines including cervical cancer screening, colorectal cancer screening, management of sexually transmitted infections, HIV prevention, headache, chronic pain, and gout. This edition also includes several new topics including coronavirus disease, trauma-informed care, vaginitis, vulvar diseases, pyelonephritis, abnormal uterine bleeding, and acne. Residents, medical students, midlevel providers, and practicing physicians in family medicine, internal medicine, pediatrics, and obstetrics and gynecology alike will find it a great resource.

Several guidelines include race as a consideration in their approaches to care. As race is a primarily social construct and purportedly scientific mechanisms to explain racial differences in outcomes are rooted in biased data, guidelines that suggest differentiating care by race should be considered with caution. Drs. Vyas, Einstein, and Jones offer a thoughtful assessment at NEJM 2020;383:847-882 (https://www.nejm.org/doi/full/10.1056/NEJMms2004740).

Although painstaking efforts have been made to find all errors and omissions, some may remain. If you find an error or wish to suggest a change, please e-mail at EditorialServices@mheducation.com.

Evidence-based guidelines such as those reviewed in this book are wonderful tools. They enable management strategies to be standardized and disseminated to a broad swath of the medical profession. At their best, they offer immediate access to the wisdom and analytical approach to data-driven medical care employed by the experts, elevating the quality of our care. But, as with any human endeavor, they are susceptible to bias and misunderstanding. While evidence-based guidelines increasingly dictate the standards for our clinical practice, the highest quality medical care will always derive from a clinician's experience, curiosity, critical thinking, compassion, and personal relationship with a patient. In that spirit, please use the tools in this book to further hone your craft.

Jacob A. David, MD, FAAFP

Screening and Prevention, Adults

This section addresses screening measures and primary prevention recommendations for adults. Specific population groups such as newborns and infants, children and adolescents, women, men, and older adults are addressed in Section 2. Unless otherwise specified, screening and prevention recommendations apply generally to an adult population at average risk.

Behavioral Health and Substance Use Disorders

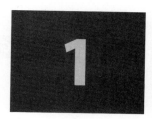

ALCOHOL USE DISORDERS

Organizations
▶ CDC 2018, USPSTF 2018

Screening Recommendations
–Screen all adults in primary care settings for alcohol misuse, including pregnant people.
–If positive, administer a brief behavioral counseling intervention and offer or refer for diagnostic assessment.

Comments
1. Screen regularly using a validated tool such as the AUDIT, CAGE, or MAST questionnaires.
2. The TWEAK, T-ACE, and 4P's Plus are designed to screen pregnant people for alcohol misuse.

Sources
–CDC. *Alcohol Screening and Brief Intervention for People Who Consume Alcohol and Use Opioids.* 2018.
–USPSTF. *JAMA.* 2018;320(18):1899-1909.
–ASAM. *Public Policy Statement on Screening for Addiction in Primary Care Settings.* 1997.

DEPRESSION

Organization
▶ USPSTF 2016

Screening Recommendations
–Screen adults for depression, including pregnant and postpartum women.
–If positive, confirm diagnosis, offer effective treatment, and ensure appropriate follow-up.

Comments
1. A positive PHQ-2 should be followed by a PHQ-9 or a similar instrument, to diagnose depression.
2. Optimal screening interval is unknown. AAP recommends screening mothers for postpartum depression at the infant's 1-, 2-, 4-, and 6-mo visits.

Source
–USPSTF. *JAMA.* 2016;315(4):380-387.

ILLICIT DRUG USE

Organization
▶ USPSTF 2020

Screening Recommendation
–Screen and implement a treatment care plan.

Comment
1. The NIH hosts a collection of screening tools at https://nida.nih.gov/nidamed-medical-health-professionals/screening-tools-resources/chart-screening-tools

Source
–USPSTF. *JAMA*. 2020;323(22):2301-2309.

TOBACCO USE

Organization
▶ AAFP 2015, USPSTF 2015

Screening Recommendations
–Screen all adults for tobacco use.
–Provide tobacco cessation interventions for those who use tobacco products.

Comment
1. Provide some type of SBIRT (Screening, Brief Intervention, and Referral to Treatment) such as:
    a. The "5-A" framework is helpful for smoking cessation counseling:
        i. Ask about tobacco use.
        ii. Advise to quit through clear, individualized messages.
        iii. Assess willingness to quit.
        iv. Assist in quitting.
        v. Arrange follow-up and support sessions.

Source
–USPSTF. *JAMA*. 2021;325(3):265-279.

Cardiovascular Disorders

2

ABDOMINAL AORTIC ANEURYSM

Population
–Men.

Organizations
▶ USPSTF 2019, Society for Vascular Surgery (SVS) 2018, Canadian Society for Vascular Surgery (CSVS) 2018, European Society for Vascular Surgery (ESVS) 2018, ACRa/AIUM/SRU 2014, NICE 2020

Screening Recommendation
–Screen once with ultrasound if of the recommended age and gender.

GUIDELINES DISCORDANT: POPULATION TO SCREEN			
Organization	**Men**	**Women**	**Women**
USPSTF	Age 65–75 y if ever smoked Selectively offer screening if no smoking hx	Do not screen if no smoking or family history of AAA Insufficient evidence to assess benefits/harms if smoker or positive family hx	Do not screen if no smoking or family history of AAA Insufficient evidence to assess benefits/harms if smoker or positive family hx
SVS	Age 65–75 y if ever smoked or first-degree relative with AAA Consider >75 y if in good health and not yet screened	Screen once age 65–75 y, if ever smoked or first-degree relative with AAA Consider screening >75 y if in good health and not yet screened	Screen once age 65–75 y, if ever smoked or first-degree relative with AAA Consider screening >75 y if in good health and not yet screened
CSVS	Age 65–80 y regardless of smoking history	Screen once age 65–80 y if ever smoked or has cardiovascular disease	Screen once age 65–80 y if ever smoked or has cardiovascular disease
ESVS	Age 65 y regardless of smoking history	Do not screen	Do not screen

GUIDELINES DISCORDANT: POPULATION TO SCREEN *(Continued)*			
Organization	**Men**	**Women**	**Women**
ACRa, AIUM, SRU	Age ≥ 65 y regardless of history ≥50 y with family history of aortic and/or peripheral vascular aneurysmal disease or personal history of aneurysmal disease	Screen age ≥ 65 y if positive cardiovascular risk factors Screen age ≥ 50 y with personal or family history of aortic and/or peripheral vascular aneurysmal disease	Screen age ≥ 65 y if positive cardiovascular risk factors Screen age ≥ 50 y with personal or family history of aortic and/or peripheral vascular aneurysmal disease
NICE	Age > 65 y with COPD, CAD/CVD/PAD, family h/o AAA, HLD, HTN, smoking (current or former)	Age ≥ 70 y with COPD, CAD/PAD/CVD, family h/o AAA, HLD, HTN, smoking (current or former)	Age ≥ 70 y with COPD, CAD/PAD/CVD, family h/o AAA, HLD, HTN, smoking (current or former)

Comment

1. Age ranges vary across guidelines based on risk tolerance and attention to cost of screening. Consider patient preference and risk tolerance when deciding who to screen.

Sources

–USPSTF. *JAMA*. 2019;322(22):2211-2218.

–*J Vasc Surg*. 2018;67(1):2-77.

–CSVS. *2018 Screening for Abdominal Aortic Aneurysms in Canada: Review and Position Statement from the Canadian Society of Vascular Surgery*. 2018.

–ESVS 2019 clinical practice guidelines on the management of abdominal aorto-iliac artery aneurysms. *Eur J Vasc Endovasc Surg*. 2018;1-97.

–ACR-AIUM-SRU. *Practice Parameter for the Performance of Diagnostic and Screening Ultrasound Examinations of the Abdominal Aorta in Adults*. 2015.

–*NICE guidelines 156*. Abdominal aortic aneurysm: diagnosis and management. 19 March 2020.

ATHEROSCLEROTIC CARDIOVASCULAR DISEASE (ASCVD), ASPIRIN THERAPY

Organizations

▶ USPSTF 2021, FDA 2016, ACC/AHA 2019

Prevention Recommendation

–Use of low-dose aspirin (75–100 mg/d) for primary prevention is controversial.

Organization	Data Supports Use for This Group	Data Does not Support Routine Use for This Group
USPSTF	Age 40–59 (and perhaps age 60–69 y): For those with 10-y ASCVD risk ≥ 10%, a low risk of bleeding and willing to take daily aspirin, consider offering as there is a small net benefit	Age < 40 or ≥ 60
FDA	None	Do not use aspirin for primary prevention of heart attack or strokes, given serious risks including intracerebral and GI bleeding
ACC/AHA	Age 40–70 y: consider for select adults at higher ASCVD risk[a] who are not at increased bleeding risk[b]	Age > 70 y or adults at increased bleeding risk

[a]A risk value is no longer given due to recent trials calling into question the value of aspirin for primary prevention. Recommend using all available risk factors when determining higher ASCVD risk.
[b]Examples of increased bleeding risk: history of previous GI or other sites bleeding, PUD, age >70, thrombocytopenia, coagulopathy, CKD, NSAID/steroid/anticoagulant use.

Comments

1. The ACC/AHA's "ABCS" of primary prevention presents risk reduction for ASCVD for mainstays of primary prevention: aspirin therapy in appropriate patients (RR 0.90), blood pressure control (RR 0.84 for CHD, 0.64 for stroke), cholesterol management (RR 0.75), and smoking cessation (RR 0.73). (*J Am Coll Cardiol.* 2017;69(12):1617-1636)
2. Aspirin for primary prevention does reduce the incidence of cardiovascular events, does not reduce mortality or nonfatal MI, and does increase bleeding risk. (*Fam Prac* 2020;37(3):290-296)
3. Risks of aspirin therapy: hemorrhagic stroke and GI bleeding (risk factors include age, male sex, GI ulcers, upper GI pain, concurrent NSAID/anticoagulant use, and uncontrolled hypertension).
4. Establish risk factors using the ACC/AHA pooled cohort equation (PCE).

Sources

–https://www.uspreventiveservicestaskforce.org/uspstf/draft-recommendation/aspirin-use-to-prevent-cardiovascular-disease-preventive-medication
–FDA. *Use of Aspirin for Primary Prevention of Heart Attack and Stroke.* 2016.
–*J Am Coll Cardiol.* 2019;74(10):e177-e232.

ATHEROSCLEROTIC CARDIOVASCULAR DISEASE (ASCVD), LIFESTYLE INTERVENTIONS

This recommendation includes adults with elevated blood pressure or known hypertension, metabolic syndrome, dyslipidemia, or estimated 10-y CVD risk > 7.5%. It does not include those with abnormal blood glucose levels, obesity, or smoking, though all persons benefit from healthy eating and physical activity behaviors.

Organizations

▶ USPSTF 2020, ESC 2016, AHA/ACC 2019

Prevention Recommendations

– Offer behavioral counseling, cognitive-behavioral strategies, and multidisciplinary/multimodal interventions to promote healthy diet and physical activity on an individualized basis.

– *Behavioral counseling:*
  - Intensive counseling with multiple contacts over extended periods of time.
  - Interventions typically take 6 to 18 mo with an estimated 6 h of contact time over a median of 12 contacts.

– *Dietary guidelines:*
  - Balance calorie intake and physical activity to achieve or maintain a healthy body weight.
  - Consume diet rich in vegetables and fruits.
  - Choose whole grain, high-fiber foods.
  - Consume fish, especially oily fish, at least twice a week.
  - Limit intake of saturated fats to <7% energy, trans fats to <1% energy, and cholesterol to <300 mg/d by:
    - Choosing lean meats and vegetable alternatives.
    - Selecting fat-free (skim), 1% fat, and low-fat dairy products.
  - Minimize intake of beverages and foods with added sugars.
  - Choose and prepare foods with little or no salt.
  - If you consume alcohol, do so in moderation.
  - Follow these Prevention Recommendations for food consumed/prepared inside *and* outside of the home.

– Recommended diets: Dietary Approaches to Stop Hypertension (DASH), USDA Food Pattern, AHA Diet, or Mediterranean diet.

– Avoid use of and exposure to tobacco products.

– Physical activity guidelines:
  - 90–180 min/wk of moderate to vigorous activity. For adults unable to meet these Prevention Recommendations, aim for some moderate- or vigorous-intensity physical activity to reduce ASCVD risk.
  - Decrease sedentary behavior.

Comments

1. There is a strong correlation between healthy diet, physical activity, and incidence of CVD.
2. Behavioral counseling has shown to have a small benefit in the absence of metabolic disorders. There is better data to support behavioral interventions for patients with obesity and adults with abnormal blood glucose. (USPSTF 2018)
3. Those who take more steps every day enjoy lower all-cause mortality. (*JAMA* 2020;323(12):1151-1160)

Sources

– *J Am Coll Cardiol.* 2019;74(10):e177-e232.
– *Eur Heart J.* 2016;37:2315-2381.

–*JAMA*. 2017:318:167-174.
–USPSTF. *JAMA*. 2020;324(20):2069-2075.
–USPSTF. *Ann Int Med*. 2015;163(11):861-869.

ATHEROSCLEROTIC CARDIOVASCULAR DISEASE (ASCVD), STATIN THERAPY

Organizations

▶ USPSTF 2016, ACC/AHA 2018, 2019, ESC/EAS 2019, CCS 2021, VA-DoD 2020

Prevention Recommendation

–A variety of guidelines exist to guide thresholds to initiate statin therapy.

GUIDELINES DISCORDANT: ASCVD PREVENTION GUIDELINES USING STATIN THERAPY					
Organization	**ACC/AHA**	**CCS**	**ESC/EAS**	**USPSTF**	**VA-DoD**
Risk estimator	PCE	Framingham	SCORE	PCE	PCE or Framingham
Treatment threshold (10-y risk)	≥7.5% age 40-–75 LDL-C ≥ 190 mg/dL age ≥ 21 *See Table 2-1 for detail*	≥20% age 40--75 FRS 10%–19.9% and LDL-C > 3.4 or non-HDL-C > 4.1 or ApoB > 1.04 Statin indicated conditions	ASCVD, DM with end-organ damage, or 3 major risk factors[a]	≥10% and 1 risk factor age 40-75	Higher risk CVD or ≥12% risk for adults > 40 y or LDL-C ≥ 190 mg/dL
Treatment Prevention Recommendations *(see Table 2-2 for statin intensity levels)*	Lifestyle ≥7.5% risk: M or H int. statin 5%–7.5% risk: M int. statin Select patients < 5% risk or age < 40 or ≥ 75 and LDL-C < 190 mg/dL: consider M int. statin	Lifestyle Maximally tolerated statin for LDL-C < 2.0 mmol/L or ApoB < 0.8 g/L or non-HDL-C < 2.6 mmol/L	Lifestyle Very high risk: Statin to reduce LDL-C ≥ 50% and < 55 mg/dL High risk: Statin to reduce LDL-C ≥ 50% and < 70 mg/dL Moderate risk: Statin to reduce LDL < 100 mg/dL Low risk: Statin to reduce LDL < 116 mg/dL	Lifestyle ≥10% risk: L to M int. statin 7.5%–10% risk: L to M int. statin for select patients	Lifestyle ≥12% risk: M int. statin 6%–12% risk: M int. statin for select patients

GUIDELINES DISCORDANT: ASCVD PREVENTION GUIDELINES USING STATIN THERAPY (Continued)					
Organization	**ACC/AHA**	**CCS**	**ESC/EAS**	**USPSTF**	**VA-DoD**
Treatment Prevention Recommendations for patients with ASCVD (secondary prevention)	≤75 y: H int. statin ≥75 y: M int. statin	H int. Maximally tolerated dose, consider adjunct if LDL-C > 1.7 mmol/L or ApoB > 0.69 g/L or non-HDL-C > 2.3 mmol/L	Maximally tolerated statin for target Goal of LDL-C ≤ 70 mg/dL or ≥ 50% reduction reasonable	No recommendation	CVD with M int. statin Higher risk CVD with H or M int. statin at either maximal dose or add ezetimibe +/− PCSK9 inhibitor

*aSevere CKD, heterozygous familial.

Sources

–USPSTF. *JAMA*. 2016;316(19):1997-2007.
–ACC/AHA. *J Am Coll Cardiol*. 2019;73(24):e285-e350.
–*Eur Heart J*. 2020;41(1):111-188.
–*Canadian J Cardiol*. 2021;37(1129-1150).
–*VA/DoD Clinical Practice Guidelines: The Management of Dyslipidemia for Cardiovascular Risk Reduction*. 2020.

Comments

1. ACC/AHA: If risk is uncertain, assess coronary artery calcium. Potential candidates for coronary artery calcium measurement include:
   a. Patients reluctant to start statin therapy, who want to understand risk/benefits.
   b. Patients who may want to know the benefits of statin therapy after discontinuation due to side effects.
   c. Older men age 55–80 or women age 60–80 with fewer risk factors, who question whether they would benefit from statin therapy.
   d. Adults age 40–55 in borderline risk group (with ASCVD risk 5%–7.5%) with other factors that increase their risk.
2. Recommend lifestyle management and drug therapy for high-risk groups.
3. In patients intolerant of statin, consider reducing dose or switching to an alternate agent unless reaction is severe. See Table 2-3 for listing of proven adverse effects of statins.
4. Consider combination of statin and nonstatin therapy (refer to Table 2-4) in select patients.
5. CCS:
   a. For Primary Prevention:
      ◦ Consider add-on therapy with ezetimibe as first-line if LDL-C > 1.9 mmol/L or ApoB > 0.7 g/L or non-HDL-C > 2.6 mmol/L on maximally tolerated statin.

TABLE 2-1 ASCVD GROUPS THAT BENEFIT FROM STATIN THERAPY

Risk Group	Statin Prescription
Age ≤ 75 y with clinical ASCVD, particularly individuals at very high risk[a]	High-intensity statin or maximal tolerated statin, with goal of reducing LDL-C by ≥50% If LDL-C on statin is still ≥70 mg/dL, consider adding ezetimibe; if still ≥70 mg/dL, consider adding PCSK9-I
Age >75 y with clinical ASCVD or already tolerating high-intensity statin	Reasonable to continue moderate- or high-intensity statin after shared decision-making
Heart failure with reduced ejection fraction attributable to ischemic heart disease with life expectancy 3–5 y and not already on a statin	Consider initiation of moderate-intensity statin to reduce occurrence of ASCVD events
Age 40–75 y with diabetes Age 40–75 y with diabetes and multiple ASCVD risk factors Age ≥ 75 y with diabetes on statin Diabetes with 10-y ASCVD risk ≥ 20% Age 20–39 y with diabetes-specific risk factors[b]	Moderate-intensity statin High-intensity statin, with goal of reducing LDL-C by ≥50% Reasonable to continue statin or initiate after shared decision-making Add ezetimibe to reduce LDL-C by ≥50% Reasonable to initiate statin

Source: ACC/AHA. *J Am Coll Cardiol.* 2019;73(24):e285-e350.
[a]Very high-risk ASCVD is history of multiple major ASCVD events or 1 major ASCVD event and multiple high-risk conditions. Major ASCVD events are ACS in past year, MI, ischemic stroke, symptomatic PAD. High-risk conditions are age ≥ 65 y, heterozygous familial hypercholesterolemia, prior CABG or PCI, diabetes, hypertension, CKD, dGFR 15–59 mL/min/1.73 m^2, smoking, LDL-C ≥ 100 mg/dL despite statin and ezetimibe, CHF.
[b]Diabetes-specific risk enhancers are: duration of diabetes type 2 ≥ 10 y or type 1 ≥ 20 y, albuminuria ≥ 30 mcg/mg Cr, eGFR < 60 mL/min/1.73 m^2, retinopathy, neuropathy, ABI < 0.9.

TABLE 2-2 STATIN INTENSITY DRUG LEVELS

High intensity (lowers LDL-C ≥ 50%)	Atorvastatin 40–80 mg Rosuvastatin 20–40 mg
Moderate intensity (lowers LDL-C 30%–49%)	Atorvastatin 10–20 mg Rosuvastatin 5–10 mg Simvastatin[a] 20–40 mg Pravastatin 40–80 mg Lovastatin 40 mg Fluvastatin XL 80 mg Fluvastatin 40 mg BID Pitavastatin 1–4 mg
Low intensity (lowers LDL-C < 30%)	Simvastatin 10 mg Pravastatin 10–20 mg Lovastatin 20 mg Fluvastatin 20–40 mg Pitavastatin 1 mg

Note: If unable to tolerate moderate- to high-intensity statin therapy, consider the use of low-intensity dosages to reduce ASCVD risk.
[a]Avoid Simvastatin 80 mg due to high risk of myopathy.

TABLE 2-3 STATIN-ASSOCIATED SIDE EFFECTS

Side Effect	Frequency	Predisposing Factors	Evidence
Myalgias (no elevation CK)	1%–10%	Age, female, low BMI, Rx interactions, HIV, renal/liver/thyroid disease, Asian descent, alcohol, exertion, trauma	RCTs, observation
Myositis/Myopathy (↑ CK)	Rare		RCTs, observation
Rhabdomyolysis (↑ CK + renal injury)	Rare		RCTs, observation
Statin-associated autoimmune myopathy	Rare		Case reports
New-onset diabetes mellitus	More frequent if risk factors	BMI ≥ 30, FBG ≥ 100 mg/dL, metabolic syndrome, A1c ≥ 6%	RCTs, meta-analyses
Liver transaminases ≥ 3× ULN	Infrequent		RCTs, observation, case reports
Memory/Cognition	Rare: no increase in 3 RCTs		Case reports
Cancer, renal, cataracts, tendon rupture, hemorrhagic stroke, lung disease, low testosterone	Unfounded		

TABLE 2-4 NONSTATIN CHOLESTEROL-LOWERING AGENTS

- In high-risk patients (clinical ASCVD, age < 75 y; LDL-C ≥ 190 mg/dL; 40- to 75-y-old with DM) who are intolerant to statins, the use of nonstatin cholesterol-lowering drugs may be considered.
- **Niacin:** Indicated for LDL-C elevation or fasting triglyceride ≥500 mg/dL; avoid with liver disease, persistent hyperglycemia, acute gout, or new-onset AF.
- **BAS:** Indicated for LDL-C elevation; avoid with triglycerides ≥ 300 mg/dL.
- **Ezetimibe:** Indicated for LDL-C elevation; when combined with statin, monitor transaminase levels.
- **Fibrates:** Indicated for fasting triglycerides ≥ 500 mg/dL. If needed, consider adding fenofibrate only to a low- or moderate-intensity statin. Avoid the addition of Gemfibrozil to statin agent due to increased risk of muscle symptoms. Avoid fenofibrate if moderate/severe renal impairment.
- **Omega-3 fatty acids:** Indicated in severe fasting triglycerides ≥ 500 mg/dL.
- **PCSK9** (proprotein convertase subtilisin kexin 9) inhibitors: FDA-approved monoclonal antibodies including alirocumab (Praluent®) and evolocumab (Repatha®). Studies have shown decrease in LDL cholesterol most notably in patients with heterozygous familial hypercholesterolemia. FOURIER trial tested evolocumab in combination with statin therapy against placebo plus statin therapy in patients with elevated cholesterol levels and existing CVD. There was a modest additional reduction in LDL and composite cardiovascular events. (*NEJM* 2017;376:1713-1722)

Source: Adapted from *J Am Coll Cardiol.* 2018;71:794-799.

b. For Secondary Prevention:
  - Recommends adjunct treatment to maximally tolerated statin be PCSK9 inhibitor (in patients with highest benefit or LDL-C > 2.2 mmol/L or ApoB > 0.8 g/L or non-HDL-C > 2.9 mmol/L) +/− ezetimibe.
  - Consider icosapent ethyl 2000 mg BID if TG is >2.4 to <5.6 mmol/L in patients already receiving maximally tolerated statin.

   c. Statin Indicated Conditions:
- LDL > 4.9 mmol/L.
- Most patients with DM: >39 y or >29 y with >14 y duration or microvascular disease.
- CKD: >49 y and eGFR < 60 mL/min/1.73m².

6. VA/DoD:
   a. For higher risk groups, shared decision making should be used regarding harms and benefits when deciding between moderate or high intensity statins.
   b. For patients needing intensified therapy: Recommends maximal dosing of statin or ezetimibe prior to PCSK9 inhibitors due to safety profile and efficacy.
   c. Recommends against using niacin or omega-3 fatty acids and against adding fibrates to statins, for primary or secondary prevention.
   d. Consider icosapent ethyl in patients on statin therapy with persistent fasting TG > 150 mg/dL for secondary prevention only.

Sources
–ACC/AHA. *J Am Coll Cardiol.* 2019;73(24):e285-e350.
–ACC/AHA. *J Am Coll Cardiol.* 2019;74(10):e177-e232.

ATHEROSCLEROTIC CARDIOVASCULAR DISEASE (ASCVD), SPECIFIC RISK FACTORS

Population
–Adults with HTN.

Organizations
▶ JNC 8 2014, AHA/ACC 2017, Hypertension Canada 2018, ESC/ESH 2018

Prevention Recommendations

GUIDELINES DISCORDANT: WHEN TO INITIATE ANTIHYPERTENSIVES	
Organization	**Guidance**
JNC 8	General population: ≥140/90 Age ≥ 60 y: ≥150/90 Age ≥ 60 y w DM, CKD: ≥140/90 *See Chapter 19 for JNC8 treatment algorithm*
AHA/ACC	10-y ASCVD risk < 10%, no CAD: ≥140/90 10-y ASCVD risk ≥ 10%, no CAD: ≥130/80
Hypertension Canada	Any risk factors or macrovascular organ damage: ≥140/90

Sources
–*JAMA.* 2014;311(5):507-520.
–*J Am Coll Cardiol.* 2018;71(19):e127-e248.
–Hypertension Canada. *Can J Cardiol.* 2018;35(5):506-525.

Population
–Adults with diabetes mellitus.

Organization
▶ ADA 2019

Prevention Recommendations
–Lifestyle interventions:

Diet: Mediterranean or DASH-style diet; reduce saturated fat, trans fat, and cholesterol intake; increase n-3 fatty acids, viscous fiber, and plant stanols/sterols.

- Weight loss: if overweight or obese.
- Physical activity.
- Smoking cessation.

–Target BP goals:
- BP < 130/80 mmHg in patients with DM, HTN, and 10-y ASCVD risk > 15%.
- BP < 140/90 mmHg in patients with DM, HTN, and 10-y ASCVD risk < 15%.

–BP interventions:
- BP > 120/80: Lifestyle modifications.
- BP ≥ 140/90: Initiate/titrate pharmacotherapy.
- BP ≥ 160/100: Initiate/titrate 2-drug regimen.

–Antihypertensives should include classes demonstrated to reduce CV events in diabetic patients: angiotensin-converting enzyme (ACE) inhibitors, angiotensin receptor blockers (ARBs), thiazide-like diuretics, dihydropyridine calcium channel blockers (CCBs).

–Urinary albumin/Cr ratio ≥ 30 mg/gCr: first-line are ACE inhibitors or ARBs at maximum tolerated dose for BP treatment.

–Statin therapy:
- All ages with 10-y ASCVD risk > 20% or multiple ASCVD risk factors, use high-intensity statin. If LDL-C is still ≥70 mg/dL, consider adding ezetimibe (preferred) or PCSK9-I.
- Age < 40 y with ASCVD risk factors, consider moderate-intensity statin.
- Age ≥ 40 y without ASCVD risk factors, consider moderate-intensity statin.

–Contraindicated in pregnancy.

–For patients who do not tolerate intended statin intensity, use maximally tolerated dose.

–Although statin use is associated with increased risk of incident diabetes, the CVD rate reduction with statins outweighed the risk of incident diabetes even for patients with the highest risk for diabetes.

–Aspirin therapy:
- Patients with ASCVD: Use aspirin (75–162 mg/d) for secondary prevention. Use clopidogrel 75 mg/d for patients with documented aspirin allergy. Consider ACE inhibitor to reduce risk of CV events. Use SGLT2 I or GLP1 A as part of diabetes regimen to reduce risk.
- Patients at increased ASCVD risk: Consider aspirin for primary prevention.

Comments
1. Avoid intensive glucose lowering in patients with a history of hypoglycemic spells, advanced microvascular or macrovascular complications, long-standing DM, or if extensive comorbid conditions are present.

2. Treat DM with BP readings of 130–139/80–89 mmHg that persist after lifestyle and behavioral therapy with ACE inhibitor or ARB agents. Multiple agents are often needed. *Administer at least one agent at bedtime.*

3. No advantage of combining ACE inhibitor and ARB in HTN Rx (ONTARGET Trial). (*N Engl J Med.* 2008;358:1547-1559)

Source

−ADA. *Diabetes Care.* 2019;42(suppl 1):S103-S123.

Population

−Adults who use tobacco.

Organizations

▶ AHA/ACC 2019, USPSTF 2015

Prevention Recommendations

−Assess for tobacco use at every health care visit.

−Strongly advise cessation in all patients who use tobacco.

−Combine behavioral interventions and US FDA-approved pharmacotherapy to maximize cessation rates.

−Recommended pharmacotherapy options for smoking cessation:

- Nicotine replacement: Patch (21, 14, 7 mg), Gum (2, 4 mg), Lozenge (2, 4 mg), Nasal spray (10 × 10 mg).
- Drug: Bupropion 150 mg SR, Varenicline (0.5, 1 mg).

Comment

1. New evidence on the health effects of passive smoking strengthens the recommendation on passive smoking. Smoking bans in public places, by law, lead to a decrease in incidence of myocardial infarction.

Sources

−AHA/ACC. *J Am Coll Cardiol.* 2019;73(24):e285-e350.

−USPSTF. *Tobacco Smoking Cessation in Adults and Pregnant Women.* 2015.

−http://rxforchange.ucsf.edu

Population

−Women at risk for ASCVD. This includes women with prior pregnancy complications including hypertensive disorders of pregnancy, gestational diabetes, preterm birth, stillbirth, LBW infant, or placental abruption.

Organizations

▶ AHA 2011, AHA 2019, CCS 2021

Prevention Recommendations

−Limit alcohol consumption to ≤1 drink daily.

−Coronary artery calcium may further define risk in low-risk women (<7.5% 10 y).

–Substantial benefit of smoking cessation in pregnant women on perinatal outcomes.

–Statin therapy may be indicated for women with prior pregnancy-related conditions based on CV age over 10-y risk calculator.

Comments

1. Estrogen plus progestin hormone therapy should not be used or continued.
2. Do not recommend antioxidants (vitamins E and C, and beta-carotene), folic acid, and B_{12} supplementation to prevent CHD.
3. Women who are reproductive age with indication for statin therapy should use hydrophilic compounds in conjunction with effective birth control.

Sources
–*J Am Coll Cardiol.* 2011;57(12):1404-1423.
–*J Am Coll Cardiol.* 2019;73(24):e285-e350.

CAROTID ARTERY STENOSIS (CAS) (ASYMPTOMATIC)

Organizations
▶ USPSTF 2021, CCF/ACR/AIUM/ASE/ASN/ICAVL/SCAI/SCCT/SIR/SVM/SVS 2012, AHA/ASA 2011, AAFP 2015, Society of Thoracic Surgeons 2013

Recommendation
–Do not screen.

Comments

1. The overall US prevalence of internal CAS of ≥70% varies from 0.5% to 1%, with increased prevalence in older adults, smokers, individuals with hypertension or heart disease. No clinically useful risk stratification tool has been found to reliably distinguish between individuals with clinically important CAS and those who do not. No evidence suggests that screening for asymptomatic CAS reduces fatal or nonfatal strokes. (*Ann Int Med.* 2014;161(5):356-362)
2. Carotid duplex ultrasonography to detect CAS > 70%: 90% sensitivity, 94% specificity. (*Ann Int Med.* 2014;161(5):356-362)
3. In 2021, USPSTF reviewed evidence since 2014 and did not change the recommendation.

Sources
–USPSTF *JAMA.* 2021;325(5):476-481.
–ACCF/ACR/AIUM/ASE/ASN/ICAVL/SCAI/SCCT/SIR/SVM/SVS. *J Am Coll Cardiol.* 2012;60(3):242-276.
–ASA/ACCF/AHA/AANN/AANS/ACR/ASNR/CNS/SAIP/SCAI/SIR/SNIS/SVM/SVS. *Circulation.* 2011;124:e54-e130.
–AAFP. *Am Fam Physician.* 2015;91(10):online.
–Choosing Wisely: Society of Thoracic Surgeons. 2013.

CHOLESTEROL AND LIPID DISORDERS

Organizations

▶ USPSTF 2016, AHA/ACC 2018, Canadian Cardiovascular Society (CCS) 2021, AACE 2017, VA/DoD 2020

Screening Recommendations

–Screen all adults within recommended age range.

GUIDELINES DISCORDANT: POPULATION TO SCREEN	
Organization	**Population**
USPSTF	Age 40–75: screen (frequency undetermined) Age 20–39: use clinical judgment as evidence is insufficient
CCS	Age 40–75 and postmenopausal women. Screen every 5 y; add lipoprotein(a) once in lifetime at initial screening
AACE	Age 45 (men) or 55 (women) through 65: screen every 1–2 y Age 20 through 45 (men) or 55 (women): screen every 5 y Age 65+: screen annually
VA/DoD	Age ≥ 40: no more frequently than every 10 y

–Use lipid data to determine risk score (ie, ASCVD risk calculator: https://tools.acc.org/ascvd-risk-estimator-plus) to determine need for primary prevention.

–Use lipid data, other levels (FPG/HgbA1c, eGFR), with Framingham Risk Score (FRS) or the Cardiovascular Life Expectancy Model (CLEM) to determine need for primary prevention. (CCS)

–Consider screening adults regardless of age with other risk factors (clinical evidence of atherosclerosis, abdominal aortic aneurysm, diabetes mellitus, arterial hypertension , cigarette smoking, stigmata of dyslipidemia-corneal arcus, xanthelasma, xanthoma), family history of premature CVD or dyslipidemia, CKD (eGFR ≤ 60), BMI ≥ 30, inflammatory diseases (RA, SLE, PsA, AS, IBD), HIV infection, erectile dysfunction, COPD, history of hypertensive disorder of pregnancy. (CCS)

Sources

–*VA/DoD Clinical Practice Guideline for the Management of Dyslipidemia for Cardiovascular Risk Reduction.* June 2020.

–*JAMA.* 2016;316(19):1997-2007.

–*Circulation.* 2019;139:e1046-e1081.

–*Can J Cardiol.* 2021 Aug;37(8):1129-1150.

–*Endocr Pract.* 2017 Apr;23(Suppl 2).

CORONARY ARTERY DISEASE

Organizations

▶ ACC/AHA 2019, ESC 2012, USPSTF 2018, VA/DoD 2020

Screening Recommendations

–For adults 40–75 y, routinely assess cardiovascular risk factors and calculate 10-y risk of ASCVD using PCEs.[1]

–For adults 20–39 y, assess traditional ASCVD risk factors at least every 4–6 y.

–For adults at borderline risk (5%–7.5% 10-y ASCVD risk) or intermediate risk (≥10% to <20% 10-y ASCVD risk), consider using additional risk-enhancing factors to guide decision making about preventive interventions. If decisions remain uncertain, it is "reasonable" to measure a coronary artery calcium score to guide risk discussion.

–For adults 20–39 y or adults 40–59 y with <7.5% 10-y ASCVD risk, consider estimating lifetime or 30-y ASCVD risk (or HeartScore screening risk score in Europe).[2]

–Insufficient evidence to recommend for or against the addition of Ankle-Brachial Index (ABI), high-sensitivity C-reactive protein (hsCRP), and coronary artery calcium score to traditional risk assessment for CVD in asymptomatic adults with no history of CVD.

–Do not offer a cardiovascular risk assessment more frequently than every 5 y, using 10-y risk calculator.

–Do not use coronary artery calcium, high-sensitivity C-reactive protein, or ABI when assessing cardiovascular risk.

–Do not screen with resting or exercise electrocardiogram (ECG), exercise treadmill test (ETT), stress echocardiogram, or electron-beam CT for coronary artery calcium.

–Do not screen with stress cardiac imaging or advanced noninvasive imaging in the initial evaluation of asymptomatic patients, unless high-risk markers are present.

–Do not perform annual stress cardiac imaging or advanced noninvasive imaging as part of routine follow-up in asymptomatic patients.

Comments

1. 10-y ASCVD risk calculator (The Pooled Cohort Equation) can be found at: http://tools.acc.org/ASCVD-Risk-Estimator-Plus/.

2. USPSTF recommends against screening asymptomatic individuals because of the high rate of false-positive results, low mortality of asymptomatic disease, and iatrogenic diagnostic and treatment risks.

Sources

–*J Am Coll Cardiol.* 2019;74(10):e177-e232.

–*Eur Heart J.* 2012;33:1635-1701.

---

[1]Use Pooled Cohort Equations to replace Framingham Risk Score. Pooled Cohort Equations incorporate age, sex, race, total cholesterol, HDL cholesterol, systolic BP, use of antihypertensive medication, and history of diabetes and/or tobacco use.
[2]HeartScore Europe incorporates age, sex, systolic BP, total cholesterol, HDL cholesterol, and history of tobacco use.

–USPSTF. *JAMA*. 2018;320(3):272-280.

–AAFP. *Clinical Preventive Service Recommendation: Cardiovascular Disease Risk*. 2018.

–USPSTF. *JAMA*. 2018;319(22):2308-2314.

–*VA/DoD Clinical Practice Guideline for the Management of Dyslipidemia for Cardiovascular Risk Reduction*. June 2020.

–Choosing Wisely: American College of Physicians. 2012. http://www.choosingwisely.org/societies/american-college-of-physicians/

–Choosing Wisely: American Academy of Family Physicians. 2013. http://www.choosingwisely.org/societies/american-academy-of-family-physicians/

–Choosing Wisely: American Society of Echocardiography. 2012. http://www.choosingwisely.org/societies/american-society-of- echocardiography/

–Choosing Wisely: American College of Cardiology. 2014. http://www.choosingwisely.org/societies/american-college-of-cardiology/

–*Ann Intern Med*. 2012;157:512-518.

–*J Am Coll Cardiol*. 2019;74(10):e177-e232.

Population

–Women.

Organization

▶ 2011 AHA

Prevention Recommendations

–Assess CVD risk in women beginning at age 20 y, identifying women at higher risk.

–There are racial/ethnic differences in risk factors, with Black and Hispanic women having a higher prevalence of hypertension and diabetes. The highest CVD morbidity and mortality occurs in Black women.

–Autoimmune diseases (systemic lupus erythematosus, rheumatoid arthritis) and preeclampsia are significant risk factors for CVD in women.

–Psychological stress (anxiety, depression) and socioeconomic disadvantages are associated with a higher CVD risk in women.

–Microvascular disease with endothelial dysfunction, also known as female pattern disease, is the etiology of ischemia in more women than men.

–Women are more likely to have atypical cardiovascular symptoms such as sudden or extreme fatigue, dyspnea, sleep disturbances, anxiety, nausea, vomiting, and indigestion.

–ACC/AHA guidelines recommend a routine exercise stress test as the initial evaluation in symptomatic women who have a good exercise capacity and a normal baseline ECG. Exercise stress perfusion study (myocardial perfusion scintigraphy [MPS]) or exercise echo should be reserved for symptomatic women with higher pretest likelihood for CAD or indeterminate routine testing.

–Women often receive less medical therapy and lifestyle counseling than men.

–After PCI procedure, women experience higher rate of complications and mortality than men.

–Management of stable CAD should be the same as in men which include ASA, beta-blocker, statin, ACE inhibitor (ejection fraction [EF] <40%), and nitrate/calcium channel blocker (CCB) for angina management.

–In microvascular disease, beta-blockers have shown to be superior to CCB for angina management. Statins, ACE inhibitors, ranolazine, and exercise can improve angina scores and endothelial dysfunction in female pattern disease.

Sources

–Moasca L, Benjamin EJ, Berra K, et al. Effectiveness-based guidelines for the prevention of cardiovascular disease in women—2011 update: a guideline from the American Heart Association. *Circulation.* 2011;123:1243-1262.

–Gulati M, Shaw LJ, Bairey Merz CN. Myocardial ischemia in women: lessons from the NHLBI wise study. *Clin Cardiol.* 2012;35:141-148.

HYPERTENSION (HTN), ADULTS

Organizations

▶ ACC/AHA 2018, ESH/ESC 2018, USPSTF 2021

Screening Recommendations

–Screen for hypertension in adults ≥ 18-y-old with office blood pressure measurement. Obtain blood pressure measurements outside of clinical setting before starting treatment.

–Screen for HTN using an average BP measurement based on ≥2 readings obtained on ≥2 occasions.

–Use single-visit BP measurement to diagnose HTN only in cases of severe BP elevation/ grade 3 HTN (≥180/110) with clear evidence of hypertension-mediated organ damage (eg, hypertensive retinopathy, LVH, vascular or renal damage). (ESH/ESC)

–Elements of proper measurement include appropriately sized cuff at the level of right atrium, while patient is seated, ≥5 min between office entry and BP measurement.

–Screen every 3–5 y for age 18–39 without risk factors.

–Screen annually at age 40+ or if risk factors are found (prior BP ≥ 130–139/85–89, obese, overweight, Black).

Comments

1. Blood pressure can be measured with programmed portable device that automatically takes BP every 20–30 min over 12–24 h, or self-measured at home 1–2 times a day or week with automated device. (USPSTF)

2. Blood pressure measurements should be taken at upper arm, while seated, after resting for 5 min. (USPSTF)

3. Corresponding BPs based on site/methods: office/clinic 140/90, home monitoring 135/85, day-time ambulatory monitoring 135/85, night-time ambulatory monitoring 120/70, 24-h ambulatory monitoring 130/80. (*J Am Coll Cardiol.* 2018;71:e127-e248)

4. Electronic (oscillometric) measurement methods are preferred to manual measurements. Routine auscultatory Office BP Measurements (OBPMs) are 9/6 mmHg higher than standardized research BPs (primarily using oscillometric devices). (*Can Pharm J.* 2015;148(4):180-186)

5. Assess global cardiovascular risk in all hypertensive patients. Informing patients of their global risk ("vascular age") improves the effectiveness of risk factor modification.

Sources
–ACC/AHA. *J Am Coll Cardiol.* 2018;71:e127-e248.
–USPSTF. *JAMA.* 2021;325(5):476-481.
–ESC/ESH. *Eur Heart J.* 2018;39:3021-3104.

Organizations

▶ ACC/AHA 2017, ESC/ESH 2018, Hypertension Canada 2018, JNC 8, ICSI 2018

Prevention Recommendations

–Persons at risk for developing HTN—family history of HTN, African ancestry, overweight or obesity, sedentary lifestyle, excess intake of dietary sodium, insufficient intake of fruits, vegetables, and potassium, excess consumption of alcohol—should undergo lifestyle changes.

–Achieve and maintain normal BMI < 25, restrict sodium intake <2 g/d, moderate alcohol consumption <14 drinks/wk for men, <8–9 drinks/wk for women, increase physical exercise 30 min/d 5–7 d/wk, emphasize smoking cessation.

–Consume diet rich in vegetables, fruit, fish, nuts, whole grains, low-fat dairy products, and unsaturated fats.

–Do not supplement calcium or magnesium for the prevention or treatment of HTN.

–For patients not at risk of hyperkalemia, increase dietary potassium intake to reduce BP.

–Recommend stress management including relaxation techniques for patients whose stress might be contributing to high BP.

Comments

1. A 10-mmHg reduction in SBP or 5-mmHg reduction in DBP would decrease all major cardiovascular events by 20%, all-cause mortality by 10–15%, stroke by 35%, coronary events by 20%, heart failure by 40%. (ESC/ESH. *Eur Heart J.* 2018;39:3021-3104)

2. For overweight patients, expect 1-mmHg reduction in SBP for every 1-kg reduction in body weight. (ACC/AHA. *J Am Coll Cardiol.* 2018;71:e127-e248)

Sources
–ACC/AHA. *J Am Coll Cardiol.* 2018;71:e127-e248.
–USPSTF. *Ann Int Med.* 2015;163(10):778-787.
–ESC/ESH. *Eur Heart J.* 2018;39:3021-3104.
–*Can J Cardiol.* 2018;34:506-525.
–*JAMA.* 2014;311(5):507-520.
–ICSI Hypertension Work Group: 2018 Commentary.

Lifestyle Modifications for Prevention of Hypertension

- Maintain a healthy body weight for adults (BMI, 18.5–24.9 kg/m²; waist circumference <102 cm for men and <88 cm for women).
- Reduce dietary sodium intake to no more than 2000 mg sodium/d (approximately 5 g of sodium chloride). Per CHEP 2015: adequate intake 2000 mg daily (all ≥ 19-y-old) (80% in processed foods; 10% at the table or in cooking); 2000 mg sodium (Na) = 87 mmol sodium (Na) = 5 g of salt (NaCl) ~1 teaspoon of table salt.
- Engage in regular aerobic physical activity, such as brisk walking, jogging, cycling, or swimming (30–60 min per session, 4–7 d/wk or 90–150 min/wk), in addition to the routine activities of daily living. Higher intensities of exercise are not more effective. Weight training exercise does not adversely influence BP. Isometric exercise, eg, hand grip 4×2 min, 1 min rest between exercises, 3 sessions/wk shown to reduce BP.
- Limit alcohol consumption to no more than 2 drinks (eg, 24 oz [720 mL] of beer, 10 oz [300 mL] of wine, or 3 oz [90 mL] of 100-proof whiskey) per day in most men and to no more than one drink per day in women and lighter-weight persons (≤14/wk for men, ≤9/wk for women).
- Maintain adequate intake of dietary potassium (≥90 mmol [3500 mg]/d). Above the normal replacement levels, do not supplement potassium, calcium, and magnesium for prevention or treatment of hypertension.
- Daily K dietary intake ≥80 mmol.
- Consume a diet that is rich in fruits and vegetables and in low-fat dairy products with a reduced content of saturated and total fat (DASH eating plan).
- Offer advice in combination with pharmacotherapy (varenicline, bupropion, nicotine replacement therapy) to all smokers with a goal of smoking cessation.
- Consider stress management as an intervention in hypertensive patients in whom stress may be contributing to BP elevation.

Sources
–CHEP 2015. http://guidelines.hypertension.ca
–*J Am Coll Cardiol.* 2018;71(19):e127-e248.

PERIPHERAL ARTERY DISEASE (PAD)

Organizations
▶ USPSTF 2018, AHA/ACC 2017

Screening Recommendations

GUIDELINES DISCORDANT: WHETHER TO SCREEN	
Organization	**Population**
USPSTF	Insufficient evidence to recommend for or against routine screening with Ankle-Brachial Index (ABI)
ACC	Consider screening with resting ABI if increased risk of PAD, despite absence of suggestive history or physical examination findings

Comments

1. Patients at increased risk of PAD:
   a. Age ≥ 65 y.
   b. Age 50–64 y, with atherosclerotic risk factors or family history of PAD.
   c. Age <50 y with diabetes mellitus and 1 additional atherosclerotic risk factor.
   d. Known atherosclerotic disease in another vascular bed.
2. Suggestive history and physical examination findings: Claudication, nonjoint-related exertional lower extremity symptoms, impaired walking function, ischemic rest pain, abnormal lower extremity pulses, vascular bruit, nonhealing lower extremity wound, lower extremity gangrene, elevation pallor, dependent rubor.

Sources
–*JAMA*. 2018;320(2):177-183.
–AHA/ACC. *Circulation*. 2017;135(12):e686-e725.

SLEEP APNEA

Organizations
▶ USPSTF 2017, AAFP 2017

Screening Recommendation
–Insufficient evidence to recommend for or against routine screening.

Sources
–USPSTF. *JAMA*. 2017;317(4):407-414.
–*Am Fam Phys*. 2017.96(2):122A-122C.

STROKE, SPECIFIC RISK FACTORS

Population
–DM.

Organization
▶ AHA/ASA 2011

Prevention Recommendations
–HgA1c goal is <6.5%.
–Blood pressure goal is <130/80 mmHg.
–Statin therapy.
–Consider ACE inhibitor or ARB therapy for further stroke risk reduction.

Comments

1. Sixfold increase in stroke in patients with DM. Short-term glycemic control does not lower macrovascular events.
2. Strokes and nonfatal strokes are reduced in diabetic patients by lower BP targets (<130/80 mmHg). In the absence of harm, this benefit appears to justify the lower BP goal.

Source

–*Stroke.* 2011;42:517-584.

Population

–Asymptomatic carotid artery stenosis (CAS).

Organizations

▶ USPSTF 2014, AHA/ASA 2014

Prevention Recommendations

–No indication for general screening for CAS with ultrasonography.

–Screen for other stroke risk factors and treat aggressively.

–ASA and statin unless contraindicated.

–Prophylactic carotid endarterectomy (CEA) for patients with high-grade (≥70%) CAS by ultrasonography when performed by surgeons with low (<3%) morbidity/mortality rates may be useful in selected cases depending on life expectancy, age, sex, and comorbidities.

–However, recent studies have demonstrated that "best" medical therapy results in a stroke rate <1%.

Comment

1. The number needed to treat (NNT) in published trials to prevent 1 stroke in 1 y in this asymptomatic group varies from 84 up to 2000. (*J Am Coll Cardiol.* 2011;57(8):e16-e94)

Sources

–USPSTF. *Carotid Artery Stenosis.* https://www.uspreventiveservicestaskforce.org/uspstf/recommendation/carotid-artery-stenosis-screening

–*Neurology.* 2011;77:751-758.

–*Neurology.* 2011;77:744-750.

–*Stroke.* 2011;42:517-584.

–*Stroke.* 2014;45:3754-3832.

Population

–Symptomatic CAS.

Organizations

▶ ASA/ACCF/AHA/AANN/AANS/ACR/CNS 2011

Prevention Recommendations

–Optimal timing for CEA is within 2 wk posttransient ischemic attack.

–CEA plus medical therapy is effective within 6 mo of symptom onset with ≥70% CAS.

–Intense medical therapy alone is indicated if the occlusion is <50%.

–Intensive medical therapy plus CEA may be considered with obstruction 50%–69%.

–Limit surgery to male patients with a low perioperative stroke/death rate (<6%) and should have a life expectancy of at least 5 y.

Comments

1. Treat asymptomatic CAS aggressively.
2. Individualize surgical intervention, guided by comparing comorbid medical conditions and life expectancy to the surgical morbidity and mortality.
3. Atherosclerotic intracranial stenosis: Use ASA in preference to warfarin.
4. Warfarin—significantly higher rates of adverse events with no benefit over ASA. (*N Engl J Med.* 2005;352(13):1305-1316)
5. Qualitative findings (embolic signals and plaque ulceration) may identify patients who would benefit from asymptomatic CEA.

Sources

–*J Am Coll Cardiol.* 2011;57(8):1002-1038.
–*Neurology.* 2005;65(6):794-801.
–*Arch Intern Med.* 2011;171(20):1794-1795.
–*Stroke.* 2011;42:227-276, 517-584.

Population

–Cryptogenic CVA.
–Hyperlipidemia.

Organizations

▶ ASA/ACCF/AHA/AANN/AANS/ACR/CNS 2011

Prevention Recommendations

–Carotid artery stenting is associated with increased nonfatal stroke frequency but this is offset by decreased risk of MI post-CEA.

–Cryptogenic CVA with patent foramen ovale (PFO) should receive ASA 81 mg/d.

Comments

1. Consider referral to tertiary center for enrollment in randomized trial to determine optimal Rx.
2. Closure I trial demonstrated no benefit at 2 y of PFO closure device over medical therapy.
3. In 2013, the PC Trial also failed to demonstrate significant benefit in reducing recurrent embolic events in patients undergoing PFO closure compared to medical therapy, at 4 y follow-up.

Sources

–*J Am Coll Cardiol.* 2011;57(8):1002-1044.
–*J Am Coll Cardiol.* 2009;53(21):2014-2018.
–*N Engl J Med.* 2012;366:991-999.
–*N Engl J Med.* 2013;368:1083-1091.

Population

–Sickle cell disease.

Organizations

▶ ASA/ACCF/AHA/AANN/AANS/ACR/CNS 2011

Prevention Recommendations

–Transfusion therapy (target reduction of hemoglobin S from a baseline of ≥90% to <30%) is effective for reducing stroke risk in those children at elevated stroke risk.

–Begin screening with transcranial Doppler (TCD) at age 2 y.

–Use transfusion therapy for patients at high-stroke risk per TCD (high cerebral blood flow velocity ≥200 cm/s).

–Frequency of screening not determined.

Sources

–*J Am Coll Cardiol.* 2011;57(8):1002-1044.

–*ASH Education Book.* 2013;2013(1):439-446.

Population

–Primary prevention in women.

Organizations

▶ ACC/ASA 2014

Prevention Recommendations

–Higher lifetime risk, third leading cause of death in women, 53.5% of new recurrent strokes occur in women.

–Sex-specific risk factors: pregnancy, preeclampsia, gestational diabetes, oral contraceptive (OC) use, postmenopausal hormone use, changes in hormonal status.

–Risk factors with a stronger prevalence in women: migraine with aura, atrial fibrillation (AF), diabetes, hypertension, depression, psychosocial stress.

Source

–*Circulation.* 2011;123:1243-1262.

Population

–OC users/menopause, postmenopausal hormone therapy.

Organization

▶ ACC/ASA 2014

Prevention Recommendations

–Stroke risk with low-dose OC users is about 1.4–2 times that of non-OC users.

–Measure BP prior to initiation of hormonal contraception therapy.

–Routine screening for prothrombotic mutations prior to initiation of hormonal contraception is not useful.

–Among OC users, aggressive therapy of stroke risk factors may be reasonable.

–Hormone therapy (conjugated equine estrogen with or without medroxyprogesterone) should not be used for primary or secondary prevention of stroke in postmenopausal women.

–Selective estrogen receptor modulators, such as raloxifene, tamoxifen, or tibolone, should not be used for primary prevention of stroke.

Source
   –*Stroke.* 2014;45:1545-1588.

SAM$_E$ TT$_2$R$_2$ Score

Sex (female)	1
Age ≥ 60	1
Medical history (≥2 comorbidities: HTN, DM, CAD/MI, PAD, CHF, history of stroke, pulmonary disease, hepatic or renal disease)	1
Treatment (rhythm control strategy) (interacting medications, eg, beta-blocker, verapamil, amiodarone)	1
Tobacco use (within 2 y)	2
Race (non-white)	2
Maximum points	8
Interpretation	Score ≥ 2 = DOAC
	Score 0–2 = VKA with TTR
	≥65%–70%

Source: Fauchier L, Angoulvant D, Lip GY. The SAM$_E$-TT$_2$R$_2$ score and quality of anticoagulation in atrial fibrillation: a simple aid to decision-making on who is suitable (or not) for vitamin K antagonists. doi: http://dx.doi.org/10.1093/europace/euv088.

TOBACCO USE

Organizations
▶ USPSTF 2021, AAFP 2015, ICSI 2014

Recommendations
   –Screen all adults for tobacco use and provide tobacco cessation interventions for those who use tobacco products.
   –For nonpregnant adults, provide FDA-approved pharmacotherapy in addition to behavioral intervention. (USPSTF)

Comments
   1. The "5-A" framework is helpful for smoking cessation counseling:
      a. Ask about tobacco use.
      b. Advise to quit through clear, individualized messages.
      c. Assess willingness to quit.
      d. Assist in quitting.
      e. Arrange follow-up and support sessions.
   2. There is insufficient evidence to assess the balance of benefits and harms of pharmacotherapy in pregnant individuals.

Sources
- AAFP. *Clinical Preventive Service Recommendation: Tobacco Use in Adults, Including Pregnant Women.* 2015.
- USPSTF. *JAMA.* 2021;325(3):265-279.
- ICSI. *Preventive Services for Adults.* 20th ed. 2014.

VENOUS THROMBOEMBOLISM (VTE) PROPHYLAXIS IN NONSURGICAL PATIENTS

Organizations
▶ ASH 2018, ACCP 2016, ACP 2011

Prevention Recommendations
- In acutely ill patients (hospitalized, not in ICU/CCU), determine risk for VTE using Padua Prediction Score or IMPROVE score (Table 2-5). (ASH)
- Consider determining risk of bleeding using IMPROVE bleeding score or risk factors (Tables 2-6 and 2-7). (ASH)
- Do not use pharmacologic prophylaxis or mechanical prophylaxis in low-risk patients.
- Use thromboprophylaxis with LMWH in acutely ill hospitalized patients at elevated risk: equivalent of enoxaparin 40 mg SQ daily; fondaparinux 2.5 mg SQ daily. Only use low-dose unfractionated heparin (UFH) 5000 units BID or TID in patients with significant renal disease. UFH has a 10-fold increased risk of heparin-induced thrombocytopenia (HIT). Women are 2.5 times likely to develop HIT compared to men. Continue for duration of hospital stay.
- If not using pharmacological prophylaxis because of bleeding risk, use mechanical (use intermittent pneumatic compression [IPC] or graduated compression stockings [GCS]).
- If unable to use pharmacologic or mechanical prophylaxis, consider aspirin.
- Do not use both pharmacological and mechanical prophylaxis together.
- Do not use DOACs for prophylaxis unless on DOAC for some other reason.
- Do not use VTE prophylaxis in chronically ill (including nursing home), outpatients with minor risk factors, or low-risk long-distance travelers (≥4 h).
- For high-risk long-distance travelers (Table 2-8): use graduated compression stockings or LMWH.

Comments
1. Routine ultrasound screening for DVT is not recommended in any group.
2. 150–200,000 deaths from VTE in the United States per year. Hospitalized patients have a VTE risk which is 130-fold greater than that of community residents. (*Mayo Clin Proc.* 2001;76:1102)
3. Neither heparin nor warfarin is recommended prophylactically for patients with central venous catheters.
4. In higher risk long-distance travelers, frequent ambulation, calf muscle exercises, aisle seat, and below-the-knee graduated compression stockings (GCS) are recommended over aspirin or anticoagulants.

TABLE 2-5 RISK FACTORS FOR VTE IN HOSPITALIZED MEDICAL PATIENTS	
Risk Factor	**Points**
Padua Predictive Scale	
Active cancer[a]	3
Previous VTE	3
Reduced mobility[b]	3
Underlying thrombophilic disorder[c]	3
Recent (<1 mo) trauma or surgery	2
Age (≥70 y)	1
Congestive heart failure (CHF) or respiratory failure	1
Acute MI or stroke	1
Acute infection or inflammatory disorder	1
Obesity (BMI ≥ 30)	1
Thrombophilic drugs (hormones, tamoxifen, erythroid-stimulating agents, lenalidomide, bevacizumab)	1
High risk: ≥4 points—11% risk of VTE without prophylaxis	
Low risk: <3 points—0.3% risk of VTE without prophylaxis	
IMPROVE VTE Risk Scale	
Previous VTE	3
Known thrombophilia	2
Lower limb paralysis	2
Active cancer	2
Immobilization ≥7 d	1
ICU/CCU stay	1
Age ≥ 60 y	1
Score	Risk of VTE
0–1	0.5%
2–3	1.5%
≥4	5.7%

[a]Local or distant metastases and/or chemotherapy or radiation in prior 6 mo.
[b]Bedrest with bathroom privileges for at least 3 d.
[c]Antithrombin, protein C/S, factor V leiden, prothrombin or antiphospholipid defects.

5. Treat hospitalized inpatients with solid tumors without additional risk factors for VTE (history of DVT, thrombophilic drugs, immobilization) with prophylactic dose LMWH.
6. Be cautious in patients with Ccr <20–30 mL/min—UFH or dalteparin (half-dose) preferred.
7. Consider adjusted LMWH dose in patients <50 kg or ≥110 kg in weight. Monitor with heparin anti-10a activity testing.

TABLE 2-6   RISK FACTORS FOR BLEEDING (*CHEST.* 2011;139:69-79)

Risk Factor[a,b]	N = % of Patients	Overall Risk
Active gastroduodenal ulcer	2.2	4.15
GI bleed <3 mo previous	2.2	3.64
Platelet count <50,000	1.7	3.37
Age ≥85 y (vs. 40 y)	10	2.96
Hepatic failure (INR[c] ≥1.5)	2	2.18
Renal failure (GFR[d] <30 mL/min)	11	2.14
ICU admission	8.5	2.10
Current cancer	10.7	1.78
Male sex	49.4	1.48

[a]Although not studied in medical patients, antiplatelet therapy would be expected to increase risk of bleeding.
[b]Go to www.outcomes-umassmed.org/IMPROVE/risk_score/vte/index.html to calculate the risk of bleeding for individual patients.
[c]International normalized ratio.
[d]Glomerular filtration rate.

TABLE 2-7 IMPROVE BLEEDING RISK SCALE

Risk Factor	Points
Renal failure (GFR 30–59)	1
Male vs. female	1
Age 40–80 y	1.5
Current cancer	2
Rheumatic disease	2
Central venous catheter	2
ICU/CCU stay	2.5
Renal failure (GFR < 30)	2.5
Hepatic failure (INR ≥ 1.5)	2.5
Age ≥ 85 y	3.5
Platelets < 50,000	4
Bleeding in last 3 mo	4
Active gastroduodenal ulcer	4.5
Score	Bleeding risk (major/any)
<7	0.4%/1.5%
≥7	4.1%/7.9%

TABLE 2-8 HEREDITARY THROMBOPHILIC DISORDERS

Disorder	% of US Population	Increase in Lifetime of Risk of Clot
Resistance to activated protein C (factor V Leiden mutation)	5–6	3×
Prothrombin gene mutation	2–3	2.5×
Elevated factor 8 (≥175% activity)	6–8	2–3×
Elevated homocysteine	10–15	1.5–2×
Protein C deficiency	0.37	10×
Protein S deficiency	0.5	10×
Antithrombin deficiency	0.1	25×
Homozygous factor V Leiden	0.3	60×

8. Inferior vena cava (IVC) filter indicated in patients with diagnosed DVT with or without pulmonary embolism (PE) who cannot be anticoagulated because of bleeding. There are no other situations where a filter has been proven to be beneficial. Do not use IVC filter prophylactically.
9. Although several studies have shown survival benefit for VTE prophylaxis in surgical patients, this has not been proven in medical patients. (*N Engl J Med.* 2011;365:2463) (*N Engl J Med.* 2007;356:1438)

Sources

–*Blood Adv.* 2018;2:3198-3225.

–American Society of Hematology 2018. *Guidelines for Management of Venous Thromboembolism: Prophylaxis for Hospitalized and Nonhospitalized Medical Patients.*

–*JAMA.* 2012;307:306.

–*Ann Intern Med.* 2011;155:625-632.

–*Chest.* 2016;149:315-352.

–http://www.uwhealth.org/files/uwheath/docs/anticoagulation/VTE

VENOUS THROMBOEMBOLISM (VTE) IN SURGICAL PATIENTS

Organization

▶ ACCP 2016

Prevention Recommendations

–Stratify surgical risk:
  • Low risk: <40 y, minor surgery,[1] no risk factors,[2] Caprini score < 2 (see Table 2-9).
  • Intermediate risk: minor surgery plus risk factors, age 40–60 y, major surgery with no risk factors, Caprini score 3–4.

[1]Eye, ear, laparoscopy, cystoscopy, and arthroscopic operations.
[2]Prior VTE, cancer, stroke, obesity, congestive heart failure pregnancy, thrombophilic medications (tamoxifen, raloxifene, lenalidomide, thalidomide, erythroid-stimulating agents).

TABLE 2-9 CAPRINI RISK STRATIFICATION MODEL

1 Point	2 Points	3 Points	5 Points
• Age 41–60 y • Minor surgery • BMI ≥251 g/m^2 • Swollen legs • Varicose veins • Pregnancy or postpartum • History of recurrent spontaneous abortion • Sepsis (<1 mo) • Lung disease • History of acute MI • Congestive heart failure (CHF) (<1 mo) • History of inflammatory bowel disease • Medical patient at bed rest	• Age 61–74 y • Arthroscopic surgery • Major open surgery ≥45 min • Laparoscopic surgery • Malignancy • Confined to bed • Immobilizing cast • Central venous catheter	• Age ≥ 75 y • History VTE • Family history of VTE • Factor V Leiden • Prothrombin gene mutation • Lupus anticoagulant • Elevated homocysteine • Other congenital or acquired thrombophilia	• Stroke (<1 mo) • Elective arthroplasty; hip, pelvis, or leg fracture • Acute spinal cord injury (<1 mo)
		Caprini score <3: low risk Caprini score 3–4: intermediate risk Caprini score ≥5: high risk	

- High risk: major surgery plus risk factors, high-risk medical patient, major trauma, spinal cord injury, craniotomy, total hip or knee arthroplasty (THA, TKA), thoracic, abdominal, pelvic cancer surgery.

–Employ preventive measures:
- Early ambulation: consider mechanical prophylaxis and IPC or GCS.
- UFH 5000 U SQ q 8–12 h should ONLY be used in patients with renal disease with a Ccr < 20–30 mL/min.
- LMWH equivalent to enoxaparin 40 mg SQ 2 h before surgery then daily or 30 mg q12h SQ starting 8–12 h postop.
- Fondaparinux 2.5 mg SQ daily starting 8–12 h postop.
- LMWH: equivalent to enoxaparin 40 mg SQ 2 h preoperative then daily or 30 mg SQ q12h starting 8–12 h postop and also use mechanical prophylaxis with IPC or GCS.
- Extend prophylaxis for as long as 28–35 d in high-risk patients. In THA, TKA ortho patients, acceptable VTE prophylaxis also includes rivaroxaban 10 mg/d, dabigatran 225 mg/d, adjusted dose warfarin, and aspirin, although LMWH is preferred. DOACs are likely to play a larger role in the future as trials continue to show superiority over warfarin. (*Ann Int Med.* 2013;159:275) (*Thromb Haemot.* 2011;105:444)
- If high risk of bleeding, use IPC alone. (*Ann Intern Med.* 2012;156:710, 720) (*JAMA.* 2012;307:294)
- Do not use UFH for prophylaxis if Ccr is ≥20 mL/min. There is a 10-fold increased risk of HIT compared to LMWH.

Comments

1. 75%–90% of surgical bleeding is structural. VTE prophylaxis adds minimally to risk of bleeding.
2. With creatinine clearance <20 to 30 mL/min UFH with partial thromboplastin time (PTT) monitoring is preferred (decrease dose if PTT is prolonged). In all other situations LMWH or DOACs are preferred to reduce the risk of HIT.
3. Patients with liver disease and prolonged international normalized ratio (INR) are still at risk for clot. Individualize risk-to-benefit ratio of VTE prophylaxis.
4. Epidural anesthesia: before placing catheter wait 18 h after daily prophylactic dose of LMWH and 24 h after prophylactic dose of fondaparinux. For patients on BID therapeutic LMWH anticoagulation or once daily LMWH, wait more than 24 h before placing epidural catheter. Patients on DOACs should hold their anticoagulation for 3–5 d. After placing or removing an epidural catheter hold on starting anticoagulation for 6–8 h.
5. Do not place prophylactic IVC filter for high-risk surgery.
6. For cranial and spinal surgery patients at low risk for VTE use mechanical prophylaxis: high-risk patients should have pharmacologic prophylaxis added to mechanical prophylaxis once hemostasis is established and bleeding risk decreased.
7. Patients at high risk of bleeding[1] with major surgery should have mechanical prophylaxis (IPC, GCS): initiate anticoagulant prophylaxis if risk is lowered.
8. Surgical patients receive indicated prophylaxis 60% of the time compared to 40% in medical patients.

Sources

−*Chest.* 2016;149:315.

−http://www.fda.gov/Drugs/ResourcesForYou/Consumers/ucm390574.htm

[1]Selected factors in the rising risk of major bleeding complications:

General risk factors: active bleeding, previous major bleed, known untreated bleeding disorder, renal or liver failure, thrombocytopenia, acute stroke, uncontrolled high BP, concomitant use of anticoagulants, or antiplatelet therapy.

Procedure-specific risk factors: major abdominal surgery—extensive cancer surgery, pancreatic-duodenectomy, hepatic resection, cardiac surgery, thoracic surgery (pneumonectomy or extended resection). Procedures where bleeding complications have especially severe consequences: craniotomy, spinal surgery, spinal trauma.

Ears, Nose, and Throat

3

ORAL CANCER

Organizations
▶ AAFP 2015, USPSTF 2013, NCCN 2018

Screening Recommendations

GUIDELINES DISCORDANT: WHETHER TO SCREEN	
Organization	**Guidance**
USPSTF, AAFP	Insufficient evidence to recommend for or against routinely screening adults for oral asymptomatic cancer
NCCN	Screen with annual clinical exam

Comment

1. Primary risk factors for oral cancer are tobacco and alcohol use. Additional risk factors include male sex, older age, use of betel quid, ultraviolet light exposure, infection with *Candida* or bacterial flora, and a compromised immune system. Recently, sexually transmitted oral human papillomavirus infection has been recognized as an increasing risk factor for oropharyngeal cancer, another subset of head and neck cancer.

Sources
–http://www.aafp.org/online/en/home/clinical/exam.html
–http://www.ahrq.gov/clinic/uspstf/uspsoral.htm
–www.nccn.org

Organization
▶ National Cancer Institute 2018

Prevention Recommendations

–Minimize Risk Factor Exposure. Risk factors include:
- Tobacco (in any form, including smokeless).
- Alcohol and dietary factors—double the risk for people who drink 3–4 drinks/d vs. nondrinkers. (*Cancer Causes Control.* 2011;22:1217)
- Betel-quid chewing. (*Cancer.* 2014;135:1433)

- Oral HPV infection—found in 6.9% of general population and found in 70%–75% of patients with oropharyngeal squamous cell cancer. (*N Engl J Med*. 2007;356:1944)
- Lip cancer—avoid chronic sun exposure and smokeless tobacco.

Comments

1. Oropharyngeal squamous cell CAs (tonsil and base of tongue) are related to HPV infection (types 16 and 18) in 75% of patients. This correlates with sexual practices, number of partners, and may be prevented by HPV vaccine. HPV (+), nonsmokers have improved cure rate by 35%–45%. (*N Engl J Med*. 2010;363:24, 82)
2. There is inadequate evidence to suggest change in diet will reduce risk of oral cancer.

Source

–https://www.cancer.gov/types/head-and-neck/hp/oral-prevention-pdq

Endocrine and Metabolic Disorders

4

CANCER

Organization
▶ ACS 2020

Prevention Recommendations
–Achieve and maintain a healthy body weight throughout life.
–Be physically active:
  • Adults should get 150–300 min of moderate-intensity physical activity/wk, or 75–150 min of vigorous-intensity physical activity/wk. Exceeding the upper limit of 300 min is optimal.
  • Children and adolescents should get at least 1 h of moderate- or vigorous-intensity activity each day.
  • Limit sedentary behavior.
–Follow a healthy eating pattern at all ages:
  • A healthy eating pattern includes foods high in nutrients, a variety of vegetables and fruits, and whole grains.
  • A healthy eating pattern limits or does not include red and processed meats, sugar-sweetened beverages, highly processed foods, and refined grain products.
–Avoid alcohol. People who choose to drink should limit consumption to no more than 1 drink/d for women and 2 drinks/d for men.

Organization
▶ ACS 2020

Prevention Recommendations
–Work at national, state, and local levels to develop, advocate for, and implement policy and environmental changes that increase access to affordable, nutritious foods; provide safe, enjoyable, and accessible opportunities for physical activity; and limit alcohol for individuals.

Source
–*CA Cancer J Clin* 2020; 70:245-271.

DIABETES MELLITUS (DM), TYPE 2 AND PREDIABETES

Organizations
▶ USPSTF 2021, ADA 2021, IDF 2017

Screening Recommendations
–Universal screen if age 45 or older.
–Screen asymptomatic adults age 35 or older who have a body mass index (BMI) ≥ 25. Consider screen at an earlier age if patient is from a population with a high prevalence of diabetes (Native American/Alaska Native, Black, Hawaiian/Pacific Islander, Hispanic/Latino) and at a lower BMI (≥ 23) if the patient is Asian American.
–Offer patients with prediabetes effective preventative interventions.
–Screen children and adolescents who are overweight (BMI ≥ 85th percentile) or obese (BMI ≥ 95th percentile) and have additional risk factor(s) after the onset of puberty or after 10 y of age, whichever occurs first.
–Screen women planning pregnancy who are overweight or have one or more risk factors for diabetes.
–Screen patients with HIV with a fiber Bragg grating (FBG) before starting antiretroviral therapy, when switching antiretroviral therapy, and 3–6 mo after starting or switching therapy.
–Screen women who were diagnosed with gestational diabetes mellitus (GDM) every 3 y.
–Screen patients with prediabetes annually for the development of diabetes.
–Screen with an FBG, 2-h plasma glucose after 75-g oral GTT, or HgbA1c.

Comments
1. Repeat screening at least every 3 y in asymptomatic adults above the age of 45.
2. Screen and treat patients with prediabetes for modifiable cardiovascular risk factors such as hypertension and dyslipidemia.
3. Risk factors for diabetes and prediabetes in asymptomatic adults:
   a. First-degree relative with diabetes.
   b. High-risk race/ethnicity (eg, African American, Latino, Native American, Asian-American, Pacific Islander).
   c. History of CVD.
   d. Hypertension (>140/90 or on meds for HTN).
   e. HDL < 35 and/or triglycerides > 250.
   f. Women with polycystic ovary syndrome (PCOS).
   g. Physical inactivity.
   h. Increased abdominal waist circumference.
   i. Clinical conditions associated with insulin resistance (eg, severe obesity, acanthosis nigricans).
4. Risk factors for diabetes and prediabetes in asymptomatic children:
   a. Maternal history of diabetes or GDM during the child's gestation.
   b. Family history of type 2 diabetes in first- or second-degree relatives.
   c. High-risk race/ethnicity (eg, African American, Latino, Native American, Asian-American, Pacific Islander).

  d. Clinical conditions associated with insulin resistance (eg, acanthosis nigricans, hypertension, dyslipidemia, polycystic ovary syndrome [PCOS], small-for-gestational-age birth weight).
5. Overweight or obese children and adolescents in whom type 2 diabetes is being considered should be tested for pancreatic autoantibodies to exclude the possibility of autoimmune type 1 diabetes.

Sources
–USPSTF. *Recommendation: Screening for Prediabetes and Type 2 Diabetes.* 2021.
–ADA. *Standards of medical care in diabetes—2021. Diabetes Care* 2021;44(1):S4-S24.
–International Diabetes Federation. *IDF Clinical Practice Recommendations for Managing Type 2 Diabetes in Primary Care.* 2017. www.idf.org/managing-type2-diabetes

Organization
▶ ADA 2020

Prevention Recommendations
–A variety of eating patterns are acceptable for persons with prediabetes or impaired glucose tolerance (IGT).[1]
–Employ intensive behavioral lifestyle intervention with a goal of sustained 7% weight loss.
–Recommend moderate physical activity such as brisk walking at least 150 min/wk. Pursue tobacco cessation.
–Consider metformin for patients at highest risk for developing diabetes (eg, BMI 35 kg/m^2 or greater, those age 60 y or younger, and women with prior GDM).
–Based on patient preference, consider technology-assisted diabetes prevention interventions (eg, SBGM) as they may be effective in preventing type 2 diabetes.
–Monitor at least annually for the development of type 2 diabetes.
–Screen for and treat modifiable risk factors for cardiovascular disease.

Comments
1. Recommendations for disease prevention:
   a. Annual influenza vaccine.
   b. Pneumococcal polysaccharide vaccine if 2 y or older with single-time revaccination when over 64 y.
   c. Hepatitis B vaccine series if unvaccinated and 19–59 y of age.
   d. Aspirin 81 mg daily for primary prevention if 10-y risk of significant CAD is at least 10% (by Framingham Risk Score); includes most men over 50 y and most women over 60 y.
2. An integrated lifestyle change program, such as the CDC's National Diabetes Prevention Program,[2] reduces the progression to diabetes by more than 50%. This intervention included 7% weight loss, reducing intake of fat and calories, exercising 150 min/wk. This is twice the benefit seen with metformin, and the benefit persisted 15 y after the initial intervention (https://www.niddk.nih.gov/about-niddk/research-areas/diabetes/diabetes-prevention-program-dpp).

---

[1]IGT, or pre-diabetes, if fasting glucose 100–125 mg/dL, 2-h glucose after 75-g anhydrous glucose load 140–199 mg/dL, or HgbA1c 5.7%–6.4%.
[2]https://www.cdc.gov/diabetes/prevention/index.html

3. Older adults with prediabetes are unlikely to ever develop diabetes (*JAMA Intern Med.* 2021;181(4):511-519)

Source
–*Diabetes Care.* 2020;43(suppl 1):S32-S36.

Organization

▶ USPSTF 2015

Prevention Recommendation

–Intensive behavioral intervention to promote healthy diet and physical activity for persons with abnormal blood glucose or BMI > 25.

Source
–*Ann Intern Med.* 2015;163(11):861-868.

OBESITY

Organizations

▶ AAFP 2012, USPSTF 2017, 2021, VA/DoD 2014

Screening Recommendations

–Screen all adults using BMI and offer intensive counseling and behavioral weight loss interventions to prevent obesity-related morbidity and mortality in adults with BMI ≥ 30.
–Consider annual measurement of waist circumference.

Comments

1 Intensive counseling involves more than one session per month for at least 3 mo.
2 Offer intensive intervention to promote weight loss in:
    a. Obese adults (BMI ≥ 30 or waist circumference ≥ 40 in. [men] or ≥ 35 in. [women]).
    b. Overweight adults (BMI 25–29.9) with an obesity-associated condition.[1]

Sources
–USPSTF. *Obesity in Adults: Screening and Management.* 2021.
–USPSTF. *Obesity in Children and Adolescents: Screening.* 2017.
–*VA/DoD Clinical Practice Guideline for Screening and Management of Overweight and Obesity,* Version 2.0. 2014.

Organizations

▶ ICSI 2013, CDC 2011

Prevention Recommendations

–Employ a team approach for weight management in all persons of normal weight (BMI 18.5–24.9) or overweight (BMI 25–29.9), including:

---

[1]HTN, DM type 2, dyslipidemia, obstructive sleep apnea, degenerative joint disease, or metabolic syndrome.

- Nutrition.
- Physical activity: 150 min of moderate-intensity aerobic exercise/wk.
- Lifestyle changes: Avoid inactivity.
- Screen for depression.
- Screen for eating disorders.
- Review medication list and assess if any medications can interfere with weight loss.
 −Ensure regular follow-up to reinforce principles of weight management.

Comments

1. Recommend 30–60 min of moderate physical activity on most days of the week.
2. Nutrition education focused on decreased caloric intake, encouraging healthy food choices and managing restaurant and social eating situations. Eat 5–6 servings of fruits and vegetables daily.
3. Weekly weight checks.
4. Encourage nonfood rewards for positive reinforcement.
5. Stress management techniques.
6. 5%–10% weight loss can produce a clinically significant reduction in heart disease risk.

Source

 −Fitch A, Everling L, Fox C, et al. *Prevention and Management of Obesity for Adults*. Bloomington, MN: ICSI; 2013.

THYROID CANCER

Organizations

▶ USPSTF 2017, American Cancer Society, NIH/National Cancer Institute 2019

Screening Recommendations

 −Do not screen asymptomatic people with ultrasound.
 −Genetic testing is recommended for patients with a family history of medullary thyroid cancer (MTC), with or without multiple endocrine neoplasia type 2 (MEN2).
 −Be aware of higher risk patients: head-and-neck radiation administered in infancy and childhood for benign (thymus enlargement, acne) or malignant conditions, which results in an increased risk beginning 5 y after radiation and continuing until >20 y later; nuclear fallout exposure (eg, Japanese survivors of atomic bombing); history of goiter; family history of thyroid disease or thyroid cancer; MEN2; female gender; Asian race.

Comments

1. Neck palpation for nodules in asymptomatic individuals has sensitivity of 15%–38% and specificity of 93%–100%. Only a small proportion of nodular thyroid glands are neoplastic, resulting in a high false-positive rate.
2. Fine-needle aspiration (FNA) is the procedure of choice for evaluation of thyroid nodules. (*Otolaryngol Clin North Am*. 2010;43:229-238; *N Engl J Med*. 2012;367:705)

Sources

 −*JAMA*. 2017;317(18):1882-1887.

–*N Engl J Med.* 2015;373:2347.

–PDQ® Screening and Prevention Editorial Board. *PDQ Thyroid Cancer Screening.* Bethesda, MD: National Cancer Institute. https://www.cancer.gov/types/thyroid/hp/thryoid-screening-pdq. Accessed April 16, 2019.

THYROID DYSFUNCTION

Organizations

▶ AAFP 2015, USPSTF 2015, ATA 2012, AACE 2012, ASRM 2015, CTF 2019

Screening Recommendations

–Insufficient evidence to recommend for or against routine screening for thyroid disease in asymptomatic adults without risk factors.

- ATA/AACE: consider screening patients older than 60, those with risk factors, and women planning pregnancy.

–CTF: do not screen asymptomatic nonpregnant adults for thyroid dysfunction.

–Evaluate adults with laboratory or radiologic abnormalities that could be caused by thyroid disease using serum TSH.

–Do not test for thyroid disease in hospitalized patients unless thyroid disease is strongly suspected.

Comments

1. Individuals with symptoms and signs potentially attributable to thyroid dysfunction require TSH testing.
2. Less than 1% of adults have subclinical hypothyroidism; outcomes data to support treatment are lacking. Subclinical hyperthyroidism detected during routine screening may be treated in select patients at high risk of cardiovascular or skeletal complications.
3. Higher risk individuals are those with autoimmune disorders (eg, type 1 diabetes), pernicious anemia, goiter, previous radioactive iodine therapy and/or head-and-neck irradiation or surgery, pituitary or hypothalamic disorders, first-degree relative with a thyroid disorder, use of medications that may impair thyroid function, and those with psychiatric disorders.
4. Thyroid function should be measured in patients with the following: substantial hyperlipidemia, hyponatremia, high-serum muscle enzymes, macrocytic anemia, pericardial or pleural effusions.
5. Consider TSH screening in infertile women attempting pregnancy.
6. Monitor TSH in patients on thyroid meds or after thyroid surgery.

Gastrointestinal Disorders

5

BARRETT ESOPHAGUS (BE)

Organization
▶ ASGE 2019

Recommendations
–Do not screen lower risk general population with gastroesophageal reflux disease (GERD).
–Screen moderate- to high-risk individuals using upper endoscopy (EGD) and biopsy.
  • Moderate risk: GERD and ≥1 other risk factor: age > 50 y, male sex, white, obesity (BMI ≥ 30), central adiposity, tobacco use.
  • High risk: family history of esophageal adenocarcinoma or BE.

Comments
1. 40% of persons with BE and esophageal cancer have no preceding GERD symptoms.
2. Treat all persons with biopsy-proven BE with proton pump inhibitor (PPI) therapy, including asymptomatic individuals.

Sources
–*Gastrointest Endosc.* 2019;90(3):335-359.
–*Am J Gastroenterol.* 2016;111(1):30-50.

CELIAC DISEASE

Organizations
▶ USPSTF 2017, AAFP 2017, ACG 2013

Recommendations

GUIDELINES DISCORDANT: POPULATION TO SCREEN	
Organization	**Population**
USPSTF, AAFP	Insufficient evidence regarding screening of asymptomatic individuals
NICE	Do not screen the general population Screen first-degree relatives of individuals with celiac disease

GUIDELINES DISCORDANT: POPULATION TO SCREEN *(Continued)*	
Organization	**Population**
ACG	Consider screening asymptomatic persons with type 1 diabetes mellitus every 1–2 y using serologic testing with IgA tissue transglutaminase antibody and total IgA level, as 3%–10% have concurrent celiac disease

Comments

1. Serologic testing and biopsy must be performed while on gluten-containing diet.
2. IgA tissue transglutaminase (TTG) antibody is the test of choice (>90% sensitivity and specificity), along with total IgA level. If equivocal TTG, perform IgA endomysial antibody test.
3. Symptoms of celiac disease include diarrhea, flatulence, and a range of extraintestinal manifestations including anemia (malabsorption of iron and folic acid), dermatitis herpetiformis (IgA deposits), abnormal liver enzymes, peripheral neuropathy or ataxia, oral findings such as aphthous ulcers or enamel defects, and osteopenia/osteoporosis. While screening is generally discouraged by guidelines, testing for celiac disease is often indicated in the evaluation of these conditions.

Sources

–USPSTF. *JAMA.* 2017;317(12):1252.
–AAFP. *Clinical Recommendations: Screening for Celiac Disease.* 2017.
–*Am J Gastroenterol.* 2013;108(5):656-676.
–NICE. *Coeliac Disease: Recognition, Assessment and Management.* 2015.
–*Am Fam Physician.* 2014 Jan 15;89(2):99-105.

COLORECTAL CANCER

Organizations

▶ AAFP 2021, USPSTF 2021, ACS 2020, ACG 2021, US Multi-Society Task Force on Colorectal Cancer (USMSTF-CC) 2017, 2020, ACP 2019, Canadian Task Force (CTF) 2016, NCCN 2021, ASCO 2019

Recommendations

–Screen all adults, with age ranges, modalities, and frequencies varying by organization.
–Adults with elevated risk are outside the scope of these recommendations.[1]

---

[1]Risk factors indicating need for earlier/more frequent screening: personal history of CRC or adenomatous polyps or hepatoblastoma, CRC or polyps in a first-degree relative age *Ann Intern Med.* 1998;128(1):900; *Am J Gastroenterol.* 2009;104:739; *N Engl J Med.* 1994;331(25):1669; 1995;332(13):861) Additional high-risk group: history of ≥30 Gy radiation to whole abdomen; all upper abdominal fields; pelvic, thoracic, lumbar, or sacral spine. Begin monitoring 10 y after radiation or at age 35 y, whichever occurs last (http://www.survivorshipguidelines.org). Screening colonoscopy in those age ≥ 80 y results in only 15% of the expected gain in life expectancy seen in younger patients. (*JAMA.* 2006;295:2357)

Organization	Ages and Frequencies	Modality
AAFP	Age 50–75 y: screen all patients Age 76–85 y: individualize screening decision	No preference
ACS, USPSTF	Age 45–75 y: screen all patients Age 76–85 y: individualize screening decision Age > 85 y: do not screen	No preference
ACG, NCCN	Age 45–75 y: screen all patients Age > 75 y: individualize	ACG: prefer colonoscopy or fecal immunochemical test (FIT)
USMSTF-CC	Age 50–75 y: screen all patients (consider starting at age 45 in Blacks) Age > 75 y: do not screen For patients with normal,[a] high-quality colonoscopy, repeat CRC screening in 10 y[a]	Prefer colonoscopy or FIT
ACP	Age 50–75 y: screen all patients Age > 75 y: do not screen	Life expectancy < 10 y: do not screen
CTF	Age 50–74 y: screen all patients	Screen with stool-based test or flexible sigmoidoscopy, not colonoscopy
ASCO	Age 50–75 y: screen all patients	No preference

[a] Colonoscopy is considered normal where no adenoma, sessile serrated adenoma/polyp or sessile serrated polyp (SSP), hyperplastic polyp (HP) ≥ 10 mm, traditional serrated adenoma (TSA), or CRC was found. Individuals with only HPs < 10 mm are considered to have normal colonoscopy.

Comments

1 Recommendations for follow-up testing after the initial colonoscopy are detailed in Table 5-1.

2 Recommendations for screening in resource-limited settings are detailed in Table 5-2.

3 USPSTF, ACG, ACS, and NCCN all recognize that evidence for initiating screening at age 45 is not as strong. USPSTF gives starting at age 45 a "B" recommendation while starting at age 50 is an "A" recommendation. ACG "recommends" starting at age 50 and "suggests" starting at age 45. Incidence of colorectal adenocarcinoma in adults 40- to 49-y-old has increased by almost 15% from 2000–2002 to 2014–2016. (*Ann Intern Med.*2021;174)

4 Acceptable screening methods[1,2,3]:

   a. Guaiac fecal occult blood test (gFOBT-guaiac based or FIT = fecal immunochemical test) annually.[4]

   b. Flexible sigmoidoscopy every 5 y with reflex colonoscopy if abnormal.

   c. FIT[5] annually plus flexible sigmoidoscopy every 10 y.

[1]A positive result on an FOBT should be followed by colonoscopy. An alternative is flexible sigmoidoscopy and air-contrast barium enema.

[2]FOBT should be performed on 2 samples from 3 consecutive specimens obtained at home. A single stool guaiac during annual physical examination is not adequate.

[3]USPSTF did not find direct evidence that a screening colonoscopy is effective in reducing CRC mortality rates.

[4]Use the guaiac-based test with dietary restriction, or an immunochemical test without dietary restriction. Two samples from each of 3 consecutive stools should be examined without rehydration. Rehydration increases the false-positive rate.

[5]Population-based retrospective analysis: risk of developing CRC remains decreased for >10 y following negative colonoscopy findings. (*JAMA.* 2006;295:2366)

TABLE 5-1 US MULTI-SOCIETY TASK FORCE RECOMMENDATIONS FOR FOLLOW-UP AFTER BASELINE SCREENING COLONOSCOPY IN AVERAGE-RISK ADULTS

	Baseline Colonoscopy	Size	Pathology	Recommended Surveillance Colonoscopy	Recommendation Strength
Normal	No adenoma, SSP, TSA, HP ≥ 10 mm, CRC; HP < 10 mm acceptable			10 y	High
Adenoma	1–2 adenomas	<10 mm	Tubular	7–10 y	Moderate
	3–4 adenomas	<10 mm	Tubular	3–5 y	Very low
	5–10 adenomas	<10 mm	Tubular	3 y	Moderate
	≥1 adenoma	≥10 mm		3 y	High
			Tubulovillous or villous histology	3 y	Moderate
			High-grade dysplasia	3 y	Moderate
	>10 adenomas			1 y	Very low
	Piecemeal resection	≥20 mm		6 mo	Moderate
Polyp	≤20 HPs in rectum or sigmoid	<10 mm		10 y	Strong
	≤20 HPs proximal to sigmoid	<10 mm		10 y	Weak
	1–2 SSPs	<10 mm		5–10 y	Weak
	3–4 SSPs	<10 mm		3–5 y	Weak
	5–10 SSPs	<10 mm		3 y	Weak
	SSP	≥10 mm		3 y	Weak
	SSP		Dysplasia	3 y	Weak
	HP	≥10 mm		3–5 y	Weak
	TSA			3 y	Weak
	Piecemeal resection of SSP	≥20 mm		6 mo	Strong

Source: USMSTF. *Gastroenterol.* 2020;158:1131-1153.

    d. Colonoscopy every 10 y.

    e. CT colonoscopy every 5 y.

5 Follow-up/surveillance colonoscopy according to findings: refer to Chapter 5 for updated USMSTF 2020 recommendations.

6 FOBT alone decreased colorectal cancer (CRC) mortality by 33% compared with those who were not screened. (*Gastroenterology.* 2004;126:1674)

Resource Setting[a]	Recommended CRC Screening Options
Basic	HSgFOBT annually (preferred) to every 2 y FIT annually (preferred) to every 2 y
Limited	HSgFOBT annually FIT annually FSIG every 5 y FSIG every 10 y *plus* FIT (preferred) or HSgFOBT annually
Enhanced	HSgFOBT annually FIT annually FSIG every 5 y FSIG every 10 y *plus* FIT (preferred) or HSgFOBT annually Colonoscopy every 10 y
Maximal	HSgFOBT annually FIT annually FSIG every 5 y FSIG every 10 y *plus* FIT (preferred) or HSgFOBT annually Colonoscopy every 10 y CT colonography FIT-DNA

TABLE 5-2 SCREENING IN HIGH-INCIDENCE SETTINGS STRATIFIED BY RESOURCE AVAILABILITY

[a]ASCO resource setting stratification:

Basic—Core, fundamental recourses/services essential for any public health/primary care system.

Limited—Second-tier resources/services intended to produce major improvements in outcomes/public health with limited financial means.

Enhanced—Third-tier resources/services that are optional but important.

Maximal—High-level/state-of-the-art resources/services associated with significantly higher cost and/or impracticality for broad use in resource-limited area.

Source: USPSTF 2021; American Society of Clinical Oncology (ASCO) Resource-Stratified Guideline for CRC screening in average-risk adults age 50–75 y in settings with high incidence of CRC. *J Global Onc.* 2019;5:1-22.

7 Accuracy of colonoscopy is operator dependent—rapid withdrawal time, poor prep, and lack of experience will increase false-negatives. (*N Engl J Med.* 2006;355:2533) (*Ann Intern Med.* 2012;156:692) (*Gastroenterology* 2015;110:72)

8 Multitargeted DNA stool testing vs. iFOBT with more cancers detected (92.3% vs. 73.8%) but more false-positives with DNA test. (*N Engl J Med.* 2014;370:1287-1306)

9 Percentage of US adults receiving some form of CRC screening increased from 44% in 1999 to 63% in 2008. The goal was 80% by 2018. (*CA Cancer J Clin.* 2015;65:30) (*Arch Intern Med.* 2011;171:647; 2012;172:575). However, the percentage increased from 58.7% in 2010 to 65.5% in 2018 (www.cdc.gov/mmwr/volumes/69/wr/mm6929a6.htm). In 2016, an estimated 134,000 new cases of CRC were diagnosed and 49,000 Americans died from CRC. Median age of diagnosis is 68. (*CA Cancer J Clin.* 2016;66:7)

10 Colonoscopy vs. iFOBT testing in CRC with similar detection of cancer, but more adenomas identified in the colonoscopy group. (*N Engl J Med.* 2012;366:687,697)

11 A normal screening colonoscopy may provide reassurance for up to 17 y. (*Ann Intern Med.* 2020;173(2):81-91)

Sources

–ACS. 2020. https://www.cancer.org/cancer/colon-rectal-cancer/detection-diagnosis-staging/acs-recommendations.html

–USPSTF. *JAMA.* 2016;315(23):2564-2575.

–AAFP. 2021. https://www.aafp.org/family-physician/patient-care/clinical-recommendations/all-clinical-recommendations/colorectal-cancer-adults.html

–ACG. *Am J Gastroenterol.* March 2021;116(3):458-479.

–ACP. *Ann Int Med.* 2019;171(9):643-654.

–USMSTF. *Gastroenterol.* 2020;158:1131-1153.

–USMSTF. *Am J Gastroenterol.* 2017;112(7):1016-1030.

–CTF. *CMAJ.* 2016;188(5):340-348.

–NCCN. 2021. https://www.nccn.org/professionals/physician_gls/pdf/colorectal_screening.pdf

–ASCO. *J Global Onc.* 2019;5:1-22.

Organizations

▶ AAFP 2018, NCCN 2020

Prevention Recommendations

–Modifiable risk factors:
- Diet:
  - Advise patients to increase consumption of fruits, nonstarchy vegetables, and whole grains. Preferentially optimize nutrition from natural food sources rather than dietary supplements.
  - Cholesterol: 2-fold increased risk of CRC with increased intake.
  - Fat: 25% increased risk of serrated polyps with increased fat intake.
  - Dairy: 15% reduced risk of CRC with >8 oz of cow's milk daily.
  - Fiber: no reduced risk of CRC or adenomatous polyps with increased fiber intake.
  - Red and processed meat: 22% increased risk of CRC with increased red and processed meat intake.
- Lifestyle:
  - Alcohol: 8% increased risk of CRC and 24% increased risk of serrated polyps. Reducing alcohol intake does not clearly lower risk for CRC or polyps.
  - Cigarettes: 114% increased risk of high-risk adenomatous polyps and CRC in current smokers.
  - Obesity: bariatric surgery associated with 27% reduced risk of CRC in obese individuals. Increased BMI is associated with increased mortality from CRC.
  - Occupational physical activity: 25% decreased risk of colon cancer and 12% decreased risk of rectal cancer.
  - Recreational physical activity: 20% decreased risk of colon cancer and 13% decreased risk of rectal cancer.

- Medications:
  - Statins: weak evidence that statin use ≥5 y is associated with decreased risk of advanced adenomatous polyps.
  - Calcium: 26% reduced risk of adenomatous polyps; 22% reduced risk of CRC in individuals taking 1400 mg daily calcium compared to 600 mg.
- Polyp removal:
  - Based on fair evidence, removal of adenomatous polyps reduces the risk of CRC, especially polyps >1 cm. (*Ann Intern Med.* 2011;154:22) (*Gastrointest Endosc.* 2014;80:471)
  - Based on fair evidence, complications of polyp removal include perforation of the colon and bleeding estimated at 7–9 events per 1000 procedures.
- Interventions without benefit:
  - Vitamin D.
  - Folic acid.
  - Antioxidants.

Sources
- *Am Fam Physician.* 2018;97(10):658-665.
- NCCN. *Colorectal Cancer Screening.* 2020:1-61.

COLORECTAL CANCER, HIGH-RISK INDIVIDUALS

Organizations
▶ USMSTF on CRC 2017, NCCN 2021, ACG 2021

Screening Recommendations
- Screen adults with family history of early CRC[1] or advanced adenoma (AA) with colonoscopy every 5 y starting at age 40 y or 10 y prior to earliest age of diagnosis of first-degree relative.
- Use Amsterdam I and II criteria to diagnose hereditary nonpolyposis CRC (HNPCC), with subsequent genetic screen for Lynch syndrome (LS).
  - Amsterdam I criteria:
    - ≥3 relatives with histologically verified CRC, one of which is a first-degree relative of the other two. Diagnosis of familial adenomatous polyposis (FAP) excluded.
    - ≥2 generations with CRC.
    - ≥1 CRC diagnosis before age 50 y.
  - Amsterdam II criteria:
    - ≥3 relatives with histologically verified HNPCC-associated cancer (colorectal, endometrial, small bowel, ureter, renal pelvis), one of which is a first-degree relative of the other two. Diagnosis of FAP excluded.
    - ≥2 generations with CRC.
    - ≥1 CRC diagnosis before age 50 y.

[1]First-degree relative diagnosed prior to age 60 or advanced adenoma in ≥2 first-degree relatives at any age.

–Lynch syndrome (LS): screening colonoscopy every 1–2 y for persons with LS or at-risk (first-degree relatives of those affected), starting at age 20–25 y, or 2–5 y before youngest age of family CRC diagnosis if diagnosed before age 25 y.

–Family CRC Type X syndrome: screening colonoscopy every 3–5 y beginning 10 y before the age at diagnosis of the youngest affected relative.

Sources
–USMSTF. *Am J Gastroenterol.* 2017;112(7):1016-1030.

–NCCN. 2021. https://www.nccn.org/professionals/physician_gls/pdf/colorectal_screening.pdf

–ACG. *Am J Gastroenterol.* March 2021;116(3):458-479.

ESOPHAGEAL CANCER

Organization
▶ ASGE 2017

Recommendations
–Follow-up intervals for biopsy-proven BE:
- No dysplasia: follow-up EGD with biopsy every 3–5 y.
- Indeterminate dysplasia: repeat EGD with biopsy in 3–6 mo after optimizing PPI therapy.
- Low-grade dysplasia: endoscopic eradication therapy or ongoing annual endoscopic surveillance.
- High-grade dysplasia: endoscopic eradication therapy.

Comments
1. In 2017, 16,940 new cases of esophageal cancer were diagnosed in the United States; 15,690 persons died from esophageal cancer.
2. There is a 4-fold incidence of esophageal adenocarcinoma compared to squamous cell carcinoma.

Source
–*Gastrointest Endosc.* 2017;85(5):889-903.

Organization
▶ AAFP 2017

Prevention Recommendations
–Minimize exposure to risk factors.

–Adenocarcinoma risk factors:
- Age 50–60 y.
- Male sex (8-fold risk).
- White race (5-fold risk).
- GERD (5- to 7-fold risk, depending on symptom frequency).
- Obesity (2.4-fold risk with BMI $\geq$ 30), particularly central adiposity.
- Smoking (2-fold risk).
- BE (premalignant).

–Squamous cell carcinoma risk factors:
- Age 60–70 y.
- Achalasia (10-fold risk).
- Smoking (9-fold risk).
- Alcohol use (3- to 5-fold risk with ≥3 drinks/d).
- Black race (3-fold risk).
- High-starch diet without fruits or vegetables.

Comments

1. Longstanding GERD associated with BE and increased risk of esophageal CA. (*PLOS.* 2014;9:e103508)
2. Radiofrequency ablation of BE with moderate or severe dysplasia may reduce risk of progression to malignancy. (*N Engl J Med.* 2009;360:2277-2288)
3. Uncertain if elimination of GERD by surgical or medical therapy will reduce the risk of esophageal adenocarcinoma although a few trials show benefit. (*Gastroenterology.* 2010;138:1297)
4. No trials in the United States have shown any benefit from the use of chemoprevention with vitamins and/or minerals to prevent esophageal cancer. (*Am J Gastroenterol.* 2014;109:1215) (*Gut.* 2016;65:548)

Source
–*Am Fam Physician.* 2017;95(1):22-28.

GASTRIC CANCER

Organization
▶ ACG 2015

Recommendations

–Do not routinely screen average-risk adults, given low incidence in the United States.
–Screen with EGD for specific high-risk subgroups.[1] For AP syndromes, start EGD screening for gastric and proximal small bowel tumors starting at age 25–30 y, with follow-up depending on the stage of duodenal polyposis.

Sources
–*Gastrointest Endosc.* 2016;84(1):18-28.
–*Am J Gastroenterol.* 2015;110(2):223-262.

Organization
▶ AAFP 2017

Prevention Recommendations

–Modifiable risk factors:

---

[1]High-risk groups include those with gastric adenomas, pernicious anemia, gastric intestinal metaplasia, Lynch syndrome, familial adenomatous polyposis, and family history of gastric cancer.

- *H. pylori*: classified as Group 1 (definite) carcinogen by World Health Organization (WHO), *H. pylori* triggers a series of inflammatory reactions leading to chronic gastritis, stomach atrophy, and early steps in the carcinogenesis sequence.
  - Screen for *H. pylori* in patients with peptic ulcer disease or gastric MALT lymphoma. (*Am J Gastroenterol.* 2007;102:1808-1825)
  - A study over 15 y showed a 40% reduction in risk of gastric cancer with *H. pylori* eradication. (*Ann Intern Med.* 2009;151:121) (*J Natl Cancer Inst.* 2012;104:488)
- Diet: increased risk with smoked foods (N-nitroso compounds), high salt diet. Decreased risk with fruit and nonstarch vegetable intake.
- Cigarette use: 60% increased risk in current male smokers and 20% increased risk in female smokers, compared to nonsmokers.
- Obesity: increased risk with BMI $\geq$ 30.
- Physical activity: 21% decreased risk.
- Male sex: 2-fold to 5-fold risk compared to women, though postmenopausal women have increased risk approaching that of men.
- First-degree relative with gastric cancer: 2.6-fold to 3.5-fold risk.

–Clinical consideration:
- Patients with hereditary susceptibility (HNPCC, e-cadherin mutation, Li–Fraumeni syndrome), pernicious anemia, atrophic gastritis, partial gastrectomy, or gastric polyps should be followed carefully for early cancer symptoms and for upper endoscopy at intervals according to risk.

Sources
–*Am Fam Physician.* 2017;95(1):22-28.
–*Gastrointest Endosc.* 2016;84(1):18-28.

HEPATOCELLULAR CARCINOMA (HCC)

Organization
▶ AASLD 2018

Screening Recommendations
–For adults with cirrhosis (Child-Pugh class A and B), screen using ultrasound with or without alfa-fetoprotein (AFP) every 6 mo to improve overall survival.
–For Child's class C cirrhosis, do not screen unless they are on a transplant waiting list, given the low anticipated survival associated with Child's class C.
–For individuals with risk factors without cirrhosis, do not screen, given significantly lower risk of HCC.

Comments
1. In 2016, there were an estimated 39,230 new diagnoses of HCC and 27,170 deaths due to this disease in the United States; 80% of HCC cases occur in persons with cirrhosis.
2. Due to low-level evidence, HCC screening is considered controversial.

3. Due to low sensitivity, AFP alone should not be used for screening unless ultrasound is not available.

Source
   –AASLD. *Hepatology*. 2018;68(2):723-750.

Organizations

▶ AASLD 2018, NCI 2019

Prevention Recommendations

–Modifiable risk factors: cirrhosis and associated risk factors:
   • Chronic hepatitis B (HBV) infection.
   • Hepatitis C (HCV) infection.
   • Extensive alcohol use.
   • Nonalcoholic steatohepatitis (NASH).
   • Hereditary hemochromatosis.
   • Primary biliary cholangitis.
   • Wilson's disease.
   • Aflatoxin B1 (fungal toxin that contaminates corn, grains, and nuts that are not stored properly).
–Prevention:
   • Vaccinate against hepatitis B.
   • Treat hepatitis C infection.
   • Achieve alcohol cessation.
   • Treat underlying risk factors as applicable.

Sources
   –AASLD. *Hepatology*. 2018;68(2):723-750.
   –NCI. *Adult Primary Liver Cancer Treatment (PDQ)*. 2019.

HEREDITARY HEMOCHROMATOSIS (HH)

Organizations

▶ ACG 2019, AASLD 2011, AAFP 2013

Recommendations

–Screen family members, particularly first-degree relatives, of patients diagnosed with HH, using iron studies and serum HFE mutation analysis.
–If evidence of active liver disease, obtain iron studies (ferritin, transferrin saturation). If abnormal, evaluate for HH.

Comments

1. HH is one of the most common genetic disorders among persons of northern European descent. There are 4 main HH categories based on which iron homeostasis proteins are affected. Screening indicated by positive family history should be tailored to specific type of HH in the family. (ACG 2019)

2. There is no established consensus regarding elevated ferritin or transferrin saturation threshold levels that would warrant further evaluation for HH. Possible threshold values are serum ferritin >200 µg/L in women and >300 µg/L in men, and transferrin saturation >45%.

3. There is fair evidence that clinically significant disease caused by hereditary hemochromatosis is uncommon in the general population. Male homozygotes for *C282Y* gene mutation have a 2-fold increase in the incidence of iron overload–related symptoms, compared with females.

4. There is poor evidence that early therapeutic phlebotomy improves morbidity and mortality in screening-detected vs. clinically detected individuals.

5. Both men and women who have a heterozygote *C282Y* gene mutation rarely develop iron overload.

6. For clinicians who choose to screen, one-time screening of non-Hispanic white men with serum ferritin level and transferrin saturation has highest yield.

Sources
–ACG. *Am J Gastroenterol.* 2019;114:1202-1218.
–AASLD. *Hepatology.* 2011;54(1):328-343.
–*Am Fam Physician.* 2013;87(3):183-190.

HEPATITIS B VIRUS (HBV) INFECTION

Organizations
▶ USPSTF 2020, CDC 2018, 2020

Recommendations
–Screen high-risk individuals using HBV surface antigen (HBsAg):
- Foreign-born persons from countries where HBV prevalence ≥2%.[1]
- US-born persons not vaccinated at birth whose parents were born in countries where HBV prevalence ≥8%.[k]
- HIV-positive persons.
- Household contacts or sexual partners of persons with HBV infection.
- Men who have sex with men.
- Persons with injection drug use.
- Hemodialysis patients. (CDC)
- Persons needing immunosuppressive therapy, immunosuppression related to organ transplantation, and immunosuppression for rheumatologic or gastroenterologic disorders. (CDC)

[1]HBV prevalence ≥2% in Africa, Asia, South Pacific, Middle East (except Cyprus and Israel), Eastern Europe (except Hungary), Malta, Spain, indigenous populations of Greenland, Alaska natives, indigenous populations of Canada, Caribbean, Guatemala, Honduras, and South America. HBV prevalence ≥ 8% in Angola, Benin, Burkina Faso, Burundi, Cameroon, Central African Republic, Congo, Côte d'Ivoire, Djibouti, Equatorial Guinea, Gabon, Gambia, Ghana, Guinea, Liberia, Malawi, Mali, Mauritania, Mozambique, Namibia, Niger, Nigeria, Senegal, Sierra Leone, Somalia, South Sudan, Sudan, Swaziland, Togo, Uganda, Zimbabwe, Haiti, Kiribati, Nauru, Niue, Papua New Guinea, Solomon Islands, Tonga, Vanuatu, Kyrgyzstan , Laos, Vietnam, Mongolia, Yemen.

- Blood, organ, plasma, semen, or tissue donors. (CDC)
- People with elevated alanine aminotransferase levels ($\geq$19 IU/L for women and $\geq$30 IU/L for men). (CDC)
- Infants born to HBV-infected mothers (HBsAg and antibody to hepatitis B surface antigen [anti-HBs] only are recommended). (CDC)

Sources
−USPSTF. *JAMA*. 2020;324(23):2415-2422.
−CDC. *MMWR Recomm Rep*. Jan 12, 2018;67(1):1−31.
−CDC. July 28, 2020, www.cdc.gov/hepatitis/hbv/hbvfaq.htm

HEPATITIS C VIRUS (HCV) INFECTION

Organizations
▶ AASLD 2020, USPSTF 2020

Recommendations
−Offer one-time universal opt-out HCV screening, using anti-HCV antibody testing with reflex HCV RNA PCR, to all adults aged 18 y or older, regardless of risk factors.
−Individuals with increased risk[1] of HCV exposure:
  - One-time HCV screening for age <18 y.
−Periodic repeat testing for all individuals as indicated.
−Annual screening for individuals who inject drugs and for men with HIV who have unprotected sex with men, including those with prior infections who were treated or cleared spontaneously.

Comments
1. Anti-HCV antibodies typically develop 2–6 mo after exposure. HCV RNA is typically reliably detectable within 2–3 wk after exposure. In patients with negative anti-HCV antibody testing, perform HCV RNA testing for suspicion of acute HCV infection, or for unexplained liver disease in an immunocompromised patient.
2. Of persons with acute hepatitis C, 15%–25% resolve their infection; of the remaining persons that develop chronic infection, 10%–20% develop cirrhosis within 20–30 y after infection, and 1%–5% develop hepatocellular carcinoma.
3. Universal HCV screening is recommended because of the opioid epidemic, high efficacy of DAA therapy, and long-term benefits of successful treatment.

Sources
−AASLD. *Hepatology*. 2020; 71(2):686-721.
−USPSTF. *JAMA*. 2020;323(10):970-975.

---

[1]Risk factors for HCV infection: injection drug use, intranasal illicit drug use, men who have sex with men, long-term hemodialysis patients, percutaneous/parenteral exposures in an unregulated setting; health care providers and public safety workers after needlestick, sharps, or mucosal exposures to HCV-infected blood; children born to HCV-infected women, history of incarceration, prior recipients of blood transfusion(s) or organ transplant, HIV infection, sexually active persons about to start preexposure prophylaxis for HIV, unexplained chronic liver disease and/or chronic hepatitis, solid organ donors and transplant recipients.

PANCREATIC CANCER

Organization
▶ USPSTF 2019

Recommendations
–Do not screen asymptomatic adults.
–No established screening guidelines in individuals with inherited genetic cancer syndromes or familial pancreatic cancer.

Comments
1. Cigarette smoking has consistently been associated with increased risk of pancreatic cancer. BRCA2 mutation is associated with a 5% lifetime risk of pancreatic cancer; blood group O with lower risk, and diabetes with a 2-fold higher risk. (*J Natl Cancer Inst.* 2009;101:424) (*J Clin Oncol.* 2009;27:433)
2. Patients with a strong family history (≥2 first-degree relatives with pancreatic cancer) should undergo genetic counseling and may benefit from interval screening with CA 19-9, CT scan, and magnetic resonance cholangiopancreatography (MRCP). (*Nat Rev Gastroenterol Hepatol.* 2012;9:445-453)

Sources
–USPSTF. *JAMA.* 2019;322(5):438-444.
–*Gastroenterology.* 2019;156(7):2024-2040.

Genitourinary Disorders

6

▼ BLADDER CANCER

Organizations
▶ AAFP 2011, USPSTF 2016

Screening Recommendation
  –Do not screen routinely for bladder cancer (CA) in adults.

Comments
  1. There is inadequate evidence to determine whether screening for bladder CA would affect mortality. Based on fair evidence, screening for bladder CA would result in unnecessary diagnostic procedures and overdiagnosis (70% of bladder CA is in situ) with attendant morbidity. (NCI 2017)
  2. Urinary biomarkers (nuclear matrix protein 22, tumor-associated antigen p300, presence of DNA ploidy) do not have significant sensitivity or specificity to be utilized in clinical practice. Microscopic hematuria leads to a diagnosis of bladder CA in only 5% of patients.
  3. Eighty-one thousand cases of bladder CA were expected in 2022 in the United States, with the majority being noninvasive (70%), but still 17,100 Americans were expected to die of bladder CA in 2017. (*Ann Inter Med.* 2010;153:461) (*Eur Urol.* 2013;63:4) (American Cancer Society. *Cancer Facts & Figures 2022.* Atlanta: American Cancer Society; 2022.)
  4. Maintain a high index of suspicion in anyone with a history of smoking (4- to 7-fold increased risk[1]), an exposure to industrial toxins (aromatic amines, benzene), therapeutic pelvic radiation, cyclophosphamide chemotherapy, a history of *Schistosoma haematobium* cystitis, hereditary nonpolyposis colon CA (Lynch syndrome), and history of transitional cell carcinoma of ureter (50% risk of subsequent bladder CA). Large screening studies in these high-risk populations have not been performed.
  5. Voided urine cytology with sensitivity of 40% but only 10% positive predictive value, urinary biomarkers (nuclear matrix protein 22, telomerase) with suboptimal sensitivity and specificity. Screening for microscopic hematuria has <10% positive predictive value.

[1]Individuals who smoke are 4–7 times more likely to develop bladder CA than individuals who have never smoked. Additional environmental risk factors: exposure to aminobiphenyls; aromatic amines; azo dyes; combustion gases and soot from coal; chlorination by-products in heated water; aldehydes used in chemical dyes and in the rubber and textile industries; organic chemicals used in dry cleaning, paper manufacturing, rope and twine making, and apparel manufacturing; contaminated Chinese herbs; arsenic in well water. Additional risk factors: prolonged exposure to urinary *S. haematobium* bladder infections, cyclophosphamide, or pelvic radiation therapy for other malignancies.

Sources
  –http://www.aafp.org/online/en/home/clinical/exam.html
  –http://www.ahrq.gov/clinic/uspstf/uspsblad.htm
  –http://www.cancer.gov

Infectious Diseases

7

COLITIS, CLOSTRIDIUM DIFFICILE

Organizations
▶ ACG 2013, CID 2018

Prevention Recommendations
–Develop antibiotic stewardship programs to minimize the frequency and duration of high-risk antibiotic therapy.
–Place patients with suspected *C. difficile* infection (CDI) preemptively on contact precautions pending the *C. difficile* test results.
–Maintain contact precautions for at least 48 h after diarrhea has resolved.
–Treat patients with CDAD in a private room.
–Perform hand hygiene before and after contact of a patient with CDI and after removing gloves with either soap or water.
–Use gloves and gowns on entry to the room of a patient with known or suspected CDI and remove gowns and gloves before leaving the patient's room.
–Prevent transmission by using single-use disposable equipment. Thoroughly clean and disinfect reusable medical equipment, preferentially with a sporicidal disinfectant. Dedicated nondisposable equipment should be kept in the patient's room.
–Disinfect environmental surfaces using an Environmental Protective Agency (EPA)–registered disinfectant with *C. difficile* sporicidal label claim or minimum chlorine concentration of 5000 ppm.
–Although there is an epidemiological association between proton pump inhibitor (PPI) use and CDI, there is insufficient evidence for discontinuation of PPIs as a measure for preventing CDI.
–Although there is moderate evidence that probiotics containing *Lactobacillus rhamnosus* GG and *Saccharomyces boulardii* decrease the incidence of antibiotic-associated diarrhea, there is insufficient data to recommend administration of probiotics for primary prevention of CDI. Still, short-term use of probiotics appears to be safe and effective when used along with antibiotics in patients who are not immunocompromised or severely ill.

Sources
–*Am J Gastroenterol.* 2013;108(4):478.
–*Clin Infect Dis.* 2018;66(7):e1-e48.
–Goldenberg JZ, et al. Probiotics for the prevention of Clostridium difficile-associated diarrhea in adults and children. *Cochrane Database Syst Rev.* 2017;12:CD006095.

ENDOCARDITIS PREVENTION

Organizations
▶ AHA 2007, AHA/ACC 2014, AHA/ACC 2017, AAPD 2014

Prevention Recommendations
- Maintain optimal oral health and hygiene. This is more important in reducing the risk of infective endocarditis (IE) than prophylactic antibiotics for dental procedures.
- There is insufficient evidence to support the use of topical antiseptics for IE prevention.
- Prevent rheumatic fever by promptly recognizing and treating streptococcal pharyngitis.
- The effectiveness of antibiotic prophylaxis in preventing IE in patients undergoing dental procedures is unknown.
- Do not use antibiotic prophylaxis for mitral valve prolapse (MVP), rheumatic heart disease (RHD), or most cases of congenital heart disease (CHD).[1]
- Offer IE prophylaxis[2] only for patients with underlying cardiac conditions (patients with prosthetic valves,[3] previous history of IE, certain cardiac transplant recipients,[4] and selected patients with CHD and residual defects) who will undergo selected dental, respiratory, GI, GU, skin, and soft tissue procedures.
  - Dental procedures: consider antibiotic prophylaxis for qualifying patients undergoing dental procedures that involve the gingival tissues or periapical region of a tooth and for those procedures that perforate the oral mucosa.
  - Respiratory procedures: consider antibiotic prophylaxis for qualifying patients undergoing invasive respiratory tract procedures that involve incision or biopsy of the respiratory mucosa.
  - GI/GU procedures: do not use antibiotic prophylaxis solely to prevent IE for GU or GI tract procedures, unless there is ongoing enterococcal infection in qualifying patients. Treat patients with an enterococcal urinary tract infection (UTI) or whose urine is colonized with *Enterococcus* with an antibiotic to eradicate enterococci from the urine prior to an elective cystoscopy or other urinary tract manipulation. If the urinary tract procedure is not elective, treat concurrently with antibiotics which are active against enterococci.

---

[1]Exceptions: (1) Unrepaired cyanotic CHD, including palliative shunts and conduits; (2) completely repaired congenital heart defect with prosthetic material or device, whether placed by surgery or by catheter intervention, during first 6 mo after the procedure; (3) repaired CHD with residual defects (eg, shunts or valvular regurgitation) at the site of or adjacent to the site of a prosthetic patch or prosthetic device.

[2]Standard prophylaxis regimen: amoxicillin (adults 2 g; children 50 mg/kg orally 1 h before procedure). If unable to take oral medications, give ampicillin (adults 2.0 g IM or IV; children 50 mg/kg IM or IV within 30 min of procedure). If penicillin-allergic, give clindamycin (adults 600 mg; children 20 mg/kg orally 1 h before procedure) or azithromycin or clarithromycin (adults 500 mg; children 15 mg/kg orally 1 h before procedure). If penicillin-allergic and unable to take oral medications, give clindamycin (adults 600 mg; children 20 mg/kg IV within 30 min before procedure). If allergy to penicillin is not anaphylaxis, angioedema, or urticaria, options for nonoral treatment also include cefazolin (1 g IM or IV for adults, 50 mg/kg IM or IV for children); and for penicillin-allergic, oral therapy includes cephalexin 2 g PO for adults or 50 mg/kg PO for children (IM, intramuscular; IV, intravenous; PO, by mouth, orally).

[3]Prosthetic cardiac valves, including transcatheter-implanted prostheses and homografts, or prosthetic material used for cardiac valve repair (annuloplasty rings, chords).

[4]Only those who develop cardiac valvulopathy.

- Skin/soft tissue procedures: consider antibiotic prophylaxis for qualifying patients undergoing surgical procedures involving infected skin, skin structure, or musculoskeletal tissue using an agent that is active against staphylococci and beta-hemolytic streptococci. Advise against body piercing.

–Arrange perioperative prophylactic antibiotics with staphylococcal coverage for patients undergoing surgery for placement of prosthetic intravascular or intracardiac materials (eg, prosthetic valves).

–Give long-term antistreptococcal prophylaxis for secondary prevention of rheumatic fever in patients with RHD, specifically mitral stenosis.

–Continue IE prophylaxis indefinitely in postcardiac transplant patients with a structurally abnormal valve.

–Do not use antibiotic prophylaxis for the following procedures and events:
  - Routine anesthetic injections through noninfected tissue.
  - Taking dental radiographs.
  - Placement of removable prosthodontic or orthodontic appliances.
  - Adjustment of orthodontic appliances or placement of orthodontic brackets.
  - Shedding of deciduous teeth.
  - Bleeding from trauma to the lips or oral mucosa.
  - Bronchoscopy without incision of the respiratory tract mucosa.
  - Diagnostic esophagogastroduodenoscopy or colonoscopy.
  - Vaginal or Cesarean delivery.
  - Hysterectomy.
  - Tattooing.
  - Coronary artery bypass graft surgery.

Comment

1. IE is much more likely to result from frequent exposure to random bacteremia associated with daily activities (eg, chewing food, tooth brushing, flossing, use of toothpicks, use of water irrigation devices) and dental disease than from bacteremia caused by a dental, GI, or GU procedure. Antibiotic prophylaxis may reduce the incidence and duration of bacteremia but does not eliminate bacteremia. Only an extremely small number of cases of IE might be prevented by antibiotic prophylaxis even if it were 100% effective.

Sources
–*Circulation*. 2007;116:1736-1754.
–Nishimura RA, et al. *J Am Coll Cardiol*. 2014;63(22):e57.
–Nishimura RA, et al. *J Am Coll Cardiol*. 2017;70(2):252-289.
–American Academy of Pediatric Dentistry. 2014;40(6):386-391.

GONORRHEA AND CHLAMYDIA

Population
–Women.

Organizations
▶ CDC 2015, AAP 2014, USPSTF 2021

Screening Recommendations
–Screen all women <25 y who are sexually active and ≥25 y if at increased risk.[1]

GUIDELINES DISCORDANT: RECOMMENDED SCREENING INTERVAL	
Organization	**Interval**
CDC, AAP	Screen annually
USPSTF	Screen when sexual history reveals new or persistent risk factors since last negative test. Insufficient data to determine universal screening interval.

Comments
1. In addition to the public health benefit of identifying and treating a communicable disease, infections in women are often asymptomatic but may lead to pelvic inflammatory disease (PID) which can lead to chronic pelvic pain, ectopic pregnancy, and infertility.
2. Women age <25 y are at highest risk for gonorrhea infection. Other risk factors that place women at increased risk include a previous gonorrhea infection, the presence of other sexually transmitted diseases (STDs), new or multiple sex partners, sex partner with concurrent partners, sex partner who has an STI, inconsistent condom use, commercial sex work, history of incarceration and drug use.

Sources
–CDC. *Sexually Transmitted Diseases Guidelines.* 2015.
–*Pediatrics.* 2014;134(1):e302.
–USPSTF. *Chlamydia and Gonorrhea: Screening.* 2021.

Population
–Young heterosexual men; nonpregnant women >25 y without risk factors.

Organizations
▶ CDC 2015, USPSTF 2014

Screening Recommendations
–Insufficient evidence for or against routine screening.
–Consider screening in high prevalence clinical settings.

Comments
1. *Chlamydia* and *Gonorrhea* are a reportable infection to the Public Health Department in every state.
2. Men are more likely than women to have symptomatic infection and are at lower risk of permanent sequelae such as infertility, making the rationale for asymptomatic screening less evident.

[1]Women age <25 y are at highest risk for gonorrhea infection. Other risk factors that place women at increased risk include a previous gonorrhea infection, the presence of other sexually transmitted diseases (STDs), new or multiple sex partners, inconsistent condom use, commercial sex work, and drug use.

Sources
- USPSTF. *Chlamydia and Gonorrhea: Screening.* 2014.
- CDC. *Sexually Transmitted Diseases Guidelines.* 2015.

Population
- Men who have sex with men.

Organization

▶ CDC 2015

Screening Recommendations
- Annual testing, regardless of condom use.
- Frequency of q 3–6 mo for high-risk activity.

Comments
1. Urine nucleic amplification acid test (NAAT) for *Chlamydia* and/or *Gonorrhea* for men who have had insertive intercourse and women with vaginal/penile intercourse.
2. NAAT of rectal swab for persons who have had receptive anal intercourse.
3. NAAT of oropharyngeal swab for persons engaged in oral sexual intercourse.

Source
- CDC. *Sexually Transmitted Diseases Treatment Guidelines.* 2015.

HERPES SIMPLEX VIRUS (HSV), GENITAL

Organizations

▶ CDC 2015, USPSTF 2016

Screening Recommendation
- Do not screen routinely for HSV with serologies.

Comment
1. In women with a history of genital herpes, routine serial cultures for HSV are not indicated in the absence of active lesions.

Sources
- *JAMA.* 2016;316(23):2525-2530.
- CDC. *Sexually Transmitted Diseases Treatment Guidelines.* 2015.

HUMAN IMMUNODEFICIENCY VIRUS (HIV)

Organizations

▶ AAFP 2013, USPSTF 2019, CDC 2015

Screening Recommendations
- Screen everyone in recommended age groups.

GUIDELINES DISCORDANT: POPULATION TO SCREEN	
Organization	**Age Range**
AAFP	18–65 y
USPSTF	15–65 y
CDC	13–64 y

–Consider screening high-risk individuals[1] of other ages.

Comments

1. Optimal screening interval is not defined.
2. Educate and counsel all high-risk patients regarding HIV testing, transmission, risk-reduction behaviors, and implications of infection.
3. If acute HIV is suspected, use plasma RNA test also.
4. False-positive results with electroimmunoassay (EIA): nonspecific reactions in persons with immunologic disturbances (eg, systemic lupus erythematosus or rheumatoid arthritis), multiple transfusions, recent influenza, or rabies vaccination.
5. Confirmatory testing is necessary using Western blot or indirect immunofluorescence assay.
6. Awareness of HIV positively reduces secondary HIV transmission risk and high-risk behavior and viral load if on highly active antiretroviral therapy (HAART). (CDC, 2006)

Sources
–AAFP. *Clinical Recommendations: HIV Infection, Adolescents and Adults.* 2013.
–CDC. *Sexually Transmitted Diseases Treatment Guidelines.* 2015.
–USPSTF. *Screening for HIV Infection.* 2019.

Organizations

▶ CDC 2021, UPSTF 2019, BHIVA/BASHH 2018

Prevention Recommendations

–Offer preexposure prophylaxis (PrEP) with effective antiretroviral therapy to adolescents and adults who are at high risk of HIV acquisition. Examples of high-risk patients include:

GUIDELINES DISCORDANT: HIGH-RISK CHARACTERISTICS FOR PREP ELIGIBILITY	
CDC	– Anal or vaginal sex in past 6 mo AND any of the following: • HIV-positive sexual partner • STI in past 6 mo (gonorrhea, chlamydia, syphilis) • History of inconsistent or no condom use – Persons who inject drugs with HIV-positive injecting partner or who share injection equipment

[1] Risk factors for HIV: men who have had sex with men after 1975; multiple sexual partners; history of intravenous drug use; prostitution; history of sex with an HIV-infected person; history of sexually transmitted disease; history of blood transfusion between 1978 and 1985; or persons requesting an HIV test.

GUIDELINES DISCORDANT: HIGH-RISK CHARACTERISTICS FOR PREP ELIGIBILITY *(Continued)*
USPSTF

- Men who have sex with men, are sexually active, and have one of the following characteristics:
  - A serodiscordant sex partner (ie, in a sexual relationship with an HIV-positive partner), unless partner has been on ART x6m and viral load <200 copies/mL
  - Inconsistently using condoms during receptive or insertive anal sex
  - Sexually transmitted infection (STI) such as syphilis, gonorrhea, or chlamydia in the past 6 mo
- Heterosexually active women and men who have one of the following characteristics:
  - A serodiscordant sex partner, unless partner has been on ART x6m and viral load <200 copies/mL
  - Inconsistently using condoms during sex with partner of unknown HIV status and is at high risk of acquiring HIV
  - STI such as syphilis, gonorrhea, or chlamydia in the past 6 mo
- Person who injects drugs and:
  - Shares use of drug injection equipment
  - Risk of sexual acquisition of HIV
- Transgender women and men who are HIV negative and have one of the following characteristics:
  - Inconsistently using condoms during receptive or insertive anal sex
  - A serodiscordant sex partner, unless partner has been on ART x6m and viral load <200 copies/mL

—Before beginning PrEP, ensure documented negative HIV Ag/Ab test within 1 wk of initial prescription, no signs/symptoms of acute HIV infection, CrCl ≥ 30 mL/min, and no contraindicated medications. If high-risk exposure in the preceding 4 wk, obtain HIV viral load.

—Obtain baseline Hepatitis B and C, syphilis, and gonorrhea and chlamydia testing at all sites of intercourse.

—Prescribe once daily emtricitabine/tenofovir disoproxil fumarate (F/TDF), up to a 90-d supply.

—For men and transgender women, consider emtricitabine/tenofovir alafenamide (F/TAF) as an alternative. (CDC)

—Consider the 2-1-1 alternate dosing schedule, only for adult men who have sex with men who prefer it to daily use:
  - Take F/TDF 2 pills 2 to 24 h before sex (closer to 24 h is preferred).
  - Take F/TDF 1 pill 24 h after the initial 2-pill dose.
  - Take F/TDF 1 pill 48 h after the initial 2-pill dose.
  - If sex on consecutive days, take 1 pill daily until 48 h after last sexual event.
  - If gap of <7 d between the last pill and the next sexual event, resume 1 pill daily.
  - If gap of ≥7 d between the last pill and the next sexual event, start again with 2 pills.
  - Prescribe no more than 30 pills without follow-up.

—Follow-up 4 wk after initiation to assess tolerance.

—Assess for HIV infection at least every 3 mo, as PrEP regimens are inadequate therapy for HIV.

—Screen for STIs and Hep C every 3–6 mo.

–Obtain renal panel every 6 mo, or every 12 mo if eGFR is >90.

–Test for pregnancy as indicated.

–If on F/TAF, assess weight and cholesterol levels annually.

Comments

1. Consider PrEP on a case-by-case basis. Although guidelines describe particular "at-risk groups," evaluate each patient as an individual and offer PrEP if risk is elevated.
2. Suggested eGFR for individuals starting TD-FTC is >60 mL/min/1.72 m^2.
3. Start individuals with eGFR <60 on a case-by-case basis.
4. Start hepatitis B vaccination in those who are nonimmune.
5. Hold PrEP if patient has symptoms suggestive of HIV and high risk of seroconversion.
6. Positive HIV test is an absolute contraindication to starting PrEP.
7. PrEP can be continued during pregnancy and breast-feeding.
8. Report information regarding use of PrEP during pregnancy to the Antiretroviral Pregnancy Registry.
9. Women using DMPA, PrEP is likely to counteract and increase in HIV acquisition. An alternative form of contraception, if available, should be offered.
10. There are no known interactions between TD-FTC and feminizing or masculinizing hormones.
11. A discussion about side effects including impact upon bone density should be held at PrEP initiation and maintenance visits.
12. In those at risk for reduced bone density, FRAX tool can guide need for DEXA scan and potential treatment.
13. Robust adherence support is required at PrEP initiation and maintenance.
14. PrEP provision should include condom provision and behavioral support.
15. TD alone can be offered to heterosexual men and women where FTC is contraindicated.

Sources

–UPSTF. *Preexposure Prophylaxis for the Prevention of HIV Infection US Preventive Services Task Force Recommendation Statement.* 2019.

–*JAMA.* 2019;321(22):2203-2213.

–*BHIVA/BASHH Guidelines on the Use of HIV Pre-exposure Prophylaxis (PrEP).* 2018.

–Centers for Disease Control and Prevention: US Public Health Service: Preexposure prophylaxis for the prevention of HIV infection in the United States—2021 Update: a clinical practice guideline. https://www.cdc.gov/hiv/pdf/risk/prep/cdc-hiv-prep-guidelines-2021.pdf. Published December 2021.

HUMAN IMMUNODEFICIENCY VIRUS (HIV), OPPORTUNISTIC INFECTIONS

Organizations

▶ CDC 2009, WHO 2018, NIH 2018

Prevention Recommendations

–See the table below (from the clinical practice guidelines at *CDC MMWR.* 2009;58(RR04);1-198).

Sources

–*CDC MMWR*. 2009;58(RR04):1-198.

–NIH. *Guidelines for the Prevention and Treatment of Opportunistic Infections in HIV-Infected Adults and Adolescents*. March 2018. https://www.cdc.gov/mmwr/preview/mmwrhtml/rr5804a1.htm

Population

–Primary prophylaxis in HIV-infected children.

Organizations

▶ CDC 2014, WHO 2018, NIH 2013

Prevention Recommendations

–See the table below (from the clinical practice guidelines at *CDC MMWR*. 2009;58(RR04):1-198).

–Antiretroviral therapy to avoid advanced immune deficiency constitutes primary prophylaxis against candidiasis, coccidioidomycosis, cryptococcosis, cryptosporidiosis, cystoisosporiasis, and giardiasis in children.

Sources

–Centers for Disease Control and Prevention. Revised Surveillance Case Definition for HIV Infection—United States, 2014. *MMWR Recomm Rep*. 2014;63(RR-03):1-10.

–NIH. *Guidelines for the Prevention and Treatment of Opportunistic Infections in HIV-Exposed and HIV-Infected Children*. November 2013.

IMMUNIZATIONS

Organization

▶ CDC 2019

Prevention Recommendation

–Immunize according to the Centers for Disease Control and Prevention (CDC) recommendations, unless contraindicated (see Chapter 33).

Sources

–CDC. *Adult Immunization Schedule*. 2019.

–CDC. *Child and Adolescent Immunization Schedule*. 2019.

PROPHYLAXIS TO PREVENT FIRST EPISODE OF OPPORTUNISTIC DISEASE AMONG HIV-INFECTED ADULTS

Pathogen	Indication	First Choice	Alternative
Pneumocystis carinii pneumonia (PCP)	CD4+ count <200 cells/µL or oropharyngeal candidiasis CD4+ <14% or history of AIDS-defining illness CD4+ count ≥200 but <250 cells/µL if monitoring CD4+ count every 3 mo is not possible and ART initiation delayed Note: Additional PCP prophylaxis is not needed if already receiving pyrimethamine/sulfadiazine for treatment/suppression of toxoplasmosis	Trimethoprim-sulfamethoxazole (TMP-SMX), 1 DS PO daily or 1 SS daily	• TMP-SMX 1 DS PO TI, *or* • Dapsone 100 mg PO daily or 50 mg PO BID, *or* • Dapsone 50 mg PO daily + pyrimethamine 50 mg PO weekly + leucovorin 25 mg PO weekly, *or* • [Dapsone 200 mg + pyrimethamine 75 mg + leucovorin 25 mg] PO weekly, *or* • Aerosolized pentamidine 300 mg via Respirgard II nebulized every month, *or* • Atovaquone 1500 mg PO daily, *or* • [Atovaquone 1500 mg + pyrimethamine 25 mg + leucovorin 10 mg] PO daily
Toxoplasma gondii encephalitis	*Toxoplasma* IgG-positive patients with CD4+ count <100 cells/µL Seronegative patients receiving PCP prophylaxis not active against toxoplasmosis should have toxoplasma serology retested if CD4+ count declines to <100 cells/µL; prophylaxis should be initiated if seroconversion occurred Note: Patients receiving primary prophylaxis for *Toxoplasma gondii* are also covered for PCP prophylaxis	TMP-SMX 1 DS PO daily	• TMP-SMX 1 DS PO TIW, *or* • TMP-SMX 1 SS PO daily, *or* • Dapsone 50 mg PO daily + pyrimethamine 50 mg PO weekly + leucovorin 25 mg PO weekly, *or* • [Dapsone 200 mg + pyrimethamine 75 mg + leucovorin 25 mg] PO weekly, *or* • Atovaquone 1500 mg PO daily, *or* • [Atovaquone 1500 mg + pyrimethamine 25 mg + leucovorin 10 mg] PO daily Note: (1) Screen for G6PD prior to administration with dapsone or primaquine (2) Screen for latent TB prior to initiating treatment with pyrimethamine

Mycobacterium tuberculosis infection (TB) (treatment of latent TB infection [LTBI])	(+) Screening test for LTBI, no evidence of active TB, and no prior treatment for active or latent TB (+) Diagnostic test for LTBI and no evidence of active TB, but close contact with a person with infectious pulmonary TB A history of untreated or inadequately treated healed TB (ie, old fibrotic lesions) regardless of diagnostic tests for LTBI and no evidence of active TB (AII)	Isoniazid (INH) 300 mg PO daily or 900 mg PO BIW by DOT + pyridoxine 25–50 mg PO daily x 9 mo For persons exposed to drug-resistant TB, selection of drugs after consultation with public health authorities	• Rifampin (RIF) 600 mg PO daily x 4 mo, or • Rifabutin (adjust dose based on concomitant ART) x 4 mo, or • [Rifapentine PO (750 mg if 32.1–49.9 kg or 900 mg if ≥50 kg) + INH 900 mg PO + pyridoxine 50 mg PO] once weekly x 12 wk (only administer rifapentine if receiving raltegravir or efavirenz-based ART regimen)
Disseminated *Mycobacterium avium* complex (MAC) disease	CD4+ count <50 cells/µL in those who are not on fully suppressive ART—after ruling out active MAC infection Not recommended for those who immediately initiate ART	Azithromycin 1200 mg PO once weekly; or clarithromycin 500 mg PO BID; or azithromycin 600 mg PO twice weekly	• Rifabutin 300 mg PO daily (dosage adjustment based on drug–drug interactions with ART); rule out active TB before starting RFB
Streptococcus pneumoniae infection	Patients who have not received any pneumococcal vaccine Patients with previous PPSV23 vaccine	PCV13 0.5 mL IM x 1, followed by 1. If CD4 ≥200 cells/µL: PPSV23 0.5 mL IM 8 wk after PCV13 2. If CD4 ≥200 cells/µL: PPV23 at least 8 wk after receiving PCV13 or after CD4 rises ≥200 cells/µL (BIII)	• PPSV23 0.5 mL IM x 1 (BII)
		If previously vaccinated with PPSV23, administer PCV13 x 1 at least 1 y after last PPSV23 If age 19–64 y and ≥5 y since first PPSV23 *or* age ≥65 y and ≥5 y since previous PPSV23, revaccinate with PPSV23 0.5 mL IM or SQ x 1	

(continued)

PROPHYLAXIS TO PREVENT FIRST EPISODE OF OPPORTUNISTIC DISEASE AMONG HIV-INFECTED ADULTS *(Continued)*			
Pathogen	**Indication**	**First Choice**	**Alternative**
Influenza A and B virus infection	All HIV-infected patients	Inactivated influenza vaccine 0.5 mL IM annually Do not use live-attenuated influenza vaccine	
Syphilis	For patients with exposure to a partner diagnosed with syphilis <90 d prior or for partners diagnosed >90 d prior with unknown serologic tests or uncertain follow-up	Benzathine penicillin G 2.4 million units IM x 1	For penicillin allergy: Doxycycline 100 mg PO BID x 14 d, *or* Ceftriaxone 1 g IM/IV daily x 8–10 d, *or* Azithromycin 2 g PO x 1 (BII) (not recommended for MSM or pregnant women)
Histoplasma capsulatum infection	CD4+ count <150 cells/μL and at high risk because of occupational exposure or live in a community with a hyperendemic rate of histoplasmosis (>10 cases/ 100 patient-y)	Itraconazole 200 mg PO daily	
Coccidioidomycosis	New positive IgM or IgG serologic test in a patient from a disease-endemic area, and CD4+ count <250 cells/μL	Fluconazole 400 mg PO daily	

Varicella-zoster virus (VZV) infection	*Preexposure prevention:* Patient with CD4+ count >200 cells/μL who have not been vaccinated, have no history of varicella or herpes zoster, or who are seronegative for VZV Note: Routine VZV serologic testing in HIV-infected adults/adolescents is not recommended *Postexposure prevention:* Close contact in susceptible persons (not vaccinated, no history of chickenpox or shingles, or VZV seronegative) with a person who has active varicella or herpes zoster	***Preexposure prevention:*** Primary varicella vaccination (Varivax), 2 doses (0.5 mL SQ) administered 3 mo apart If vaccination results in disease because of vaccine virus, treat with acyclovir *Postexposure prevention:* Varicella-zoster immune globulin (VZIG) 125 IU/10 kg (maximum of 625 IU) IM, administered as soon as possible within 10 d after exposure Note: VZIG can be obtained only under a treatment IND (1-800-843-7477, FFF Enterprises) No need to redose if patient receives monthly IVIG >400 mg/kg with last dose within previous 3 wk	*Preexposure prevention:* VZV-susceptible household contacts of susceptible HIV-infected persons should be vaccinated to prevent potential transmission of VZV to their HIV-infected contacts *Alternative postexposure prevention* (not studied in the HIV population): • Preemptive acyclovir 800 mg PO 5x/d for 5–7 d • Valacyclovir 1 g PO TID x 5–7 d • Varicella vaccines should be delayed >72 h after administration of antivirals • These two alternatives have not been studied in the HIV population
Human papillomavirus (HPV) infection	Patients age 13–26 y	HPV recombinant vaccine 9 valent (types 6, 11, 16, 18, 31, 33, 45, 52, 58) 0.5 mL IM at 0, 1–2, and 6 mo	Consider additional vaccination with recombinant 9-valent vaccine for patients who completed vaccination with recombinant bivalent or quadrivalent series (unclear who benefits or how cost-effective this is)
Hepatitis A virus (HAV) infection	HAV-susceptible patients with chronic liver disease, or who are injection-drug users, or men who have sex with men	Hepatitis A vaccine 1 mL IM x 2 doses—at 0 and 6–12 mo Reassess IgG antibody response 1 mo after vaccination; revaccinate nonresponders when CD4 count >200 cells/μL	If susceptible to both HAV and HBV, combined vaccine (Twinrix) 1 mL IM as a 3-dose series (0, 1, and 6 mo) or 4-dose series (day 0, day 7, day 21–30, and 12 mo)

(continued)

PROPHYLAXIS TO PREVENT FIRST EPISODE OF OPPORTUNISTIC DISEASE AMONG HIV-INFECTED ADULTS (*Continued*)

Pathogen	Indication	First Choice	Alternative
Hepatitis B virus (HBV) infection	No evidence of prior exposure to HBV (anti-HBs <10 IU/mL) should be vaccinated with HBV vaccine, including patients with CD4+ count <200 cells/µL Vaccinate early before CD4 falls <350 cells/µL Patients with CD4 <200 cells/µL may not respond to vaccination; consider delayed revaccination Vaccine nonresponders (anti-HBs <10 1–2 mo after vaccine series)	HBV vaccine IM (Engerix-B 20 µg/mL or Recombivax HB 10 µg/mL) at 0, 1, and 6 mo or 0, 1, 2, and 6 mo or Vaccine conjugated to CpG (Heplisav-B) IM at 0 and 1 mo (2-dose series can only be used if both doses are Heplisav-B) *or* Combined HAV and HBV vaccine (Twinrix) 1 mL IM as a 3-dose (0, 1, and 6 mo) or 4-dose series (days 0, 7, 21–30, and 12 mo) If anti-HBs ≤10 IU/mL after 1–2 mo from receipt of the vaccine, revaccinate with additional 4-dose series; consider delayed revaccination until sustained increase in CD4 count on ART *Patients with isolated anti-HBc:* Vaccinate x 1 standard dose of HBV. If anti-HBs <100 IU in 1–2 mo, vaccinate with full series and retest anti-HBs	Some experts recommend doses of double dose of either HBV vaccine
	Vaccine nonresponders: Defined as anti-HBs <10 IU/mL 1 mo after a vaccination series For patients with low CD4+ count at the time of first vaccination series, certain specialists might delay revaccination until after a sustained increase in CD4+ count with ART (CIII)	Revaccinate with a second vaccine series (BII)	Consider double doses of either HBV vaccine (BI)

Malaria	Travel to disease-endemic area	Recommendations are the same for HIV-infected and noninfected patients. One of the following three drugs is usually recommended, depending on location: atovaquone/ proguanil, doxycycline, or mefloquine. Refer to the following website for the most recent recommendations based on region and drug susceptibility: http://www.cdc.gov/malaria/	
Penicilliosis (talaromycosis)	Patients with CD4 <100 cells/µL who have extended exposure to rural areas of Thailand, Vietnam, or Southern China (BI)	Itraconazole 200 mg PO daily	Fluconazole 400 mg PO once weekly

BID, twice daily; BIW, two times weekly; DS, double strength; IM, intramuscular; PO, by mouth; SS, single strength; SQ, subcutaneous; TIW, three times weekly.

INFLUENZA, CHEMOPROPHYLAXIS

Organizations

▶ IDSA 2018, CDC 2011, AAP 2016

Prevention Recommendations

The following situations warrant chemoprophylaxis:

–Children at high risk for complications who cannot receive vaccine, or within 2 wk of receiving vaccine.

–Family members or health care providers who are unimmunized and likely to have ongoing exposure to high-risk or unimmunized children younger than 24 mo of age.

–Supplement vaccination in high-risk immunocompromised children.

–Consider preexposure antiviral chemoprophylaxis for adults and children aged ≥3 mo at highest risk of influenza complications as soon as influenza activity is detected in the community, in the absence of an outbreak.

- Continue chemoprophylaxis for the duration of the influenza season when influenza vaccination is contraindicated, unavailable, or expected to have low effectiveness.
  ◦ Anaphylactic hypersensitivity to prior influenza vaccine.
  ◦ Acute febrile illness.
  ◦ History of Guillain–Barré syndrome (GBS) within 6 wk of a previous influenza vaccination.
  ◦ Persons who are severely immunocompromised.
  ◦ Recipients of hematopoietic stem cell transplant in the first 6–12 mo posttransplant.
  ◦ Lung transplant recipients.
- Short-term chemoprophylaxis is indicated for unvaccinated adults and children aged ≥3 mo during periods of influenza activity.
  ◦ Promptly administer inactivated influenza vaccine in conjunction with chemoprophylaxis in patients in whom influenza vaccination is expected to be effective.
  ◦ Consider chemoprophylaxis for health care personnel and others who are in close contact with persons at high risk of developing influenza complications (but who cannot take antiviral chemoprophylaxis) when influenza vaccination is contraindicated or unavailable.

–Start postexposure antiviral chemoprophylaxis no later than 48 h for asymptomatic adults and children aged ≥3 mo who are

- At high risk of developing complications from influenza (eg, severely immunocompromised persons) and for whom influenza vaccination is contraindicated, unavailable, or expected to have low effectiveness, after household exposure to influenza.
- Unvaccinated household contacts of a person at very high risk of complications from influenza (eg, severely immunocompromised persons).
- Exposed residents of an extended-care facility or hospitalized patients during an institutional outbreak, regardless of influenza vaccination history.

- Unvaccinated staff in whom prophylaxis is indicated based on their underlying conditions or those of their household members (duration: throughout outbreak).
- Staff who received inactivated influenza vaccine during an institutional outbreak (duration: 14 d postvaccination).

Comments

1. Influenza vaccination is the best way to prevent influenza.
2. Antiviral chemoprophylaxis is not a substitute for influenza vaccination.
3. Agents for chemoprophylaxis of influenza A (H1N1) and B: inhaled zanamivir or oral oseltamivir.
4. Children at high risk of complications include those with chronic diseases such as asthma, diabetes, cardiac disease, immune suppression, and neurodevelopmental disorders.

Sources

–Uyeki T, et al. *Clinical Practice Guidelines by the Infectious Diseases Society of America: 2018 Update on Diagnosis, Treatment, Chemoprophylaxis, and Institutional Outbreak Management of Seasonal Influenza.* CID 2018.
–CDC. https://www.cdc.gov/flu/professionals/antivirals/summary-clinicians.htm

INFLUENZA, VACCINATION

Organizations

▶ CDC 2020, AAP 2018

Prevention Recommendations

–Vaccinate for influenza yearly in all persons age >6 mo.
–All children age 6 mo to 8 y should receive 2 doses of the vaccine (>4 wk apart) during their first season of vaccination.
–The live-attenuated influenza vaccine (Flumist quadrivalent) should not be used due to low efficacy.
–Offer vaccines before onset of influenza activity (by end of October, if possible) and continue vaccinations as long as influenza virus circulates and vaccine is available.
–High-dose vaccine is more effective for adults ≥65-y-old.
–Influenza vaccine is contraindicated only if history of severe allergic reaction is found. Egg allergy is not a contraindication, though persons with history of severe reaction should be monitored after receiving the vaccine.
–Do not vaccinate persons who have experienced GBS within 6 wk of a previous influenza vaccine if not at higher risk for influenza complications. Consider influenza chemoprophylaxis as an alternative. Benefits of influenza vaccination might outweigh risks for certain persons with a history of GBS who are also at higher risk for severe complications from influenza.
–Do not vaccinate with live-attenuated influenza vaccine (LAIV) in children (1) younger than 2 y; (2) with a moderate-to-severe febrile illness; (3) with an amount of nasal congestion that would notably impede vaccine delivery; (4) aged 2 through 4 y with a history of recurrent wheezing or a wheezing episode in the previous 12 mo; (5) with asthma; (6) who have received

other live-virus vaccines within the previous 4 wk; (7) who have an immunodeficiency or who are receiving immunosuppressive therapies; (8) who are receiving aspirin or other salicylates; (9) with any condition that can compromise respiratory function or the handling of secretions or can increase the risk for aspiration, such as neurodevelopmental disorders, spinal cord injuries, seizure disorders, or neuromuscular abnormalities; (10) children taking an influenza antiviral medication (oseltamivir, zanamivir, or peramivir) until 48 h after stopping the influenza antiviral therapy; (11) with chronic underlying medical conditions that may predispose them to complications after wild-type influenza infection.

Comment

1. Highest-risk groups for influenza complications are:
   a. Pregnant women.
   b. Children age 6 mo to 5 y.
   c. Adults age $\geq$50 y.
   d. Persons with chronic medical conditions or who are immunocompromised.[1]
   e. Pregnant females or women who will be pregnant during the influenza season or breast-feeding.
   f. Residents of extended-care facilities.
   g. Morbidly obese (BMI >40) persons.
   h. Health care personnel.
   i. Household contacts of persons with high-risk medical conditions or caregivers of children age <5 y or adults age >50 y.
   j. Children and adolescents receiving long-term aspirin therapy.
   k. American Indians or Alaska Natives.
   l. People with a history of influenza-associated encephalopathy.

Sources

–*Pediatrics*. 2018;142(4):e2018-2367.

–Grohskopft L, et al. Prevention and Control of Seasonal Influenza with Vaccines: Recommendations of the Advisory Committee on Immunization Practices—United States, 2018–19 Influenza Season. *CDC MMWR*. 2018;67(3):1-20.

SEXUALLY TRANSMITTED INFECTIONS

Organization

▶ UPSTF 2020

Prevention Recommendations

–Employ behavioral counseling for all sexually active adolescents and adults at increased risk for STIs.

---

[1]Chronic heart, lung, renal, liver, hematologic, cancer, metabolic, neuromuscular or neurodevelopmental, or seizure disorders, severe cognitive dysfunction, diabetes, HIV infection, or immunosuppression.

  –Population at risk: Patients diagnosed with an STI within the past year, not consistently using condoms, having multiple sex partners or having a partner(s) at high risk for STIs, belonging to a population that has a high STI prevalence (such as persons seeking STI testing or attending an STI clinic, sexual and gender minorities, persons living with HIV, persons with injection drug use, persons who exchange sex for money or drugs, persons who have recently been in a correctional facility, and some racial/ethnic minority groups).

  –Provide behavioral counseling to sexually active adolescents and to adults at increased risk:
   • Deliver counseling in person, refer patients to outside counseling services, or inform patients about media-based interventions
   • Interventions that include group counseling, involve more than 120 min of counseling, and are delivered over several sessions have the strongest effect in preventing STIs:
     ◦ Counseling interventions shorter than 30 min delivered in a single session may also be effective
   • Provide information on common STIs and STI transmission; aim to increase motivation or commitment to safer sex practices; and provide training in condom use, communication about safer sex, problem solving, and other pertinent skills.

Source
  –*JAMA*. 2020;324(7):674-681.

SYPHILIS

Organizations
▶ USPSTF 2016, AAFP 2016, CDC 2015

Screening Recommendation
  –Screen all high-risk[1] persons.

Comments
  1. A nontreponemal test (Venereal Disease Research Laboratory [VDRL] test or rapid plasma reagent [RPR] test) should be used for initial screening.
  2. All reactive nontreponemal tests should be confirmed with a fluorescent treponemal antibody absorption (FTA-ABS) test.
  3. Syphilis is a reportable disease in every state.

Sources
  –*JAMA*. 2016;315(21):2321-2327.
  –AAFP. *Clinical Recommendations: Syphilis*. 2016.
  –CDC. *Sexually Transmitted Diseases Treatment Guidelines*. 2015.

[1]High risk includes commercial sex workers, persons who exchange sex for money or drugs, persons with other STDs (including HIV), sexually active homosexual men, and sexual contacts of persons with syphilis, gonorrhea, *Chlamydia*, or HIV infection.

SURGICAL SITE INFECTIONS

Organization
▶ NICE 2020

Prevention Recommendations

– Offer patients and caregivers:
- Clear, consistent information and advice throughout all stages of their care including risks of surgical site infections, what is being done to reduce them, and how they are managed.
- Information and advice on how to care for their wound after discharge.
- Information and advice about how to recognize a surgical site infection and who to contact if they are concerned.
- Always inform patients after their operation if they have been given antibiotics.

– Preoperative phase:
- Advise patients to shower or have a bath using soap, either the day before, or on the day of, surgery.
- Consider nasal mupirocin in combination with a chlorhexidine body wash before procedures in which *Staphylococcus aureus* is a likely cause of a surgical site infection. (This should be locally determined and taken into account: type of procedure, individual patient risk factors, increased risk of side effects in preterm infants, and potential impact of infection.)
- Do not use mechanical bowel preparation routinely to reduce the risk of surgical site infection.

– Antibiotic prophylaxis:
- Give antibiotic prophylaxis to patients before clean surgery involving the placement of a prosthesis or implant, clean-contaminated surgery, or contaminated surgery.
- Do not use antibiotic prophylaxis routinely for clean nonprosthetic uncomplicated surgery.
- Use the local antibiotic formulary and always take into account the potential adverse effects when choosing specific antibiotics for prophylaxis.
- Give antibiotic treatment (in addition to prophylaxis) to patients having surgery on a dirty or infected wound.
- Inform patients before the operation, whenever possible, if they will need antibiotic prophylaxis, and afterwards if they have been given antibiotics during their operation.

– Postoperative phase:
- Use an aseptic nontouch technique for changing or removing surgical wound dressings.
- Use sterile saline for wound cleansing up to 48 h after surgery
- Advise patients that they may shower safely 48 h after surgery.
- Use tap water for wound cleansing after 48 h if the surgical wound has separated or has been surgically opened to drain pus.

- Use topical antimicrobial agents for wound healing by primary intention.
- Do not use topical antimicrobial agents for surgical wounds that are healing by primary intention to reduce the risk of surgical site infection. Dressings for wound healing by secondary intention.
- Do not use Eusol and gauze, or moist cotton gauze or mercuric antiseptic solutions to manage surgical wounds that are healing by secondary intention.
- Use an appropriate interactive dressing to manage surgical wounds that are healing by secondary intention.
- Ask a tissue viability nurse (or another health care professional with tissue viability expertise) for advice on appropriate dressings for the management of surgical wounds that are healing by secondary intention.
- When surgical site infection is suspected by the presence of cellulitis, either by a new infection, or an infection caused by treatment failure, give the patient an antibiotic that covers the likely causative organisms. Consider local resistance patterns and the results of microbiological tests in choosing an antibiotic.

Source

−www.nice.org.uk/guidance/ng125

Disorders of the Musculoskeletal System

8

BACK PAIN, LOW

Organizations

▶ AAFP 2004, USPSTF 2004

Prevention Recommendation

–Insufficient evidence for or against interventions to prevent low-back pain in adults in primary care settings.

Comments

1. Insufficient evidence to support back strengthening exercises, mechanical supports, or increased physical activity to prevent low-back pain.
2. Meta-analyses in *Lancet*. 2018;391:2368-2383, *Am J Epidemiol*. 2018;187(5):1093-1101, and *JAMA Intern Med*. 2016;176(2):199-208:
   a. Exercise alone or exercise in combination with education is effective for preventing low-back pain.
   b. Education alone, back belts, and shoe insoles are not effective.
   c. Exercises that were studied and shown to be effective are a combination of strengthening with either stretching or aerobic exercise, 2–3 times/wk.

Sources
   –AAFP. *Clinical Recommendations: Low Back Pain*. 2004.
   –USPSTF. *Low Back Pain*. 2004.

OSTEOPOROSIS

Organizations

▶ Osteoporosis International 2014, ACOG 2014

Prevention Recommendations

–Counsel on the risk of osteoporosis and fractures.
–Diet with adequate calcium and vitamin D (respectively):
   • Age 9–18 y: 1300 mg/d and 600 U/d.
   • Age 19–50 y: 1000 mg/d and 600 U/d.
   • Age 51–70 y: 1200 mg/d and 600 U/d (1000 mg/d for men 50–70 y).
   • Age ≥71 y: 1200 mg/d and 800–1000 U/d with dietary supplements if needed.

–Regular weight-bearing and muscle-strengthening exercise.

–Assess risk factors for falls and offer modifications (eg, home safety, balance training, vitamin D deficiency, CNS depressant medications, antihypertensive medication monitoring, vision correction).

–Target a serum vitamin D level of 20 ng/mL.

–Tobacco cessation.

–Avoid excess alcohol intake.

–In patients with low bone mass (T-score on screening DXA scan of ≤2.5), consider pharmacologic therapy—see Chapter 27, section: Osteoporosis.

Comment

1. A single DXA is likely sufficient, as serial screens don't add meaningfully to prognosis. (*JAMA Intern Med.* 2020;180(9):1232-1240)

Sources

–*Osteoporos Int.* 2014: doi:10.1007/s00198-014-2794-2

–*Obstet & Gyn.* 120(3):718-734.

–*Am Fam Phys.* 2015;92(4):261-268.

OSTEOPOROSIS, GLUCOCORTICOID-INDUCED

Population

–Adults with glucocorticoid-induced osteoporosis.

Organization

▶ ACR 2017

Prevention Recommendations

–Offer all patients receiving glucocorticoid therapy education and assess risk factors for osteoporosis annually.

–Use FRAX calculator to place patients at low risk, medium risk, or high risk for major osteoporotic fracture. Use FRAX with BMD testing every 1–3 y if never treated for osteoporosis, every 2–3 y during treatment if on high-dose glucocorticoids, osteoporosis fracture at least 18 mo after osteoporosis treatment, poor medication compliance, or other osteoporosis risk factors present, and every 2–3 y after completion of osteoporosis treatment.

–If glucocorticoid treatment is expected to last >3 mo, recommend:

- Weight-bearing or resistance training exercises.
- Smoking cessation.
- Limit alcoholic drinks to 1–2 per day.
- Calcium 1000–1200 mg/d.
- Vitamin D 600–800 IU/d.
- Fall risk assessment.
- Annual 25-OH vitamin D.
- Baseline and annual height measurement.

- Assessment of prevalent fragility fractures.
- X-rays of spine.
- Assessment of degree of osteoporosis medication compliance, if applicable.

–For adults ≥40 y + glucocorticoid use >3 mo:
  - Low-risk group.
    - Optimize calcium/vitamin D intake and lifestyle modifications over treatment with bisphosphonates, teriparatide, denosumab, or raloxifene.
  - Moderate- and high-risk groups.
    - Treat with oral bisphosphonate over calcium/vitamin D alone. Oral bisphosphonate preferred over IV bisphosphonates, teriparatide, denosumab, or raloxifene.

–For adults <40 y + glucocorticoid use >3 mo:
  - Low-risk group.
    - Optimize calcium/vitamin D intake and lifestyle modifications over bisphosphonates.
  - Moderate- to-high-risk groups.
    - Treat with an oral bisphosphonate over calcium/vitamin D alone, or IV bisphosphonates, teriparatide, or raloxifene.

Comments

1. Clinical factors that may increase the risk of osteoporotic fracture estimated by FRAX calculator:
   a. BMI <21 kg/m^2.
   b. Parental history of hip fracture.
   c. Current smoking.
   d. ≥3 alcoholic drinks/d.
   e. Higher glucocorticoid doses or cumulative dose.
   f. IV pulse glucocorticoid use.
   g. Declining central bone mineral density measurement.
2. In women of childbearing potential, first line in those indicated for osteoporosis treatment is oral bisphosphonates. Second line is teriparatide.

Source

–ACR. American College of Rheumatology guideline for the prevention and treatment of glucocorticoid-induced osteoporosis. *Arthritis Rheumatol.* 2017;69:1521-1537.

Organization

▶ ACR 2017

Prevention Recommendations

–Assess clinical fracture risk within 6 mo of starting GC treatment.
–Include history of dose and duration of steroids, falls, fractures, frailty.
–High risk of fracture: malnutrition, weight loss/low body weight, hypogonadism, hyperparathyroidism, thyroid disease, family hx hip fracture, alcohol use, smoking.

-For adults ≥40 y, use FRAX to assess risk (https://www.shef.ac.uk/FRAX/tool.jsp).[1]
-For adults <40 y with hx osteoporotic (OP) fracture or high risk, perform bone mineral density testing.
-For adults taking >.5 mg/d prednisone, FRAX risk increases by 15% for major OP fracture and 20% for hip fracture.
-High fracture risk: hx OP fracture, T-score ≤-2.5 (postmenopausal or male ≥50 y), FRAX 10-y risk OP fracture ≥20% or hip fracture ≥3%.
-Moderate fracture risk: FRAX 10-y risk OP fracture 10%–19% or hip fracture 1%–3% (or if <40 y Z-score <-3 or ≥10% bone loss over 1 y and continued GC ≥7.5 mg/d for ≥6 mo).
-Low fracture risk: lower FRAX risk.
-Adults taking prednisone ≥2.5 mg/d for ≥3 mo: calcium (1000–1200 mg/d), vitamin D (600–800 U/d), healthy diet, normal weight, no smoking, exercise, alcohol ≤1–2 drinks/d.
-Adults at low risk of fracture: Ca, VitD, lifestyle as above.
-Adults at moderate or high risk of fracture: add oral bisphosphonate.
-If GC treatment continued, reassess risk every 12 mo.
-Continue bisphosphonate treatment for 5 y if continues to be at moderate-to-high risk or continues to take GC.
-Treat with another class of OP medication (teriparatide or denosumab) or IV bisphosphonate if malabsorption of oral form, if fracture after 18 mo of oral bisphosphonate, ≥10% bone loss after 1 y, or continue to be moderate-to-high risk after 5 y.

Source
-*Arthritis Rheumatol.* 2017:69(8):1521-1537.

VITAMIN D DEFICIENCY

Organizations
▶ USPSTF 2021, Endocrine Society 2011

Screening Recommendations
-Insufficient evidence to screen for vitamin D deficiency in community dwelling, nonpregnant asymptomatic adults.
-Screen with serum 25-hydroxyvitamin D level in patients at risk[2] for deficiency.

---

[1]The FRAX calculator reports significantly lower fracture risk for female patients identified as Black, Asian, or Hispanic with identical risk factors to those of a white patient. This could have the effect of delaying intervention with osteoporosis therapy. (*N Engl J Med.* 2020;383(9):874-882)
[2]Indications for screening include rickets, osteomalacia, osteoporosis, CKD, hepatic failure, malabsorption syndromes, hyperparathyroidism, certain medications (anticonvulsants, glucocorticoids, AIDs drugs, antifungals, cholestyramine), African-American and Hispanic race, pregnancy, and lactation, older adults with history of falls or nontraumatic fractures, BMI > 30, and granulomatous diseases.

Comments

- –The USPSTF's review showed that treating Vitamin D deficiency does not improve cancer risk, diabetes risk, fracture risk or death in community-dwelling adults, and that other outcomes lacked sufficient data.
- –Treating Vitamin D deficiency has been considered in the care of other chronic disorders, but insufficient evidence exists. Vitamin D's effect on conditions including pregnancy, depression, diabetes, COPD, asthma, hypertension, and nonspecific pain has been assessed without definitive evidence of benefit.

Sources

- –*J Clin Endocrinol Metab.* 2011;96(7):1911-1930.
- –*JAMA.* 2021;325(14):1436-1442
- –*Am Fam Physician.* 2018 Feb 15;97(4):254-260.

Pulmonary Disorders

9

CHRONIC OBSTRUCTIVE PULMONARY DISEASE (COPD)

Organization
▶ USPSTF 2016

Screening Recommendation
–Do not screen asymptomatic adults for COPD.

Comments
1. Detection while asymptomatic doesn't alter disease course or improve outcomes.
2. Several symptom-based questionnaires have high sensitivity for COPD.
3. In symptomatic patients (ie, dyspnea, chronic cough, or sputum production with a history of exposure to cigarette smoke or other toxic fumes), diagnostic spirometry to measure FEV1/FVC ratio is indicated.

Source
–*JAMA*. 2016;315(13):1372-1377.

LUNG CANCER

Organizations
▶ USPSTF 2021, ACCP 2021, NCCN 2020

Screening Recommendations
–Screen for lung cancer annually with low-dose chest CT in older adults who have a significant smoking history.
–Use the Tammemagi lung cancer risk calculator when weighing risk factors other than smoking history, a score >1.3% 6-y risk is considered sufficient risk to pursue screening. (NCCN)
–Stop screening if a person has not smoked for 15 y, or if they develop a significant medical problem that would limit ability to receive treatment for an early stage lung cancer.
–Do not screen routinely with chest x-ray and/or sputum cytology.
–Only screen if a highly skilled support team is available to evaluate CT scans, schedule appropriate follow-up, and perform lung biopsies safely when indicated.

GUIDELINES DISCORDANT: POPULATION TO SCREEN	
Organization	**Age Range**
USPSTF	Age 50–80 y, 20 pack-year history
ACCP	Age 55–77 y, or 50–80 with 20 pack-year
NCCN	Age 55–77 y Age ≥50 if there are additional cancer risk factors in addition to a ≥20 pack-year smoking history

Comments

1. Risk assessment for lung cancer:
   a. Cigarette smoking (20-fold increased risk). Medication and counseling together are better than either alone to increase cessation rates.
   b. Second-hand smoke exposure, according to NCCN, is not a sufficient risk factor for lung cancer to warrant a screening recommendation with LDCT. It is a highly variable exposure risk. However, it should be considered in conjunction with other risk factors. The Tammemagi lung cancer risk calculator can be used to assess risk.
   c. Family history of lung cancer in first-degree relatives.
   d. Pulmonary disease history (COPD or pulmonary fibrosis).
   e. Documented radon gas exposure (can be measured in the home), severe air pollution. Air pollution increases risk of lung cancer by 40% with highest pollution exposure. (*Am J Respir Crit Care Med.* 2006;173:667)
   f. Occupational exposures (silica, asbestos, arsenic, nickel, chromium, coal smoke, soot, diesel fumes).
2. If a pulmonary nodule is found on LDCT, the characterization of the nodule—solid, part-solid, nonsolid, multiple nonsolid—will determine what size nodule screens positive. NCCN guidelines discuss appropriate follow-up imaging, procedures, and referrals.
3. If coronary arterial calcification is detected on chest CT, its presence may be a marker of atherosclerosis. Further evaluation is recommended if it is reported as severe. (*J Am Coll Radiol.* 2018;15:1087-1096)
4. Reducing overall risk:
   a. Smokers who quit gain 13% reduction in risk of all-cause mortality and 21% reduction in risk of lung cancer mortality in first 5 y. The excess risk decreases to that of a never-smoker ~20 y after quitting on average; however, for lung cancer it takes ~30 y. (*JAMA.* 2008;299(17):2037-2047)
   b. No evidence that vitamin E, tocopherol, retinoids, vitamin C, or beta-carotene in any dose reduces the risk of lung cancer. (*Ann Inter Med.* 2013;159:824)
   c. Minimize indoor exposure to radon (can be measured in home), especially if smoker. Avoid occupational exposures (asbestos, arsenic, nickel, chromium, beryllium, and cadmium).

Sources
–https://www.uspreventiveservicestaskforce.org/Page/Document/UpdateSummaryFinal/lung-cancer-screening

–*J Natl Compr Canc Netw.* 2018;16:412-441.

–https://www.cancer.org/health-care-professionals/american-cancer-society-prevention-early-detection-guidelines/lung-cancer-screening-guidelines.html

–*Chest*. 2018;153(4):954-985. https://www.ncbi.nlm.nih.gov/pubmed/29374513

–National Comprehensive Cancer Network Guidelines Version 1.2020, Lung Cancer Screening. https://www.nccn.org/professionals/physician_gls/

–*PLOS Med*. 2014;11:1-13.

Renal Disorders

10

Organizations
▶ NICE 2019, VA/DoD 2019, KDIGO 2012

Prevention Recommendations
–General care of the acutely ill patient.
- In the absence of hemorrhagic shock, use isotonic crystalloids rather than colloids for intravascular volume expansion.
- Do not use diuretics to prevent or treat acute kidney injury (AKI) except in the management of volume overload.
- Do not use low-dose dopamine in either the prevention or treatment of AKI.
- Use vasopressors in addition to fluids for management of vasomotor shock with or at risk for AKI.

–Adults receiving intravenous iodinated contrast.
- Consider IV volume expansion to at-risk adults, including those with:
  ◦ CKD with eGFR <30 mL/min.
  ◦ Heart failure.
  ◦ Age 75 y or older.
  ◦ History of renal transplant.
  ◦ Use of a large volume of contrast medium.
  ◦ Intra-arterial administration of contrast medium with first-pass renal exposure.
- Consider temporarily stopping ACE inhibitors and ARBs in adults having iodine-based contrast media if they have chronic kidney disease with an eGFR less than 40 mL/min.
- Inconsistent evidence for N-acetylcysteine use to prevent contrast-induced nephropathy.

–Consult a pharmacist to assist with drug dosing in adults or children at risk for AKI.

Comments
1. AKI is defined as any of the following:
   a. The increase in SCr by ≥0.3 mg/dL over 48 h.
   b. Increase in SCr to ≥1.5 times baseline within the past 7 d.
   c. Urine volume < 0.5 mL/kg/h for 6 h.

Sources
- –NICE. *Acute Kidney Injury: Prevention, Detection and Management of Acute Kidney Injury up to the Point of Renal Replacement Therapy.* London, UK: National Institute for Health and Care Excellence (NICE); 2019. https://www.nice.org.uk/guidance/ng148
- –VA/DoD. *Clinical Practice Guideline for the Management of Chronic Kidney Disease in Primary Care.* Washington, DC: Department of Veterans Affairs, Department of Defense; 2019.
- –Kidney Disease Improving Global Outcomes (KDIGO). *KDIGO Clinical Practice Guideline for Acute Kidney Injury: Kidney International Supplements*; March 2012;2(1).

KIDNEY DISEASE, CHRONIC (CKD)

Organizations

▶ USPSTF 2012, ACP 2013, AAFP 2014, NICE 2014, VA/DoD 2019

Screening Recommendations

GUIDELINES DISCORDANT: WHETHER TO SCREEN	
Organization	**Guidance**
USPSTF	Insufficient evidence to recommend for or against routine screening
ACP, AAFP, NICE	Do not screen adults unless they have symptoms or risk factors[a]
VA/DoD	For patients at risk for CKD,[b] periodically obtain SCr, eGFR, urinalysis, and spot uACR; periodicity of screening is not defined

[a] DM, HTN, CVD, structural renal disease, nephrolithiasis, benign prostatic hyperplasia (BPH), multisystem diseases with potential kidney involvement (eg, systemic lupus erythematosus [SLE]), FH of stage 5 CKD or hereditary kidney disease, or personal history of hematuria or proteinuria.

[b] DM, HTN, cardiac disease/CHF, or vascular disease, systemic illness such as SLE, HIV, gout, urinary tract abnormalities, history of AKI, proteinuria, family history of kidney disease, age > 60 y, and ethnicities associated with increased risk (eg, African-Americans, Hispanics, Native Americans).

Comments

1. Diagnose CKD if either of the following present for >3 mo:
   a. Markers of kidney damage such as albuminuria > 30 mg/g, urinary sediment abnormalities, electrolyte abnormalities due to tubular disorders, histologic abnormalities, structural abnormalities by imaging, or kidney transplantation.
   b. GFR < 60 mL/min/1.73 m^2.
2. Monitor glomerular filtration rate (GFR) at least annually in people who are prescribed drugs known to be nephrotoxic.[1]
3. Do not test for proteinuria in adults taking an ACE inhibitor or ARB, regardless of diabetes status.

Sources
- –USPSTF. *Chronic Kidney Disease (CKD): Screening.* 2012.
- –AAFP. *Clinical Recommendations: Chronic Kidney Disease.* 2014.

---

[1]Examples: calcineurin inhibitors, lithium, or nonsteroidal anti-inflammatory drugs (NSAIDs).

–*Ann Intern Med.* 2013;159(12):835.

–NICE. *Early Identification and Management of Chronic Kidney Disease in Adults in Primary and Secondary Care.* London, UK: NICE; 2014.

–Kidney Disease Improving Global Outcomes (KDIGO). *KDIGO 2012 Clinical Practice Guideline for the Evaluation and Management of Chronic Kidney Disease.* 2013;3(1).

Disorders of the Skin

ORAL CANCER

Organizations

▶ AAFP 2015, USPSTF 2013, NCCN 2018

Screening Recommendations

GUIDELINES DISCORDANT: WHETHER TO SCREEN	
Organization	**Guidance**
USPSTF, AAFP	Insufficient evidence to recommend for or against routinely screening adults for oral asymptomatic cancer
NCCN	Screen with annual clinical exam

Comment

1. Primary risk factors for oral cancer are tobacco and alcohol use. Additional risk factors include male sex, older age, use of betel quid, ultraviolet light exposure, infection with *Candida* or bacterial flora, and a compromised immune system. Recently, sexually transmitted oral human papillomavirus infection has been recognized as an increasing risk factor for oropharyngeal cancer, another subset of head-and-neck cancer.

Sources

–http://www.aafp.org/online/en/home/clinical/exam.html
–http://www.ahrq.gov/clinic/uspstf/uspsoral.htm
–www.nccn.org

Organization

▶ National Cancer Institute 2018

Prevention Recommendations

–Minimize risk factor exposure. Risk factors include:

- Tobacco (in any form, including smokeless).
- Alcohol and dietary factors—double the risk for people who drink 3–4 drinks/d vs. nondrinkers. (*Cancer Causes Control.* 2011;22:1217)
- Betel-quid chewing. (*Cancer.* 2014;135:1433)
- Oral HPV infection—found in 6.9% of general population and found in 70%–75% of patients with oropharyngeal squamous cell cancer. (*N Engl J Med.* 2007;356:1944)
- Lip cancer—avoid chronic sun exposure and smokeless tobacco.

Comments

1. Oropharyngeal squamous cell CAs (tonsil and base of tongue) are related to HPV infection (types 16 and 18) in 75% of patients. This correlates with sexual practices, number of partners, and may be prevented by HPV vaccine. HPV (+), nonsmokers have improved cure rate by 35%–45%. (*N Engl J Med.* 2010;363:24, 82)
2. There is inadequate evidence to suggest change in diet will reduce risk of oral cancer.

Source

–https://www.cancer.gov/types/head-and-neck/hp/oral-prevention-pdq

PRESSURE ULCERS

Organizations

▶ NICE 2014, ACP 2015

Prevention Recommendations

–In adults with impaired mobility, assess risk for in both outpatient and inpatient settings (eg, the Braden Scale in adults and Braden Q Scale in children).
–Educate patient, family, and caregivers regarding the causes and risk factors of pressure ulcers.
–Use compression stockings cautiously in patients with lower extremity arterial disease. Avoid thigh-high stockings when compression stockings are used.
–Move patients with caution. Avoid dragging patient when moving and lubricate or powder bed pans prior to placing under patient.
–Minimize pressure on skin, especially areas with bony prominences.
  • Turn patient side-to-side every 2 h.
  • Pad areas over bony prominences.
  • Pad skin-to-skin contact.
  • Use heel protectors or place pillows under calves.
  • Consider a bariatric bed for patients weighing over 300 lb.
  • Consider high-specification foam (not air) mattress for high-risk patients admitted to secondary care or who are undergoing surgery.
–Manage moisture.
  • Moisture barrier protectant on skin.
  • Frequent diaper changes.
  • Scheduled toileting.
  • Treat candidiasis if present.
  • Consider a rectal tube for stool incontinence with diarrhea.
–Maintain adequate nutrition and hydration.
–Keep the head of the bed at or >30-degree elevation.

Comments

1. Outpatient risk assessment for pressure ulcers:
   a. Is the patient bed or wheel chair bound?

b. Does the patient require assistance for transfers?

c. Is the patient incontinent of urine or stool?

d. Any history of pressure ulcers?

e. Does the patient have a clinical condition placing the patient at risk for pressure ulcers?
   i. DM.
   ii. Peripheral vascular disease.
   iii. Stroke.
   iv. Polytrauma.
   v. Musculoskeletal disorders (fractures or contractures).
   vi. Spinal cord injury.
   vii. Guillain–Barré syndrome.
   viii. Multiple sclerosis.
   ix. CA.
   x. Chronic obstructive pulmonary disease.
   xi. Coronary heart failure.
   xii. Dementia.
   xiii. Preterm neonate.
   xiv. Cerebral palsy.

f. Does the patient appear malnourished?

g. Is equipment in use that could contribute to ulcer development (eg, oxygen tubing, prosthetic devices, urinary catheter)?

Sources

–National Clinical Guideline Centre. *Pressure Ulcers: Prevention and Management of Pressure Ulcers*. London, UK: National Institute for Health and Care Excellence; 2014.

–*Ann Intern Med.* 2015;162(5):359-369.

SKIN CANCER

Organization

▶ USPSTF 2016

Screening Recommendations

–Insufficient evidence to assess the balance of benefits and harms of visual skin examination by a clinician to screen for skin cancer in adults.[1,2]

[1]Clinicians should remain alert for skin lesions with malignant features when examining patients for other reasons, particularly patients with established risk factors. Risk factors for skin cancer include evidence of melanocytic precursors (atypical moles), large numbers of common moles (>50), immunosuppression, any history of radiation, family or personal history of skin cancer, substantial cumulative lifetime sun exposure, intermittent intense sun exposure or severe sunburns in childhood, freckles, poor tanning ability, and light skin, hair, and eye color.

[2]Consider educating patients with established risk factors for skin cancer (see above) about signs and symptoms suggesting skin cancer and the possible benefits of periodic self-examination. Alert at-risk patients to significance of asymmetry, border irregularity, color variability, diameter > 6 mm, and evolving change in previous stable mole. All suspicious lesions should be biopsied (excisional or punch, not a shave biopsy). (*Ann Intern Med.* 2009;150:188) (USPSTF; ACS; COG)

–Counsel children, adolescents, and young adults age 10–24 y who have fair skin, to minimize exposure to ultraviolet radiation to reduce the risk of skin cancer.

Comments

1. Benefits and harms:
   a. *Benefits:* Basal and squamous cell carcinomas are the most common types of cancer in the United States and represent the vast majority of all cases of skin cancer; however, they rarely result in death or substantial morbidity, whereas melanoma skin cancer has notably higher mortality rates. In 2016, an estimated 76,400 US men and women developed melanoma and 10,100 died from the disease.
   b. *Harms:* Potential for harm clearly exists, including a high rate of unnecessary biopsies, possibly resulting in cosmetic or, more rarely, functional adverse effects, and the risk of overdiagnosis and overtreatment.
   c. Direct evidence on the effectiveness of screening in reducing melanoma morbidity and mortality is limited to a single fair-quality ecologic study with important methodological limitations.
   d. Twenty-eight million people in the United States use UV indoor tanning salons, increasing risk of squamous, basal cell cancer, and malignant melanoma. (*J Clin Oncol.* 2012;30:1588)
   e. Clinical features of increased risk of melanoma (family history, multiple nevi previous melanoma) are linked to sites of subsequent malignant melanoma, which may be helpful in surveillance. (*JAMA Dermatol.* 2017;153:23)
   f. There are no guidelines for patients with familial syndromes (familial atypical mole and melanoma [FAM-M]), although systematic surveillance is warranted.[1]

Sources
–*JAMA.* 2016;316:429.
–http://www.ahrq.gov/clinic/uspstf/uspsskca.htm

Organization

▶ USPSTF 2018

Prevention Recommendations

–Counsel to minimize UV exposure for people age 6 mo to 24 y with light skin types.
–Offer selective counseling to adults over 24 y with light skin types.
–Insufficient evidence to recommend skin self-exam.

▶ National Cancer Institute 2019

–Avoid sunburns and tanning booths,[2] especially severe blistering sunburns at a younger age.

Comments

1. Use sunscreen (SPF 15) and protective clothing, spend limited time in the sun, avoid indoor tanning and blistering sunburn in adolescents and young adults.

---

[1]Consider dermatologic risk assessment if family history of melanoma in ≥2 blood relatives, presence of multiple atypical moles, or presence of numerous actinic keratoses.
[2]Indoor tanning may account for 450,000 cases of skin cancer and 10,000 melanomas each year (*JAMA Dermatol.* 2014;150:390).

2. Phenotypic risk factors (fair skin) include ivory or pale skin color, light eye color, red or blond hair, freckles, or easily sunburned skin.

3. Nicotinamide (Vitamin B$_3$) shows promise in preventing skin cancers but further studies are required. (*J Invest Dermatol.* 2012;132:1498)

4. Chemopreventive agents (beta carotene, isoretinoin, selenium, and celecoxib) have not shown prevention of new skin cancers in randomized clinical trials. (*Arch Dermatol.* 2000;136:179)

Sources

–*JAMA.* 2018;319(11):1134-1142.

–http://www.cancer.gov/types/skin/hp/skin-prevention-pdq

Specific Populations

This section contains guidance for screening and primary prevention for specific populations. Chapters are dedicated to issues unique to newborns and infants, children and adolescents, women, men, and older adults. Unless otherwise noted, the recommendations apply to average-risk people. When gender is specified, the guidelines typically refer to gender assignment at birth.

Newborns and Infants

12

ANEMIA

Organizations
▶ USPSTF 2015, AAFP 2015, AAP 2010

Screening Recommendations

GUIDELINES DISCORDANT: WHETHER TO SCREEN ROUTINELY FOR ANEMIA	
Organization	**Guidance**
AAFP, USPSTF	Insufficient evidence to recommend for or against screening infants and newborns Consider selective screening in high-risk children*a* with malnourishment, low birth weight, or symptoms of anemia
AAP	Universal screening of Hgb at 12 mo

a Includes infants living in poverty, Blacks, Native Americans, Alaska natives, immigrants from developing countries, preterm and low-birth-weight infants, infants whose principal dietary intake is unfortified cow's milk or soy milk, bottle feeding beyond 1 y, having a mom who is currently pregnant, living in an urban area and having less than 2 servings per day of iron-rich foods (iron-fortified breakfast cereals or meats).

Comments
1. If anemic, measure ferritin, C-reactive protein, and reticulocyte hemoglobin content. Reticulocyte hemoglobin content is a more sensitive and specific marker than is serum hemoglobin level for iron deficiency.
2. One-third of patients with iron deficiency will have a hemoglobin level >11 g/dL.
3. Use of transferring receptor 1 (TfR_1) assay as screening for iron deficiency is under investigation.

Sources
–AAFP. *Clinical Recommendations: Iron Deficiency Anemia.* 2015.
–USPSTF. *Iron Deficiency in Young Children: Screening.* 2015.
–*Pediatrics.* 2010;126(5):1040-1050.

CONGENITAL HEART DISEASE

Organization
▶ AAP 2011

Screening Recommendation
–All newborns should have pulse oximetry screening for critical congenital heart disease (CCHD) at ≥24 h of life but prior to discharge home from the hospital.

Comment
1. Obtain oxygen saturations in the right hand and in one foot.

Source
–AAP. *Endorsement of HHS Recommendation for Pulse Oximetry Screening for CCHD*. 2012.

DEVELOPMENTAL DYSPLASIA OF THE HIP (DDH)

Population
–Infants.

Organizations
▶ AAP 2017, AAFP 2017

Screening Recommendations
–Examine newborn and continue periodic surveillance physical exam for DDH including length discrepancy, asymmetric thigh or buttock creases, performing Ortolani test, and observing for limited abduction.
–Obtain ultrasound for "high-risk" infants 6 wk to 6 mo of age: history of breech presentation, family history, parenteral concern, history of clinical hip instability on exam, or history of lower extremity swaddling.
–Consider radiography after 4 mo of age in high-risk infants without physical exam findings or any child with positive physical exam findings.
–Refer to orthopedics if unstable or dislocated hip in physical exam. Referral does not require imaging.

Comment
1. There is evidence that screening leads to earlier identification; however, 60%–80% of the hips of newborns identified as abnormal or suspicious for DDH by physical examination, and >90% of those identified by ultrasound in the newborn period, resolve spontaneously, requiring no intervention.

Sources
–*Pediatrics*. 2016;138(6):e20163107.
–*Am Fam Physician*. 2017;96(3):196-197.

GROWTH ABNORMALITIES

Organizations
▶ CDC 2010, AAP 2010

Screening Recommendation
–Use the 2006 World Health Organization (WHO) international growth charts for children age < 24 mo.

Comments
1. The Centers for Disease Control and Prevention (CDC) and American Academy of Pediatricians (AAP) recommend the WHO as opposed to the CDC growth charts for children age < 24 mo.
2. The CDC growth charts should still be used for children age 2–19 y.
3. This recommendation recognizes that breast-feeding is the recommended standard of infant feeding, and therefore the standard against which all other infants are compared.

Sources
–CDC. Use of World Health Organization and CDC growth charts for children aged 0–59 mo in the United States. *MMWR*. 2010;59 (No. RR-9):1-15.
–*AAP News*. 2010;31(11).

GONORRHEA, OPHTHALMIA NEONATORUM

Organization
▶ USPSTF 2019

Prevention Recommendation
–Give all newborns prophylactic ocular topical medication against gonococcal ophthalmia neonatorum.

Comments
1. Erythromycin 0.5% ointment is the only agent available in the United States for this application.
2. Canadian Paediatric Society recommends against universal prophylaxis, given incomplete efficacy of erythromycin, rarity of the condition, and disruption in maternal-infant bonding. Instead, they recommend screening mothers for gonorrhea and chlamydia infection and, if infected with gonorrhea at the time of delivery, treating the infant with ceftriaxone. (*Paediatr Child Health*. 2015;20:93-96)

Source
–USPSTF. *Ocular Prophylaxis for Gonococcal Ophthalmia Neonatorum*. 2019.

HEARING IMPAIRMENT

Organizations
▶ AAP 1999, USPSTF 2008

Screening Recommendation
–Universal screening of all newborn infants for hearing loss.

Comments
1. Screening should be performed before 1 mo of age. Those infants who do not pass the initial screening should undergo audiologic and medical evaluation before 3 mo of age.
2. Screening involves either a 1-step or a 2-step process. The 2-step process includes otoacoustic emissions (OAEs) followed by auditory brainstem response (ABR) in those who fail the OAE test. The 1-step process uses either OAE or ABR testing.

Sources
–*Pediatrics.* 1999;103(2).
–*Pediatrics.* 2008;122(1).

HEMOGLOBINOPATHIES

Organizations
▶ AAFP 2010, USPSTF 2007

Screening Recommendation
–Screen all newborns for hemoglobinopathies (including sickle cell disease).

Comments
1. Screening for sickle cell disease is mandated in all 50 states and the District of Columbia.
2. Infants with sickle cell anemia should receive prophylactic Penicillin starting at 2 mo of age and pneumococcal vaccinations at recommended intervals.

Sources
–http://www.guideline.gov/content.aspx?id=38619
–http://www.uspreventiveservicestaskforce.org/uspstf07/sicklecell/sicklers.htm

IMMUNIZATIONS, INFANTS AND CHILDREN

Organization
▶ Advisory Committee on Immunization Practices (ACIP) 2017

Prevention Recommendations
–Immunize infants and children based on the 2018 immunization schedule.

–Centers for Disease Control (CDC), the American Academy of Pediatrics (AAP), the American Academy of Family Physicians (AAFP), and the American College of Obstetricians and Gynecologists (ACOG) have approved the schedule.

Source
  –*MMWR Morb Mortal Wkly Rep.* 2018;67:156-157.

NEWBORN SCREENING

Organization
▶ ICSI 2013

Screening Recommendation
  –Perform a metabolic screening test prior to hospital discharge for all newborns.

Comment
  1. The newborn screen should be performed after 24 h of age. Infants who receive their newborn screen before 24 h of age should have it repeated before 2 wk of age.

Source
  –ICSI. *Preventive Services for Children and Adolescents.* 19th ed. 2013.

PHENYLKETONURIA (PKU)

Organizations
▶ Advisory Committee on Heritable Disorders in Newborns and Children 2015, USPSTF 2008

Screening Recommendations
  –PKU screening is mandated in all 50 states.
  –Three main methods are used to screen for PKU in the United States: Guthrie Bacterial Inhibition Assay (BIA), automated fluorometric assay, tandem mass spectrometry.

Comments
  1. If infant is tested within 24 h of birth, testing should be repeated in 2 wk.
  2. Optimal screening time for premature infants and infants with illnesses is within 7 d of birth, and in all cases before discharge from nursery.
  3. If screening is positive, implement phenylalanine restrictions immediately after birth to prevent the neurodevelopmental effects of PKU.

Sources
  –Advisory Committee on Heritable Disorders in Newborns and Children. 2015.
  –USPSTF. *Phenylketonuria in Newborns: Screening.* 2008.

SUDDEN INFANT DEATH SYNDROME (SIDS)

Organization

▶ AAP 2016

Prevention Recommendations

–Place their infants to sleep on their backs.
–Use a firm sleep surface without soft objects or loose bedding.
–Breastfeed.
–For the first 6–12 mo, infants should sleep in parents' room (but not in parents' bed).
–Avoid smoke exposure, alcohol and illicit drug use, overheating.

Comments

1. Stomach and side sleeping have been identified as major risk factors for SIDS.
2. Pacifiers may be protective.

Source

–*Pediatrics.* 2016;138(5):e20162938.

THYROID DISEASE

Organizations

▶ AAFP 2015, ATA 2020, AACE 2012, ASRM 2015, CTF 2019

Screening Recommendation

–Screen all newborns for congenital hypothyroidism.

Sources

–Advisory Committee on Heritable Disorders in Newborns and Children. 2015.
–*Am Fam Phys.* 2015;91(11).
–*Endocr Pract.* 2012;18(6):988.
–*Ann Intern Med.* 2015;162(9):641-650.
–*ASRM.* 2015;104(3):545-553.
–*CMAJ.* 2019;191:E1274-E1280.
–van Trotsenburg AS et al. 2020 Congenital hypothyroidism: A 2020 consensus guidelines update An ENDOEuropean Reference Network (ERN) initiative endorsed by the European Society for Pediatric Endocrinology and the European Society for Endocrinology. Thyroid. Epub 2020 Dec 3. PMID: 33272083.

Children and Adolescents

13

ALCOHOL ABUSE AND DEPENDENCE

Organizations
▶ AAFP 2010, USPSTF 2018, ICSI 2010

Screening Recommendation
–Insufficient evidence to recommend for or against screening or counseling interventions to prevent or reduce alcohol misuse by adolescents.

Comments
1. AUDIT and CAGE questionnaires have not been validated in children or adolescents.
2. Screen using a tool designed for adolescents, such as the CRAFFT, BSTAD, or S2BI.
3. Reinforce not drinking and driving or riding with any driver under the influence.
4. While behavioral counseling has been proven to be beneficial in adults, data do not support its benefit in adolescents.
5. Ask about friends' alcohol use.

Sources
–USPSTF. *Unhealthy Alcohol Use in Adolescents and Adults: Screening and Behavioral Counseling Interventions.* 2018.
–https://www.icsi.org/guidelines__more/catalog_guidelines_and_more/catalog_ guidelines/
–*Ann Fam Med.* 2010;8(6):484-492.

ASTHMA

Population
–Children.

Organization
▶ Global Initiative for Asthma (GINA) 2021

Prevention Recommendations
–Advise pregnant women and parents of young children not to smoke.
–Treat vitamin D deficiency in pregnant women.
–Encourage vaginal delivery.
–Minimize use of broad-spectrum antibiotics during the first year of life.

Comments

1. Environmental exposures such as automobile exhaust and dust mites are associated with higher rates of asthma, while others (household pets and farm animals) may be protective. Avoiding tobacco smoke and air pollution is protective, but allergen avoidance measures have not been shown to be effective in primary prevention.
2. Public health interventions to reduce childhood obesity, increase fruit and vegetable intake, improve maternal-fetal health, and reduce socioeconomic inequality would address major risk factors. (*Lancet*. 2015;386:1075-1085)
3. Maternal intake of allergenic food likely decreases the risk of allergy and asthma in offspring.
4. Breast-feeding is generally advisable, but not for the specific purpose of preventing allergies and asthma.
5. Obesity in pregnancy is associated with asthma development in children, but data is lacking on safety and efficacy of weight loss efforts during pregnancy.

Source

–Global Initiative for Asthma. Global Strategy for Asthma Management and Prevention, 2021. www.ginasthma.org.

ATHEROSCLEROTIC CARDIOVASCULAR DISEASE (ASCVD)

–See "CHOLESTEROL AND LIPID DISORDERS" for screening recommendations

Organization

▶ NIH/NHLBI 2012

Prevention Recommendations

Lifestyle Interventions

–If LDL or TG elevated, refer to a registered dietitian for family medical nutrition therapy:
- 25%–30% of calories from fat.
- ≤7% from saturated fat.
- ~10% from monounsaturated fat.
- <200 mg/d of cholesterol.
- Avoid trans fats as much as possible.

–Consider psyllium can be added to a low-fat, low-saturated-fat diet as cereal enriched with psyllium at a dose of 6 g/d for children 2–12 y, and 12 g/d for those >12 y.

–Decrease sugar intake by replacing simple with complex carbohydrates and eliminating sugar sweetened beverages.

–Increase dietary fish to increase omega-3 fatty acids.

–Recommend physical activity (as in all children). Age 5–10, 1 h/d of moderate-to-vigorous physical activity and <2 h/d of sedentary screen time. Age 11–21, 1 h/d of moderate-to-vigorous activity with vigorous intensity 3 d/wk, with <2 h of screen time with quality programming daily.

Pharmacologic Therapies

–Consider medication therapy if:

- Birth–10 y: Only with severe primary hyperlipidemia (homozygous familial hypercholesterolemia, primary hypertriglyceridemia with TG ≥ 500 mg/dL) or a high-risk condition or evident cardiovascular disease; all under the care of a lipid specialist.
- 10–21 y: Average 2 LDL measurements 2 wk–3 mo apart and consider statin if
  ○ 160–189 mg/dL with positive family hx or 1 high-level or 2 moderate-level risk factors.
  ○ 130–159 mg/dL with 2 high-level risk factors or 1 high-level and 2 moderate-level risk factors.

Source

–Expert Panel on Integrated Guidelines for Cardiovascular Health and Risk Reduction in Children and Adolescents. *Pediatrics*. 2011;128(5):S213-S258. https://www.nhlbi.nih.gov/files/docs/peds_guidelines_sum.pdf

ATTENTION-DEFICIT/HYPERACTIVITY DISORDER

Organizations

▶ AAFP 2016, AAP 2019, NICE 2018

Screening Recommendations

–Do not screen routinely.

–Initiate an evaluation for ADHD for any child 4–18 y who presents with academic or behavioral problems and symptoms of inattention, hyperactivity, or impulsivity. Diagnosis requires that the child meets DSM-V criteria[1] and direct supporting evidence from parents or caregivers and classroom teacher.

–Screen for comorbid conditions, including emotional or behavioral conditions (eg, anxiety, depression, oppositional defiant disorder, conduct disorders, substance use), developmental conditions (eg, learning and language disorders, autism spectrum disorders), and physical conditions (eg, tics, sleep apnea).

Comments

1. Stimulant prescription rates continue to rise. (*Lancet*. 2016; 387(10024):1240-1250)
2. Current estimates are that 7.2% of children/adolescents meet criteria for ADHD. (*Pediatrics*. 2015;135(4):e994)
3. The U.S. Food and Drug Administration (FDA) approved a "black box" warning regarding the potential for cardiovascular side effects of ADHD stimulant drugs. (*N Engl J Med*. 2006;354:1445)

Sources

–AAFP. *Clinical Recommendation: ADHD in Children and Adolescents*. 2016.

[1]The DSM-5 criteria define 4 dimensions of ADHD: (1) attention-deficit/hyperactivity disorder primarily of the inattentive presentation (ADHD/I) (314.00 [F90.0]); (2) attention-deficit/hyperactivity disorder primarily of the hyperactive-impulsive presentation (ADHD/HI) (314.01 [F90.1]); (3) attention-deficit/hyperactivity disorder combined presentation (ADHD/C) (314.01 [F90.2]); and (4) other specified and unspecified ADHD (314.01 [F90.8]).

–AAP. *Clinical Practice Guideline for the Diagnosis, Evaluation, and Treatment of Attention-Deficit/Hyperactivity Disorder in Children and Adolescents.* 2019.

–NICE. *Attention Deficit Hyperactivity Disorder: Diagnosis and Management.* 2018. nice.org.uk/guidance/ng87

AUTISM SPECTRUM DISORDER

Organizations
▶ USPSTF 2016, AAP 2014

Screening Recommendations

GUIDELINES DISCORDANT: WHETHER TO PERFORM ROUTINE AUTISM SCREENING	
Organization	**Guidance**
USPSTF	Insufficient evidence for or against routine screening
AAP	Screen with autism-specific tool at 18 mo and 24 mo

Comments

1. M-CHAT is the most commonly used screening tool (see Chapter 33).
2. Listen and respond to concerns raised by caregivers; signs may be identifiable by 9 mo of age.
3. Prevalence is 1 in 68; 4.5:1 male:female ratio. (*MMWR Surveill Summ.* 2016;65(3):1-23)

Sources
–*JAMA.* 2016;315(7):691-696.
–*Pediatrics.* 2006;118(1):405.
–*Pediatrics.* 2014;135(5):e1520.

CELIAC DISEASE

Organizations
▶ USPSTF 2017, AAFP 2017, NICE 2015

Screening Recommendations

–Do not screen the asymptomatic general population, as insufficient evidence exists regarding screening of asymptomatic people.

–Screen first-degree relatives of people with celiac disease. (NICE)

–Rule out celiac disease using serologic testing as part of the evaluation of the following signs, symptoms, or associated conditions: persistent unexplained abdominal or gastrointestinal symptoms, faltering growth, prolonged fatigue, unexpected weight loss, severe or persistent mouth ulcers, unexplained iron, vitamin B12 or folate deficiency, type 1 diabetes, autoimmune thyroid disease, irritable bowel syndrome (in adults). (NICE)

Comments

1. Patients must continue a gluten-containing diet during diagnostic testing.
2. IgA tissue transglutaminase (TTG) is the test of choice (>90% sensitivity/specificity), along with total IgA level.
3. IgA endomysial antibody test is indicated if the TTG test is equivocal.
4. Avoid antigliadin antibody testing.
5. Consider serologic testing for any of the following: Addison disease; amenorrhea; autoimmune hepatitis; autoimmune myocarditis; chronic immune thrombocytopenic purpura (ITP); dental enamel defects; depression; bipolar disorder; Down syndrome; Turner syndrome; epilepsy; lymphoma; metabolic bone disease; chronic constipation; polyneuropathy; sarcoidosis; Sjögren syndrome; or unexplained alopecia.

Sources

–AAFP. *Clinical Recommendation: Screening for Celiac Disease.* 2017.
–*JAMA.* 2017;317(12):1252.
–NICE. *Coeliac Disease: Recognition, Assessment and Management.* 2015.

CHOLESTEROL AND LIPID DISORDERS

Organizations

▶ USPSTF 2016, NLA 2011

Screening Recommendations

GUIDELINES DISCORDANT: WHETHER TO SCREEN	
Organization	**Guidance**
USPSTF	Insufficient evidence to recommend for or against routine universal lab screening
AHA, NHLBI	Selectively screen with fasting lipid panel patients age >2 y with concerning personal or family history[a] Universal screening in adolescents regardless of FH between age 9 and 11 y and again between age 18 and 21 y

[a]Obesity, hypertension, diabetes, smoking hx, or parent age < 55 y with coronary artery disease, peripheral arterial disease, cerebrovascular disease, or hyperlipidemia.

–In familial hypercholesterolemia, screen at age 9–11 y with a fasting lipid panel or nonfasting non-HDL-C. If non-HDL-C ≥ 145 mg/dL, perform fasting lipid panel. (USPSTF)
–Genetic screening for familial hypercholesterolemia is generally not needed for diagnosis or clinical management.
–Cascade screening: testing lipid levels in all first-degree relatives of diagnosed familial hypercholesterolemia patients.

Comments

1. Childhood drug treatment of dyslipidemia lowers lipid levels but effect on childhood or adult outcomes is uncertain.
2. Lifestyle approach is recommended starting after age 2 y.
3. Fasting lipid profile is the recommended screening tool. If within normal limits, repeat testing in 3–5 y is recommended.

Sources

–*J Clin Lipidol.* 2011;5:S1-S8.
–*JAMA.* 2016;316:625-633.
–*Circulation.* 2007;115:1947-1967.
–NHLBI. *Expert Panel on Integrated Guidelines for Cardiovascular Health and Risk Reduction in Children and Adolescents.* 2012.

DENTAL CARIES

Organizations

▶ USPSTF 2014, AAP 2014, AAFP 2014, Bright Futures Oral Health Guide

Prevention Recommendations

–Clean infant gums with clean, soft, damp cloth once daily.
–Apply fluoride varnish to the primary teeth of all infants and children starting at the age of primary teeth eruption. (See Table 13-1.)
–Supplement with oral fluoride starting at age 6 mo where water supply is fluoride deficient (≤0.6 mg/L). (See Table 13-2 for dosing.)

Comments

1. Fluoride mouthwash used regularly by children under 16 reduces risk of dental caries by >25%. (*Cochrane Database Syst Rev.* 2016;7:CD002284)
2. The CDC's My Water's Fluoride resource provides county-level information on content of fluoride in the water system. https://nccd.cdc.gov/DOH_MWF/
3. Brush infant teeth with a smear of fluoridated toothpaste at eruption of first tooth twice per day up to age 3. Children aged 3–6 y should brush with a pea-sized amount of fluoridated toothpaste twice daily; parents should be brushing child's teeth once daily until age 7.
4. Caries risk assessment tool can be found at: https://www.aapd.org/globalassets/media/policies_guidelines/bp_cariesriskassessment.pdf

Sources

–AAFP. *Clinical Recommendation.* 2014.
–*Pediatrics.* 2014;133(5):s1-s10.

TABLE 13-1 CLINICAL RECOMMENDATIONS FOR USE OF PROFESSIONALLY APPLIED OR PRESCRIPTION-STRENGTH, HOME-USE TOPICAL FLUORIDE AGENTS FOR CARIES PREVENTION IN PATIENTS AT ELEVATED RISK OF DEVELOPING CARIES

Age Group or Dentition Affected	Professionally Applied Topical Fluoride Agent	Prescription-Strength, Home-Use Topical Fluoride Agent
Younger than 6 y	2.26% fluoride varnish at least every 3 to 6 mo (**In Favor**)	
6–18 y	2.26% fluoride varnish at least every 3 to 6 mo (**In Favor**) or 1.23% fluoride (acidulated phosphate fluoride [APF]) gel for 4 min at least every 3 to 6 mo (**In Favor**)	0.09% fluoride mouthrinse at least weekly (**In Favor**) or 0.5% fluoride gel or paste twice daily (**Expert Opinion For**)
Older than 18 y	2.26% fluoride varnish at least every 3 to 6 mo (**Expert Opinion For**) or 1.23% fluoride (APF) gel for at least 4 min every 3 to 6 mo (**Expert Opinion For**)	0.09% fluoride mouthrinse at least weekly (**Expert Opinion For**) or 0.5% fluoride gel or paste twice daily (**Expert Opinion For**)
Adult Root Caries	2.26% fluoride varnish at least every 3 to 6 mo (**Expert Opinion For**) or 1.23% fluoride (APF) gel for 4 min at least every 3 to 6 mo (**Expert Opinion For**)	0.09% fluoride mouthrinse daily (**Expert Opinion For**) or 0.5% fluoride gel or paste twice daily (**Expert Opinion For**)

Additional Information:
   Patients at low risk of developing caries may not need additional topical fluorides other than over-the-counter fluoridated toothpaste and fluoridated water.

Source: Reproduced with permission from Weyant RJ, Tracy SL, Anselmo T (tracy), et al. Topical fluoride for caries prevention. *J Am Dent Assoc.* 2013;144(11):1279–1291.

TABLE 13-2 RECOMMENDED FLUORIDE SUPPLEMENTATION BY AGE AND FLUORIDE LEVEL IN COMMUNITY WATER SUPPLY

Age	Fluoride Level in Drinking Water < 0.3 ppm	Fluoride Level in Drinking Water 0.3–0.6 ppm
6 mo–3 y	0.25 mg/d	None
3–6 y	0.5 mg/d	0.25 mg/d
6–16 y	1.0 mg/d	0.5 mg/d

Source: Adapted from Table 1 in CDC MMWR. 2001;50(RR14):1-42. https://www.cdc.gov/mmwr/preview/mmwrhtml/rr5014a1.htm

DEPRESSION

Organizations
▶ USPSTF 2016, AAP 2021

Screening Recommendations
–Insufficient evidence to recommend for or against routine screening of children age 7–11.

–Screen all adolescents (age 12+) for major depressive disorder (MDD).

–Have systems in place to ensure accurate diagnosis, appropriate psychotherapy, and adequate follow-up.

Comments
1. Screen in primary care clinics with the Patient Health Questionnaire for Adolescents (PHQ-A) (73% sensitivity; 94% specificity) or the Beck Depression Inventory-Primary Care (BDI-PC) (91% sensitivity; 91% specificity). See Chapter 33.
2. Treatment options include pharmacotherapy (fluoxetine and escitalopram have FDA approval for this age group), psychotherapy, collaborative care, psychosocial support interventions, and CAM approaches.
3. SSRI may increase suicidality in some adolescents, emphasizing the need for close follow-up.

Sources
–*Ann Intern Med.* 2016;164(5):360-366.

–Hagan JF, Shaw JS, Duncan PM, eds. *Bright Futures: Guidelines for Health Supervision of Infants, Children, and Adolescents.* 4th ed. American Academy of Pediatrics; 2017; updated 2021.

DIABETES

Organization
▶ ADA 2012

Screening Recommendations
–Screen all children at risk for DM type 2 beginning at age 10 or start of puberty.

–"At risk" is defined as overweight (BMI or weight for height > 85th percentile) plus two of the following:
  - Family history of DM type 2.
  - Asian, Black, Hispanic, Native American, or Pacific Islander.
  - Maternal history of DM or GDM.
  - Signs of insulin resistance (acanthosis nigricans, hypertension, dyslipidemia, polycystic ovary syndrome, small-for-gestational age birth weight).

–Repeat screening every 3 y if negative.

Source
–*Diabetes Care* 2021;44(Suppl. 1):S15-S33.

FAMILY VIOLENCE AND ABUSE

Organization
▶ USPSTF 2018

Screening Recommendation
–Insufficient evidence to recommend for or against routine screening of parents or guardians for the physical abuse or neglect of children.

Comments
1. All providers should be aware of physical and behavioral signs and symptoms associated with abuse and neglect, including burns, bruises, and repeated suspect trauma.
2. CDC publishes a toolkit of assessment instruments: https://www.cdc.gov/violence prevention/pdf/ipv/ipvandsvscreening.pdf

Source
–USPSTF. *Interventions to Prevent Child Maltreatment*. 2018.

Organizations
▶ WHO 2010, USPSTF 2019

Prevention Recommendations

GUIDELINES DISCORDANT: INTERVENTIONS TO PREVENT CHILDHOOD ABUSE	
Organization	**Population**
WHO	Institute school-based programs that emphasize preventing dating violence
USPSTF	Current evidence is insufficient to assess the balance of benefits and harms of primary care interventions to prevent child maltreatment

Comment
1. Interventions with possible but not proven efficacy include:
   a. School-based programs that teach children to recognize and avoid sexually abusive situations.
   b. Empowerment and relationship skills training for women.
   c. Programs that change social and cultural gender norms.

Sources
–World Health Organization. *Preventing Intimate Partner and Sexual Violence against Women*. 2010.
–USPSTF. *Interventions to Prevent Child Maltreatment*. 2019.

HEPATITIS B VIRUS (HBV) INFECTION

Organizations
▶ USPSTF 2020, CDC 2018, 2020

Recommendations
–Screen high-risk individuals using HBV surface antigen (HBsAg):
- Foreign-born persons from countries where HBV prevalence ≥2%.[1]
- US-born persons not vaccinated at birth whose parents were born in countries where HBV prevalence ≥8%.[k]
- HIV-positive persons.
- Household contacts or sexual partners of persons with HBV infection.
- Men who have sex with men.
- Persons with injection drug use.
- Hemodialysis patients. (CDC)
- Persons needing immunosuppressive therapy, immunosuppression related to organ transplantation, and immunosuppression for rheumatologic or gastroenterologic disorders. (CDC)
- Blood, organ, plasma, semen, or tissue donors. (CDC)
- People with elevated alanine aminotransferase levels (≥19 IU/L for women and ≥30 IU/L for men). (CDC)
- Infants born to HBV-infected mothers (HBsAg and antibody to hepatitis B surface antigen [anti-HBs] only are recommended). (CDC)

Sources
–USPSTF. *JAMA.* 2020;324(23):2415-2422.
–CDC. *MMWR Recomm Rep.* 2018;67(1):1–31.
–CDC. 2020. www.cdc.gov/hepatitis/hbv/hbvfaq.htm

HUMAN IMMUNODEFICIENCY VIRUS (HIV)

Organizations
▶ AAFP 2013, USPSTF 2019, CDC 2015

Screening Recommendations
–Screen everyone in the recommended age range.
–Consider screening high-risk individuals[2] of other ages.

---

[1]HBV prevalence ≥2% in Africa, Asia, South Pacific, Middle East (except Cyprus and Israel), Eastern Europe (except Hungary), Malta, Spain, indigenous populations of Greenland, Alaska natives, indigenous populations of Canada, Caribbean, Guatemala, Honduras, and South America. HBV prevalence ≥ 8% in Angola, Benin, Burkina Faso, Burundi, Cameroon, Central African Republic, Congo, Côte d'Ivoire, Djibouti, Equatorial Guinea, Gabon, Gambia, Ghana, Guinea, Liberia, Malawi, Mali, Mauritania, Mozambique, Namibia, Niger, Nigeria, Senegal, Sierra Leone, Somalia, South Sudan, Sudan, Swaziland, Togo, Uganda, Zimbabwe, Haiti, Kiribati, Nauru, Niue, Papua New Guinea, Solomon Islands, Tonga, Vanuatu, Kyrgyzstan , Laos, Vietnam, Mongolia, and Yemen.
[2]High-risk: multiple current sexual partners, new partner, inconsistent condom use, sex while under influence of drugs/alcohol, sex in exchange for money/drugs.

GUIDELINES DISCORDANT: POPULATION TO SCREEN

Organization	Guidance
AAFP	Age 18–65 y
USPSTF	Age 15–65 y
CDC	Age 13–64 y

Comments

1. HIV testing should be voluntary and must have a verbal consent to test. Patients may "opt out" of testing.
2. Educate and counsel all high-risk patients regarding HIV testing, transmission, risk-reduction behaviors, and implications of infection.
3. If acute HIV is suspected, also use plasma RNA test.
4. False-positive results with electroimmunoassay (EIA): nonspecific reactions in persons with immunologic disturbances (eg, systemic lupus erythematosus or rheumatoid arthritis), multiple transfusions, recent influenza, or rabies vaccination.
5. Confirmatory testing is necessary using Western blot or indirect immunofluorescence assay.
6. Awareness of HIV positively reduces secondary HIV transmission risk and high-risk behavior and viral load if on highly active antiretroviral therapy (HAART). (CDC 2006)

Sources

–AAFP. *Clinical Recommendations: HIV Infection, Adolescents and Adults.* 2013.
–CDC. *Sexually Transmitted Diseases Treatment Guidelines.* 2015.
–USPSTF. *Screening for HIV Infection.* 2019.

HYPERTENSION (HTN), CHILDREN AND ADOLESCENTS

Organizations

▶ AAP 2017, NHLBI 2012, AAFP 2018, USPSTF 2020

Screening Recommendations

GUIDELINES DISCORDANT: SCREENING FOR BLOOD PRESSURE

Organization	Guidance
USPSTF	Insufficient evidence to support screening for high blood pressure in children and adolescents, as balance of benefits and harms cannot be determined
AAP, AAFP, NHLBI	Measure BP only at preventative visits for children age ≥3[a] y. Measure BP at each encounter for children age ≥3 y who have obesity, renal disease, h/o aortic arch obstruction or coarctation, diabetes, or are taking medications known to raise blood pressure

[a] In children age <3 y, conditions that warrant BP measurement include: prematurity, very low birth weight, or neonatal complications; congenital heart disease; recurrent urinary tract infections (UTIs), hematuria, or proteinuria; renal disease or urologic malformations; familial hypercholesterolemia of congenital renal disease; solid-organ transplant; malignancy or bone marrow transplant; drugs known to raise BP; systemic illnesses; and increased intracranial pressure.

Comments

1. Hypertension: average systolic blood pressure (SBP) or diastolic blood pressure (DBP) ≥ 95th percentile for gender, age, and height on 3 or more occasions. See Table 13-3 and Chapter 33 for more detail.
2. Counsel children and adolescents who have been diagnosed with hypertension regarding lifestyle modifications including diet and physical activity.
3. Prescribe pharmacologic therapy to children and adolescents who fail lifestyle modifications.
4. USPSTF concludes that the evidence to support screening for high blood pressure in children and adolescents is insufficient and that the balance of benefits and harms cannot be determined.

Sources

−*Pediatrics.* 2017;140(3):e2017-e1904.
−NHLBI. *Expert Panel on Integrated Guidelines for Cardiovascular Health and Risk Reduction in Children and Adolescents.* 2012.
−NHLBI. *A Pocket Guide to Blood Pressure Management in Children.* 2012.
−AAFP. *High Blood Pressure in Children and Adolescents.* 2018.
−USPSTF. *Screening for High Blood Pressure in Children and Adolescents.* 2020.

ILLICIT DRUG USE

Organizations

▶ USPSTF 2020, ICSI 2014, AAP 2021

Screening Recommendation

−Insufficient evidence to recommend for or against routine screening for illicit drug use.

GUIDELINES DISCORDANT: WHETHER TO SCREEN	
Organization	**Guidance**
USPSTF	Insufficient evidence to recommend for or against routine screening for illicit drug use
AAP	Perform risk assessment beginning at age 11 using CRAFFT tool[a] and take appropriate follow-up action if positive

[a] http://crafft.org/

Sources

−*ICSI Preventive Services for Adults.* 20th ed. 2014.
−USPSTF. *Screening for Unhealthy Drug Use.* 2020.
−Hagan JF, Shaw JS, Duncan PM, eds. *Bright Futures: Guidelines for Health Supervision of Infants, Children, and Adolescents.* 4th ed. American Academy of Pediatrics; 2017, updated 2021.

TABLE 13-3 CUTOFFS FOR PEDIATRIC STAGE 1 HYPERTENSION

Age		1	2	3	4	5	6	7	8	9	10	11	12	13+	14	15	16	17
Female	SBP	105	109	110	112	113	114	115	117	118	120	124	126	127	127	128	128	128
	DBP	62	66	69	71	73	74	75	75	75	76	77	79	81	82	82	82	82
Male	SBP	105	108	109	110	112	114	116	117	119	121	128	128	131	134	135	137	138
	DBP	57	61	64	68	71	73	74	75	77	78	78	79	81	84	85	86	87

Source: American Association of Pediatrics, Vol.140(3), e20171904.

Organization
▶ USPSTF 2020

Prevention Recommendation
–Current evidence is insufficient to assess the balance of benefits and harms of primary care-based behavioral counseling interventions to prevent illicit drug use, including nonmedical use of prescription drugs in children, adolescents, and young adults.

Source
–USPSTF. *Primary Care-Based Interventions to Prevent Illicit Drug Use in Children, Adolescents, and Young Adults.* 2020

IMMUNIZATIONS, INFANTS AND CHILDREN

Organization
▶ CDC 2018

Prevention Recommendation
–Immunize infants and children according to the CDC recommendations unless contraindicated (see Chapter 33).

Sources
–CDC. *Child and Adolescent Schedule.*
–CDC. *Catch-Up Immunization Schedule.*

INFLUENZA, CHEMOPROPHYLAXIS

Organizations
▶ CDC 2021, AAP 2021

Prevention Recommendations
The following situations warrant chemoprophylaxis:
–Children at high risk for complications who cannot receive vaccine, or within 2 wk of receiving vaccine.
–Family members or health care providers who are unimmunized and likely to have ongoing exposure to high-risk or unimmunized children younger than 24 mo of age.
–Unimmunized staff and children in an institutional setting during an outbreak.
–Postexposure prophylaxis for close contacts of infected person who are at high risk of complications if less than 48 h since exposure.
–Consider as supplement to vaccine if immune compromised.

Comments
1. Influenza vaccination is the best way to prevent influenza.
2. Antiviral chemoprophylaxis is not a substitute for influenza vaccination.

3. Agents for chemoprophylaxis of influenza A (H1N1) and B: zanamivir or oseltamivir.
4. Children at high risk of complications include those with chronic diseases such as asthma, diabetes, cardiac disease, immune suppression, and neurodevelopmental disorders.
5. If child <3 mo, use of oseltamivir for chemoprophylaxis is not recommended unless situation is judged critical due to limited data in this age group.

Sources

–Recommendations for Prevention and Control of Influenza in Children, 2021–2022. *Pediatrics.* 2021;148(4):e2021053744.

INFLUENZA, VACCINATION

Organizations

▶ CDC 2021, AAP 2021

Prevention Recommendations

–Give seasonal influenza vaccine to all persons age > 6 mo.
–If age 6 mo to 8 y, give 2 doses of the vaccine (>4 wk apart) during their first season of vaccination.

Comment

1. Highest-risk groups for influenza complications are:
   a. Pregnant women.
   b. Children age 6 mo to 5 y.
   c. Adults age > 50 y.
   d. Persons with chronic medical conditions.[1]
   e. Residents of extended-care facilities.
   f. Morbidly obese (BMI > 40) persons.
   g. Health care personnel.
   h. Household contacts of persons with high-risk medical conditions or caregivers of children age < 5 y or adults age > 50 y.
   i. Children and adolescents receiving long-term aspirin therapy.
   j. American Indians or Alaska Natives.

Sources

–Recommendations for Prevention and Control of Influenza in Children, 2021–2022. *Pediatrics.* 2021;148(4):e2021053744.
–CDC. https://www.cdc.gov/vaccines/hcp/acip-recs/vacc-specific/flu.html

---

[1]Chronic heart, lung, renal, liver, hematologic, cancer, neuromuscular, or seizure disorders, severe cognitive dysfunction, diabetes, HIV infection, or immunosuppression.

LEAD POISONING

Organizations

▶ AAFP 2006, USPSTF 2019, CDC 2000, AAP 2000

Screening Recommendations

–Insufficient evidence to recommend for or against routine screening in asymptomatic children at increased risk.[1]

–Do not screen asymptomatic children at average risk.

Comments

1. CDC recommends that children who receive Medicaid benefits should be screened unless high-quality, local data demonstrates the absence of lead exposure among this population.
2. Screen at ages 1 and 2 y, or by age 3 y if a high-risk child has never been screened.
3. The threshold for elevated blood lead is 5 μg/dL. (CDC. *Low Level Lead Exposure Harms Children: A Renewed Call for Primary Prevention.* 2012)
4. CDC personal risk questionnaire (http://www.cdc.gov/nceh/lead/publications/screening.htm):
   a. Does your child live in or regularly visit a house (or other facility, eg, daycare) that was built before 1950?
   b. Does your child live in or regularly visit a house built before 1978 with recent or ongoing renovations or remodeling (within the last 6 mo)?
   c. Does your child have a sibling or playmate who has or did have lead poisoning?

Sources

–USPSTF. *Elevated Blood Lead Levels in Childhood and Pregnancy: Screening.* 2019.
–*Pediatrics.* 1998;101(6):1702.
–Advisory Committee on Childhood Lead Poisoning Prevention. Recommendations for blood lead screening of young children enrolled in Medicaid: targeting a group at high risk. *CDC MMWR.* 2000;49(RR14):1-13.
–AAFP. *Clinical Recommendations: Lead Poisoning.* 2006.

MOTOR VEHICLE INJURY

Organization

▶ ICSI 2013

Screening Recommendation

–Ask about car seats, booster seats, seat belt use, helmet use while riding motorcycles.

---

[1]Child suspected by parent, health care provider, or Health Department to be at risk for lead exposure; sibling or playmate with elevated blood lead level; recent immigrant, refugee, or foreign adoptee; child's parent or caregiver works with lead; household member uses traditional folk or ethnic remedies or cosmetics or who routinely eats food imported informally from abroad; residence near a source of high lead levels.

Comment

1. One study demonstrated a 21% reduction in mortality with the use of child restraint systems vs. seat belts in children age 2–6 y involved in motor vehicle collisions. (*Arch Pediatr Adolesc Med.* 2006;160:617-621)

Source

–ICSI. *Preventive Services for Children and Adolescents.* 19th ed. 2013.

Prevention Recommendations

–Ask the family about the use of car seats, booster seats, and seat belts.
–Ask children and adolescents about helmet use in recreational activities.

Comments

1. Head injury rates are reduced by approximately 75% in motorcyclists who wear helmets compared with those who do not.
2. Properly used child restraint systems can reduce mortality up to 21% compared with seat belt usage in children age 2–6 y.
3. All infants and toddlers should ride in a rear-facing car safety seat until they are age 2 or until they have met the max height or weight allowed by car seat manufacturer.

Source

–ICSI. *Preventive Services for Children and Adolescents.* 19th ed. 2013.

OBESITY

Organizations

▶ USPSTF 2017, VA/DoD 2014

Screening Recommendation

–Screen for obesity in children aged 6 y and older and adolescents using BMI and refer patients with age- and sex-specific BMI ≥ 95th percentile to comprehensive, intensive behavioral interventions to promote weight loss.

Sources

–USPSTF. *Obesity in Children and Adolescents: Screening.* 2017.
–VA/DoD Clinical Practice Guideline for Screening and Management of Overweight and Obesity, Version 2.0. 2014.

Organizations

▶ USPSTF 2017, Endocrine Society 2017, WHO 2020

Prevention Recommendations

–Offer obese children (age 6+) intensive counseling and behavioral interventions to promote improvement in weight status.
–Encourage at least an average or 60 min/d of moderate-to-vigorous intensity, mostly aerobic, physical activity, across the week.

–Foster healthy sleep patterns.

–Limit the amount of time spent being sedentary, particularly the amount of recreational screen time.

–5%–10% weight loss can produce a clinically significant reduction in heart disease risk.

Comments

1. Avoid the consumption of calorie-dense, nutrient-poor foods (eg, juices, soft drinks, "fast food" items, and calorie-dense snacks). Consume whole fruits rather than juices.
2. Control calorie intake by portion control.
3. Reduce saturated dietary fat intake for children age > 2 y.
4. Increase dietary fiber, fruits, and vegetables.
5. Eat regular, scheduled meals and avoid snacking.
6. Limit television, video games, and computer time to 2 h daily.

Sources

–USPSTF. *Obesity in Children and Adolescents: Screening*. 2017.

–World Health Organization 2020 guidelines on physical activity and sedentary behavior.

–*J Clin Endocrinol Metab*. 2017;102(3):709-757.

Organizations

▶ ICSI 2013, CDC 2011

Prevention Recommendations

–Employ a team approach for weight management in all persons of normal weight (BMI 18.5–24.9) or overweight (BMI 25–29.9), including:

- Nutrition.
- Physical activity; 150 min of moderate-intensity aerobic exercise/wk.
- Lifestyle changes; avoid inactivity.
- Screen for depression.
- Screen for eating disorders.
- Review medication list and assess if any medications can interfere with weight loss.

–Ensure regular follow-up to reinforce principles of weight management.

Comments

1. Recommend 30–60 min of moderate physical activity on most days of the week.
2. Nutrition education focused on decreased caloric intake, encouraging healthy food choices, and managing restaurant and social eating situations. Eat 5–6 servings of fruits and vegetables daily.
3. Weekly weight checks.
4. Encourage nonfood rewards for positive reinforcement.
5. Stress management techniques.
6. 5%–10% weight loss can produce a clinically significant reduction in heart disease risk.

Source

–Fitch A, Everling L, Fox C, et al. *Prevention and Management of Obesity for Adults*. Bloomington, MN: ICSI; 2013.

OTITIS MEDIA

Organization

▶ AAP 2013

Prevention Recommendations

–Do not use prophylactic antibiotics to reduce the frequency of episodes of AOM in children with recurrent AOM.

–Exclusive breast-feeding for at least the first 6 mo of life.

–Vaccinate all children to prevent bacterial AOM with pneumococcal and influenza vaccines.

–Avoid tobacco exposure.

Source

–*Pediatrics.* 2013;131(3):e964-e999.

SCOLIOSIS

Organizations

▶ AAFP 2013, USPSTF 2017

Screening Recommendation

–Insufficient evidence to assess the balance of benefits and harms of screening for adolescent idiopathic scoliosis in children and adolescents age 10–18.

Sources

–AAFP. *Choosing Wisely: Scoliosis in Adolescents.* 2013.

–USPSTF. *Screening for Adolescents Idiopathic Scoliosis.* 2017.

SEXUALLY TRANSMITTED INFECTIONS (STIS)

Organization

▶ USPSTF 2014

Prevention Recommendation

–Employ high-intensity behavioral counseling to prevent STIs for all sexually active adolescents at increased risk for STIs. Include basic information about STIs, condom use, communication about safe sex, problem solving, and goal setting.

Source

–USPSTF. *Sexually Transmitted Infections.* 2014.

SPEECH AND LANGUAGE DELAY

Organizations
▶ AAFP 2015, USPSTF 2015

Screening Recommendations

GUIDELINES DISCORDANT: SCREENING FOR SPEECH AND LANGUAGE DELAY	
AAFP, USPSTF	Evidence is insufficient to recommend for or against routine use of brief, formal screening instruments in primary care to detect speech and language delay in children up to age 5 y
AAP	Screen using validated test during well child checks at 9, 18, and 24/30 mo

Comments
1. Fair evidence suggests that interventions can improve the results of short-term assessments of speech and language skills; however, no studies have assessed long-term consequences.
2. In a study of 9000 toddlers in the Netherlands, 2-time screening for language delays reduced the number of children who required special education (2.7% vs. 3.7%) and reduced deficient language performance (8.8% vs. 9.7%) at age 8 y. (*Pediatrics*. 2007;120:1317)
3. Studies have not fully addressed the potential harms of screening or interventions for speech and language delays, such as labeling, parental anxiety, or unnecessary evaluation and intervention.
4. Insufficient evidence to recommend a specific test, but parent-administered tools are best (eg, Communicative Development Inventory, Infant-Toddler Checklist, Language Development Survey, Ages and Stages Questionnaire).

Sources
–AAFP. *Clinical Recommendation: Speech and Language Delay*. 2015.
–*Pediatrics*. 2015;136(2):e474-e481.
–*Pediatrics*. 2006;118(1):405.
–*Pediatrics*. 2015;136(2):e448.

SUICIDE RISK

Organization
▶ AAP 2016

Screening Recommendation
–Ask questions about suicidal thoughts in routine history taking throughout adolescence.

Source
–*Pediatrics*. 2016; 138 (1): e20161420. Suicide and Suicide Attempts in Adolescents.

TOBACCO USE

Organization

▶ USPSTF 2020

Screening Recommendation

−Provide interventions including education or brief counseling to prevent the initiation of tobacco use.

Comment

1. The efficacy of counseling to prevent tobacco use in children and adolescents is uncertain.
2. Screen for use of any tobacco product including but not limited to cigarettes, cigars, hookah tobacco, smokeless tobacco products, vapes, e-cigarettes, hookah pens, and other electronic nicotine delivery systems.

Source

−USPSTF. *JAMA.* 2020;323(16):1590-1598.

Organizations

▶ AAFP 2013, USPTF 2020

Prevention Recommendation

−Provide interventions, including education or brief counseling, to prevent initiation of tobacco use among school-aged children and adolescents.

Comment

1. The efficacy of counseling to prevent tobacco use in children and adolescents is of moderate net benefit.

Source

−USPSTF. *Primary Care Interventions for Prevention and Cessation of Tobacco Use in Children and Adolescents.* 2020.

−https://www.aafp.org/family-physician/patient-care/clinical-recommendations/all-clinical-recommendations/tobacco-use-children.html

TRAUMATIC BRAIN INJURY

Organization

▶ CDC 2018

Prevention Recommendations

−Do not routinely image patients to diagnose mild traumatic brain injury (mTBI).
−Use validated, age-appropriate symptom scales to diagnose mTBI.
−Assess evidence-based risk factors for prolonged recovery.
−Provide patients with instructions on return to activity customized to their symptoms.
−Counsel patients to return gradually to non-sports activities after no more than 2−3 d of rest.

Source

–Centers for Disease Control and Prevention. *Guideline on the Diagnosis and Management of Mild Traumatic Brain Injury Among Children.* 2018.

TUBERCULOSIS, LATENT

Organizations

▶ USPSTF 2016, CDC 2010

Screening Recommendation

–Screen by tuberculin skin test (TST) or interferon-gamma release assay (IGRA) if increased risk of tuberculosis. Frequency of testing is based on likelihood of further exposure to TB and level of confidence in the accuracy of the results.

Comments

1. Risk factors include birth or residence in a country with increased TB prevalence and residence in a congregate setting (shelters, correctional facilities).
2. Typically, a TST is used to screen for latent TB.
3. IGRA is preferred if:
    a. Testing persons who have a low likelihood of returning to have their TST read.
    b. Testing persons who have received a bacille Calmette–Guérin (BCG) vaccination.

Sources

–*JAMA.* 2016;316(9):962-969.
–*CDC MWWR.* 2010;59(RR-5).

VISUAL IMPAIRMENT

Organization

▶ USPSTF 2017

Screening Recommendations

–Screen vision for all children 3–5 y at least once to detect amblyopia.
–Insufficient evidence for vision screening in children <3 y of age.

Comment

1. May screen with a visual acuity test, a stereoacuity test, a cover–uncover test, and the Hirschberg light reflex test.

Sources

–USPSTF. *Vision Screening in Children Aged 6 Months to 5 Years.* 2017.
–*JAMA.* 2017;318(9):836-844.

Pregnant Patients

14

ANEMIA

Organizations
▶ USPSTF 2015, AAFP 2014, ACOG 2008, CDC 1998

Screening Recommendation
–Consider screening all patients with hemoglobin or hematocrit at first prenatal visit.

Comments
1. Insufficient evidence to recommend for or against routine screening for iron deficiency anemia (IDA) in pregnant patients to prevent adverse maternal or birth outcomes. Insufficient evidence to recommend for or against use of iron supplements for nonanemic pregnant patients. (USPSTF, 2015)

2. When acute stress or inflammatory disorders are not present, a serum ferritin level is the most accurate test for evaluating IDA. Among patients of childbearing age, a cutoff of 30 ng/mL has sensitivity of 92%, specificity of 98%. (*Blood.* 1997;89:1052-1057)

3. Oral iron is first-line therapy for IDA in pregnancy. IV iron is preferred choice (after 13th wk) for those who have oral iron intolerance. Cobalamin and folate deficiency should be excluded. (*Blood.* 2017;129:940-949)

4. A growing body of evidence suggests that oral iron in single doses on alternating days is associated with better absorption and adherence (due to reduced side effects) compared to daily dosing or split doses on alternating days. (*Lancet Haematol.* 2017;4(11):e524; Tolkien et al. *PLoS One.* 2015;10(2):e0117383)

5. Decision to transfuse should be based on the hemoglobin, clinical context, and patient preferences. May be appropriate in severe anemia (<7 mg/dL according to WHO) in whom a 2-wk delay in Hb rise with oral iron may result in significant morbidity.

Sources
–USPSTF. https://www.uspreventiveservicestaskforce.org/
–*Ann Intern Med.* 2015;163:529-536.
–ACOG. *Obstet Gynecol.* 2008;112(1):201.
–CDC. *MMWR Morb Mortal Wkly Rep.* 1998;47(RR-3):1.
–*Am Fam Physician.* 2014;89(3):199-208.

BACTERIAL VAGINOSIS

Organization

▶ USPSTF 2020

Screening Recommendations

–Do not screen routinely.

–Insufficient evidence to recommend for or against routine screening for patients at high risk[1] for preterm delivery.

Source

–USPSTF. *Bacterial Vaginosis in Pregnant Persons to Prevent Preterm Delivery: Screening.* 2020.

BACTERIURIA, ASYMPTOMATIC

Organizations

▶ IDSA 2019, USPSTF 2019, AAFP 2006, ACOG/AAP 2017

Screening Recommendations

–Screen for bacteriuria with urine culture at first prenatal visit or at 12–16 wk gestation.

–Treat pregnant patients who have asymptomatic bacteriuria with antimicrobial therapy for 4–7 d.

Comment

1. Treating bacteriuria in pregnancy with antibiotics reduces the risk of pyelonephritis and low birth weight.

Sources

–USPSTF. *Asymptomatic Bacteriuria in Adults: Screening.* 2019.

–*Am Fam Physician.* 2006;74(6):985-990.

–*Clin Infect Dis.* 2019;68(10):e83-e110.

–American Academy of Pediatrics, American College of Obstetricians and Gynecologists. *Guidelines for Perinatal Care.* 8th ed. Elk Grove Village, Illinois and Washington, DC: AAP/ACOG, 2017:159-160.

---

[1]Risk factors: African-American race or ethnicity, body mass index less than 20 kg/m^2, previous preterm delivery, vaginal bleeding, shortened cervix <2.5 cm, pelvic infection, bacterial vaginosis.

CESAREAN SECTION, PRIMARY

Organization
▶ ACOG 2012, WHO 2018

Prevention Recommendations
–Induce labor only for medical indications. If induction is performed for nonmedical reasons, ensure that gestational age is >39 wk and cervix is favorable. (ACOG)

–Do not diagnose failed induction or arrest of labor until sufficient time[1] has passed. (ACOG)

–Consider intermittent auscultation rather than continuous fetal monitoring if heart rate is normal. (ACOG)

–Implement prenatal education programs including childbirth training, nurse-led relaxation, couple-based support, and psychoeducation. (WHO)

–Consider mandatory second opinion for cesarean section decisions. (WHO)

–Give timely feedback to health care professionals regarding cesarean section decision-making. (WHO)

Comment
1. If fetal heart rate variability is moderate, other factors have little association with fetal neurologic outcomes. For more on this and other related information on fetal monitoring, see Macones GA, Hankins GD, Spong CY, et al. The 2008 National Institute of Child Health and Human Development Workshop report on electronic fetal monitoring: update on definitions, interpretation, and research guidelines. *Obstet Gynecol.* 2008;112:661.

Sources
–*Obstet Gynecol.* 2012;120(5):1181.

–World Health Organization. *WHO Prevention Recommendations Non-Clinical Interventions to Reduce Unnecessary Cesarean Sections.* 2018.

CESAREAN SECTION, REPEAT

Organizations
▶ AAFP 2014, ACOG 2017

Prevention Recommendations
–Attempting a vaginal birth after cesarean (VBAC) is safe and appropriate for most patients.

–Encourage and facilitate planning for VBAC. If necessary, refer to a facility that offers trial of labor after cesarean (TOLAC).

---

[1]Failed induction: inability to generate contractions every 3 min and cervical change after 24 h of oxytocin administration and rupture of membranes, if feasible. Arrest of labor, first stage: 6 cm dilation, membrane rupture, and 4 h of adequate contractions or 6 h of inadequate contractions without cervical change. Arrest of labor, second stage: no descent or rotation for 4 h (nulliparous woman with epidural), 3 h (nulliparous woman without epidural or multiparous woman with epidural), or 2 h (multiparous woman without epidural).

Comments

1. Provide counseling, encouragement, and facilitation for a planned VBAC so that patients can make informed decisions. If planned VBAC is not locally available, offer patients who desire it referral to a facility or clinician who offers the service.
2. Obtain informed consent for planned VBAC, including risk to patient, fetus, future fertility, and the capabilities of local delivery setting.
3. Develop facility guidelines to promote access to planned VBAC and improve quality of care for patients who elect TOLAC.
4. Assess the likelihood of planned VBAC as well as individual risks to determine who is an appropriate candidate for TOLAC.
5. A calculator for probability for successful VBAC is available here[1]: https://mfmunetwork.bsc.gwu.edu/PublicBSC/MFMU/VGBirthCalc/vagbirth.html

Sources

–AAFP. *Clinical Prevention Recommendation: Vaginal Birth after Cesarean.* 2014.
–*Obstet Gynecol.* 2017;130(5):1167-1169.

CHLAMYDIA AND GONORRHEA

Organizations

▶ CDC 2021, AAFP 2012, AAP/ACOG 2017

Screening Recommendations

–Screen all patients age <25-y-old at first prenatal visit.
–Screen patients age ≥25 with risk factors.
–Retest those <25-y-old or age ≥25 with risk factors in the third trimester.
–If infection detected, obtain test of cure 3–4 wk after treatment.
–If chlamydia detected during first trimester, repeat within 3–6 mo or retest in third trimester.

Sources

–CDC. *Sexually Transmitted Diseases Treatment Guidelines.* 2021.
–*Am Fam Physician.* 2012;86(12):1127-1132.
–AAP & ACOG. *Guidelines for Perinatal Care.* 8th ed. 2017.

---

[1]Note that, while certain racial groups are documented to have poorer VBAC outcomes, the inclusion of race as a factor in the VBAC score may have the practical effect of dissuading women of color from attempting TOLAC because their clinician perceives their probability of success to be lower. As no biological basis for the difference has been identified, structural racism likely explains the disparity in outcomes, an effect propagated by the use of the VBAC risk calculator to determine appropriateness of TOLAC. (*NEJM* 2020;383(9):874-882)

DIABETES MELLITUS, GESTATIONAL (GDM)

Organizations
▶ USPSTF 2021, ACOG 2018

Screening Recommendations
–Screen for gestational diabetes mellitus in asymptomatic pregnant patients.

–Perform 1-h glucose screening test with 50-g anhydrous glucose load between 24 and 28 gestational wk. Use a cutoff value of either 135 or 140 mg/dL.

–Perform a 3-h glucose tolerance test if the 1-h glucose screening test is abnormal. Use either the Carpenter and Coustan criteria or the National Diabetes Data Group criteria.

–Perform early screening for undiagnosed diabetes, preferably at the initiation of prenatal care, in overweight and obese patients with additional diabetic risk factors, including those with a prior history of GDM.

–Screen all patients with GDM for overt diabetes 6–12 wk postpartum.

Comments
1. Insufficient evidence to support screening for gestational diabetes prior to 24 gestational wk.
2. Insufficient evidence to define the optimal frequency of blood glucose testing in patients with GDM. Based on the data available, consider glucose monitoring 4 times a day, once fasting and again after each meal.
3. Criteria for GDM by 75-g 2-h OGTT if any of the following are abnormal:
   a. Fasting ≥ 92 mg/dL (5.1 mmol/L).
   b. 1 h ≥ 180 mg/dL (10.0 mmol/L).
   c. 2 h ≥ 153 mg/dL (8.5 mmol/L).
4. Criteria for GDM by 100-g 3-h OGTT:
   a. Carpenter–Coustan:
      i. Fasting ≥ 95 mg/dL (5.3 mmol/L).
      ii. 1 h ≥ 180 mg/dL (10.0 mmol/L).
      iii. 2 h ≥ 155 mg/dL (8.6 mmol/L).
      iv. 3 h ≥ 140 mg/dL (7.8 mmol/L).
   b. National Diabetes Data Group:
      i. Fasting ≥ 105 mg/dL (5.8 mmol/L).
      ii. 1 h ≥ 190 mg/dL (10.6 mmol/L).
      iii. 2 h ≥ 165 mg/dL (9.2 mmol/L).
      iv. 3 h ≥ 145 mg/dL (8.0 mmol/L).
5. A1c screening has lower sensitivity than OGTT and is not recommended as a sole screening tool for GDM.

Sources
–USPSTF. *Gestational Diabetes Mellitus: Screening.* 2021.

–ACOG. *Gestational Diabetes Mellitus.* Washington, DC: American College of Obstetricians and Gynecologists (ACOG); 2018 (ACOG practice bulletin; no. 190).

DIABETES MELLITUS (DM), TYPE 2

Organizations

▶ ADA 2019, ACOG 2018

Screening Recommendations

–Screen for undiagnosed DM type 2 at first prenatal visit if risk factors for DM are present.[1]

–For all other patients, screen according to published guidelines (see section "Diabetes Mellitus, Gestational").

Comment

1. Diagnose preexisting diabetes if:
   a. Fasting glucose ≥ 126 mg/dL.
   b. 2-h glucose ≥ 200 mg/dL after 75-g glucose load.
   c. Random glucose ≥ 200 mg/dL with classic hyperglycemic symptoms.
   d. Hemoglobin A1c ≥ 6.5%.

Sources

–*Diabetes Care* 2018;41(suppl 1).

–*Obstet Gynecol.* 2018;131(2):e49.

FETAL ANEUPLOIDY

Organization

▶ ACOG 2020

Screening Recommendations

–Offer screening to all patients, ideally during first prenatal visit. The decision should be reached through informed patient choice, including discussion of sensitivity, positive screening and false-positive rates, and risks/benefits of diagnostic testing (amniocentesis and chorionic villous sampling).

–Cell-free DNA is the most sensitive and specific screening test for the common fetal aneuploidies. Nevertheless, it has the potential for false-positive and false-negative results and is not a substitute for diagnostic testing.

–For all patients with a positive screening test result for fetal aneuploidy, offer genetic counseling and a comprehensive ultrasound evaluation with an opportunity for diagnostic testing to confirm results.

–For patients with a positive serum analyte screening test result who want to avoid a diagnostic test, offer cell-free DNA screening as a follow-up test. Inform patients that this approach may delay definitive diagnosis and will fail to identify some fetuses with chromosomal abnormalities.

---

[1]Immigrants from Asia, Africa, South Pacific, Middle East (except Israel), Eastern Europe (except Hungary), the Caribbean, Malta, Spain, Guatemala, and Honduras.

Comment

1. Risk of chromosomal anomaly by maternal age at term:
   a. 20-y-old: 1 in 525.
   b. 30-y-old: 1 in 384.
   c. 35-y-old: 1 in 178.
   d. 40-y-old: 1 in 62.
   e. 45-y-old: 1 in 18.

Source

–Screening for fetal chromosomal abnormalities. *ACOG Practice Bulletin 226.* 2020;136(4).

Organization

▶ American College of Radiology 2021

Screening Recommendations

–The following choices of imaging to screen for fetal anomalies are usually appropriate:
- Low risk:
  ○ US pregnant uterus transabdominal anatomy scan.
- High risk:
  ○ US pregnant uterus transabdominal detailed scan.
- Soft markers detected on ultrasound:
  ○ US pregnant uterus transabdominal detailed scan.
  ○ US pregnant uterus transabdominal follow-up.
- Major anomalies detected on ultrasound:
  ○ US pregnant uterus transabdominal detailed scan.
  ○ MRI fetal without IV contrast.
  ○ US echocardiography fetal.
  ○ US pregnant uterus transabdominal follow-up.

Source

–*J Am Coll Radiol.* 2021;18:S189-S198.

GROUP B STREPTOCOCCAL (GBS) DISEASE

Organizations

▶ AAP 2019, ACOG 2020

Screening Recommendations

–Screen all patients between 36 0/7 and 37 and 6/7 gestational wk for GBS colonization with a vaginal–rectal swab.

–Patients with GBS bacteriuria/UTI in the current pregnancy OR with prior infant affected by GBS disease are considered colonized and do not require further testing.

Comments

1. Even patients planning a C-section benefit from GBS screening, in case of premature rupture of membranes.
2. Culture results are valid for 5 wk and include births up to 41 and 0/7 wk.
3. Repeat GBS screening is reasonable if the initial test was negative and gestation extends beyond 41 and 0/7 wk.

Prevention Recommendations

–Give intrapartum antibiotic prophylaxis (IAP) to prevent early-onset invasive GBS disease in high-risk pregnancies: positive GBS culture, GBS bacteriuria during pregnancy, or history of previous GBS-infected newborn.

–If a woman presents in labor with unknown GBS colonization status this pregnancy but has a history of GBS in a prior pregnancy or has gestational age less than 37 weeks, offer IAP.

–Do not give IAP if a cesarean delivery is performed with intact membranes and before the onset of labor.

–Consider penicillin allergy testing for all patients with a history of penicillin allergy, particularly those that are suggestive of being IgE mediated, or of unknown severity, or both.

Comments

1. Penicillin G is the agent of choice for IAP.
2. Ampicillin is an acceptable alternative to penicillin G.
3. Use cefazolin if the patient has a penicillin allergy that does not cause anaphylaxis, angioedema, urticaria, or respiratory distress.
4. Use clindamycin[1] or vancomycin if the patient has penicillin allergy that causes anaphylaxis, angioedema, urticaria, or respiratory distress.

Sources

–ACOG committee opinion. *Prevention of Group B Streptococcal Early-Onset Disease in Newborns.* 2020.

–*Pediatrics.* 2019;144(2):e20191881; doi:https://doi.org/10.1542/peds.2019-1881

HEPATITIS B VIRUS INFECTION

Organizations

▶ USPSTF 2019, CDC 2020, AAP/ACOG 2017, AAFP 2010

Screening Recommendations

–Screen all patients with HBsAg at their first prenatal visit.

–Retest at admission for delivery if >1 sex partner in the previous 6 mo, recent/current IVDU, evaluation/treatment of STI.

---

[1]Use clindamycin if isolate is sensitive to both clindamycin and erythromycin. If not, use vancomycin.

Comments

1. Breast-feeding is not contraindicated in patients with chronic HBV infection if the infant has received hepatitis B immunoglobulin (HBIG)-passive prophylaxis and vaccine-active prophylaxis.
2. All pregnant patients who are HBsAg-positive should be reported to the local Public Health Department to ensure proper follow-up.
3. Immunoassays for HBsAg have sensitivity and specificity >98%. (*MMWR*. 1993;42:707)

Sources

–*Ann Intern Med*. 2009;150(12):874-876.
–ACOG/CDC. *Screening and Referral Algorithm for Hepatitis B Virus (HBV) Infection Among Pregnant Patients*. 2020.
–AAP & ACOG. *Guidelines for Perinatal Care*. 8th ed. 2017.
–*Am Fam Physician*. 2010;81(4):502-504.
–CDC. *Sexually Transmitted Diseases Treatment Guidelines*. 2015.

HEPATITIS C VIRUS (HCV) INFECTION, CHRONIC

Organizations

▶ ACOG 2021, CDC 2020

Screening Recommendation

–Screen all pregnant patients during each pregnancy for hepatitis C regardless of risk factors.[1]

Comments

1. Route of delivery has not been shown to influence rate of vertical transmission of HCV infection. Reserve cesarean sections for obstetric indications only.
2. Breast-feeding is not contraindicated in patients with chronic HCV infection.
3. HCV RNA testing should be performed for:
   a. Positive HCV antibody test result in a patient.
   b. When antiviral treatment is being considered.
   c. Unexplained liver disease in an immunocompromised patient with a negative HCV antibody test result.
   d. Suspicion of acute HCV infection.
4. Seroconversion may take up to 3 mo.
5. Of persons with acute hepatitis C, 15%–25% resolve their infection; of the remaining, 10%–20% develop cirrhosis within 20–30 y after infection, and 1%–5% develop hepatocellular carcinoma.

---

[1]HCV risk factors: HIV infection; sexual partners of HCV-infected persons; persons seeking evaluation or care for STDs, including HIV; history of injection-drug use; persons who have ever been on hemodialysis; intranasal drug use; history of blood or blood component transfusion or organ transplant prior to 1992; hemophilia; multiple tattoos; children born to HCV-infected mothers; and health care providers who have sustained a needlestick injury.

6. Patients testing positive for HCV antibody should receive a nucleic acid test to confirm active infection. A quantitative HCV RNA test and genotype test can provide useful prognostic information prior to initiating antiviral therapy. (*JAMA.* 2007;297:724)

Sources
  −American College of Obstetricians and Gynecologists (ACOG) Practice Advisory. *Screening for Hepatitis C Infection.* 2021.
  −CDC Screening Recommendations and Reports. *Hepatitis C Screening Among Adults.* 2020;69(2):1-17.

HERPES SIMPLEX VIRUS (HSV), GENITAL

Organizations
▶ CDC 2015, USPSTF 2016

Screening Recommendation
  −Do not screen routinely for HSV with serologies.

Comments
1. In patients with a history of genital herpes, routine serial cultures for HSV are not indicated in the absence of active lesions.
2. Patients who develop primary HSV infection during pregnancy have the highest risk for transmitting HSV infection to their infants.

Sources
  −*JAMA.* 2016;316(23):2525-2530.
  −CDC. *Sexually Transmitted Diseases Treatment Guidelines.* 2015.

HUMAN IMMUNODEFICIENCY VIRUS (HIV)

Organizations
▶ AAFP 2019, USPSTF 2019, ACOG 2018, CDC 2015

Screening Recommendations
  −Screen all pregnant patients for HIV as early as possible during each pregnancy, using an opt-out approach.
  −Repeat HIV testing in third trimester for patients in areas with high HIV incidence or prevalence.
  −Offer rapid HIV screening to patients in labor who were not tested earlier in pregnancy or whose HIV is undocumented. If rapid HIV test is reactive, initiate antiretroviral prophylaxis immediately while waiting for supplemental test results.

Comment

1. Rapid HIV antibody testing during labor identified 34 HIV-positive patients among 4849 patients with no prior HIV testing documented (prevalence: 7 in 1000). Eighty-four percent of patients consented to testing. Sensitivity was 100%, specificity was 99.9%, positive predictive value was 90%. (*JAMA.* 2004;292:219)

Sources

–AAFP. *Screening for HIV Infection; Screening Recommendation Statement.* 2019.
–USPSTF. *Screening for HIV infection.* 2019.
–CDC. *Sexually Transmitted Diseases Treatment Guidelines.* 2015.
–ACOG. Committee Opinion: Committee on Obstetric Practice and HIV Expert Work Group. *Obstet Gynecol.* 2018.

INTIMATE PARTNER VIOLENCE

Organizations

▶ USPSTF 2018, ACOG 2012

Screening Recommendation

–Screen all pregnant patients for intimate partner violence.

Comments

1. Screening for intimate partner violence has the most robust evidence during pregnancy and the postpartum period.
2. Pregnant patients may be at increased risk of intimate partner violence compared to their nonpregnant peers.
3. Validated interventions include home-visit interventions for psychosocial supports and brief counseling and referral to violence prevention organizations.

Sources

–*JAMA.* 2018;320(16):1678-1687.
–*Obstet Gynecol.* 2012;119(2):412-417.

LEAD POISONING

Organizations

▶ USPSTF 2019, CDC 2000, AAP 2000, ACOG 2012

Screening Recommendations

–Do not screen universally.
–Insufficient evidence to recommend for or against routine screening for patients at increased risk.[1]

---

[1]Important risk factors for lead exposure in pregnant patients include recent immigration, pica practices, occupational exposure, nutritional status, culturally specific practices such as the use of traditional remedies or imported cosmetics, and the use of traditional lead-glazed pottery for cooking and storing food.

–For pregnant patients with blood levels of 5 µg/dL or higher, sources of lead exposure should be identified and patients should receive counseling.

   • Maternal or umbilical cord blood lead levels should be measured at delivery.

Comment

1. Symptoms of lead poisoning are generally nonspecific: constipation, abdominal pain, anemia, headache, fatigue, myalgias and arthralgias, anorexia, sleep disturbance, difficulty concentrating, and hypertension, among others. Test blood lead levels if these symptoms are present in the setting of increased risk.

Sources

–USPSTF. *Screening for Elevated Blood Lead Levels in Children and Pregnant Patients.* 2019.

–Ettinger, A, Wengrovitz, A, eds. *Guidelines for the Identification and Management of Lead Exposure in Pregnant and Lactating Women.* US Dept of Health and Human Services. 2010.

–*Obstet Gynecol.* 2012;120:416-420.

NEURAL TUBE DEFECTS

Organizations

▶ USPSTF 2016, AAFP 2016, ACOG 2017

Prevention Recommendation

–People should take a daily supplement containing 400–800 µg of folic acid if planning or capable of pregnancy.

Sources

–*Obstet Gynecol.* 2017;130:e279-e290 (lww.com).

–https://journals.lww.com/greenjournal/Fulltext/2017/12000/Practice_simplein_No__187__ Neural_Tube_Defects.41.aspx

–*JAMA.* 2017;317(2):183-189. https://www.uspreventive servicestaskforce.org/Page/Document/ Prevention RecommendationStatement Final/folic-acid-for-the-prevention-of-neural-tube-defects-preventive-medication

–AAFP. *Clinical Prevention Recommendation.* https://www.aafp.org/patient-care/clinical-Prevention Recommendations/all/neural-tube-defects.html

POSTPARTUM DEPRESSION

Organization

▶ USPSTF 2019

Prevention Recommendations

–Refer those at increased risk of perinatal depression to counseling interventions.

–No accurate screening tool to identify those at risk. Consider providing counseling to patients with 1 or more of the following risk factors: history of depression, current depressive symptoms, certain socioeconomic risk factors such as low income or adolescent or single parenthood, recent intimate partner violence, or mental health–related factors.

Source

–https://jamanetwork.com/journals/jama/fullarticle/2724195

POSTPARTUM HEMORRHAGE

Organization

▶ ACOG 2017

Prevention Recommendations

–Give uterotonic medications to all patients during the third stage of labor.
- Oxytocin 10 IU, IV, or IM is first choice.
- Methylergometrine or oral/rectal misoprostol is an alternative.

–Perform uterine massage.

–Use controlled cord traction to remove the placenta.

Comment

1. ACOG defines maternal hemorrhage as cumulative blood loss of $\geq$1000 mL or blood loss accompanied by signs or symptoms of hypovolemia within 24 h after birth.

Source

–*Obstet Gynecol.* 2017;183(130):e168-e186.

PREECLAMPSIA

Organization

▶ USPSTF 2017

Screening Recommendation

–Screen with blood pressure measurements throughout pregnancy.

Comments

1. Screening for protein with urine dipstick has low accuracy.
2. Diagnose preeclampsia if blood pressure is $\geq$140/90 $\times$2, 4 h apart, after 20 wk gestation AND there is proteinuria ($\geq$300 mg/dL in 24 h or protein:creatinine ratio $\geq$0.3, or protein dipstick $\geq$1+), thrombocytopenia, renal insufficiency, impaired liver function, pulmonary edema, or cerebral/visual symptoms.

Source

–*JAMA.* 2017;317(16):1661-1667.

Organizations

▶ USPSTF 2021, ACOG 2018

Prevention Recommendation

–Start aspirin 81 mg/d between 12 and 16 wk of gestation if ≥1 major risk factor for preeclampsia. Continue until delivery.

Comments

1. Major risk factors: personal history of preeclampsia, multifetal gestation, chronic hypertension, DM, renal disease, autoimmune disease.
2. In patients at high risk for preeclampsia, ACOG recommends initiating aspirin as late as 28 wk and continuing until delivery.

Sources

–*Ann Intern Med.* 2014;161:819-826.
–ACOG. *Committee Opinion on Low Dose Aspirin Use During Pregnancy.* 2018.

PRETERM BIRTH

Organization

▶ ACOG 2021

Prevention Recommendations

–Do not use maintenance tocolytics to prevent preterm birth.
–Do not give antibiotics for the purpose of prolonging gestation or improving neonatal outcome in preterm labor with intact membranes.
–In patients with prior spontaneous preterm delivery, start progesterone therapy between 16 and 24 wk gestation.
–Consider cerclage placement to improve preterm birth outcomes in patients with prior spontaneous preterm delivery <34 wk, current singleton pregnancy, short cervical length (<25 mm) before 24 wk gestation.
–Consider antenatal corticosteroids at 22 0/7 wk to 23 6/7 wk of gestation if neonatal resuscitation is planned and after appropriate counseling.
–Give antenatal corticosteroids between 24 0/7 wk and 25 6/7 wk.

Comments

1. No evidence to support the use of prolonged tocolytics for patients with preterm labor.
2. No evidence to support strict bed rest for the prevention of preterm birth.
3. The positive predictive value of a positive fetal fibronectin test or a short cervix for preterm birth is poor in isolation.
4. Do not give antenatal corticosteroids if less than 22 wk gestational age due to lack of evidence to suggest benefit.

Source

–*Obstet Gynecol.* 2012;120(4):964-973.

–*ACOG Practice Advisory.* Use of Antenatal Corticosteroids at 22 Weeks of Gestation. 2021.

RH D ALLOIMMUNIZATION

Organizations

▶ AAFP 2014, USPSTF 2007, ACOG 2017

Screening Recommendations

–Order ABO type and Rh D antibody testing for all pregnant patients at their first prenatal visit.

–Repeat Rh D antibody testing for all unsensitized Rh D-negative patients at 24–28 wk gestation.

Comment

1. Rh D antibody testing at 24–28 wk can be skipped if the biologic father is known to be Rh D-negative.

Sources

–AAFP. *Update on Prenatal Care.* 2014.

–*Obstet Gynecol.* 2017;13:e57-e70.

–http://www.uspreventiveservicestaskforce.org/3rduspstf/rh/rhrs.htm

Organization

▶ ACOG 2018

Prevention Recommendations

–For unsensitized Rh D-negative patients, give anti-D immune globulin at 28 wk gestation.

- Repeat after delivery, within 72 h, if infant is confirmed to be Rh D positive.
- Other situations to give anti-D immune globulin to an unsensitized Rh D-negative patient:
  ◦ External cephalic version.
  ◦ Uterine evacuation for molar pregnancy.
  ◦ First trimester miscarriage with instrumentation.[1]
  ◦ Ectopic pregnancy.
  ◦ Antenatal hemorrhage after 20 wk gestation.
  ◦ Abdominal trauma.
  ◦ Fetal death in second or third trimester
  ◦ First trimester miscarriage ("consider").

–Repeat antibody screen before giving anti-D immune globulin.

Source

–*Obstet Gynecol.* 2018;131:e8.

---

[1]ACOG suggests that clinicians "consider" giving immune globulin in any first trimester miscarriage in a patient who is unsensitized and Rh D-negative. While the risk of alloimmunization is quite low, the consequence is great.

SURGICAL SITE INFECTIONS (SSI)

Organizations
▶ Cochrane Database of Systematic Reviews 2014, ACOG 2018

Prevention Recommendations
–Treat remote infections prior to elective operations.

–Do not shave incision site unless hair interferes with operation. If necessary, remove hair immediately before operation with clippers.

–Control serum blood glucose levels and avoid perioperative hyperglycemia.

–Instruct patients to shower or bathe (full body) at least the night before abdominal surgery.

–Prepare the surgical site preoperatively with an alcohol-based agent unless contraindicated.

–Use a vaginal preparation with povidone-iodine solution immediately prior to uterine or vaginal surgery.

–Give prophylactic IV antibiotics preoperatively within 60 min of skin incision as opposed to administration after cord clamping.

Comments
1. A vaginal prep prior to cesarean section reduces the incidence of postpartum endometritis. This benefit was especially true for patients in active labor or with rupture membranes.

2. The incidence of maternal infectious morbidity is decreased (RR 0.54) when prophylactic antibiotics are administered preoperatively as opposed to after cord clamping.

Sources
–*Obstet Gynecol.* 2018;131:e172-e189.

–http://www.cochrane.org/CD007892/PREG_vaginal-cleansing-before-cesarean-delivery-to-reduce-post-cesarean-infections

SYPHILIS

Organizations
▶ CDC 2015, AAFP 2019, USPSTF 2018, WHO 2017, AAP/ACOG 2017

Screening Recommendations
–Screen all pregnant patients at the first prenatal visit.

–Screen again at 28 gestational wk if high risk[1] or previously untested.
  • Use a nontreponemal test (Venereal Disease Research Laboratory [VDRL] test or rapid plasma reagent [RPR] test) for initial screening.

[1]High-risk features include elevated community prevalence, concomitant HIV infection, and past incarceration or sex work.

Comments

1. Confirm all reactive nontreponemal tests with a fluorescent treponemal antibody absorption (FTA-ABS) test.
2. If high risk, consider testing a third time at the time of delivery.
3. Syphilis is a reportable disease in every state.

Sources

–CDC. *Sexually Transmitted Diseases Treatment Guidelines*. 2015.
–USPSTF. *JAMA*. 2018;320(9):911-917.
–WHO. *Syphilis Screening and Treatment for Pregnant Woman*. 2017.
–https://www.aafp.org/patient-care/clinical-Screening Recommendations/all/syphilis.html.
–American Academy of Pediatrics; American College of Obstetricians and Gynecologists. *Guidelines for Perinatal Care*. 8th ed. Elk Grove Village, IL: American Academy of Pediatrics; American College of Obstetricians and Gynecologists; 2017.

THROMBOEMBOLISM IN PREGNANCY

Organization

▶ ACOG 2018

Prevention Recommendations

–Consider thromboprophylaxis for patients at increased risk of thromboembolism.
–There is not sufficient evidence for routine prophylaxis in pregnancy.
–No risk assessment tool has been sufficiently validated, but risk factors include personal history of thrombosis, thrombophilia, cesarean delivery, obesity, hypertension, autoimmune disease, heart disease, sickle cell disease, multiple gestations, and preeclampsia.

THYROID DISEASE

Organizations

▶ ATA 2017, AAFP 2014

Screening Recommendations

–Insufficient evidence to recommend for or against routine screening of all patients.
–Obtain TSH levels at confirmation of pregnancy if:
  • A history or current symptoms of thyroid dysfunction.
  • Known thyroid antibody positivity or presence of a goiter.
  • History of head or neck radiation or prior thyroid surgery.
  • Age > 30 y.
  • Autoimmune disorders.
  • History of pregnancy loss, preterm delivery, or infertility.
  • Multiple prior pregnancies.

- Family history of thyroid disease.
- BMI $\geq$ 40 kg/m^2.
- Use of amiodarone or lithium, or recent administration of iodinated radiologic contrast.
- Residing in an area of known moderate-to-severe iodine insufficiency.

Sources
- *Thyroid.* 2017;27(3):315.
- *Am Fam Physician.* 2014;89(4):273-278.

TOBACCO USE

Organizations
▶ AAFP 2015, USPSTF 2015, ICSI 2014

Screening Recommendation
- Screen all pregnant patients for tobacco use and provide pregnancy-directed counseling and literature for those who smoke.

Comment
1. The "5-A" framework is helpful for smoking cessation counseling:
   a. Ask about tobacco use.
   b. Advise to quit through clear, individualized messages.
   c. Assess willingness to quit.
   d. Assist in quitting.
   e. Arrange follow-up and support sessions.

Sources
- AAFP. *Clinical Preventive Service Screening Recommendation: Tobacco Use.* 2015.
- USPSTF. *Tobacco Smoking Cessation in Adults, Including Pregnant Patients: Behavioral and Pharmacotherapy Interventions.* 2015.
- ICSI. *Preventive Services for Adults.* 20th ed. 2014.

WEIGHT GAIN IN PREGNANCY

Organization
▶ USPSTF 2021

Prevention Recommendation
- Provide behavioral counseling interventions aimed at promoting healthy weight gain and preventing excess gestational weight gain in pregnancy to all pregnant patients.

Comments

1. The Institute of Medicine recommends the following for weight gain in pregnancy; 1.1–4.4 lbs are expected in the first trimester, with the rest of the gain to follow.
   a. BMI < 18.5: 28–40 lbs.
   b. BMI 18.5–24.9: 25–35 lbs.
   c. BMI 25–29.9: 15–25 lbs.
   d. BMI ≥ 30: 11–20 lbs.

Sources

–*JAMA*. 2021;325(20):2087-2093. doi:10.1001/jama.2021.6949

–Institute of Medicine. *Weight Gain During Pregnancy: Reexamining the Guidelines*. Washington, DC. National Academies Press; 2009.

Women

15

BREAST CANCER

Organizations
▶ USPSTF 2016, ACS 2016, NCCN 2019, ACP 2019, ACOG 2017, WHO 2014

Screening Recommendations
–See below.

GUIDELINES DISCORDANT: SCREENING AGE AND INTERVAL FOR BREAST CANCER SCREENING					
	Consider Screening[a]	**Screen Regularly**	**Screening Frequency**	**Stop Screening**	**Include Breast Exam?**
USPSTF 2016	40–49 y	50–75 y	Every 2 y	Inconclusive data age > 75 y	Screen "with or without"
ACS 2016	40–44 y	≥45 y	Every year until 54 y, then every 1–2 y	Life expectancy <10 y	"Do not use"
NCCN 2019		40–80 y	Every year	>80 y	Yes
ACP 2019	40–49 y	50–74 y	Every 2 y	≥75 y or life expectancy <10 y	"Should not use"
ACOG 2017	40–49 y	50–75 y	Every 1–2 y	>75 y with shared decision-making	"May be offered"
WHO 2014	40–49 only in well-resourced settings	50–75 y	Every 2 y	75 y	Only in low-resource settings

[a]Each guideline within this category makes a statement for this age group supporting an assessment of risk, often relying heavily upon family history, and eliciting patient preference to guide a discussion of risks and benefits to determine whether to screen.

Comments

1. Harms and benefits of mammography screening:

   a. *Benefits:* Based on fair evidence, screening mammography in women age 40–70 y decreases breast cancer mortality. The benefit is higher in older women (reduction in risk of death in women age 40–49 y = 15%–20%, 25%–30% in women age ≥ 50 y) but still remains controversial. (*BMJ.* 2014;348:366) (*Ann Intern Med.* 2009;151:727)

   b. *Harms:* Based on solid evidence, screening mammography may lead to potential harm by overdiagnosis (indolent tumors that are not life threatening) and unnecessary biopsies for benign disease. It is estimated that 20%–25% of diagnosed breast cancers are indolent and unlikely to be clinically significant. (*CA Cancer J Clin.* 2012;62:5) (*Ann Intern Med.* 2012;156:491)

   c. Clinical breast exam does not improve breast cancer mortality (*Br J Cancer.* 2003;88:1047) and increases the rate of false-positive biopsies. (*J Natl Cancer Inst.* 2002;94:1445)

   d. Twenty-five percent of breast cancers diagnosed before age 40 y are attributable to *BRCA1* or *2* mutations.

   e. The sensitivity of annual screening of young (age 30–49 y) high-risk women with magnetic resonance imaging (MRI) and mammography is superior to either alone, but MRI is associated with a significant increase in false positives. (*Lancet.* 2005;365:1769) (*Lancet Oncol.* 2011;378:1804)

   f. Computer-aided detection in screening mammography appears to reduce overall accuracy (by increasing false-positive rate), although it is more sensitive in women age < 50 y with dense breasts. (*N Engl J Med.* 2007;356:1399)

   g. Digital mammography and film screen mammography have equal accuracy in women 50- to 79-y-old, but digital is more accurate in women 40- to 49-y-old. (*Ann Intern Med.* 2011;155:493)

   h. Estimated 252,710 new cases of invasive breast cancer (63,400 with DCIS) are expected in 2017, with 40,600 expected deaths. (NCI 2017)

   i. It is estimated that 1.6 million breast biopsies are performed each year in the United States with the overwhelming majority having benign disease. (*JAMA.* 2015;313:1122)

2. Continued controversy over screening:

   a. The Canadian National Breast Screening study that began in 1980 found no survival benefit for mammography in 40- to 59-y-old women, but many experts in the United States consider the study to be flawed because of its design. (*BMJ.* 2014;348:g366) (*N Engl J Med.* 2014;370:1965)

   b. A meta-analysis (*JAMA.* 2014;311:1327) found an overall reduction of 19% in breast cancer mortality (15% for women in their forties and 32% for women in their sixties). They were concerned about overdiagnosis and other potential harms of screening including false-positive findings and unnecessary biopsies. (*N Engl J Med.* 2016;375:1438)

   c. Recent trials have led to an increase in further screening studies based on the predicted individual risk of breast cancer occurrence. These also include a history of lobular carcinoma in situ, atypical hyperplasia, or history of breast cancer (invasive and DCIS). (*Ann Intern Med.* 2016;165:700, 737)

Sources

–http://www.cancer.org

–*Ann Intern Med.* 2016;164:279.
–*Ann Intern Med.* 2019;170:547.
–*CA Cancer J Clin.* 2016;66:95.
–*JAMA.* 2015;314:1599.
–*Obstet Gynecol.* 2017;130:241.
–https://www.who.int/cancer/publications/mammography_screening/en/
–www.nccn.org (Guidelines Version 1.2019).

Organizations

▶ NCCN 2019, USPSTF 2019

Prevention Recommendations

–If a woman is at high risk secondary to a strong family history or very early onset of breast or ovarian cancer, offer genetic counseling.

–Lifestyle (NCCN):

- Limit alcohol consumption. Four drinks per day increases relative risk 1.32.
- Exercise: at least 150 min/wk of moderate intensity, or at least 75 min/wk of vigorous aerobic physical activity.
- Weight control. Relative risk 2.8 if weight >82 kg vs. <59 kg.
- Breast-feeding. Relative risk decreases 4% for every year of breast-feeding.
- Pregnancy. Pregnancy <20 y carries 50% risk reduction vs. first pregnancy after age 35. Each pregnancy reduces risk 7%.
- Combined estrogen/progesterone therapy (≥3–5 y duration of use raises incidence by 26%).

Sources

–www.nccn.org. NCCN Guidelines Version 1.2019. Breast Cancer Risk Reduction.
–*JAMA.* 2019;322:857.

BREAST CANCER, HIGH-RISK PATIENTS

Organizations

▶ ACS 2017, NCCN 2019

Screening Recommendations

–Annual mammogram and MRI.

GUIDELINES DISCORDANT: WHEN TO START SCREENING	
Organization	**Population**
ACS	Start at age 30 y
NCCN	Start 10 y prior to the youngest family member; not prior to 30 y for mammogram and 25 y for MRI

–Clinical encounter every 6–12 mo to begin when identified as being at increased risk; referral to genetic counseling if not already done.

Comments

1. ACS considers high risk to be one of the following: Lifetime risk of breast cancer 20%–25% or greater (according to risk assessment tools), known as *BRCA1* or 2 mutation, first-degree relative (parent, brother, sister, or child) with a *BRCA1* or *BRCA2* gene mutation and unknown personal BRCA status, history of radiation therapy to the chest between the ages of 10 and 30 y, Li–Fraumeni syndrome, Cowden syndrome, or Bannayan–Riley–Ruvalcaba syndrome, or first-degree relatives with one of these syndromes.
2. NCCN considers high risk to be a lifetime risk of breast cancer >20% based on personal and family history (utilize Gail model, BRCAPRO model, or Tyrer–Cuzick model) and genetic predisposition (*BRCA1* or 2), PALB 2, CHEK 2 (http://www.cancer.gov/bcrisktool/).
3. *BRCA2*-related breast cancer is more like sporadic BC with 75% of patients with hormonal receptor positivity and significant decrease in aggressive growth. Only 15% of *BRCA2* patients will develop ovarian cancer with the average time of onset being in the mid-fifties.
4. One in forty Ashkenazi Jewish men and women carry a deleterious *BRCA1* or 2 gene (BRCA1 185del AG, 5382inse mutations, and BRCA2 6174delT mutation).
5. Some experts believe all men and women of Ashkenazi descent should be tested for these three genes, even with no personal or family history of malignancy. (*N Engl J Med*. 2016;374:454)
6. Risk-reducing bilateral mastectomy in *BRCA1* and 2 mutation carriers results in a 90% risk reduction in incidence of breast cancer and a 90% rate of satisfaction among patients who underwent risk-reducing surgery at 10-y follow-up. (*N Engl J Med*. 2001;345:159) (*JAMA*. 2010;304:967)

Sources

–*CA Cancer J Clin*. 2015;65:30.
–*N Engl J Med*. 2015;372:2353.
–*J Clin Oncol*. 2016;34:1882.
–*JAMA*. 2012;307:1394.
–*J Clin Oncol*. 2016;34:1840.
–*JAMA*. 2019;322:652.

Organizations

▶ NCCN 2019, USPSTF 2019

Prevention Recommendations

–If a woman is at high risk secondary to a strong family history or very early onset of breast or ovarian cancer, offer genetic counseling.
–Risk-reducing agents for high-risk patients (NCCN):
  • Discuss relative and absolute risk reducing with tamoxifen, raloxifene, or aromatase inhibitors.
  • Treatment with tamoxifen for 5 y reduced breast CA risk by 40%–50%. (*Ann Intern Med*. 2013;159:698-718). Meta-analysis shows RR = 2.4 (95% confidence interval [CI], 1.5–4.0) for endometrial CA and 1.9 (95% CI, 1.4–2.6) for venous thromboembolic events.

- Raloxifene has similar effect and risk as tamoxifen, except no reduction in noninvasive tumor and no increased risk of endometrial CA or cataracts. (*Lancet.* 2013;381:1827)
- Aromatase inhibitor use as a prevention of breast cancer will reduce the risk of developing breast cancer by 3%–5% (*Lancet.* 2014;383:1041). Harmful effects include decreased bone mineral density and increased risk of fracture, hot flashes, increased falls, decreased cognitive function, fibromyalgia, and carpal tunnel syndrome but no life-threatening side effects.

–Contraindications to tamoxifen or raloxifene: history of deep vein thrombosis, pulmonary embolus, thrombotic stroke, transient ischemic attack, or known inherited clotting trait.

–Contraindications to tamoxifen, raloxifene, and aromatase inhibitors: current pregnancy or pregnancy potential without effective nonhormonal method of contraception. Common and serious adverse effects of tamoxifen, raloxifene, or aromatase inhibitors with emphasis on age-dependent risks.

–Risk-reducing surgery for high-risk patients (NCCN):
- Consider risk-reducing mastectomy only in women with a genetic mutation conferring a high risk for breast cancer, a compelling family history, or possibly with prior thoracic radiation therapy at <30 y of age.
- Reduces risk of breast cancer as much as 90%.
- Approximately 6% of high-risk women undergoing bilateral mastectomies were dissatisfied with their decision after 10 y. Regrets about mastectomy were less common among women who opted not to have breast reconstruction.
- If no compelling family history of breast cancer, the value of risk-reducing mastectomy in women with deleterious mutations in other genes associated with a 2-fold or greater risk for breast cancer (based on large epidemiologic studies) is unknown.
- Prophylactic salpingo-oophorectomy in BRCA-positive women decreases breast cancer incidence by up to 50%. Perform in BRCA 1 patients at 35 y of age and in BRCA 2 patients at >40 y.

–For women age ≥ 35 y at increased risk of breast cancer and low risk for medication effects, prescribe tamoxifen, raloxifene, or aromatase inhibitors. Of these, only tamoxifen is used in premenopausal women. (USPSTF)

–No single risk tool is endorsed, but NCI Breast Cancer Risk Assessment Tool (bcrisktool. cancer.gov) and Breast Cancer Surveillance Consortium Risk Calculator (tools.bcsc-ccc.org/ bc5yearrisk/calculator.htm) are noted to be modeled after US populations. (USPSTF)

–A 5-y risk of >3% may be considered "high risk." (USPSTF)

–Do not use these medications if risk is not increased. (USPSTF)

Sources

–www.nccn.org. NCCN Guidelines Version 1.2019. Breast Cancer Risk Reduction.

–*JAMA.* 2019;322:857.

BREAST CANCER—MUTATIONS IN *BRCA* GENES

Organizations

▶ USPSTF 2019, NCCN 2019

Screening Recommendations

–Use a risk assessment tool to establish risk for women with family or personal history of breast, ovarian, tubal, or peritoneal cancer or *BRCA1* or *2* gene mutation. (USPSTF)

–Suggested screening tools include:

- Ontario Family History Assessment Tool.
- Manchester Scoring System (https://jmg.bmj.com/content/42/7/e39).
- Referral Screening Tool (https://www.breastcancergenescreen.org/).
- Pedigree Assessment Tool.
- 7-Question Family History Screening Tool (https://pubmed.ncbi.nlm.nih.gov/19682358/).
- International Breast Cancer Intervention Study instrument (https://ibis.ikonopedia.com/).
- BRCAPRO.

–Refer for genetic counseling if risk is increased.

–Do not screen with a risk assessment tool in the absence of suggestive history.

–Screen patients without cancer who have a family history of a deleterious *BRCA1* and *2* gene mutation. (NCCN)

- Test only for the known mutation, not a full genetic evaluation.
- If strong family history (FH) but unable to test family member with cancer (not alive or unavailable to be tested) then do full genetic evaluation. A strong FH includes:
  ○ Two primary breast cancers in a single close relative (first-, second-, and third-degree relatives).
  ○ Two breast cancer primaries on same side of family with at least one diagnosis occurring in a patient <50 y.
  ○ Ovarian cancer or male breast cancer at any age.
- Start screening 10 y prior to diagnosis of youngest family member but not before age 30.

–Screen patients with breast, ovarian, pancreas, and prostate cancer who have one of the following conditions (NCCN):

- A known mutation in a cancer susceptibility gene within a family.
- Early age onset of breast cancer (<50 y).
- Triple negative (ER-PR-, Her2-) breast cancer diagnosed in <60-y-old.
- An individual of Ashkenazi Jewish descent with breast, ovarian, or pancreatic cancer at any age.
- All women with ovarian cancer (epithelial and nonmucinous) at any age should be tested for *BRCA1* and *2* mutations.

CERVICAL CANCER

Organizations
▶ ACOG 2021, ACS 2020, USPSTF 2018

Screening Recommendations

GUIDELINES DISCORDANT: SCREENING FOR CERVICAL CANCER, AGE < 25 AT AVERAGE RISK	
Organization	Guidance
ACS	Do not screen
USPSTF, ACOG	Screen with cytology alone every 3 y in women aged 21–29

GUIDELINES DISCORDANT: SCREENING FOR CERVICAL CANCER, AGE 25–65 AT AVERAGE RISK	
Organization	Guidance
ACS	Screen with primary HPV test alone every 5 y
	Alternately, consider screening with HPV and cytology "co-testing" every 5 y or cytology alone every 3 y
USPSTF, ACOG	Women aged 30–65 y: screen with cytology alone every 3 y, every 5 y with hrHPV testing alone, or every 5 y with co-testing

–Do not screen patients older than 65 y who have had adequate prior screening with negative results (2 consecutive, negative primary human papillomavirus [HPV] tests, or 2 negative co-tests, or 3 negative cytology tests within the past 10 y, with the most recent test occurring within the past 3–5 y).

–Do not screen those without a cervix and without a history of CIN2 or more severe diagnosis in the past 25 y.

Comments

1. The United States is in a transition period moving from cytology to HPV testing, but cytology will continue to play a role in the near future, either alone or as part of co-testing, as practice patterns and access to primary HPV testing continue to evolve. (*CA Cancer J Clin* 2020;70:321-346)

2. Cervical CA is causally related to infection with HPV (almost all cases are caused by persistent infection with either HPV-16 or HPV-18 genotypes).

3. Immunocompromised women (organ transplantation, chemotherapy, chronic steroid therapy, or human immunodeficiency virus [HIV]) should be tested twice during the first year after initiating screening and annually thereafter. (*CA Cancer J Clin.* 2011;61:8) (*Ann Intern Med.* 2011;155:698)

4. Women age < 30 y with a history of cervical CA or in utero exposure to diethylstilbestrol (DES) should indefinitely continue average-risk screening protocol.

5. HPV vaccination of young women is now widely recommended. The vaccine is effective at preventing invasive cervical cancer, especially when given before age 17. (*N Engl J Med.* 2020;383(14):1340-1348)

6. Long-term use of oral contraceptives may increase risk of cervical CA in women who test positive for cervical HPV DNA. (*Lancet.* 2002;359:1085)

7. Smoking increases risk of cervical CA 4-fold. (*Am J Epidemiol.* 1990;131:945)

8. *Benefits:* Based on solid evidence, regular screening of appropriate women with the Pap test reduces mortality from cervical CA. Screening is effective when started at age 21. *Harms:* Based on solid evidence, regular screening with the Pap test leads to additional diagnostic procedures and treatment for low-grade squamous intraepithelial lesions (LSILs), with uncertain long-term consequences on fertility and pregnancy. Harms are greatest for younger women, who have a higher prevalence of LSILs. LSILs often regress without treatment. False-positives in postmenopausal women are a result of mucosal atrophy. (NCI 2008)

9. In a study of 43,000 women ages 29–61 with both HPV DNA and cervical cytology, co-testing every 5 y found that the cumulative incidence of cervical cancer in women negative for both tests at baseline was 0.01% at 9 y and 0.07% after 14 y. (*BMJ.* 2016;355:4924)

10. The risk of developing invasive cervical CA is 3–10 times greater in women who have not been screened. (*CA Cancer J Clin.* 2017;67:106)

Sources

–http://www.cancer.org
–http://www.survivorshipguidelines.org
–*CA Cancer J Clin.* 2020:1-26.
–*N Engl J Med.* 2013;369:2324.
–https://www.uspreventiveservicestaskforce.org/Page/Document/RecommendationStatementFinal/cervical-cancer-screening2. 2018.
–https://www.acog.org/clinical/clinical-guidance/practice-advisory/articles/2021/04/updated-cervical-cancer-screening-guidelines

Organizations

▶ ACOG 2021, ACS 2020, USPSTF 2018

Prevention Recommendations

–Screen for and treat high-grade precancerous cervical lesions to prevent the progression to cervical cancer.
–Vaccinate girls and boys routinely with the HPV vaccine.

Comment

1. Minimize risk factor exposure:

   a. HPV infection[1]: Abstinence from sexual activity; condom and/or spermicide use (RR, 0.4), HPV vaccination per CDC schedule.

---

[1]Methods to minimize risk of HPV infection include abstinence from sexual activity and the use of barrier contraceptives and/or spermicidal gel during sexual intercourse.

b. **HPV-16/HPV-18 vaccination**[1]: Reduces incidence and persistent infections with efficacy of 91.6% (95% CI, 64.5–98.0) and 100% (95% CI, 45–100), respectively; duration of efficacy is not yet known; impact on long-term cervical CA rates also unknown but likely to be significant. Two doses of vaccine if 9- to 14-y-old, 3 doses if 15- to 26-y-old. Shared decision-making for those age 27–45 but strong focus on preteen vaccination due to minimal public health benefit at later ages. (*Lancet.* 2009;374:1975) (*N Engl J Med.* 2015;372:711, 775) (ACIP 2020). Also will likely decrease risk of other HPV-driven malignancies (oropharynx and anal CA).

c. Cigarette smoke (active or passive): Increased risk of high-grade cervical intraepithelial neoplasia (CIN) or invasive cancer 2- to 3-fold among HPV-infected women.

d. High parity: HPV-infected women with 7 or more full-term pregnancies have a 4-fold increased risk of squamous cell CA of the cervix compared with nulliparous women.

e. Long-term use of oral contraceptives (>5 y): Increases risk by 3-fold. Longer use related to even higher risk.

Sources

–https://www.uspreventiveservicestaskforce.org/Page/Document/RecommendationStatementFinal/cervical-cancer-screening2. 2018.

–http://www.cancer.org

–https://www.acog.org/clinical/clinical-guidance/practice-advisory/articles/2021/04/updated-cervical-cancer-screening-guidelines

ENDOMETRIAL CANCER

Organization

▶ ACS 2008

Screening Recommendations

–Do not screen postmenopausal women routinely.

–Inform women about risks and symptoms of endometrial CA and strongly encourage them to report any unexpected bleeding or spotting. This is especially important for women with an increased risk of endometrial CA (history of unopposed estrogen therapy, tamoxifen therapy, late menopause, nulliparity, infertility or failure to ovulate, obesity, diabetes, or hypertension).

Comments

1. *Benefits:* There is inadequate evidence that screening with endometrial sampling or transvaginal ultrasound (TVU) decreases mortality. *Harms:* Based on solid evidence, screening with TVU will result in unnecessary additional exams because of low specificity. Based on solid evidence, endometrial biopsy may result in discomfort, bleeding, infection, and, rarely, uterine perforation. (NCI 2008)

---

[1]On June 8, 2006, the US Food and Drug Administration (FDA) announced approval of Gardasil, the first vaccine developed to prevent cervical CA, precancerous genital lesions, and genital warts caused by HPV types 6, 11, 16, and 18. The vaccine is approved for use in females age 9–26 y (http://www.fda.gov). A bivalent vaccine, Cervarix, is also FDA approved with activity against HPV subtypes 16 and 18. (*N Engl J Med.* 2006;354:1109-1112)

2. Presence of atypical glandular cells on Pap test from postmenopausal (age > 40 y) women not taking exogenous hormones is abnormal and requires further evaluation (TVU and endometrial biopsy). Pap test is not sensitive for endometrial screening.

3. Endometrial thickness of <4 mm on TVU is associated with low risk of endometrial CA. (*Am J Obstet Gynecol.* 2001;184:70)

4. Most cases of endometrial CA are diagnosed as a result of symptoms reported by patients (uterine bleeding), and a high proportion of these cases are diagnosed at an early stage and have high rates of cure. Type II endometrial CA accounts for 15% of patients. Histology is serous or clear cell. Five-year survival is 55% vs. 85% for endometrial Type I cancer. (NCI 2008) (*Lancet.* 2016;387:1094)

5. Tamoxifen use for 5 y raises the risk of endometrial CA 2- to 3-fold, but CAs are low stage, low grade, with high cure rates. (*J Natl Cancer Inst.* 1998;90:1371)

6. In 2022, there will be an estimated 65,950 new cases of endometrial cancer diagnosed with 12,550 deaths. The mean age at diagnosis is 60 y.

Source

–http://www.cancer.org

Prevention Recommendation

–Evidence-based guidelines do not address prevention of endometrial cancer in average-risk women.

Comments

1. Unopposed estrogen: a significant risk factor for the development of uterine cancer. Unopposed estrogen use in postmenopausal women for 5 or more years more than doubled the risk of endometrial CA compared to women who did not use estrogen. Other significant events from unopposed estrogen use include stroke (39% relative increase) and pulmonary embolus (34% relative increase). (*Lancet.* 2005;365:1543) (*JAMA.* 2004;291:1701)

2. Combined estrogen and progesterone: use of oral contraceptives for 4 y reduces the risk of endometrial CA by 56%; 8 y, by 67%; and 12 y, by 72%, but will increase risk of breast cancer by 26%.

3. Obesity: risk increases 1.59-fold for each 5 kg/m^2 change in body mass, but there is insufficient evidence to conclude that weight loss decreases incidence of endometrial cancer.

4. Exercise: regular exercise (2 h/wk) with 38%–48% decrease in risk.

5. Tamoxifen: use for >2 y has a 2.3- to 7.5-fold increased risk of endometrial CA (usually stage I—95% cure rate with surgery).

6. Parity: nulliparous women have a 35% increased risk of endometrial CA. Breast-feeding also reduces risk.

7. Endometrial hyperplasia and atypia: 50% go on to develop uterine cancer. Most often occurs in women over 50-y-old. (*Gynecol.* 1995;5:233)

OVARIAN CANCER

Organizations
▶ USPSTF 2018, ACOG 2017, ACS 2017, ACR 2010, AAFP 2017

Screening Recommendations
−Do not screen asymptomatic women at average risk[1] routinely.

−Beware of symptoms of ovarian CA that can be present in early stage disease (abdominal, pelvic, and back pain; bloating and change in bowel habits; urinary symptoms). (*Ann Intern Med.* 2012;157:900-904) (*J Clin Oncol.* 2005;23:7919) (*Ann Intern Med.* 2012;156:182)

Comments
1. Transvaginal ultrasound and CA-125 are useful to evaluate signs and symptoms of ovarian cancer.

2. Risk factors: age > 60 y; low parity; personal history of endometrial, colon, or breast CA; family history of ovarian CA; and hereditary breast/ovarian CA syndrome. Use of oral contraceptives for 5 y decreases the risk of ovarian CA by 50%. (*JAMA.* 2004;291:2705)

3. *Benefits:* There is inadequate evidence to determine whether routine screening for ovarian CA with serum markers such as CA-125 levels, TVU, or pelvic examinations would result in a decrease in mortality from ovarian CA. *Harms:* Problems have been lack of specificity (positive predictive value) and need for invasive procedures to make a diagnosis. Based on solid evidence, routine screening for ovarian CA would result in many diagnostic laparoscopies and laparotomies for each ovarian CA found. (NCI 2008) (*JAMA.* 2011;305:2295)

4. In addition, cancers found by screening have not consistently been found to be lower stage. (*Lancet Oncol.* 2009;10:327)

5. A large United Kingdom trial assessing multimodal screening strategy (annual CA-125, risk of ovarian CA algorithm [ROLA], transvaginal ultrasound) vs. annual ultrasound vs. usual care: >200,000 women recruited (age 50–74) found no mortality reduction at average of 16 y F/U. (*Lancet.* 2021;397(10290):2182-2193)

6. If a woman is newly diagnosed with ovarian cancer, she should be tested for BRCA1 or 2 at any age—if positive, family members should be tested for that specific gene mutation and undergo genetic counseling.

Sources
−*JAMA.* 2018;319(6);588-594.

−*Obstet Gynecol.* 2017;130(3):e146-e149.

−*CA Cancer J Clin.* 2017;67(2):100-121.

−*Ultrasound Q.* 2010;26(4):219-223.

−https://www.aafp.org/patient-care/clinical-recommendations/all/ovarian-cancer.html

---

[1]Lifetime risk of ovarian CA in a woman with no affected relatives is 1 in 70. If 1 first-degree relative has ovarian CA, lifetime risk is 5%. If 2 or more first-degree relatives have ovarian CA, lifetime risk is 7%. Women with 2 or more family members affected by ovarian cancer have a 3% chance of having a hereditary ovarian CA syndrome. If BRCA1 mutation, lifetime risk of ovarian CA is 45%–50%; if BRCA2 mutation, lifetime risk is 15%–20%. Lynch syndrome = 8%–10% lifetime risk of ovarian CA.

Population

–Women whose family history is associated with an increased risk for deleterious mutations in *BRCA1* or *2* genes.[1]

Organizations

▶ USPSTF 2013, NCCN 20122, ACOG 2017

Screening Recommendations

–Do not routinely screen.
–Refer for genetic counseling and evaluation for *BRCA* testing.

Comments

1. Screening with CA-125, transvaginal ultrasound, and pelvic exam have not been shown to improve survival rate.

Sources

–NCCN guideline version 1.2022. https://www.nccn.org
–*Obstet Gynecol.* 2017;130:e110-126.
–http://www.ahrq.gov/clinic/uspstf/uspsbrgen.htm

Population

–High-risk patients with known or suspected *BRCA1* or *2* mutations.

Organizations

▶ ACOG 2009, NCCN 2022

Screening Recommendations

–Encourage patient to undergo risk-reducing salpingo-oophorectomy (RRSO) between age 35 and 40 and upon completion of childbearing.
–If pt opts against RRSO, consider screening with CA-125 and transvaginal ultrasound at age 30–35 y.

Sources

–NCCN guideline version 1.2022. https://www.nccn.org
–http://www.ahrq.gov/clinic/uspstf/uspsbrgen.htm

Prevention Recommendations

–Evidence-based guidelines do not address prevention of ovarian cancer in average-risk women.

Comments

Risk factors for ovarian cancer:

a. Postmenopausal use of unopposed estrogen replacement will lead to a 3.2-fold increased risk of ovarian cancer after >20 y of use.
b. Talc exposure and use of fertility drugs have inadequate data to show increased risk of ovarian cancer—remains controversial.

---

[1]USPSTF recommends against routine referral for genetic counseling or routine BRCA testing of women whose family history is not associated with increased risk for deleterious mutation in *BRCA1* or *2* genes.

c. Obesity and height: elevated BMI including during adolescence associated with increased mortality from ovarian cancer. (*J Natl Cancer Inst.* 2003;95:1244). Taller women with higher risk of ovarian cancer. RR of ovarian cancer per 5 cm increase in height is 1.07.

Approaches to reduce risk:

a. Oral contraceptives: 5%–10% reduction in ovarian cancer per year of use, up to 80% maximum risk reduction. Increased risk of deep venous thrombosis (DVT) with oral contraceptive pill (OCP). The risk amounts to about 3 events per 10,000 women per year; increased breast CA risk among long-term OCP users of about 1 extra case per 100,000 women per year.

b. Tubal ligation decreases the risk of ovarian cancer (30% reduction).

c. Breast-feeding associated with an 8% decrease in ovarian cancer with every 5 mo of breast-feeding.

PELVIC EXAMINATIONS

Organizations

▶ AAFP 2017, ACP 2014, USPSTF 2017, ACOG 2012

Screening Recommendations

GUIDELINES DISCORDANT: WHETHER TO PERFORM ROUTINE SCREENING PELVIC EXAMS IN ASYMPTOMATIC PATIENTS	
Organization	**Guidance**
AAFP, ACP	Do not perform routine screening pelvic examinations
USPSTF	Insufficient evidence to recommend for or against
ACOG	Screen all women age 21+ with annual pelvic exam

Comments

1. Pelvic examination remains a necessary component of evaluation for many complaints.
2. Tradition and patient or physician experience may support an annual exam. Outcome data does not, though the data also does not clearly refute the exam.
3. Potential harms associated with screening include overdiagnosis, fear/anxiety/embarrassment, discomfort, and additional diagnostic procedures.

Sources

–AAFP. *Clinical Recommendation: Screening Pelvic Exam.* 2017.
–*Ann Intern Med.* 2014;161(1):67-72.
–*JAMA.* 2017;317(9):947-953.
–*Obstet Gynecol.* 2012;120:421-424.

TRICHOMONAS

Organization

▶ CDC 2015

Screening Recommendation

–Consider screening women in high-prevalence settings (STD clinics, correctional facilities) and at increased risk (multiple sex partners, commercial sex, illicit drug use, history of STD).

Population

–Persons with HIV.

Organization

▶ CDC 2015

Screening Recommendation

–Screen sexually active women with HIV at first visit and at least annually thereafter. Refer to Table 15-1 for details.

Source

–CDC. *Sexually Transmitted Diseases Treatment Guidelines.* 2015. https://www.cdc.gov/std/tg2015/trichomoniasis.htm

TABLE 15-1 CERVICAL CANCER SCREENING RECOMMENDATIONS		
	American Cancer Society (ACS) 2020, American College of Obstetricians and Gynecologists (ACOG) 2021	**US Preventive Services Task Force (USPSTF) 2018**
When to start screening[a]	Age 25. Do not screen <25 y regardless of the age of onset of sexual activity or other risk factors	Age 21. Do not screen patients <21 y[b]
Statement about annual screening	Women of any age should not be screened annually by any screening method	Individuals and clinicians can use the annual Pap test screening visit as an opportunity to discuss other health problems and preventive measures. Individuals, clinicians, and health systems should seek effective ways to facilitate the receipt of recommended preventive services at intervals that are beneficial to the patient. Efforts also should be made to ensure that individuals are able to seek care for additional health concerns as they present

TABLE 15-1 CERVICAL CANCER SCREENING RECOMMENDATIONS *(Continued)*		
	American Cancer Society (ACS) 2020, American College of Obstetricians and Gynecologists (ACOG) 2021	**US Preventive Services Task Force (USPSTF) 2018**
Cytology (conventional or liquid-based)[c]		
21–29 y of age	Not recommended <25 y	Every 3 y
30–65 y of age	Every 3 y[d]	Every 3 y *(A recommendation)*
HPV co-test (cytology + HPV test administered together)		
21–29 y of age	Start at age 25 y, primary HPV[e] test alone every 5 y (preferred) Co-testing every 5 y or cytology alone every 3 y are acceptable options	Recommend against HPV co-testing in women aged <30 y
30–65 y of age	Primary HPV test alone every 5 y (preferred) Co-testing every 5 y or cytology alone every 3 y are acceptable options	For women who want to extend their screening interval, HPV co-testing every 5 y is an option
Primary hrHPV testing[f] (as an alternative to co-testing or cytology alone)[g]	For women aged 25–65 primary HPV testing every 5 y is the preferred screening strategy[h, i]	Every 5 y for women 30–65 y of age
When to stop screening	Individuals with a cervix who are >65 y, no history of CIN2+ within the past 25 y, and who have documented negative prior screening	Aged >65 y with adequate screening history[j] and are not otherwise at high risk for cervical cancer[k]

(Continued)

TABLE 15-1　CERVICAL CANCER SCREENING RECOMMENDATIONS *(Continued)*

	American Cancer Society (ACS) 2020, American College of Obstetricians and Gynecologists (ACOG) 2021	**US Preventive Services Task Force (USPSTF) 2018**
When to screen after age 65 y	Aged >65 y without documentation of prior screening should continue screening until criteria for cessation are met as noted above	Women aged >65 y who have never been screened, do not meet the criteria for adequate prior screening, or for whom the adequacy of prior screening cannot be accurately accessed or documented[l] Routine screening[m] should continue for at least 20 y after spontaneous regression or appropriate management of a high-grade precancerous lesion, even if this extends screening past age 65 y. Certain considerations may support screening in women aged >65 y who are otherwise considered high risk (such as women with a high-grade precancerous lesion or cervical cancer, women with in utero exposure to diethylstilbestrol, or women who are immunocompromised)
Screening post-hysterectomy	Individuals without a cervix and without a history of CIN 2 or a more severe diagnosis in the past 25 y or cervical cancer ever should not be screened	Recommend against screening in women who have had a hysterectomy (with removal of the cervix)[n]
Screening among those immunized with HPV vaccine	Women at any age with a history of HPV vaccination should be screened according to the age-specific recommendations for the general population	The possibility that vaccination might reduce the need for screening with cytology alone or in combination with HPV testing is not established. Given these uncertainties, women should continue to be screened regardless of vaccination status

TABLE 15-1 CERVICAL CANCER SCREENING RECOMMENDATIONS

	American Cancer Society (ACS) 2020, American College of Obstetricians and Gynecologists (ACOG) 2021	US Preventive Services Task Force (USPSTF) 2018

HPV = human papillomavirus; CIN = cervical intraepithelial neoplasia; AIS = adenocarcinoma in situ; hrHPV = high-risk HPV.

[a]These recommendations do not address special, high-risk populations who may need more intensive or alternative screening. These special populations include women with a history of CIN2, CIN3, or cervical cancer, women who were exposed in utero to diethylstilbestrol, women who are infected with HIV, or women who are immunocompromised (such as those who have received solid organ transplants).

[b]Since cervical cancer is believed to be caused by sexually transmissible human papillomavirus infections, women who have not had sexual exposures (eg, virgins) are likely at low risk. Women aged >21 y who have not engaged in sexual intercourse may not need a Pap test depending on circumstances. The decision should be made at the discretion of the women and her physician. Women who have had sex with women are still at risk of cervical cancer. Ten to fifteen percent of women aged 21–24 y in the United States report no vaginal intercourse (Saraiya M, Martinez G, Glaser K, et al. *Obstet Gynecol*. 2009;114(6):1213-1219. doi: 10.1097/AOG.0b013e3181be3db4). Providers should also be aware of instances of nonconsensual sex among their patients.

[c]Conventional cytology and liquid-based cytology are equivalent regarding screening guidelines, and no distinction should be made by test when recommending next screening.

[d]There is insufficient evidence to support longer intervals in women aged 30–65 y, even with a screening history of negative cytology results.

[e]All ACOG references to HPV testing are for high-risk HPV testing only. Tests for low-risk HPV should not be performed.

[f]Primary hrHPV testing is defined as a stand-alone test for cervical cancer screening without concomitant cytology testing. It may be followed by other tests (like a Pap) for triage. This test specifically identifies HPV 16 and HPV 18, while concurrently detecting 12 other types of high-risk HPVs.

[g]Because of equivalent or superior effectiveness, primary hrHPV screening can be considered as an alternative to current US cytology-based cervical cancer screening methods. Cytology alone and co-testing remain the screening options specifically recommended in major guidelines.

[h]More experience and data analysis pertaining to the primary hrHPV screening will permit a more formal ACS evaluation.

[i]Primary hrHPV screening should begin 3 y after the last negative cytology and should not be performed only 1 or 2 y after a negative cytology result at 23–24 y of age.

[j]Adequate negative prior screening results are defined as 2 consecutive, negative primary HPV tests, or 2 negative co-tests, or 3 negative cytology tests within the past 10 y, with the most recent test occurring within the past 3–5 y, depending on the test used.

[k]Once screening is discontinued it should not resume for any reason, even if a woman reports having a new sexual partner.

[l]Women older than age 65 y who have never been screened, women with limited access to care, minority women, and women from countries where screening is not available may be less likely to meet the criteria for adequate prior screening.

[m]Routine screening is defined as screening every 5 y using co-testing (preferred) or every 3 y using cytology alone (acceptable).

[n]Unless the hysterectomy was done as a treatment for cervical precancer or cancer.

Men

16

PROSTATE CANCER

Organizations
▶ USPSTF 2018, AUA 2018, ACS 2016, EAU 2017, NCCN 2019

Screening Recommendations

GUIDELINES DISCORDANT: APPROACH TO SCREENING FOR PROSTATE CANCER					
Organization	**AUA**	**USPSTF**	**ACS**	**EAU**	**NCCN**
Screening age, general population	Age 55–69, only if patient opts in after discussion of potential benefits and harms of screening: small potential benefit of reducing chance of dying from prostate cancer vs. overdiagnosis, overtreatment, and treatment complications		Age 50+ if ≥10-y life expectancy; discuss risks and benefits	Data is lacking to determine appropriate screening age. Consider screening if pt prefers and has 10–15 y life expectancy	Age 45–75 after discussion of risks and benefits. Consider in age 75+ if healthy, especially if not screened prior
Screening age, high-risk populations	Consider at age 40–55 if first-degree family history, BRCA-1 and 2, or African American	Inadequate evidence to assess for mortality benefit from early screening in high-risk groups	Age 45 if first-degree relative dx before age 65 y or African American; age 40 if multiple first-degree relatives affected at early age	Age 45 if positive family history, if African American,	Age 40–75 y if African ancestry, germline mutations that increase prostate cancer risk, or suspicious family history
Preferred screening method, if elected	PSA alone		PSA and digital rectal exam (DRE)	Not defined	PSA; "strongly consider" DRE

GUIDELINES DISCORDANT: APPROACH TO SCREENING FOR PROSTATE CANCER *(Continued)*					
Organization	**AUA**	**USPSTF**	**ACS**	**EAU**	**NCCN**
Frequency of screening, if elected	insufficient evidence to recommend a screening interval	PSA ≥ 2.5 ng/mL: annual PSA < 2.5 ng/mL: q2 y	Optimal interval unknown. Propose risk-adapted strategy based on initial PSA: q2 years if PSA > 1 ng/mL at age 40 or > 2 ng/mL at age 60. Otherwise delay at least 8 years	PSA < 1 ng/mL: q2–4 y PSA 1–3 ng/mL: q1–2 y PSA > 3 ng/mL and or suspicious DRE: needs further evaluation	

Comments

1. Prevalence: there are 220,800 new cases of prostate cancer and 27,500 deaths expected in 2017. In the United States the lifetime risk of being diagnosed with prostate cancer is approximately 11%, and the lifetime risk of dying of prostate cancer is 2.5%.

2. 75% of men with PSA > 3 ng/mL will have no cancer on subsequent biopsy. More than 10% of men screened will have a false-positive PSA elevation if tested annually for 4 y and >5% will undergo a negative biopsy. (AUA 2018)

3. There is good evidence that PSA can detect early-stage prostate CA (2-fold increase in organ-confined disease at presentation with PSA screening), but mixed and inconclusive evidence that early detection improves health outcomes or mortality. Two long-awaited studies add to the confusion. A US study of 76,000 men showed increased prostate CA in screened group, but no reduction in risk of death from prostate CA. A European study of 80,000 men showed a decreased rate of death from prostate CA by 20% but significant overdiagnosis (there was no difference in overall death rate). To prevent 1 death from prostate CA, 1410 men needed to be screened, and 48 cases of prostate CA were found. Patients older than age 70 y had an increased death rate in the screened group. (*N Engl J Med.* 2009;360:1310, 1320) (*N Engl J Med.* 2012;366:981, 1047) These 2 very large studies set the framework for new PC guidelines. The US study (prostate, lung, colorectal, and ovarian cancer screening trial) showed no evidence for overall survival benefit from PSA screening and postulated that many patients with low-grade cancers were treated aggressively, leading to morbidity and mortality. Subsequent evaluation found that approximately 90% of patients in the control arm had undergone PSA testing during the course of the trial. This fact makes the trial result uninterpretable. The European study found that PSA screening did reduce prostate-specific mortality by 20%. In this trial 781 men needed to be invited to screening to prevent 1 death. What should be the response to this new data? First, we can improve survival by recognizing low-risk patients to be followed by active surveillance and not exposed to treatment until evidence of disease progression. Recognized high-risk patients (African-Americans and men with first-degree

relatives with prostate cancer) should be screened early and frequently. Average-risk men can be screened by PSA twice between the ages of 45 and 55 and if the PSA is 0.70 ng/mL, their risk of lethal prostate cancer is quite low. Guideline groups are presently working on new guidelines for PC screening to minimize overtreatment of this disease but at the same time screening a higher risk population for aggressive prostate cancer at a stage that can be treated with conservative intent. (*N Engl J Med.* 2017;376:1285) (*J Clin Oncol.* 2016;34:2705-2711, 3481-3491, 3499-3501)

4. *Benefit:* Insufficient evidence to establish whether a decrease in mortality from prostate CA occurs with screening by DRE or serum PSA. *Harm:* Based on solid evidence, screening with PSA and/or DRE detects some prostate CAs that would never have caused important clinical problems. Based on solid evidence, current prostate CA treatments result in permanent side effects in many men, including erectile dysfunction and urinary incontinence. (NCI 2008)

5. Men with localized, low-grade prostate CAs (Gleason score 2–4) have a minimal risk of dying from prostate CA during 20 y of follow-up (6 deaths per 1000 person-years) (*JAMA.* 2005;293:2095) (*N Engl J Med.* 2014;370:932)

6. Many physicians continue to screen African-American men and men with a strong FH of prostate cancer despite the guidelines. (*J Urol.* 2002;168:483) (*J Natl Cancer Inst.* 2000;92:2009) (*JAMA.* 2014; 311:1143) African-American men have double risk of prostate cancer and a >2-fold risk of prostate cancer–specific death. These patients and those with first-degree relatives < 65 y with prostate cancer are at high enough risk to justify PSA screening until a definitive study of this population is available. (*JAMA.* 2014;311:1143)

7. Increase in prostate cancer distant metastases at diagnosis in the United States over the last 3 y. (*JAMA Oncol.* 2016;2:1657)

8. Radical prostatectomy (vs. watchful waiting) reduces disease-specific and overall mortality in patients with early stage prostate CA. (*N Engl J Med.* 2011;364:1708) This benefit was seen only in men age > 65 y. Active surveillance for low-risk patients is safe and increasingly used as an alternative to radical prostatectomy. (*J Clin Oncol.* 2010;28:126) (*Ann Intern Med.* 2012;156:582) A gene signature profile reflecting virulence and treatment responsiveness in prostate CA is now available. (*J Clin Oncol.* 2008;26:3930) (*J Natl Compr NNetr.* 2016;14:659)

9. PSA velocity (>0.5–0.75 ng/y rise) is predictive for the presence of prostate CA, especially with a PSA of 4–10. (*Eur Urol.* 2009;56:573)

10. Multiparametric MRI scanning is emerging as a tool for more accurate detection of early prostate cancer as well as distinguishing indolent from high-grade cancers. (*J Urol.* 2011;185:815) (*Nat Rev Clin Oncol.* 2014;11:346)

11. PSA screening is confounded by the morbidity and mortality associated with the treatment of prostate cancer. Molecular profiling that can stratify patients into high-risk and low-risk groups is a critical need for individualized adaptive therapies, which could minimize toxicity and maximize benefit from there in many patients (oncotype, Decipher, and Polaris are now available to look at molecular profiling).

Sources

–USPSTF. 2018.

https://www.uspreventiveservicestaskforce.org/Page/Document/UpdateSummaryFinal/prostate-cancer-screening1

–*JAMA.* 2018;319(18):1901-1913.

–Eur. Urol. 2017;71:618-629.

–https://www.auanet.org/guidelines/prostate-cancer-early-detection-guideline

–NCCN Guidelines. Version 1.2022. NCCN.org.

–http://www.cancer.org

Prevention Recommendations

–No evidence-based guidelines exist to guide recommendations for the prevention of prostate cancer.

Comments

1. Diet: High dietary fat intake does not increase risk for prostate CA but is associated with more aggressive cancers and shorter survivals.
2. Medications:
   a. Finasteride: Decreased 7-y prostate CA incidence from 25% (placebo) to 18% (finasteride), but no change in mortality. Trial participants report reduced ejaculate volume (47%–60%); increased erectile dysfunction (62%–67%); increased loss of libido (60%–65%); increased gynecomastia (3%–4.5%).
   b. Dutasteride: Absolute risk reduction of 22.8%. No difference in prostate CA-specific or overall mortality. Concern raised by mild increase in more aggressive cancers in patients on dutasteride (Gleason score of 7–10). (*N Engl J Med.* 2010;302:1192; 2013;369:603)
3. Vitamins and minerals:
   a. Vitamin E/alfa-tocopherol—inadequate data—one study showed a 17% increase in prostate CA with vitamin E alone. (*JAMA.* 2011;306:1549)
   b. Selenium—no study shows benefit in reducing risk of prostate CA.
   c. Lycopene—largest trials to date show no benefit. (*Am J Epidemiol.* 2010;172:566)

TESTICULAR CANCER

Organizations

▶ AAFP 2008, USPSTF 2011

Screening Recommendation

–Do not screen routinely. Be aware of risk factors for testicular CA[1]: previous testis CA (2%–3% risk of second cancer), cryptorchid testis, family history of testis CA, HIV (increased risk of seminoma), and Klinefelter syndrome.

Comments

1. Benefits: Based on fair evidence, screening would not result in appreciable decrease in mortality, in part because therapy at each stage is so effective.

---

[1]Patients with history of cryptorchidism, orchiopexy, family history of testicular CA, or testicular atrophy should be informed of their increased risk for developing testicular CA and counseled about screening. Such patients may then elect to be screened or to perform testicular self-examination. Adolescent and young adult males should be advised to seek prompt medical attention if they notice a scrotal abnormality. (USPSTF, 2011)

2. Harms: Based on fair evidence, screening would result in unnecessary diagnostic procedures and occasional removal of a noncancerous testis. (NCI 2011)

3. In 2016 approximately 8850 men in the United States were diagnosed with testicular cancer but only 400 men died of this disease. Worldwide there are approximately 72,000 cases and 9000 deaths annually. (*CA Caner J Clin.* 2017;67:7)

4. There is a 3- to 5-fold increase in testis cancer in white men vs. other ethnicity. (*N Engl J Med.* 2007;356:1835; 2014;371:2005)

Sources

–http://www.aafp.org/online/en/home/clinical/exam.html

–http://www.ahrq.gov/clinic/uspstf/uspstest.htm

Older Adults

17

ATRIAL FIBRILLATION

Organization
▶ USPSTF 2018

Recommendation
–Insufficient evidence to assess benefits/harms of routine ECG screening for atrial fibrillation in asymptomatic adults over age 65.

Source
–*JAMA.* 2018;320(5):478-484.

CARE DEPENDENCY

Organization
▶ WHO 2019

Screening Recommendations
–Screen older adults for declines in intrinsic capacity: cognitive decline, mobility limitations, malnutrition, visual impairment, hearing loss, and depressive symptoms. (Refer to appendix "WHO: ICOPE Screening Tool" in Chapter 33.)
–Further evaluate and pursue care pathways for potential limitations.

Prevention Recommendations
–Cognitive decline:
  • Evaluate with tools such as Mini-Cog,[1] Montreal cognitive assessment,[2] mini-mental state examination,[3] or general practitioner assessment of cognition.[4]
  • Optimize malnutrition, delirium, polypharmacy, cerebrovascular disease, depressive symptoms.
  • Prevent further decline with multimodal exercise and cognitive stimulation.
  • Optimize smoking cessation, hypertension, and diabetes.

[1]http://mini-cog.com/wp-content/uploads/2015/12/Universal-Mini-Cog-Form-011916.pdf
[2]https://www.mocatest.org
[3]https://www.parinc.com/products/pkey/237
[4]http://gpcog.com.au/index/downloads

- Environment: assess need for social care, provide personal care and support with activities of daily living (ADL), give advice to maintain independent toileting, assess for caregiver burden, develop social care and support plan.
- Mobility:
  - If abnormal Chair Rise Test (cannot rise from chair 5 times in 14 s without using arms), perform Short Physical Performance Battery.[1]
  - If SPPB score is normal or mildly limited, consider a multimodal exercise program such as Vivifrail.[2]
  - Optimize polypharmacy, osteoarthritis, osteoporosis, frailty, and pain.
  - Environment: assess fall risk in physical environment, adapt home for fall prevention, consider assistive device, and identify safe space for walking.
- Nutrition:
  - Environment: overcome barriers to good nutrition, encourage family and social dining, arrange assistance with preparation of food.
- Vision:
  - Optimize hypertension, diabetes, and steroid use.
  - Environment: adapt home with lighting and contrasting colors to prevent falls, and remove hazards from walking path.
- Hearing:
  - If abnormal audiology, provide hearing age or refer to hearing specialist if severe or atypical (ear pain, drainage, dizziness, otitis media, unilateral).
  - Environment: emotional support, auditory aids for phone and doorbell.
- Depression:
  - If depressive symptoms, offer cognitive behavioral therapy, multimodal exercise, and mindfulness practice.
  - If significant depression, consider specialized care.
  - Optimize polypharmacy, anemia, malnutrition, thyroid disease, and pain.
  - Environment: strengthen social support, minimize stressors, promote daily activities, and work against loneliness.

Source
- WHO. *Integrated Care for Older People (ICOPE): Guidance for Person-Centred Assessment and Pathways in Primary Care.* Geneva: World Health Organization; 2019 (WHO/FWC/ALC/19.1).

---

[1]http://hdcs.fullerton.edu/csa/research/documents/sppbinstructions_scoresheet.pdf
[2]http://www.vivifrail.com/resources

DEMENTIA

Organizations
▶ USPSTF 2020, CTFPHC 2019, AAN 2021, ACR 2020

Screening Recommendations

GUIDELINES DISCORDANT: ROUTINE SCREENING FOR COGNITIVE IMPAIRMENT	
Organization	**Guidance**
USPSTF	Insufficient evidence to recommend for or against routine screening for cognitive impairment or dementia
CTFPHC	Do not screen asymptomatic adults for cognitive impairment
AAN/Alzheimer Association	Assess for cognitive impairment only when a patient or close contact voices concern about memory or impaired cognition. Use a validated assessment tool, and do not dismiss the concern as normal aging

Comments

1. False-positive rate for screening is high, and treatment interventions do not show consistent benefits.
2. Early recognition of cognitive impairment allows clinicians to anticipate problems that patients may have in understanding and adhering to recommended therapy and help patients and their caregivers anticipate and plan for future problems related to progressive cognitive decline.
3. Of pts with mild cognitive impairment (MCI), 6%–25% annually progress to dementia or Alzheimer disease.
4. Good evidence supports use of MME, Memory Impairment Screen, and neuropsychological batteries.
5. To meet Medicare Annual Wellness Visit requirement of screening for cognitive impairment, use a validated screening instrument rather than subjective report of memory concerns.
6. Monitor MCI over time and recommend exercise.

Sources
–*Neurology*. 2018;90:126-135.
–*CMAJ*. 2016;188(1):37-46. http://www.cmaj.ca/content/188/1/37
–*JAMA*. 2020;323(8):757-763.

Organization
▶ WHO 2019

Prevention Recommendations
–Recommend physical activity to adults with normal cognition and with MCI.
–Recommend the Mediterranean diet to adults with normal cognition or MCI.

–Pursue tobacco cessation.

–If harmful alcohol use, pursue reduction in use.

–Manage hypertension and diabetes according to existing guidelines.

–Do not recommend vitamin B, E, polyunsaturated fatty acids, or multicomplex supplementation to prevent cognitive decline.

–There is insufficient data to recommend for or against social activity, but it has other connections to good health so should be encouraged.

–There is insufficient data to recommend antidepressant medications to preserve cognition, though they may be otherwise indicated to treat depression.

–There is insufficient data to recommend hearing aids to preserve cognition, though they may be otherwise indicated.

Comments

1. The following recommendations have low- or very low-quality evidence, but may be considered:
   a. Cognitive training for older adults with normal cognition or MCI.
   b. Interventions for obesity midlife.
   c. Manage dyslipidemia.

Source

–WHO. *Risk Reduction of Cognitive Decline and Dementia: WHO Guidelines.* Geneva: World Health Organization; 2019.

DRIVING RISK

Organization

▶ AAN 2019

Prevention Recommendation

–Assess patients with dementia for the following characteristics that place them at increased risk for unsafe driving (Clinical Dementia Rating Scale):

- Caregiver's assessment that the patient's driving ability is marginal or unsafe.
- History of traffic citations and motor vehicle collisions.
- Self-reported situational avoidance.
- Reduced driving mileage (<60 miles/wk).
- Self-reported situational avoidance.
- Mini-Mental Status Exam score ≤24.
- Aggression or impulsivity.
- Alcohol, medications, sleep disorders, visual impairment, motor impairment.

Sources

–*Neurology.* 2010 ;74(16):1316; Reaffirmed 2022

–https://www.aan.com/Guidelines/home/GuidelineDetail/396

FALLS IN THE ELDERLY

Organizations

▶ NICE 2020, AAOS 2001, AGS 2010, British Geriatrics Society 2001, NFPCG/Public Health England 2017

Screening Recommendation

–In persons >65, ask yearly about falls.

Sources

–NICE. *Falls in Older People: Assessing Risk and Prevention.* June 2013, published 2020.

–2010 AGS/BGS Clinical Practice Guideline: Prevention of Falls in Older Persons. http://www.americangeriatrics.org/files/documents/health_care_pros/Falls.Summary.Guide.pdf

–*Public Health England/National Falls Prevention Coordination Group.* 2017. Falls and Fracture Consensus Statement, Supporting Commissioning for Prevention.

Organizations

▶ USPSTF 2018, Cochrane Database of Systematic Reviews 2012

Prevention Recommendations

–Do not give vitamin D supplementation to community-dwelling older adults without vitamin D deficiency or osteoporosis for fall prevention.

–Recommend vitamin D supplementation to elderly patients in care facilities. This reduces the rate of falls by 37%.

–Recommend home-hazard modification (eg, adding nonslip tape to rugs and steps, provision of grab bars, etc.) for all homes of persons age >65 y.

–Recommend exercise interventions to prevent falls including group and home-based programs as well as balance and strength training.

–Selectively offer a multifactorial assessment and management approach in community-dwelling older adults at increased risk for falls.

–Pursue cataract surgery if indicated, foot wear assessment with customized insoles and foot/ankle exercises in people with disabling foot pain, and pacemaker if carotid sinus hypersensitivity.

Comments

1. 30%–40% of all community-dwelling persons age >65 y fall at least once a year.
2. Falls are the leading cause of fatal and nonfatal injuries among persons age >65.
3. A review and modification of chronic medications, including psychotropic medications, is important although not proven to reduce falls. Please refer to appendix "Vulnerable Seniors: Preventing Adverse Drug Events" in Chapter 33 for Beers List of potentially problematic medications.
4. Public Health England (2017): Older adults should aim for at least 150 min of moderate activity or 75 min of vigorous activity per week. Strength/balance training is recommended at least 2 d/wk. Extended sedentary periods should be minimized.

5. Persons 65 and older that are admitted to hospital should be considered for a multifactorial assessment for fall risk during hospital stay.

6. Individuals are at increased risk if they report at least 2 falls in the previous year, or 1 fall with injury. Risk factors: Intrinsic: lower-extremity weakness, poor grip strength, balance disorders, functional and cognitive impairment, visual deficits. Extrinsic: polypharmacy (≥ 4 prescription medications), environment (poor lighting, loose carpets, lack of bathroom safety equipment).

7. A fall prevention clinic appears to reduce the number of falls among the elderly. (*Am J Phys Med Rehabil.* 2006;85:882)

8. Effective exercise interventions include supervised individual and group classes and physical therapy.

9. Multifactorial interventions include initial assessment of modifiable fall risk factors (balance, vision, postural blood pressure, gait, medication, environment, cognition, psychological health) and interventions (nurses, clinicians, physical/occupational therapy, dietitian/nutritionist, CBT, education, medication management, urinary incontinence management, environmental modification, social/community resources, referral to specialist "ophthalmologist, neurologist, etc.").

10. All who report a single fall should be observed as they stand up from a chair without using their arms, walk several paces, and return (see "Functional Assessment Screening in the Elderly," Chapter 33). Those demonstrating no difficulty or unsteadiness need no further assessment. Those who have difficulty or demonstrate unsteadiness, have ≥ 1 fall, or present for medical attention after a fall should have a fall evaluation.

11. Free "Tip Sheet" for patients from AGS: http://www.healthinaging.org/public_education/falls_tips.php.

12. Of US adults age ≥ 65 y, 15.9% fell in the preceding 3 mo; of these, 31.3% sustained an injury that resulted in a doctor visit or restricted activity for at least 1 d. (*MMWR Morb Mortal Wkly Rep.* 2008;57(9):225)

Sources
–USPSTF. *Falls Prevention in Older Adults: Counseling and Preventive Medication.* 2018.
–Cochrane Collaborative. *Interventions for Preventing Falls in Older People in Care Facilities and Hospitals.* 2012; 2018
–Public Health England. *Falls and Fracture Consensus Statement: Supporting Commissioning for Prevention.* 2012; 2017

FAMILY VIOLENCE AND ABUSE

Organization
▶ USPSTF 2018

Screening Recommendations
–Insufficient evidence to recommend for or against routine screening of all older or vulnerable adults for abuse and neglect.

–Screen for intimate partner violence in women of reproductive age and provide or refer women who screen positive to ongoing support services.

Comments

1. All clinicians should be aware of physical and behavioral signs and symptoms associated with abuse and neglect, including burns, bruises, and repeated suspect trauma.
2. CDC publishes a toolkit of assessment instruments: https://www.cdc.gov/violence prevention/pdf/ipv/ipvandsvscreening.pdf

Source

–Screening for intimate partner violence, elder abuse, and abuse of vulnerable adults. *JAMA*. 2018;320(16):1678-1787.

HEARING LOSS

Organizations

▶ USPSTF 2021, UK NSC 2021, ASHA 2006

Screening Recommendations

GUIDELINES DISCORDANT: SCREENING FOR HEARING LOSS IN ASYMPTOMATIC ADULTS AGE >50 Y	
Organization	**Recommendation**
USPSTF	Insufficient evidence to recommend for or against screening for hearing loss
UK NSC	Do not screen
ASHA	Screen once per decade and every 3 y after age 50

Comment

1. Increasing age is the most important risk factor for hearing loss.

Sources

–Screening for hearing loss in older adults. *JAMA*. 2021;325(12):1196-1201. doi:10.1001/jama.2021.2566
–https://view-health-screening-recommendations.service.gov.uk/hearing-loss-adult/
–*Audiol Today*. 2006;18(5):1-44.

HORMONE REPLACEMENT THERAPY TO PREVENT CHRONIC CONDITIONS

Organization
▶ USPSTF 2017

Prevention Recommendations
–Do not use combined estrogen and progestin to prevent chronic conditions, including osteoporosis, coronary artery disease, breast cancer, and cognitive impairment.
–If h/o hysterectomy, do not use estrogen to prevent chronic conditions, including osteoporosis, coronary artery disease, breast cancer, and cognitive impairment.

Source
–*JAMA.* 2017;318(22):2224-2233.

Comment
1. This recommendation does not apply to women under the age of 50 y who have undergone a surgical menopause and require estrogen for hot flashes and vasomotor symptoms.

Source
–*JAMA.* 2017;318(22):2224-2233.

OSTEOPOROSIS

Organizations
▶ USPSTF 2018, ACPM 2009, ACOG 2021, NAMS 2021, AACE 2020, NOF 2005, Endocrine Society 2012

Screening Recommendation
–Screen women age ≥65 y, or younger women at increased risk,[1] routinely using dual-energy X-ray absorptiometry (DXA) of the hip and lumbar spine. (Gold Standard Method)

GUIDELINES DISCORDANT: WHETHER TO SCREEN OLDER MEN FOR OSTEOPOROSIS	
Organization	**Guidance**
USPSTF	Insufficient evidence to recommend for or against routine osteoporosis screening
NOF, ACPM, Endocrine Society	Age ≥ 70 y: screen routinely using bone mineral density (BMD) Age 50–69: consider screening men with risk factors

[1]Several tools are available to assess osteoporosis risk: the Simple Calculated Osteoporosis Risk Estimation (SCORE), Osteoporosis Risk Assessment Instrument (ORAI), Osteoporosis Index of Risk (OSIRIS), and the Osteoporosis Self-Assessment Tool (OST).

Comments

1. USPSTF specifically defines "increased risk" as having a fracture risk equivalent to that of a 65-y-old white woman.
2. The optimal screening interval is unclear, but should not be more frequent than every 2 y.
3. ACOG: If FRAX score does not suggest treatment, DXA should be repeated every 15 y if T-score ≥1.5, every 5 y if T-score is −1.5 to −1.99, and annually if T-score is −2.0 to −2.49.
4. Ten-year risk for osteoporotic fractures can be calculated for individuals by using the FRAX tool (http://www.shef.ac.uk/FRAX/).
5. Quantitative ultrasonography of the calcaneus predicts fractures of the femoral neck, hip, and spine as effectively as does DXA. May be used in reduced resource settings.
6. The criteria for treatment of osteoporosis rely on DXA measurements.

Sources

–Screening for osteoporosis to prevent fractures. *JAMA*. 2018;318(24):2521-2531.
–*Osteoporosis*. Washington, DC: ACOG; 2012. (ACOG practice bulletin; no. 129).
–*Menopause*. 2021;28(9):973.
–*Endocr Pract*. 2020;26(Suppl 1).
–*Am J Prev Med*. 2009;36(4):366-375.
–Screening for osteoporosis to prevent fractures. *JAMA*. 2018;318(24):2521-2531.
–*Am J Prev Med*. 2009;36(4).
–*Osteoporos Int*. 2014;25(10):2359-2381.
–Osteoporosis in men: an Endocrine Society Clinical Practice Guideline. *J Clin Endocrinol Metab*. 2012;97(6):1802-1822.

OSTEOPOROTIC HIP FRACTURES

Organization

▶ USPSTF 2018

Prevention Recommendations

–Screen for osteoporosis in women age 65+ according to guidelines and intervene when indicated (see Chapter 27, section "Osteoporosis," for intervention guidelines).
–Do not supplement daily with ≤00 IU vitamin D and ≤1000 mg calcium for primary prevention of fractures, as there is insufficient evidence for benefit from higher doses.

Comments

1. Insufficient evidence for vitamin D and calcium supplementation for anyone for the primary prevention of fractures.
2. These recommendations do not apply to individuals with history of osteoporotic fractures, increased risk for fall, diagnosis of osteoporosis, or vitamin D deficiency.

Sources

–*JAMA*. 2018;319(24):2521-2531.
–uspreventitiveservicestaskforce.org
–*JAMA*. 2018;319(15):1592-1599.

Organization

▶ USPSTF 2017

Prevention Recommendations

–Do not routinely use combined estrogen and progestin for the prevention of chronic conditions including osteoporotic fractures.

–In postmenopausal women who have had a hysterectomy, do not use estrogen routinely to prevent chronic conditions including osteoporotic fractures.

Comment

1. The results of studies including the WHI and the Heart and Estrogen/Progestin Replacement Study reveal that hormone therapy (HT) probably reduces osteoporotic hip and vertebral fractures and may decrease the risk of colon CA; however, HT may lead to an increased risk of breast CA, stroke, cholecystitis, dementia, and venous thromboembolism. HT does not decrease the risk of coronary artery disease.

Source

–*JAMA*. 2017;318(22):2224-2233.

VISUAL IMPAIRMENT, GLAUCOMA, OR CATARACT

Organizations

▶ USPSTF 2016, ICSI 2014, AAO 2020

Screening Recommendation

GUIDELINES DISCORDANT: WHETHER TO SCREEN FOR VISUAL IMPAIRMENT	
Organization	**Guidance**
USPSTF	Insufficient evidence to recommend for or against visual acuity screening or glaucoma screening in older adults
ICSI	Age ≥65 y: test vision objectively (Snellen chart)
AAO	Age ≥ 65 y: examination by an ophthalmologist every 1–2 y

Comment

1. Adults with no signs or risk factors for eye disease should have a baseline comprehensive eye exam at age 40. Those with no signs or risk factors aged 40–54 should be examined by an ophthalmologist every 2–4 y, then every 1–3 y at age 55–64.

2. Increase frequency for adults at risk for glaucoma (African-American and Hispanic).

3. Smoking is a risk factor for many ocular diseases—recommend smoking cessation.

Sources

–Screening for impaired visual acuity in older adults. *JAMA*. 2016;315(9):908-914.

–ICSI. *Preventive Services for Adults*. 20th ed. 2014.

–AAO Policy Statement. *Frequency of Ocular Examinations*. 2020.

Management

Behavioral Health Disorders

18

ACUTE PSYCHIATRIC ILLNESS

Population
–Adult patients presenting to emergency department with psychiatric symptoms.

Organization
▶ ACEP 2017

Recommendations
–Do not obtain routine laboratory testing. Medical history, examination, and previous psychiatric diagnoses should guide testing.
–Do not routinely order neuroimaging studies in the absence of focal neurological deficits.
–Do not use risk assessment tools in isolation to identify low-risk adults who are safe for ED discharge if they present with suicidal ideations.

Source
–Nazarian DJ, Broder JS, Thiessen ME, Wilson MP, Zun LS, Brown MD; American College of Emergency Physicians. Clinical policy: critical issues in the diagnosis and management of the adult psychiatric patient in the emergency department. *Ann Emerg Med.* 2017;69(4):480-498.

ALCOHOL USE DISORDERS

Population
–Adults.

Organizations
▶ USPSTF 2018, APA 2018

Recommendations
–For patients identified with an alcohol use disorder, provide a brief intervention and schedule follow-up via SBIRT (Screening Brief Intervention, and Referral to Treatment) model.
–Refer all patients with life-threatening withdrawal such as seizure or delirium tremens to a hospital for admission.
–Refer more stable outpatients to a behavioral therapy such as the IOP (Intensive Outpatient Program), an RTC (residential treatment center), or a Sober Living facility.
–Recommend prophylactic thiamine for all harmful alcohol use or alcohol dependence.

–Refer suitable patients with decompensated cirrhosis for consideration of liver transplantation once they have been sober from alcohol for ≥3 mo.

–Recommend pancreatic enzyme supplementation for chronic alcoholic pancreatitis with steatorrhea and malnutrition.

Comments

1. Assess all patients for a coexisting psychiatric disorder (dual diagnosis).
2. Use disorder-focused psychosocial intervention for patients with alcohol dependence.
3. Consider adjunctive pharmacotherapy under close supervision for alcohol dependence:
   a. Naltrexone and Acamprosate have the best evidence (COMBINE Trial).
   b. Consider gabapentin or topiramate if patient has not responded to above.

Sources

–*JAMA.* 2018;320(18):1899-1909.
–*Am J Psychiatr.* 2018;175(1):86-90.

ALCOHOL WITHDRAWAL

Population

–Adults treated in an ambulatory setting.

Organization

▶ ASAM 2020

Recommendations

–Assess risk for complicated withdrawal. Consider use of Prediction of Alcohol Withdrawal Severity Scale (PAWWS) or Luebeck Alcohol-Withdrawal Risk Scale (LARS). If elevated risk, arrange for inpatient level of care or a specialized ambulatory facility with extended on-site monitoring.

–Assess for medical comorbidities, pregnancy, mental disorders (GAD7, PHQ9). Consider labs including CBC, CMP, hepatitis panel, HIV, and tuberculosis.

–Arrange for daily check in with nurse or medical assistant for up to 5 d following cessation.

–Monitor severity with a validated instrument, and transfer to a higher level of monitoring if multiple doses of medication do not resolve agitation/tremor, severe signs/sxs such as hallucinations, syncope or seizure, comorbid conditions worsen, patient is oversedated, returns to alcohol use, or unstable vital signs.

–Advise a daily multivitamin and noncaffeinated fluids. Consider oral thiamine 100 mg PO daily for 3–5 d.

–Treat mild withdrawal (CIWA score < 10) with either supportive care or medication. Treat moderate withdrawal (CIWA score 10–18) with medication. Higher CIWA scores should prompt transfer to higher level of care.

–Use benzodiazepines as first-line therapy.

–Carbamazepine and gabapentin are alternatives if benzodiazepines are contraindicated, or may be used as adjuncts along with valproic acid (caution in hepatic disease).

–Offer a symptom triggered approach using Clinical Institute Withdrawal Assessment of Alcohol Scale, Revised (CIWA-Ar) if patient or caregiver can reliably monitor symptoms and follow guidance. Otherwise offer a front-load dosing under supervision or employ a fixed-dose schedule.

- Sample symptom-triggered schedule with chlordiazepoxide:
  - If front-loading, give 50–100 mg PO q1–2h until CIWA-Ar < 10.
  - 25–100 mg PO q4–6h when CIWA-Ar ≥ 10.
  - Consider additional doses as needed.
- Sample fixed-dose schedule with chlordiazepoxide:
  - If front-loading, give 50–100 mg PO q1–2h for 3 doses then begin schedule.
  - Day 1: 25–100 mg PO q4–6h.
  - Day 2: 25–100 mg PO q6–8h.
  - Day 3: 25–100 mg PO q8–12h.
  - Day 4: 25–100 mg PO qHS.
  - Day 5: optional 25–100 mg PO qHS.

–Do not treat alcohol withdrawal with alcohol, baclofen, or magnesium.

Comment

1. Risk factors associated with complicated withdrawal include history of alcohol withdrawal delirium or alcohol withdrawal seizure; prior withdrawal episodes; comorbidities (especially TBI); age > 65y; long duration of heavy and regular alcohol consumption; marked autonomic hyperactivity on presentation; benzodiazepines or barbiturates dependence. There is no universal agreement on which factors associated with increased patient risk are most predictive.

Source

–ASAM Clinical Practice Guideline on Alcohol Withdrawal Management. *J Addict Med.* 2020 Sep/Oct;14(5):376-392.

ANXIETY

Population

–Adults.

Organization

▶ NICE 2020

Recommendations

–Recommend cognitive behavioral therapy for generalized anxiety disorder (GAD).

–Consider sertraline first if drug treatment is needed.

–If sertraline is ineffective, recommend a different selective serotonin reuptake inhibitor (SSRI) or selective noradrenergic reuptake inhibitor (SNRI).

–Avoid long-term benzodiazepine use or antipsychotic therapy for GAD.

Source

–NICE. *Generalised Anxiety Disorder and Panic Disorder in Adults: Management* (CG113). 2021.

ATTENTION-DEFICIT HYPERACTIVITY DISORDER (ADHD)

Population
–Children age 4–18 y.

Organizations
▶ AAP 2019, NICE 2019

Recommendations
–Consider children with ADHD as children with special health care needs.

–Stress the value of a balanced diet, good nutrition, and regular exercise for children, young people, and adults with ADHD.

–Do not use drug treatment for preschool children with ADHD. Use parent- or teacher-administered behavior therapy.

–Obtain a second opinion or refer to a tertiary service if ADHD symptoms are not controlled on one or more stimulants and one nonstimulant.

GUIDELINES DISCORDANT: ROLE OF DRUG THERAPY FOR ADHD IN CHILDREN	
AAP	– For children age 6–18 y, first-line treatment is with FDA-approved medications for ADHD ± behavior therapy – Methylphenidate is reserved for severe refractory cases
NICE	– Do not use drug treatment as the first-line treatment for school-age children and young people with ADHD – Consider it only in those with severe symptoms and impairment or for those with moderate levels of impairment who have refused nondrug interventions – Where drug treatment is considered appropriate, methylphenidate, atomoxetine, and dexamfetamine are recommended, within their licensed indications, as options for the management of ADHD in children and adolescents

Comments
1. Essential to assess any child with ADHD for concomitant emotional, behavioral, developmental, or physical conditions (eg, mood disorders, tic disorders, seizures, sleep disorders, learning disabilities, or disruptive behavioral disorders).

2. For children 6–18 y, evidence is best to support stimulant medications and less strong to support atomoxetine, ER guanfacine, and ER clonidine for ADHD.

Sources
–*AAP Clinical Practice Guideline for the Diagnosis, Evaluation, and Treatment of Attention-Deficit/Hyperactivity Disorder in Children and Adolescents.* October 2019.

–NICE. *Attention Deficit Hyperactivity Disorder: Diagnosis and Management* (NG87). 2019.

Population
–Adults.

Organization

▶ NICE 2018

Recommendations

–For adults with ADHD, drug treatment should be the first-line treatment.
  • Following a decision to start drug treatment in adults with ADHD, lisdexamfetamine or methylphenidate should normally be tried first.
  • Atomoxetine or dexamfetamine should be considered in adults unresponsive or intolerant to an adequate trial of methylphenidate.
–Obtain a second opinion or refer to a tertiary service if ADHD symptoms are not controlled on one or more stimulants and one nonstimulant.
–Do not offer any of the following medications for ADHD without advice from a tertiary ADHD service:
  • Guanfacine for adults.
  • Atypical antipsychotics in addition to stimulants for people with ADHD or coexisting pervasive aggression, rages, or irritability.

Source

–NICE. *Attention Deficit Hyperactivity Disorder: Diagnosis and Management* (NG87). 2019.

AUTISM SPECTRUM DISORDERS

Population

–Children and young adults.

Organization

▶ NICE 2017

Recommendations

–Consider autism for regression in language or social skills in children <3 y.
–Consider clinical signs of possible autism in the context of a child's overall development and account for cultural variations.
–Refer to a specialist for an autism evaluation if any of the following signs of possible autism:
  • Language delay.
  • Regression in speech.
  • Echolalia.
  • Unusual vocalizations or intonations.
  • Reduced social smiling.
  • Rejection of cuddles by family.
  • Reduced response to name being called.
  • Intolerance of others entering into their personal space.
  • Reduced social interest in people or social play.

- Reduced eye contact.
- Reduced imagination.
- Repetitive movements like body rocking.
- Desire for unchanged routines.
- Immature social and emotional development.

Source

−NICE. *Autism Spectrum Disorder in Under 19s: Recognition, Referral and Diagnosis* (CG128). 2017.

DEPRESSION

Population
−Children and adolescents.

Organizations
▶ USPSTF 2016, NICE 2019

Recommendations
−Use SSRIs, psychotherapy, or combined therapy to decrease symptoms of major depressive disorder in adolescents age 12–18 y. (USPSTF)
−Insufficient evidence to support screening and treatment of depression in children age 7–11 y. (USPSTF)
−Use behavioral support and treatment (NICE):
  - 5–11 y: Consider CBT.
  - 12–18 y: CBT.

Comment
1. Good evidence showed that SSRIs may increase absolute risk of suicidality in adolescents by 1%–2%. Therefore, SSRIs should be used only if close clinical monitoring is possible.
2. Fluoxetine is approved by the FDA for treatment of MDD in children aged 8 y or older, and escitalopram is approved for treatment of MDD in adolescents aged 12–17 y.

Sources

−USPSTF. *Depression in Children and Adolescents: Screening.* 2016.
−NICE. *Depression in Children and Young People: Identification and Management.* 2019.

EATING DISORDERS

Population
–Adults and children with eating disorders.

Organizations
▶ APA 2010, NICE 2017

Recommendations
–Establish a therapeutic alliance.
–Use a multidisciplinary approach with a psychiatrist, dietician, social worker, and physician.
–Consider the following components in the initial evaluation:
  • A thorough history and physical examination.
  • Assessment of the social history.
  • An evaluation of the height and weight history.
  • Any family history of eating disorders or mental health disorders.
–Assess attitude of eating, exercising, and appearance.
–Assess for suicidality.
–Assess for substance abuse.
–Recommend cognitive behavioral therapy (CBT).
–Provide acute medical care (including emergency admission) for people with an eating disorder who have severe electrolyte imbalance, severe malnutrition, severe dehydration or signs of incipient organ failure.
–Recommend nutritional rehab for seriously underweight patients.
–Recommend nasogastric tube feeding over parenteral nutrition for patients not meeting caloric requirements with oral feeds alone.
–Recommend psychosocial rehab for patients with both anorexia nervosa and bulimia nervosa.
–Consider Prozac, which is a preferred agent, to prevent relapse during maintenance phase of bulimia nervosa.
–Consider the following labs:
  • CBC.
  • Chemistry panel.
  • TSH.
–Consider the following additional testing:
  • Bone mineral densitometry if amenorrhea for more than 6 mo.
  • Dental evaluation for history of purging.

Sources
–APA. *Practice Guidelines for the Treatment of patients with Eating Disorders*, 3rd ed. 2010.
–NICE. *Eating Disorders: Recognition and Treatment* (NG69). 2017.

OPIOID USE DISORDER

Population
–Adults.

Organizations
▶ ASAM 2020, US Dept Health and Human Services 2004

Recommendations
–Obtain medical history to assess for concomitant medical conditions including infectious diseases (TB, HIV, hepatitis), acute trauma, and pregnancy. Assess mental health status, possible psychiatric disorders, past and current substance use, and social and environmental factors.

–Include CBC, liver function tests, hepatitis C, HIV, and urine drug testing in initial lab evaluation. Consider testing for STIs and TB. Offer hepatitis B vaccination if appropriate.

–Consider use of clinical scales that measure withdrawal symptoms, like the Clinical Opioid Withdrawal Scale (COWS).

–Choose medications to manage opioid withdrawal, including methadone, buprenorphine, and naltrexone, rather than abrupt cessation. Consider non-narcotic medications like clonidine, benzodiazepines, loperamide, acetaminophen or NSAIDs, and ondansetron to target specific opioid withdrawal symptoms.

–Provide psychosocial treatment for patients on opioid agonist treatment.

–Physicians prescribing outpatient medication-assisted opioid therapy with buprenorphine must complete training compliant with the Drug Use disorder Treatment Act of 2000.

–Consider patients to be candidates for buprenorphine therapy if they want treatment, have no contraindications, can be expected to be compliant, provide informed consent, and are willing to follow safety precautions.

–Consider alternatives to office-based buprenorphine if patients use high doses of benzodiazepines, alcohol, or other CNS depressants; have significant untreated psychiatric disease; have frequently relapsed despite maintenance therapy previously; have previously had poor response to buprenorphine; have significant medical illness.

–Use buprenorphine/naloxone combination for maintenance in most patients rather than buprenorphine monotherapy.

–For buprenorphine induction, consider office-based, home, or microdosing induction protocols.

–If transitioning from methadone to buprenorphine, taper methadone to 30–40 mg or less per day at least 1 wk prior to induction, and wait at least 24 h after last dose of methadone before beginning the induction process.

–Monitor for diversion by testing for buprenorphine and metabolites, counting pills, accessing the Prescription Drug Monitoring Program and arranging frequent visits (weekly at onset of therapy).

Sources
–The ASAM National Practice Guideline for the Treatment of Opioid Use Disorder. https://www. asam.org/Quality-Science/quality/2020-national-practice-guideline

–McNicholas L. *Clinical Guidelines for the Use of Buprenorphine in the Treatment of Opioid Addiction*. Rockville, MD: U.S. Department of Health and Human Services; 2004. https://www.samhsa.gov/medication-assisted-treatment/training-materials-resources/buprenorphine-waiver

PREGNANCY, SUBSTANCE ABUSE

Population
–Pregnant or postpartum patients using alcohol or illicit drugs.

Organizations
▶ WHO 2014, ASAM 2020, CMQCC 2020

Recommendations
–Ask all pregnant women about their use of alcohol and other illicit drugs at prenatal visits.
–Offer a brief intervention and individualized care to all pregnant women using alcohol or drugs.
–Refer pregnant women with alcohol or cocaine or methamphetamine abuse to a detoxification center.
  • Women with opioid use disorder should continue a structured opioid maintenance program with either methadone or buprenorphine.
  • Women with a benzodiazepine use disorder should gradually wean the dose.
–Encourage mothers with a substance abuse history to breast-feed unless the risks outweigh the benefits.
–Carefully monitor and treat infants of substance abusing mothers.

Sources
–The ASAM National Practice Guideline for the Treatment of Opioid Use Disorder. https://www.asam.org/Quality-Science/quality/2020-national-practice-guideline http://www.who.int/substance_abuse/activities/pregnancy_substance_use/en/
–California Maternal Quality Care Collaborative Opiate Use Disorder Toolkit. https://www.cmqcc.org/qi-initiatives/mother-baby-substance-exposure-initiative

POSTTRAUMATIC STRESS DISORDER (PTSD)

Population
–Adults.

Organizations
▶ VA 2017, NICE 2018

Recommendations
–For suspected PTSD, determine DSM criteria, acute risk of harm to self or others, functional status, medical history, treatment history, and relevant family history.

–Establish a risk management and safety plan as part of initial treatment planning if there is a risk of harm to self or others.

–Do not offer psychologically focused debriefing for the prevention or treatment of PTSD.

–Treat PTSD initially with individual, manualized trauma-focused psychotherapy.

–When trauma-focused psychotherapy is unavailable or not preferred, use pharmacotherapy or other psychotherapy. Recommended medications include sertraline, paroxetine, fluoxetine, or venlafaxine.

Sources

–https://www.healthquality.va.gov/guidelines/MH/ptsd/

–nice.org.uk/guidance/ng116

TOBACCO ABUSE, SMOKING CESSATION

Population

–Adults, including pregnant women who smoke tobacco.

Organizations

▶ USPSTF 2015, AAFP 2015, ACOG 2017

Recommendations

–Offer nicotine replacement therapy, bupropion, and/or varenicline:

- Bupropion SR 150 mg daily × 3 d then 150 mg bid. Initiate 1–2 wk prior to quit. Continue for 7–12 wk up to 6 mo.
- Varenicline 0.5 mg qd for 3 d, then 0.5 mg bid for 4 d, then 1.0 mg PO bid. Continue for 12 or 24 wk.

–Current evidence is insufficient to recommend electronic nicotine delivery systems for tobacco cessation in adults, including pregnant women.

–Current evidence is insufficient to assess the benefits and harms of pharmacotherapy interventions for tobacco cessation in pregnant women.

Sources

–USPSTF. *Tobacco Smoking Cessation in Adults, Including Pregnant Women: Behavioral and Pharmacotherapy Interventions.* 2015.

–*Am Fam Physician.* 2016;93(10).

–ACOG. https://www.acog.org/Clinical-Guidance-and-Publications/Committee-Opinions/Committee-on-Obstetric-Practice/Smoking-Cessation-During-Pregnancy

TOBACCO CESSATION TREATMENT ALGORITHM

Five As:
1. Ask about tobacco use
2. Advise to quit through clear, personalized messages
3. Assess willingness to quit
4. Assist in quitting,[a] including referral to Quit Lines (eg, 1-800-NO-BUTTS)
5. Arrange follow-up and support

[a] Physicians can assist patients to quit by devising a quit plan, providing problem-solving counseling, providing intratreatment social support, helping patients obtain social support from their environment/friends, and recommending pharmacotherapy for appropriate patients. Use caution in recommending pharmacotherapy in patients with medical contraindications, those smoking <10 cigarettes per day, pregnant/breast-feeding women, and adolescent smokers. As of March 2005, Medicare covers costs for smoking cessation counseling for those who (1) have a smoking-related illness; (2) have an illness complicated by smoking; or (3) take a medication that is made less effective by smoking (http://www.cms.hhs.gov).
Source: Fiore MC, Jaén CR, Baker TB, et al. *Treating Tobacco Use and Dependence: Quick Reference Guide for Clinicians*. Rockville, MD: U.S. Department of Health and Human Services. Public Health Service; 2008 (http://www.ahrq.gov/legacy/clinic/tobacco/tobaqrg.pdf).

MOTIVATING TOBACCO USERS TO QUIT

Five Rs:
1. Relevance: personal
2. Risks: acute, long term, environmental
3. Rewards: have patient identify (eg, save money, better food taste)
4. Road blocks: help problem-solve
5. Repetition: at every office visit

TRAUMA-INFORMED CARE

Population
–Women.

Organization
▶ ACOG 2021

Recommendations
–Recognize the prevalence and effect of trauma on patients and the health care team and incorporate trauma-informed approaches to delivery of care.
–Become familiar with the trauma-informed model of care and strive to universally implement a trauma-informed approach across all levels of practice with close attention to avoiding stigmatization and prioritizing resilience.
–Build a trauma-informed workforce by training clinicians and staff on how to be trauma-informed.
–Create a safe, physical, and emotional environment for patients and staff.
–Implement universal screening for current trauma and a history of trauma.

CORE CONCEPTS IN TRAUMA-INFORMED CARE

The Four "Rs" (SAMHSA):

Realize the widespread effect of trauma and understand potential paths for recovery

Recognize the signs and symptoms of trauma in clients, families, staff, and others involved with the system

Respond by fully integrating knowledge about trauma into policies, procedures, and practices

Seek to actively resist retraumatization

Four Cs—Skills in Trauma-Informed Care

Calm: Pay attention to how you are feeling while caring for the patient. Breathe and calm yourself to help model and promote calmness for the patient and care for yourself

Contain: Ask the level of detail of trauma history that will allow patient to maintain emotional and physical safety, respect the time frame of your interaction, and will allow you to offer patients further treatment

Care: Remember to emphasize, for patient and yourself, good self-care and compassion

Cope: Remember to emphasize, for patient and yourself, coping skills to build upon strength, resiliency, and hope

Source: Modified from Kimberg L, Wheeler M. Trauma and trauma-informed care. In: Gerber MR, ed. *Trauma-Informed Healthcare Approaches: A Guide for Primary Care.* Cham, Switzerland: Springer; 2019:25-56.

Source

–ACOG Committee Opinion No. 825. Caring for patients who have experienced trauma. *Obstet Gynecol.* 2021;137(4):e94-e99.

Cardiovascular Disorders

ABDOMINAL AORTIC ANEURYSM (AAA)

Population
–Adults with AAA found by screening, incidental finding on imaging, or diagnosed once symptomatic (abdominal pain and/or back pain, cardiovascular collapse, loss of consciousness, pulsatile abdominal mass).

Organizations
▶ NICE 2020, ESC 2014, ACC/AHA 2011

Recommendations

Surveillance
–Offer surveillance without intervention if AAA diameter < 5.5 cm and slow growth < 1 cm/y.
–If size 4.5–5.4 cm, repeat imaging in 3 mo.
–If 3.0–4.4 cm, repeat imaging in 1 mo.
–In patients with small AAA, monitor with imaging at the following frequencies:
  • Every 4 y for AAA 2.5–2.9 cm diameter.
  • Every 3 y for AAA 3.0–3.9 cm diameter.
  • Every 2 y for AAA 4.0–4.4 cm diameter.
  • Every year for AAA ≥ 4.5 cm diameter.

Pharmacologic Therapy
–Target modifiable risk factors that hasten AAA growth or rupture. No nonsurgical interventions primarily prevent AAA from growing with or without subsequent rupture.
–Smoking is a risk factor for rupture. Provide cessation counseling and medications to all patients with AAA, as cessation slows the growth. Duration of smoking is more significant than quantity smoked.
–HTN is a risk factor for AAA rupture. Use beta-blockers as first-line treatment if HTN is a comorbid condition.
–Otherwise, treat other modifiable risk factors for expansion (CAD, PAD, HLD) as usual with guideline-directed medical therapy.
–Nonmodifiable risk factors include size of aneurysm, age, female gender, cardiac/renal transplant.
–Consider statins and ACE-inhibitors to reduce complications.
–Consider beta-blockers to reduce the rate of growth. (ACC)

GUIDELINES DISCORDANT: BLOOD PRESSURE GOALS IN AAA	
Organization	**Guidance**
ACC/AHA	<130/80[a]
ESC	<140/90

[a] Per the 2017 ACC/AHA guideline for HTN management. *Hypertension*. 2018;71(6):e13-e115.

Surgical Therapy

–Indication for repair:
- Symptomatic.
- Asymptomatic > 4.0 cm in diameter growing >1 cm/y.
- Asymptomatic and ≥5.5 cm in diameter.

–Indication for referral urgency:
- If symptomatic but nonruptured, urgent referral to vascular specialist.
- If asymptomatic >5.5 cm, see vascular specialist in 2 wk.
- If asymptomatic 3.0–5.4 cm, see vascular specialist in 3 mo.

–Repair ruptured AAA emergently. Can give TXA to slow blood loss.

–Give beta-blockers perioperatively to reduce cardiac risk and mortality from AAA repair.

–In patients who are good surgical candidates, recommend open repair or endovascular aortic repair (EVAR). EVAR is preferential for women, men > 70-y-old, and patients with abdominal copathology (multiple abdominal adhesions due to prior open abdominal surgeries or large abdominal wall defects).

–Open surgery has a better benefit/harm ratio for men < 70-y-old. For open surgery, consider both epidural and general anesthesia.

–EVAR requires closer long-term surveillance than open repair. Monitor for vascular leak, stability of the excluded aneurysm sac, graft position, and need for further intervention.

–Monitor for compartment syndrome after repair of ruptured AAA.

Comments

1. Studies of beta-blockers and rate of expansion have produced contradictory data. 2013 ESC HTN guidelines suggest using them as first line for HTN and AAA, but data doesn't strongly support their use outside of HTN.

Risk Factors for Developing AAA

1. Age > 60 y. About 1 person in 1000 develops an AAA between the ages of 60 and 65.
2. Smoking. The risk is directly related to number of years smoking and decreases in the years following smoking cessation.
3. Men develop AAA 4–5 times more often than women.
4. Ethnicity. More common in the white population.
5. History of CHD, PAD, HTN, and hypercholesterolemia.
6. Family history of AAA. Accentuates the risks associated with age and gender. The risk of developing an aneurysm among brothers of a person with a known aneurysm who are >60 y of age is as high as 18%.

Risk Factors for AAA Expansion

1. Age > 70 y, cardiac or renal transplant, previous stroke, severe cardiac disease, tobacco use.

Risk Factors for AAA Rupture

1. Aneurysms expand at an average rate of 0.3–0.4 cm/y.
2. The annual risk of rupture based upon aneurysm size is estimated as follows:
   a. <4.0 cm diameter = <0.5%.
   b. Between 4.0 and 4.9 cm diameter = 0.5%–5%.
   c. Between 5.0 and 5.9 cm diameter = 3%–15%.
   d. Between 6.0 and 6.9 cm diameter = 10%–20%.
   e. Between 7.0 and 7.9 cm diameter = 20%–40%.
   f. ≥8.0 cm diameter = 30%–50%.
3. Aneurysms that expand rapidly (>0.5 cm over 6 mo) are at high risk of rupture.
4. Growth tends to be more rapid in smokers and less rapid in patients with peripheral artery disease or diabetes mellitus.
5. The risk of rupture of large aneurysms (≥5.0 cm) is significantly greater in women (18%) than in men (12%).
6. Other risk factors for rupture: cardiac or renal transplant, decreased forced expiratory volume in 1 s, higher mean BP, larger initial AAA diameter, current tobacco use.

Sources

–*NICE guidelines 156.* Abdominal aortic aneurysm: diagnosis and management. 19 March 2020.

–Hirsch AT, Haskal ZJ, Hertzer NR, et al. ACC/AHA guidelines for the management of patients with peripheral arterial disease (lower extremity, renal, mesenteric, and abdominal aortic). *J Vasc Inter Radiol.* 2006;17:1383-1398.

–Rooke TW, Hirsch AT, Misra S, et al. 2011 ACCF/AHA focused update of the guideline for the management of patients with peripheral artery disease (updating the 2005 guideline). *JACC.* 2011;58(19):2020-2045.

–Erbel R, Aboyans V, Boileau C, et al. 2014 ESC guidelines on the diagnosis and treatment of aortic diseases. Document covering acute and chronic aortic diseases of the thoracic and abdominal aorta of the adult. The Task Force for the diagnosis and treatment of aortic disease of the European Society of Cardiology (ESC). *Eur Heart J.* 2014;35:2873-2926. doi:10.1093/eurheartj/ehu281.

ANAPHYLAXIS

Population

–Children and adults.

Organizations

▶ NICE 2011, EACCI 2014

Recommendations

–Obtain blood samples for mast cell tryptase testing at onset and after 1–2 h.

–Administer epinephrine (1:1000) 0.01 mg/kg (maximum 0.5 mg) SC; repeat as necessary IM every 15 min.

–If circulatory instability, place patient supine with lower extremities raised and give intravenous saline 20 mL/kg bolus.

–Give inhaled beta-2 agonists and glucocorticoids for wheezing or signs of bronchoconstriction.

–Consider H1- and H2-blockers for cutaneous signs of anaphylaxis.

–Observe all people ≥16 y suspected of having an anaphylactic reaction for at least 6–12 h before discharge.

–Admit all children younger than age 16 y suspected of having an anaphylactic reaction for observation.

–Refer all patients treated for an anaphylactic reaction to an allergy specialist.

–Prescribe an epinephrine injector (eg, EpiPen).

Comment

1. Anaphylaxis is a severe, life-threatening, generalized hypersensitivity reaction. It is characterized by the rapid development of:
   a. Airway edema.
   b. Bronchospasm.
   c. Circulatory dysfunction.

Sources

–http://www.nice.org.uk/nicemedia/live/13626/57474/57474.pdf

–http://www.guideline.gov/content.aspx?id=48690

ATRIAL FIBRILLATION (AF), RATE AND RHYTHM CONTROL

Population

–All adults with AF.

Organizations

▶ NICE 2021, AHA/ACC/HRS 2019, ESC 2018, ACCP 2018

Recommendations

–If hemodynamically unstable with AF or atrial flutter for <48 h, use electric or pharmacologic cardioversion urgently. Anticoagulate (heparin or dabigatran/argatroban; consider DOAC if CHA_2DS_2-VASC = 0 (men) or 1 (women)) as soon as possible and continue for at least 4 wk.

–If hemodynamically stable, obtain rate control. Pursue rhythm control only if symptoms persist after rate control or rate control is unsuccessful.

Management of Rate

–Acutely slow the rate to <110 bpm with IV beta-blocker or calcium channel blocker (Table 19-1).

–For chronic rate control, use beta-blocker or nondihydropyridine calcium channel in both persistent and paroxysmal AF. If unsuccessful or contraindicated, consider amiodarone (ACC/AHA) or digoxin (ESC).

TABLE 19-1   RATE CONTROL THERAPY IN ATRIAL FIBRILLATION

Class	Beta-Blockers	Calcium Channel Blockers	Cardiac Glycosides	Antiarrhythmics
Acute rate control i.v. therapy	Metoprolol 2.5–10 mg i.v. bolus Esmolol 0.5 mg/kg i.v. bolus over 1 min, then 0.05–0.23 mg/kg/min. Repeat prn.	Diltiazem 15–25 mg i.v. bolus, then 0.75–1.5 mg over 24 h in divided doses Verapamil 2.5–20 mg i.v. bolus Repeat prn. Digoxin 0.4–0.6 mg i.v. bolus	Digoxin 0.5 mg i.v. bolus, then	Amiodarone 300 mg i.v. over 30–60 min, preferably via CVC. May follow with 900 mg i.v. over 2 h
Long-term rate control oral therapy	Metoprolol 100–200 mg total daily dose Carvedilol 3.125–50 mg bid Bisoprolol 1.25–20 mg daily	Diltiazem 180–360 mg total daily dose Verapamil 120–360 mg total daily dose	Digoxin 0.0625–0.25 mg daily dose Digoxin 0.05–0.3 mg daily dose	Amiodarone 200 mg daily
Side effects	Most common reported adverse symptoms are lethargy, headache, peripheral edema, upper respiratory tract symptoms, gastrointestinal upset, and dizziness. Adverse effects include bradycardia, atrioventricular block, and hypotension	Most common reported adverse symptoms are dizziness, mobilize, lethargy, headache, hot flushes, gastrointestinal upset, and edema. Adverse effects include bradycardia, atrioventricular block, and hypotension (prolonged hypotension possible with verapamil)	Most common reported adverse symptoms are gastrointestinal upset, dizziness, blurred vision, headache, and rash. In toxic states (serum level > 2 ng/mL), digoxin is proarrhythmic and can aggravate heart failure, particularly with coexistent hypokalemia	Hypotension, bradycardia, nausea, QT prolongation, pulmonary toxicity, skin discoloration, thyroid dysfunction, corneal deposits, and cutaneous reaction with extravasation
Comments	Bronchospasm is rare—in cases of asthma use beta-1 selective agents (avoid carvedilol). Contraindicated in acute cardiac failure and a history of severe bronchospasm	Use with caution in combination with beta-blockers. Reduce dose with hepatic impairment and start with smaller dose in renal impairment. Contraindicated in LV failure with pulmonary congestion or LVEF <40%	High plasma levels are associated with increased risk of death. Check renal function before starting; adapt dose in patients with CKD. Contraindicated in patients with accessory pathways, ventricular tachycardia, and hypertrophic cardiomyopathy with outflow tract obstruction	Suggested as adjunctive therapy in patients where heart rate control cannot be achieved using combination therapy

AF, atrial fibrillation; CKD, chronic kidney disease; i.v., intravenous; LV, left ventricular; LVEF, left ventricular ejection fractions.

Source: From Kirchhof P, Benussi S, Kotecha D, et al. 2020 ESC Guidelines for the diagnosis and management of atrial fibrillation developed in collaboration with the European Association for Cardio-Thoracic Surgery (EACTS) The Task Force for the diagnosis and management of atrial fibrillation of the European Society of Cardiology (ESC) Developed with the special contribution of the European Heart Rhythm Association (EHRA) of the ESC, *Eur Heart Journal* 2020, 42(5):373-498. doi: 10.1093/eurheartj/ehaa612. Reprinted by permission of Oxford University Press on behalf of the European Society of Cardiology.

–If asymptomatic and LVEF is preserved, titrate medication to a resting heart rate <110.

–If symptomatic at HR <110, titrate medication to a resting heart rate <80.

–If rate and/or rhythm control strategies fail, consider AV nodal ablation and pacemaker placement.

Management of Rhythm

–For chronic rhythm control, use dronedarone, flecainide, propafenone, or sotalol.

–Avoid amiodarone for long-term antiarrhythmic unless concomitant heart failure (HF), given considerable side effect profile.

–Avoid flecainide or propafenone if evidence of ischemic or structural heart disease.

–Consider catheter ablation of AF as initial rhythm-control strategy,[1] or after failure of an antiarrhythmic medication. Only offer ablation if patients can be anticoagulated for at least 8 wk after procedure.

–Consider AF catheter ablation in selected patients with symptomatic AF and HF with reduced left ventricular (LV) ejection fraction (HFrEF), as it may lower mortality rate and reduce hospitalization for HF.

–Consider antiarrhythmic drug treatment for 3 mo after left atrial ablation.

Comments

1. AF guidelines apply to patients with atrial flutter as well.
2. Risk factors for AF include age > 60, CKD, COPD, valvular heart disease, OSA, tobacco use, MI, HF, hyperthyroidism, obesity, HTN, and heavy alcohol use.
3. ACC/AHA definitions of AF:
   a. Paroxysmal: Terminates within 7 d of onset.
   b. Persistent: Sustained continuously >7 d.
   c. Long-standing persistent: Sustained continuously >12 mo.
   d. Permanent: Declared once patient and physician decide to stop trying to restore sinus rhythm.
   e. Nonvalvular: Mitral stenosis, prosthetic valve, or mitral valve repair absent.
4. Expected ventricular heart rate (HR) in untreated AF is between 110 and 210 beats/min.
   a. If HR < 110 beats/min, atrioventricular (AV) node disease present.
   b. If HR > 220 beats/min, preexcitation syndrome (WPW) present.
5. Holter monitor best measures the adequacy of the chronic HR control. In acute medical conditions when the patient has noncardiac illness (ie, pneumonia), the resting HR may be allowed to increase to simulate physiologic demands (mimic HR if sinus rhythm was present). (ESC recommends HR target <110 beats/min; CCS recommends <100 beats/min; ACCF/AHA/HRS recommends HR target <110 beats/min only if EF > 40%.)
6. Choosing Wisely: American Society of Echocardiography (2013) recommends against transesophageal echocardiography to detect cardiac sources of embolization if a source has been identified and patient management will not change. (http://www.choosingwisely.org/sourcessocieties/american-society-of-echocardiography/)

---

[1]ESC guidelines observe that if ablation is done in expert centers, ablation reduces recurrence rate much more than antiarrhythmics for paroxysmal AF. The long-term benefit is less certain for persistent AF.

7. Various studies (AFFIRM, RACE, PIAF, STAF, etc.) have failed to show quality of life difference for rhythm control vs. rate control. Rhythm control is more likely to be effective in symptomatic patients who are younger with minimal heart disease, few comorbid conditions, and recent onset of AF.

Sources
–*JACC.* 2014;64(21):2246-2280. http://www.onlinejacc.org/content/64/21/2246
–*Eur Heart J.* 2016;37:2893-2962.
–*Eur Heart J.* 2018;39(16):1330-1393. https://academic.oup.com/eurheartj/article/39/16/1330/4942493
–2019 AHA/ACC/HRS Focused Update of the 2014 AHA/ACC/HRS. *Guideline for the Management of Patients with Atrial Fibrillation.*

Population
–Adults with HF with reduced ejection fraction (HFrEF).

Organizations
▶ AHA/ACC/HRS 2014, ESC 2016, NICE 2021

Recommendations
–Acutely, avoid calcium channel blockers in patients with LV ejection fraction <40%. Use only beta-blockers and digoxin as rate controllers in HFrEF because of the negative inotropic potential of verapamil and diltiazem.
–Long term, choose amiodarone rather than other antiarrhythmics in patients with HF. Otherwise do not choose amiodarone for AF without HFrEF for long-term antiarrhythmic because of side-effect profile.
–Consider catheter ablation to restore LV function in AF patients with HFrEF, though further data are still needed.

Sources
–*JACC.* 2014;64(21):2246-2280. http://www.onlinejacc.org/content/64/21/2246
–*Eur Heart J.* 2016;37:2893-2962.
–*NICE guideline 196.* Atrial fibrillation: diagnosis and management. 2021.

Population
–Adults with AF and HF with preserved ejection fraction (HFpEF).

Organizations
▶ AHA/ACC/HRS 2014, ESC 2016

Recommendations
–It may be difficult to separate symptoms that are due to HF from those due to AF.
–Focus on the control of fluid balance and concomitant conditions such as hypertension and myocardial ischemia.

Sources
–*JACC.* 2014;64(21):2246-2280. http://www.onlinejacc.org/content/64/21/2246
–*Eur Heart J.* 2016;37:2893-2962.

Population

–Patients with AF and acute transient ischemic attack (TIA) or ischemic stroke.

Organization

▶ ESC 2016

Recommendations

–When to start oral anticoagulation:
  • TIA: 1 d after acute event.
  • Mild stroke (NIHSS <8): 3 d after acute event.
  • Moderate stroke (NIHSS 8–15): evaluate hemorrhagic transformation by CT or MRI at day 6, then start OAC 6 d after acute event.
  • Severe stroke (NIHSS >16): evaluate hemorrhagic transformation.

Source

–*Eur Heart J.* 2016;37:2893-2962.

ATRIAL FIBRILLATION (AF), STROKE PREVENTION

Population

–Adults with AF.

Organizations

▶ AAFP 2017, AHA/ACC 2019, ESC 2015

Prevention Recommendations

–Discuss risk of stroke and bleeding with patients considering anticoagulation. Estimate stroke risk with CHA_2DS_2-VASc score (see Table 19-2). Estimate bleeding risk with HAS-BLED or ORBIT (see Tables 19-3 and 19-4).

–Identify low-risk AF patients who do not require antithrombotic therapy (CHA_2DS_2VASc score, 0 for men, 1 for women).[1] Offer oral anticoagulant (OAC) to patients with at least 1 risk factor (except when the only risk is being a woman). Address patient's individual risk of bleeding (BP control, discontinuing unnecessary medications such as ASA or nonsteroidal anti-inflammatory drugs). (AHA/ACC)

–Prescribe chronic anticoagulation unless low stroke risk ($CHADS_2 < 2$) or specific contraindications, in which case antiplatelet therapy is indicated.

–Choose non-vitamin K antagonists (NOACs; apixaban, dabigatran, edoxaban, or rivaroxaban) over warfarin, except for patients with severe mitral stenosis, mechanical heart valves, or in the first 3 mo after bioprosthetic valve replacement. See Table 19-5 for more information about choice of NOAC.

–Do not give dual treatment with anticoagulant and antiplatelet therapy.

[1]Major risk factors: Previous stroke, TIA, systemic embolism, age ≥75. Other relevant risk factors: HF or LVEF ≤40%, HTN, DM, female sex, age 65–74, vascular disease. (*JAMA.* 2001;285:2864-2870)

TABLE 19-2 STROKE RISK STRATIFICATION WITH THE CHADS$_2$ AND CHA$_2$DS$_2$-VASc SCORES	
Adjusted Stroke Rate (% per year)	
CHADS$_2$ score acronym[a]	
0	1.9
1	2.8
2	4.0
3	5.9
4	8.5
5	12.5
6	18.2
CHA$_2$DS$_2$-VASc score acronym[b]	
0	0
1	1.3
2	2.2
3	3.2
4	4.0
5	6.7
6	9.8
7	9.6
8	6.7
9	15.20

[a]C, CHF; H, hypertension; A, age >75 y; D, diabetes mellitus; S, history of stroke or TIA.
[b]C, CHF; H, hypertension; A, age 65–74 y; D, diabetes mellitus; S, history of stroke or TIA; V, vascular disease; A, age 75 y or older; S, female sex.

–For patients with AF who have mechanical valves, use warfarin with an international normalized ratio (INR) target of 2–3 or 2.5–3.5, depending on the type and location of prosthesis. (AHA/ACC)

–For patients with nonvalvular AF with a history of stroke, TIA or CHA$_2$DS$_2$VASc ≥2, use oral anticoagulation: warfarin (INR: 2–3) or direct oral anticoagulants (DOACs) (novel oral anticoagulation agents)—see treatment. (AHA/ACC)

–In patients treated with warfarin, perform INR weekly until INR is stable and at least monthly when INR is in range and stable. (AHA/ACC)

–Following coronary revascularization (PCI or surgical) in patients with CHA$_2$DS$_2$VASc ≥2, use clopidogrel without aspirin alongside OAC. (AHA/ACC)

TABLE 19-3 HAS-BLED BLEEDING RISK SCORE FOR WARFARIN THERAPY

HAS-BLED scoring system

Hypertension: 1 point for SBP >160

Abnormal renal function: 1 point for each, up to 2 points max:
  – Presence of chronic dialysis or renal transplantation or serum creatinine ≥2.6 mg/dL and abnormal liver function
  – Chronic hepatic disease or biochemical evidence of significant hepatic derangement
  – Bilirubin >2× upper limit of normal, in association with glutamic-oxaloacetic transaminase [GOT]/glutamic-pyruvic transaminase [GPT] >3× upper limit normal

Stroke: 1 point if positive history

Bleeding: 1 point if history of bleeding or predisposition

Labile INR: 1 point if INRs volatile or elevated

Elderly: 1 point if age >65y

Drugs or alcohol: 1 point for concomitant antiplatelets/NSAIDS, and 1 point for alcohol abuse

Risk of spontaneous major bleeding within 1 y

HAS-BLED score	0	1	2	3	4	5	6+
Bleeds per 100 pt-years	1.13	1.02	1.88	3.74	8.7	12.5	Not quantified

Source: Adapted from Camm AJ, Kirchhof P, Lip GYH, et al. Guidelines for the management of atrial fibrillation: The Task Force for the Management of Atrial Fibrillation of the European Society of Cardiology (ESC). *Eur Heart J.* 2010;31(19): 2369-2429, doi:10.1093/eurheartj/ehq278.

Interrupting and Bridging Anticoagulation
  – Bridge therapy with unfractionated heparin or LWMH only for patients with AF and mechanical heart valve undergoing procedures that require interruption of warfarin. Otherwise, bridging is not required.
  – When switching from vitamin K antagonist (warfarin) to non-vitamin K antagonist, start the NOAC as soon as the INR is <2.0. If INR 2.0–2.5, start NOAC the following day. If INR ≥2.5, recheck INR in 1–3 d.
  – When switching from non-vitamin K antagonist to warfarin, administer both concomitantly until the INR is in the therapeutic range.

	CHADS$_2$	Points	CHA$_2$DS$_2$-VASc	Points
C	Congestive heart failure	1	Congestive heart failure (or left ventricular systolic dysfunction [LVEF] ≤40%)	1
H	Hypertension (blood pressure [BP] consistently >140/90 mmHg or treated hypertension [HTN] on medication)	1	Hypertension (BP consistently >140/90 mmHg or treated HTN on medication)	1
A	Age ≥75 y	1	Age ≥75 y	2
D	Diabetes mellitus	1	Diabetes mellitus	1
S2	Prior stroke or transient ischemic attack (TIA)	2	Prior stroke or TIA or thromboembolism	2
V			Vascular disease (eg, coronary artery disease, peripheral artery disease, myocardial infarction [MI], aortic plaque)	1
A			Age 65–74 y	1
Sc			Sex category (ie, female gender)	1
Max.		6		9

TABLE 19-4 THROMBOEMBOLIC RISK SCORES IN NONVALVULAR ATRIAL FIBRILLATION

Comments

1. Average stroke rate in patients with risk factors is approximately 5% per year.
2. Adjusted-dose warfarin and antiplatelet agents reduce absolute risk of stroke.
3. Women have a higher prevalence of stroke than men.
4. Women have unique risk factors for stroke, such as pregnancy, hormone therapy, and higher prevalence of hypertension in older ages.
5. In patients age 80+, a lower dose of edoxaban (15 mg daily) reduces stroke risk. (*N Engl J Med.* 2020;383(18):1735–1745)

Sources

−*Am Fam Physician.* 2017;96(5):332-333.

−*Circulation.* 2014;130(23):e199-e267.

−*JAMA.* 2015;313(19):1950-1962.

−2019 AHA/ACC/HRS Focused Update of the 2014 AHA/ACC/HRS. *Guideline for the Management of Patients with Atrial Fibrillation.*

TABLE 19-5 DOAC COMPARISON CHART

	Warfarin	Dabigatran	Rivaroxaban	Apixaban	Edoxaban
Molecular target	Vitamin-dependent clotting factor	Thrombin	Factor Xa	Factor Xa	Factor Xa
Dosing in AF	Once daily	Twice daily	Once daily	Twice daily	Once daily
Time to peak plasma concentration (min)	240	85–150	30–180	30–120	30–60
Time to peak effect (h)	96–120	2	2–3	1–2	1–2
Half-life (h)	40	14–17	5–9 (increased to 11–13 in elderly)	8–15	9–11
Renal clearance	<1%	80%	33%	25%	35%
Hepatic excretion		20%	66%	75% (hepatic-biliary-intestinal)	65%
Food and drug interactions	Foods rich in vitamin K, substrates of CYP2C9, CYP3A4, and CYP1A2	Strong P-gp inhibitors and inducers	Strong CYP3A4 inducers, strong inhibitors of both CYP3A4 and P-gp	Strong inhibitors and inducers of CYP3A4 and P-gp	Strong P-gp inhibitors
Creatinine clearance below which drug is contraindicated	n/a	<30 mL/min	<15 mL/min	<15 mL/min	<30 mL/min (Japan)

Sources: Reproduced with permission from Lau YC, Lip GY. Which drug should we use for stroke prevention in atrial fibrillation? *Curr Opin Cardiol.* 2014;29(4):293-300.

BRADYCARDIA

Population
–Adults.

Organization
▶ ACC/AHA/HRS 2018

Recommendations
–Consider evaluating for and treating sleep apnea if nocturnal bradycardia.
–Consider evaluating for structural heart disease including acute myocardial infarction.

–Evaluate for systemic conditions that may contribute such as medications (many antihypertensives, antiarrhythmics and psychoactive medications), rheumatologic conditions and inflammatory disorders, physical conditioning, carotid sinus hypersensitivity, syncope disorders, sleep, increased intracranial pressure, hypothyroidism, and sleep apnea.

–Give atropine for sinus node disease causing bradycardia with symptoms or hemodynamic instability.

–If bradycardia is caused by medication, use a reversal agent (10% calcium chloride or gluconate for calcium channel blocker overdose, glucagon or high-dose insulin for beta-blocker overdose, and digoxin antibody fragment for digoxin overdose).

–Use transcutaneous pacing for patients who remain hemodynamically unstable after medical therapy.

–Refer for pacemaker regardless of symptoms for second-degree Mobitz type II, high-grade AV block or third-degree AV block without reversible etiology.

–Refer for pacemaker if symptomatic from bradycardia with other etiologies that are not reversible.

–There is no minimum duration of pause that indicates the need for pacemaker, but rather the correlation between the pause and symptoms.

Comment

1. Sinus bradycardia occurs in 15%–20% of patients with acute MI, especially if it involves the RCA as it supplies the SA node. (*Circulation.* 1972;45:703)

Source

–*JACC.* 2018;74(4):e51-e156.

CAROTID ARTERY DISEASE

Organizations

▶ AHA/ASA 2014, 2021; SVS 2021

Recommendations

–Give daily aspirin and statin for atherosclerosis of the extracranial carotid and/or vertebral arteries.

–Use antihypertensives to maintain BP <140/90 for patients with hypertension and asymptomatic extracranial carotid and/or vertebral atherosclerosis.

–If ischemic stroke or TIA and moderate (50-69%) or severe (≥70%) stenosis, refer for revascularization procedure. (AHA/ASA)

- If severe stenosis, choose carotid artery stenting (CAS) or endarterectomy (CEA), provided perioperative morbidity/mortality risk <6%. If age 70+, consider CEA over CAS. If anatomy increases risk of CEA, choose CAS.
- If moderate stenosis, refer for CEA, provided perioperative morbidity/mortality risk <6%.

–For patients undergoing CAS, use dual antiplatelet therapy (aspirin 81–325 mg daily and clopidogrel 75 mg daily) preprocedure and for a minimum of 30 d after.

–For patients undergoing CEA, use aspirin alone preprocedure and continue indefinitely postoperatively.

GUIDELINES DISCORDANT: CAROTID ENDARTERECTOMY IN ASYMPTOMATIC PATIENTS WITH SEVERE (≥70%) STENOSIS	
AHA/ASA	Consider referring for carotid endarterectomy (CEA) if risk of perioperative stroke, MI, and death is <3%, though data is lacking to compare outcomes to medical management
SVS	Choose CEA plus medical management over medical therapy alone for low surgical risk patients

Comment

1. Don't recommend CEA for asymptomatic carotid artery stenosis unless the complication rate is <3% (https://www.choosingwisely.org/clinician-lists/american-academy-neurology-cea-for-asymptomatic-carotid-stenosis/).

Sources
–*Stroke.* 2014;45:3754-3832.
–*Stroke.* 2021;52:e364-e467.
–*J Vasc Surg.* 2022;75:4S-22S.

CORONARY ARTERY DISEASE (CAD)

Population
–Patients with known or suspected coronary disease experiencing angina.

Organizations
▶ ACCF/AHA/ACP/AATS/PCNA/SCAI/STS 2012, 2014

Recommendations
–Classify patients presenting with angina pectoris as stable or unstable.
–Obtain resting ECG with all symptoms of chest pain (typical or atypical in nature).
–Choose exercise treadmill test if the baseline ECG is normal, the patient can exercise, and the pretest likelihood of coronary disease is intermediate (10%–90%).
–If unable to perform an exercise treadmill and the pretest likelihood is >10%, choose either a nuclear myocardial perfusion imaging study (MPI) or exercise echocardiogram.
–Repeat exercise and imaging studies when there is a change in clinical status or if needed for exercise prescription.
–Consider coronary computed tomography angiogram (CTA) in patients with an intermediate pretest probability of CAD (FRS) in whom symptoms persist despite prior normal testing, with equivocal stress tests, or in patients who cannot be studied otherwise. Coronary CTA is not indicated if known moderate or severe coronary calcification or in the presence of prior stents.
–Obtain an echocardiogram to assess resting LV function and valve disease in patients with suspected CAD, pathological Q waves, presence of HF, or ventricular arrhythmias.
–Treat patients who have stable coronary disease with:
  • Lifestyle guidance (diet, weight loss, smoking cessation, and exercise education).
  • Blood pressure control per JNC guidelines.

- Associated risk factor assessment: Presence of chronic kidney disease and psychosocial factors such as depression, anxiety, and poor social support have been added to the classic risk factors.
- ASA 75–162 mg daily, moderate-dose statin.

–Treat chronic angina in CAD by either increasing O2 supply to heart muscle (nitrates and CCBs) or by decreasing the muscles' O2 demand (BB, CCB, ranolazine, ivabradine). BB and CCB are first line. If these are contraindicated, poorly tolerated, or insufficient then long-acting nitrates and ranolazine can be used.

–Consider coronary angiography in patients who survive sudden cardiac death, who have high-risk noninvasive test results (large areas of silent ischemia are often associated with malignant ventricular arrhythmias) and in whom anginal symptoms cannot be controlled with optimal medical therapy.[1]

–Coronary bypass grafting surgery (CABG) is preferred to angioplasty in diabetic patients with multivessel disease (FREEDOM trial 2012).

Sources

–*Circulation.* 2020;141:e779-e806.
–*Circulation.* 2014 Nov 4;130(19):1749-1767.
–*Circulation.* 2012;126(25):3097-3137.

Population

–Patients with CAD and elevated cardiac troponin level.

Organization

▶ ACC 2012

Recommendations

–Elevated troponin levels are an imperfect diagnostic test and are dependent upon the probability of underlying CAD.

–Establish pretest probability and global risk scores (TIMI, GRACE, PERSUIT) to determine the significance of elevated troponin levels.

–Clinical factors that establish a high pretest probability include a history of typical angina, typical ECG changes consistent with ischemia (ST-segment changes), history of established coronary risk factors, or the history of known CAD.

–Elevated troponin levels in patients with high pretest probability of CAD (typical chest pain and ECG changes of ischemia) have a predictive accuracy of ≥95% to establish acute coronary syndrome.

---

[1]Coronary angiography is useful in patients with presumed SIHD who have unacceptable ischemic symptoms despite GDMT (guideline-determined medical therapy) and who are amenable to, and candidates for, coronary revascularization. Coronary angiography is reasonable to define the extent and severity of CAD in patients with suspected SIHD whose clinical characteristics and results of noninvasive testing (exclusive of stress testing) indicate a high likelihood of severe IHD and who are amenable to, and candidates for, coronary revascularization. Coronary angiography is reasonable in patients with suspected symptomatic SIHD who cannot undergo diagnostic stress testing, or have indeterminate or nondiagnostic stress tests, when there is a high likelihood that the findings will result in important changes to therapy. Coronary angiography might be considered in patients with stress test results of acceptable quality that do not suggest the presence of CAD when clinical suspicion of CAD remains high and there is a high likelihood that the findings will result in important changes to therapy.

–Elevated troponin levels in patients with low pretest probability of CAD (atypical chest pain and nonspecific ECG changes) have a predictive accuracy of only 50% to establish ACS.

–Use global risk scores to further establish the role of early conservative vs. early invasive therapy in patients with elevated troponin levels and a high pretest probability.

–Cardiac causes for elevated troponin levels include ACS, coronary spasm or embolism, cocaine or methamphetamine use, stress cardiomyopathy, congestive HF, myocarditis or pericarditis, trauma, infiltrative diseases, postprocedure (ablation, electric shock, coronary bypass surgery, and postcoronary angioplasty).

–Noncardiac causes for elevated troponin levels include pulmonary embolus, renal failure, stroke, sepsis, drug toxicity (anthracycline), and hypoxia.

Source

–Newby LK, Jesse RL, Babb JD, et al. ACCF 2012 expert consensus document of practical clinical considerations in the interpretation of troponin elevations: a report of the American College of Cardiology Foundation task force on Clinical Expert Consensus Documents. *J Am Coll Cardiol.* 2012;60:2427-2463.

Population

–Patients with stable coronary disease experiencing unstable angina or non-ST elevation MI (NSTEMI).

Organizations

▶ ACC/AHA 2014, ESC 2015

Recommendations

–Include in initial evaluation an ECG, cardiac troponin I or T levels (obtained at symptom onset and 3–6 h later, with levels beyond 6 h if EKG or clinical presentation suggests a high probability of ACS), and assess prognosis with risk scores such as TIMI[1] or GRACE.[2]

–Give sublingual nitroglycerin q5min ×3 for ongoing ischemic pain. Use IV nitroglycerin for persistent ischemia, HF, or hypertension.

–Give dual antiplatelet therapy in likely or definite NSTE-ACS. Aspirin (162–325 mg, non-enteric-coated) and clopidogrel (300–600 mg loading dose, then maintenance) or ticagrelor (180 mg loading dose, then maintenance). After stabilization, consider dual antiplatelet therapy (clopidogrel or ticagrelor in addition to aspirin) "up to" 12 mo if not stented, and for "at least" 12 mo if stented.

–Anticoagulate, in addition to dual antiplatelet therapy. Use unfractionated heparin, enoxaparin, or fondaparinux. The strongest evidence supports enoxaparin.

–Give oral beta-blockers in the first 24 h, unless signs of HF, low output state, risk factors for cardiogenic shock, or other contraindications to beta-blockade. If contraindicated or if ischemia persists despite beta-blockers and nitrates, give nondihydropyridine calcium channel blocker.

---

[1]TIMI Risk Score predicts 30-d and 1-y mortality in ACS (mortality rises at TIMI = 3–4). 1 point each for age ≥65, ≥3 risk factors for CAD, known CAD, ST changes on EKG (≥0.5 mm), active angina (≥2 episodes in past 24 h), aspirin in past 7 d, elevated cardiac marker.
[2]GRACE risk model predicts in-hospital and postdischarge mortality or MI. Downloadable tool: http://www.outcomes-umassmed.org/grace/

–If patients are already on beta-blockers with normal LVEF or stable reduced LVEF, continue home dose of long-acting metoprolol succinate, carvedilol, or bisoprolol.

–Block the renin-angiotensin-aldosterone system with an ACE inhibitor. Continue after stabilization if LVEF < 40%, HTN, DM, or stable CKD.

–Start or continue high-intensity statin, unless contraindicated, and continue indefinitely.

–Give supplemental oxygen if SaO_2 <= 90% or respiratory distress.

–Give IV morphine for analgesia if anti-ischemic medications have been maximized. Do not give NSAIDs.

–After stabilization, continue aspirin (81–325 mg/d) indefinitely.

Sources

–*Eur Heart J.* 2016;37(3):267-315. https://academic.oup.com/eurheartj/article/37/3/267/2466099

–*J Am Coll Cardiol.* 2014;64(24):e139-e228. http://content.onlinejacc.org/article.aspx?articleid=1910086

–*J Am Coll Cardiol.* 2016;68(10):1082-1115. http://content.onlinejacc.org/article.aspx?articleid=2507082

Population

–Patients with stable coronary disease experiencing ST Elevation MI (STEMI).

Organizations

▶ ACC/AHA 2013, ESC 2012, NICE 2013

Recommendations

–Draw serum biomarkers, but do not wait for results to initiate reperfusion therapy.

–Elect PCI rather than fibrinolysis for all patients with STEMI if an experienced team is available within 120 min of first medical contact.

–Give aspirin (162–325 mg) and a loading dose of an ADP-receptor inhibitor (clopidogrel 600 mg, prasugrel 60 mg, or ticagrelor 180 mg) as early as possible.

–Anticoagulate with unfractionated heparin (UFH), enoxaparin, or bivalirudin. A glycoprotein IIb/IIIa inhibitor (abciximab, eptifibatide, tirofiban) may be added to UFH.

–If hypertensive or with ongoing ischemia, give beta-blocker at presentation.

–If PCI is not available, treat instead with fibrinolytics. Give a loading dose of clopidogrel (300 mg; 75 mg if >75 y of age) with aspirin. Anticoagulate with heparin, enoxaparin, or fondaparinux until hospital discharge (minimum 48 h, up to 8 d) or until revascularization is performed. Give fibrinolytic therapy within 30 min of hospital arrival. It is most useful if ischemic symptoms started within the past 12 h and is a reasonable choice between 12 and 24 h if there is evidence of ongoing ischemia or a large area of myocardium at risk. Transfer to a PCI-capable facility if fibrinolysis fails.

–Give patients who have undergone PCI for STEMI dual antiplatelet therapy for 1 y. Continue aspirin indefinitely. Initiate beta-blockers within 24 h of admission, high-intensity statin, and if LVEF <40% an ace inhibitor or angiotensin receptor blocker.

Sources

–*J Am Coll Cardiol.* 2013;61(4). https://www.guideline.gov/summaries/summary/39429?

–*Eur Heart J.* 2012;33(20):2569-619. https://www.guideline.gov/summaries/summary/39353?

–National Institute for Health and Care Excellence (NICE); 2013:28. https://www.guideline.gov/summaries/summary/47019?

–*J Am Coll Cardiol.* 2016;68(10):1082-1115. http://content.onlinejacc.org/article.aspx?articleid=2507082

Population

–Patients with stable coronary disease experiencing sexual dysfunction.

Organization

▶ AHA/Princeton Consensus Panel 2013

Recommendations

–Patients with CAD with angina pectoris should undergo full medical evaluation prior to partaking in sexual activity. Patients should be able to perform 3–5 metabolic equivalents (METs) on a treadmill or climb 2 flights of stairs or walk briskly without angina before engaging in sexual activity.

–After uncomplicated MI if no symptoms on mild-to-moderate activity exist >1 wk, patient may resume sexual activity.

–After angioplasty, sexual activity is reasonable within 1 wk if the radial groin site is healed.

–After coronary bypass, sexual activity is reasonable after 6–8 wk, being limited by the sternal healing or pain.

–Sexual activity is contraindicated in patients with angina at low effort, refractory angina, or unstable angina.

–Nitrate therapy is contraindicated with phosphodiesterase 5 (PDE5) inhibitor therapy. Following sildenafil (Viagra) or vardenafil (Levitra) at least 24 h must elapse before nitrates can be started; ≥48 h if tadalafil (Cialis) is used.

–Beta-blockers, calcium channel blockers, and Ranolazine are not contraindicated; however, they may exacerbate erectile dysfunction.

Sources

–Schwartz BG, Kloner RA. Clinical cardiology: physician update: erectile dysfunction and cardiovascular disease. *Circulation.* 2011;123:98-101.

–Nehra A, Jackson G, Martin Miner, et al. The Princeton III consensus recommendations for the management of erectile dysfunction and cardiovascular disease. *Mayo Clin Proc.* 2012;87:766-778.

–Kloner RA, Henderson L. Sexual function in patients with chronic angina pectoris. *Am J Cardiol.* 2013;111:1671-1676.

Population

–Patients with CAD and AF.

Organization

▶ ACC/AHA/ESC 2014

Recommendations

–Consider use of triple anticoagulation therapy with aspirin, clopidogrel, and warfarin in AF patients at high risk of thromboembolism and recent coronary stent placement, balancing the risk of thrombotic vs. bleeding events. If the bleeding risk is high but the AF thromboembolic risk is low, dual antiplatelet therapy may be preferred. See Table 19-6 for a summary of anticoagulation strategies.

–Choose bare-metal stents if triple anticoagulation therapy is required. Reserve drug-eluting stents for high-risk clinical or anatomic situations (diabetic patients or if the coronary lesions are unusually long, totally occlusive, or in small blood vessels) if triple anticoagulation therapy is required.

–Dual antiplatelet therapy with clopidogrel (75 mg/d) and ASA (81 mg/d) is the most effective therapy to prevent coronary stent thrombosis.

–If dual antiplatelet or triple anticoagulation therapy, give prophylactic GI therapy with an H2-blocker (except cimetidine) or PPI agent. If considering omeprazole (Prilosec), review the risk-to-benefit ratio because of its possible interference with clopidogrel function.

Comments

1. Triple anticoagulation therapy is the most effective therapy to prevent both coronary stent thrombosis and the occurrence of embolic strokes in high-risk patients. However, the addition of warfarin to DAPT increases the bleeding risk by 3.7-fold. Therefore, awaiting a definitive clinical trial (WOEST trial), perform a risk stratification of patients to evaluate the thrombo-embolic potential of AF vs. the bleeding potential. The HAS-BLED (see Table 19-3) bleeding risk score is the best measure of bleeding risk. A high risk of bleeding is defined by a score >3.

Sources

–*Circulation.* 2014;130(23).

–*Eur Heart J.* 2010;31:2369-2429.

–*BMJ.* 2008;337:a840.

–*Chest.* 2011;139:981-987.

–*J Am Coll Cardiol.* 2008;51:172-208; 2009;54:95-109; 2010;56:2051-2066; 2011;57:1920-1959.

CORONARY ARTERY DISEASE: STENT THERAPY USE OF TRIPLE ANTICOAGULATION TREATMENT

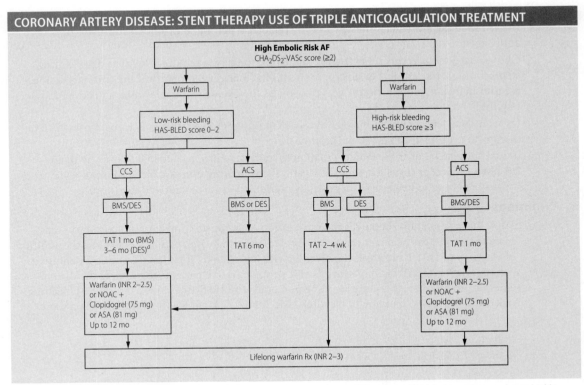

ACS, acute coronary syndrome; AF, atrial fibrillation; ASA, aspirin; BMS, bare-metal stent; CCS, patient with chronic coronary syndrome (stable coronary artery disease); DES, drug eluting stent; INR, international normalized ratio; Rx, therapy [warfarin (INR 2–2.5) + aspirin (81 mg daily) + clopidogrel (75 mg daily)]; TAT, triple anticoagulation therapy.

[a]DES stents if sirolimus, everolimus, or tacrolimus require 3-mo dual platelet therapy (ASA plus clopidogrel). If DES stent is paclitaxel, 6-mo dual therapy is required.

Sources: European Heart Rhythm Association; European Association for Cardio-Thoracic Surgery, Camm AJ, Kirchhof P, Lip GY, et al. Guidelines for the management of atrial fibrillation: the Task Force for the Management of Atrial Fibrillation of the European Society of Cardiology (ESC). *Eur Heart J.* 2010;31:2369-2429. Lip GY. Managing the anticoagulated patient with atrial fibrillation at high risk of stroke who needs coronary intervention. *BMJ.* 2008;337:a840. Rubboli A, Kovacic JC, Mehran R, Lip GY. Coronary stent implantation in patients committed to long-term oral anticoagulation: successfully navigating the treatment options. *Chest.* 2011;139:981-987. King SB III, Smith SC Jr, Hirshfeld JW Jr, et al. 2007 focused update of the ACC/AHA/SCAI 2005 guideline update for percutaneous coronary intervention: a report of the American College of Cardiology/American Heart Association Task Force on Practice guidelines. *J Am Coll Cardiol.* 2008;51:172-208. January CT, Wann LS, Alpert JS, et al. 2014 AHA/ACC/HRS Guideline for the Management of Patients with Atrial Fibrillation. *Circulation.* 2014. http://circ.ahajournals.org/content/early/2014/04/10/CIR.0000000000000041. Wright RS, Anderson JL, Adams CD, et al. 2011 ACCF/AHA focused update of the Guidelines for the Management of Patients with Unstable Angina/Non-ST-Elevation Myocardial Infarction (updating the 2007 guideline): a report of the American College of Cardiology Foundation/American Heart Association Task Force on Practice Guidelines developed in collaboration with the American College of Emergency Physicians, Society for Cardiovascular Angiography and Interventions, and Society of Thoracic Surgeons. *J Am Coll Cardiol.* 2011;57:1920-1959. Abraham NS, Hlatky MA, Antman EM, et al. ACCF/ACG/AHA. ACCF/ACG/AHA 2010 expert consensus document on the concomitant use of proton pump inhibitors and thienopyridines: a focused update of the ACCF/ACG/AHA 2008 expert consensus document on reducing the gastrointestinal risks of antiplatelet therapy and NSAID use. A Report of the American College of Cardiology Foundation Task Force on Expert Consensus Documents. *J Am Coll Cardiol.* 2010;56:2051-2066. Holmes DR Jr, Kereiakes DJ, Kleiman NS, Moliterno DJ, Patti G, Grines CL. Combining antiplatelet and anticoagulation therapies. *J Am Coll Cardiol.* 2009;54:95-109.

TABLE 19-6 ANTITHROMBOTIC STRATEGIES FOLLOWING CORONARY ARTERY STENTING IN PATIENTS WITH AF AT MODERATE-TO-HIGH THROMBOEMBOLIC RISK (IN WHOM ORAL ANTICOAGULATION THERAPY IS REQUIRED)

Hemorrhagic Risk	Clinical Setting	Stent Implanted	Anticoagulation Regimen
Low or intermediate (eg, HAS-BLED score 0–2)	Elective	Bare metal	1 mo: triple therapy of VKA (INR 2.0–2.5) + aspirin ≤100 mg/d + clopidogrel 75 mg/d Up to 12th mo: combination of VKA (INR 2.0–2.5) + clopidogrel 75 mg/d (or aspirin 100 mg/d) Lifelong: VKA (INR 2.0–3.0) alone
	Elective	Drug eluting	3 (-olimus[a] group) to 6 (paclitaxel) mo: triple therapy of VKA (INR 2.0–2.5) + aspirin ≤100 mg/d + clopidogrel 75 mg/d Up to 12th mo: combination of VKA (INR 2.0–2.5) + clopidogrel 75 mg/d (or aspirin 100 mg/d) Lifelong: VKA (INR 2.0–3.0) alone
	ACS	Bare metal/drug eluting	6 mo: triple therapy of VKA (INR 2.0–2.5) + aspirin ≤100 mg/d + clopidogrel 75 mg/d Up to 12th mo: combination of VKA (INR 2.0–2.5) + clopidogrel 75 mg/d (or aspirin 100 mg/d) Lifelong: VKA (INR 2.0–3.0) alone
High (eg, HAS-BLED score ≥3)	Elective	Bare metal[b]	2–4 wk: triple therapy of VKA (INR 2.0–2.5) + aspirin ≤100 mg/d + clopidogrel 75 mg/d Lifelong: VKA (INR 2.0–3.0) alone
	ACS	Bare metal[b]	4 wk: triple therapy of VKA (INR 2.0–2.5) + aspirin ≤100 mg/d + clopidogrel 75 mg/d Up to 12th mo: combination of VKA (INR 2.0–2.5) + clopidogrel 75 mg/d[c] (or aspirin 100 mg/d) Lifelong: VKA (INR 2.0–3.0) alone

[a]Sirolimus, everolimus, and tacrolimus.

[b]Drug-eluting stents should be avoided as far as possible, but, if used, consideration of more prolonged (3–6 mo) triple antithrombotic therapy is necessary.

[c]Combination of VKA (INR 2.0–3.0) + aspirin ≤100 mg/d (with PPI, if indicated) may be considered as an alternative.

Source: Reproduced with permission from Lip GY, Huber K, Andreotti F, et al. Management of antithrombotic therapy in atrial fibrillation patients presenting with acute coronary syndrome and/or undergoing percutaneous coronary intervention/ stenting. *Thromb Haemost.* © Georg Thieme Verlag KG. 2010;103(1):13-28.

Population

–Patients with CAD and Type 2 Diabetes Mellitus.

Organization

▶ AHA 2020

Recommendations

–Use an A1c goal of <8.0–8.5.

–The use of different medications to attain a glycemic goal can affect CAD-related endpoints. See Table 19-7.

–Antiplatelet therapy: Data is insufficient to give a definitive recommendation.

–Hypertension: BP goals based on combination of comorbidities:
- T2DM + HTN + CAD <140 / <90.
- T2DM + HTN + CAD + stroke risk <130 / <80.
- T2DM + HTN + CAD + CKD/microalbuminuria <130 / <80.

–Benefits/risks of antihypertensive classes in T2DM and CAD:
- ACEi/ARBs: first line. Reduce first and recurrent cardiovascular events; reduce progression of microalbuminuria.
- Long-acting thiazide-like (chlorthalidone/indapamide): second-line option. Increase serum glucose slightly by decreasing insulin sensitivity but unclear if of clinical significance. Has cardiovascular benefit.
- Dihydropyridine CCBs (amlodipine): second-line option. Has cardiovascular benefit and is antianginal.
- Aldosterone antagonists (spironolactone): third-line option. Important in comorbid LV dysfunction or prior MI.
- Beta-blockers: Do not reduce mortality in CAD after 30 days. Can be used in T2DM if there is concurrent chronic angina or if need another agent. Not all beta-blockers have equal benefit. Use carvedilol, labetolol, or nebivolol for vasodilatory effect and neutrality in T2DM. Instead, metoprolol and atenolol will reduce demand but cause peripheral vasoconstriction, which increases insulin resistance and increases LDL.

–Lipids: Use statins for all with CAD and DM.
- If LDL is >70 despite high-intensity statin, consider ezetimibe or PCSK9 inhibitors (evolocumab or alirocumab) for additional risk reduction in death, MI, stroke, or hospitalization.
- If triglycerides are >135 despite statins, consider addition of Icosapent Ethyl 2g bid which has been shown to decrease cardiovascular death, MI, stroke, CABG, unstable angina.

–Smoking: Stop smoking. The weight gain in T2DM from cessation does not undo the drop in risk of major cardiac event.

–Diet: Recommend a Mediterranean diet with extra virgin olive oil or mixed nuts saw benefit for reduction in major cardiac events or stroke.

–Activity: Recommend 150 min/wk of moderate to vigorous physical activity. Refer to cardiac rehabilitation after the first major cardiac event, as the intervention has been shown to be preventative of future cardiac events if tailored to T2DM.

–Weight loss: Diet and exercise have modest benefit in CAD and T2DM. Liraglutide has been shown to decrease weight (see Table 19-7) and improve CAD outcomes. Bariatric surgery has been shown to better control CAD risk factors (glycemic control, LDL, triglycerides, HTN) but not necessarily to improve CAD endpoints.

TABLE 19-7 DIABETES MEDICATIONS WITH CARDIOVASCULAR BENEFITS

Drug Class	Specific Drugs and Trials	Risk/Benefit for CAD	Effect in Diabetes
SGLT2 inhibitors	Empagliflozin (EMPA-REG) Canagliflozin (CANVAS) Dapagliflozin (DECLARE-TIMI)	–Decreases major cardiac events –Decreases CHF hospitalizations –Decreases blood pressure slightly –Less CKD progression –Contributes to weight loss	–No hypoglycemia risk –Stop medication if at risk for amputation, Fournier's gangrene, bone fractures, and euglycemic DKA
GLP1 agonists	Liraglutide (LEADER) Lixasenatide (ELIXA) Semaglutide (SUSTAIN-6) Exenatide (EXCEL)	–Overall recommended for decreasing major cardiac events –Contributes more to weight loss than SGLT2i –More variety within the class for CAD benefit in recent research: • Liraglutide and semaglutide decrease major cardiac events • Exenatide and lixisenatide are neutral	–No hypoglycemia risk –Stop medication if at risk for gastroparesis, pancreatitis, or CrCl <30 mL/min (use caution if 30–50 mL/min)
Metformin		–Benefit is possible	–No hypoglycemia –Stop in CrCl < 30 mL/min –Monitor for anemia and B12 deficiency
DPP4 inhibitors	Saxagliptin (SAVOR-TIMI) Alogliptin (EXAMINE) Sitaliptin (TECOS) Linagliptin (CAROLINA)	–Neutral CAD effect –Weight loss neutral –Saxagliptin and alogliptin may contribute to CHF hospitalization	–No hypoglycemia –Stop in gastroparesis and pancreatitis –Monitor for URI symptoms
Insulin		–Neutral CAD effect –Can cause weight gain	–Can cause hypoglycemia
Sulfonylureas	Glimepiride (CAROLINA)	–Neutral CAD effect –Can cause weight gain	–Can cause hypoglycemia
Thiazolidinediones	Pioglitazone (PROactive, IRIS) Rosiglitazone (RECORD)	–Likely CAD benefit –Need to monitor/stop for CHF, esp. if using with insulin –Can cause weight gain	–No hypoglycemia –Stop if risk for bone fractures

Comments

1. Intensive glycemic control A1C < 6.0%–7.0% has not been shown to decrease major cardiac events, though glycemic control <7.0% does show some benefit for microvascular consequences of diabetes such as blindness, microalbuminuria, ESRD, and distal neuropathies.

2. T2DM is a generalized prothrombotic state, especially when exacerbated by CKD. Responsiveness to DAPT may be impaired. Clopidogrel alone may be reasonable compared to aspirin alone in T2DM w/ prior MI, ischemic stroke, or PAD. At this time, large trials have not shown benefit when antithrombotic regimens are adjusted based on platelet function testing.

3. 70%–80% of patients with T2DM also have HTN. This increases the risk of MI, stroke, and all-cause mortality. Intensive control of systolic blood pressure in this group <130 decreases risk of stroke, but has no benefit in decreasing coronary events. There are increased risks of adverse events in too much control of HTN in CAD.

4. The ACCORD trial demonstrated that 30% of T2DM need 2 antihypertensives, 39% of T2DM need 3 antihypertensives.

5. Statins have significant benefit in primary and secondary CAD prevention and patients with T2DM. Studies have shown that statins can cause small increase in incident T2DM, but the risk is lower than with thiazides or nonvasodilating BB; the protective benefit of statins in T2DM is more substantive and favors administration.

6. Stress: Patients with T2DM have increased risk for stress and depression. This has been shown to increase risk of stroke. Stress in T2DM has been shown to increase risk of major cardiac event. The mechanisms are unknown. It is unknown if decreasing stress/depression then resolves the increased risk.

Source

–Arnold SV, Bhatt DL, Barsness GW, et al.; on behalf of the American Heart Association Council on Lifestyle and Cardiometabolic Health and Council on Clinical Cardiology. Clinical management of stable coronary artery disease in patients with type 2 diabetes mellitus: a scientific statement from the American Heart Association. *Circulation.* 2020;141:e779–e806.

HEART FAILURE

HEART FAILURE STAGING

Stage A: Patients with hypertension, atherosclerotic disease, diabetes mellitus, metabolic syndrome, or those using cardiotoxins or having a family history of cardiomyopathy

Stage B: Patients with previous MI, LV remodeling including LVH and low EF, or asymptomatic valvular disease

Stage C: Patients with known structural heart disease; shortness of breath and fatigue, reduced exercise tolerance

Stage D: Patients who have marked symptoms at rest despite maximal medical therapy (eg, those who are recurrently hospitalized or cannot be safely discharged from the hospital without specialized interventions)

Source: Adapted from the American College of Cardiology, American Heart Association, Inc. *Circulation.* 2017. doi:10.1161/CIR.0000000000000509.

Population
–Adults with HF.

Organizations
▶ ACC/AHA 2013, 2017, NICE 2018

Recommendations

Assessment

–Classify HF as reduced or preserved ejection fraction:

- Heart failure with reduced ejection fraction (HFrEF), referred to as systolic heart failure, when LVEF ≤40%.
- Heart failure with preserved ejection fraction (HFpEF), referred to as diastolic dysfunction, when LVEF >40%.

–Diagnosing HF:

- Measure N-terminal pro-B-type natriuretic peptide.
- If BNP >2000 ng/L, obtain transthoracic echo within 6 wk (of note, other causes of high BNP include age over 70 y, LVH, tachycardia, RV overload, hypoxemia, pulmonary embolism, renal dysfunction, COPD, DM, and cirrhosis).
- If BNP <400 in an untreated person, HF is less likely (of note, obesity, African or African-Caribbean family origin, or treatment with diuretics can reduce levels of BNP).

–Obtain CXR, blood tests (renal function, thyroid function, liver function, lipid profile, A1c, complete blood count), urine analysis, and peak flow or spirometry. Identify prior cardiac or noncardiac disease that may lead to HF. For patients at risk of developing HF (Stage A/B), natriuretic peptide biomarker–based screening (BNP or NT-pro-BNP) and optimizing GDMT can help prevent the development of LV dysfunction (systolic or diastolic) or new-onset HF.

–Obtain history to include diet or medicine nonadherence; current or past use of alcohol, illicit drugs, and chemotherapy; or recent viral illness.

–If idiopathic dilated cardiomyopathy, obtain a three-generational family history to exclude familial disease.

–Consider risk score evaluation to help predict outcomes, chronic HF—Seattle Heart Failure Model. (http://depts.washington.edu/shfm/)

–Identify the patient's present activity level and desired post-treatment level.

–Assess the patient's volume status, orthostatic BP changes, height and weight, and body mass index.

–Control hypertension and lipid disorders in accordance with contemporary guideline to lower the risk of HF. Control or avoid other risk factors.

–In initial blood work, measure N-terminal pro-brain natriuretic peptide (NT-pro-BNP) or BNP levels to support clinical judgment for diagnosis, especially if diagnosis is uncertain. Also include CBC, chemistry panel, lipid profile, troponin I level, and TSH level.

–Obtain 12-lead ECG.

–Obtain 2D echocardiogram to determine the systolic function, diastolic function, valvular function, and pulmonary artery pressure.

–In patients with angina or significant ischemia, perform coronary arteriography unless the patient is not eligible for surgery.

Management

–If volume overloaded, initiate diuretic therapy and salt restriction. Diuretics do not improve long-term survival, but improve symptoms and short-term survival. Once euvolemic and symptoms have resolved, carefully wean dosage as an outpatient to lowest dose possible to prevent electrolyte disorders and activation of the renin-angiotensin system.

–Give ACE inhibitor or ARB or ARNI (ARB plus a neurolysin inhibitor, such as valsartan/sacubitril) early in the initial course if ejection fraction reduced to decrease afterload. Titrate dosage every 2 wk to target dose in clinical studies as BP allows. Measure renal function and electrolytes 1–2 wk after each change.

–In patients with chronic symptomatic HFrEF NYHA Class II or III who tolerate an ACE inhibitor or ARB, replace with an ARNI to further reduce morbidity and mortality.

–Add beta-blockers (specifically carvedilol, sustained release metoprolol succinate, or bisoprolol) to reduce morbidity and mortality. These beta-blockers improve survival the most in systolic HF. Start with low dose, and titrate dosage gradually to heart rate 65–70 beats/min.

–Start aldosterone antagonist in patients with moderate or severe symptoms (NYHA Class II–IV) and reduced ejection fraction. Creatinine should be <2.5 mg/dL in men and <2 mg/dL in women, and the potassium should be <5 mEq/L.

–Consider ivabradine to reduce HF hospitalization in select patients: symptomatic stable chronic HFrEF (EF <35%) at least 4 wk removed from exacerbation on optimal medical therapy including optimal dosing of ACE inhibitor and beta-blocker at maximal tolerated dose in sinus rhythm with resting HR >70.

–Use the combination of hydralazine and nitrates to improve outcomes in African-Americans with moderate-to-severe HF with decreased ejection fraction, in addition to optimal therapy.[1] If ACE inhibitor or ARB agent is contraindicated, hydralazine and nitrates may be used as alternative therapy.

–Consider digoxin if severe or worsening HFrEF despite optimal first-line therapies.

–Statins are not beneficial as adjunctive therapy when prescribed solely for the diagnosis of HF. In all patients with a recent or remote hx of CAD, CVA, PAD, or hyperlipidemia, use statins according to guidelines.

–Discontinue anti-inflammatory agents, diltiazem, and verapamil.

–Nutritional supplements are not useful therapy for patients with current or prior symptoms of systolic dysfunction (HFrEF).

–Avoid calcium channel blockers in the routine treatment for patients with HFrEF.

–Recommend exercise training, which is beneficial in HF patients with decreased ejection fraction (systolic dysfunction) or preserved ejection fraction (diastolic dysfunction) once therapy is optimized.

[1]Race-based recommendations for specific therapies are controversial, in part because the definition of racial groups is not standardized. This guidance comes from a study that looked at patients identified as Black with NYHA Class III or IV HF. All were given standard therapies, and the groups were randomized to add either placebo or isosorbide dinitrate + hydralazine. Mortality rate, admission rate, and quality life were significantly worse in the placebo group. (*N Engl J Med.* 2004; 351:2049-2057)

–Refer for intracardiac cardiac defibrillator to obtain secondary survival benefit in patients who survive cardiac arrest, ventricular fibrillation, or hemodynamically significant ventricular tachycardia.

–Refer for intracardiac cardiac defibrillator to obtain primary survival benefit in patients with ischemic or nonischemic cardiomyopathy with EF ≤35% with New York Heart Association (NYHA) class II or III. The patient should be stable on GDMT (guideline-determined medical therapy) optimal chronic medical HF therapy and at least 40 d post-MI and have a life expectancy of at least 1 y.

–Consider biventricular heart pacemaker (CRT) in refractory HF with ejection fraction equal to or less than 35% with NYHA class II and III or ambulatory class IV on GDMT. The rhythm should be sinus, with a QRS ≥150 ms, ± LBBB.

–Do not administer long-term anticoagulation therapy in patients with chronic systolic function while in sinus rhythm in the absence of AF, a prior thromboembolic event, or cardioembolic source.

–Maintain blood pressure less than 130/80 mmHg.

–In HF patients with preserved systolic function (diastolic dysfunction), randomized data on therapy are lacking. The goal is to control blood volume (diuretic), keep systolic blood pressure <130 mmHg (beta-blocker, ACE inhibitor, ARB agent, or diuretic), slow heart rate (beta-blocker), and treat coronary artery ischemia. Whether beta-blockers, ACE inhibitors, ARB agents, or aldosterone antagonists improve survival independently is yet to be proven.

–Give all patients comprehensive written discharge instruction. Emphasize diet, weight monitoring, medicine, and salt adherence. Discuss activity along with education of symptoms of worsening HF.

–During an HF hospitalization, consider obtaining a predischarge natriuretic peptide level (BNP or NT-pro-BNP) to establish a postdischarge prognosis.

–Arrange postdischarge appointment with physician and health care team with attention to information on discharge medications.

Comments

1. Lifetime risk of developing HF for Americans ≥40-y-old is 20%.
2. Overall mortality is 50% in 5 y; varies with HF stage:
   a. Stage B: 5-y mortality 4%.
   b. Stage C: 5-y mortality 25%.
   c. Stage D: 5-y mortality 80%.

Sources

–ACCF/AHA 2017 Guidelines. *Circulation.* 2017. doi: 10.1161/CIR.0000000000000509.

–*N Engl J Med.* 2012.

–WARCET Trial; American Academy of Family Physicians; American Academy of Hospice and Palliative Medicine; American Nurses Association; American Society of Health-System Pharmacists; Heart Rhythm Society; Society of Hospital Medicine, Bonow RO, Ganiats TG, Beam CT, et al. ACCF/AHA/AMA-PCPI 2011 performance measures for adults with heart failure: a report of the American College of Cardiology Foundation/American Heart Association Task Force on Performance Measures and the American Medical Association-Physician Consortium for Performance Improvement. *J Am Coll Cardiol.* 2012;59(20):1812-1832.

–Yancy CW, Jessup M, Bozkurt B, et al. 2013. ACCF/AHA guideline for the management of heart failure: a report of the American College of Cardiology Foundation/American Heart Association Task Force on practice guidelines. *Circulation.* 2013;128:e240-e327.

HYPERLIPIDEMIA

The risk assessment and management of ASCVD risk factors, including hyperlipidemia, is detailed in Chapter 2: Cardiovascular Disorders.

HYPERTENSION

Population
–All adults.

Organizations
▶ ACC/AHA 2017, JNC8 2014, ESC/ESH 2018, ASH 2014, CHEP 2015

Recommendations
–Initiate lifestyle modification including structured exercise and dietary adjustments including lower sodium diet and efforts at weight loss if overweight or obese.

–Consider overall cardiovascular risk in patients with hypertension and evaluate need for primary prevention measures for ASCVD including smoking cessation, aspirin, and statin.

GUIDELINES DISCORDANT: WHEN TO INITIATE TREATMENT FOR HYPERTENSION	
Organization	**Guidance**
ACC/AHA	BP 120–129/<80: lifestyle changes, follow-up 3–6 mo BP 130–139/80–89, 10-y ASCVD risk ≥10%: lifestyle changes and medications, follow-up 1 mo BP 130–139/80–89, 10-y ASCVD risk <10%: lifestyle changes and medications, follow-up 3–6 mo BP ≥140/90: lifestyle changes and medications, follow-up 1 mo
ACC/AHA	BP ≥140/90 mmHg in the general population age <60-y-old BP ≥150/90 mmHg in general population age ≥60-y-old

GUIDELINES DISCORDANT: WHEN TO INITIATE TREATMENT FOR HYPERTENSION

Organization	Guidance
ESC/ESH	BP 130–139/85–89: lifestyle modification (salt restriction <5 g/d, alcohol intake <14 drinks/wk for men and <8 drinks/wk for women, increasing fruits/vegetables/fish/nuts/olive oil in diet, controlling BMI, regular physical activity, and smoking cessation BP 140–159/90–99: lifestyle modification; medications if high cardiovascular risk, hypertension-mediated organ damage, or persistent elevation after 3–6 mo lifestyle changes BP 160+/100+: lifestyle modification and drug therapy
ASH	BP <150/90 mmHg in patients ≥80-y-old BP <140/90 mmHg in patients 60- to 79-y-old BP <140/90 mmHg or <130/80 mmHg (if tolerated), in patients <50-y-old
CHEP	BP ≥160/100 mmHg in patients without macrovascular target organ damage or other CV risk factors BP ≥140/90 mmHg in patients with macrovascular target organ damage or high cardiovascular risk SBP >160 mmHg in elderly (≥60 y)

GUIDELINES DISCORDANT: TREATMENT TARGETS IN HYPERTENSION

Organization	Guidance
ACC/AHA	<130/80 for CVD or 10-y ASCVD risk ≥10%; consider <130/80 for all
JNC8	BP <140/90 mmHg in patients <60-y-old BP <150/90 mmHg in patients ≥60-y-old If BP cannot be reached within 1 mo, increase the dose of the initial drug or add a second and then third drug from the recommended classes
ESC/ESH	Target <140/90 in all patients Target SBP<150 in patients >65 y If tolerating 140/90, target SBP 120–129 if <65 y and 130–139 if ≥65 y
CHEP	BP <140/90 mmHg in the general population SBP <150 mmHg in the elderly (≥60 y) SBP <140 mmHg in the elderly with cerebrovascular disease (history of CVA/TIA) Caution in elderly patients who are frail and in patients with CAD and have low DBP <60 mmHg

GUIDELINES DISCORDANT: CHOICE OF ANTIHYPERTENSIVE AGENTS

Organization	Guidance
ACC/AHA	First line: thiazide diuretics, calcium channel blockers ACE inhibitors, and angiotensin receptor blockers Begin therapy with two drugs initially if desired BP reduction is more than 20/10 mmHg
ACC/AHA	Initial treatment should include a thiazide-type diuretic, CCB, ACEI, or ARB In the general Black[a] population, initial treatment should include a thiazide-type diuretic or CCB
ESC/ESH	Start with combination pill including ACE inhibitor (ACEi) or angiotensin receptor blocker (ARB) plus a calcium channel blocker (CCB) or diuretic. Consider using a single agent in older/frailer patients or those with mild elevations If not controlled with initial therapy, switch to a three-drug combination pill including ACEi/ARB + CCB + diuretic If not controlled on three drugs, add spironolactone, diuretic, alpha-blocker or beta-blockers and consider further investigation for resistant hypertension
ASH	In patients <60-y-old initiate with ACEI/ARB. If uncontrolled, add CCB or thiazide. If needed, add spironolactone, centrally acting agents, and beta-blockers In non-Black patients ≥60-y-old initiate with CCB or thiazide. If needed, add spironolactone, centrally acting agents, and beta-blockers In Black patients initiate with CCB or thiazide. If unable to control BP, add ACEI/ARB. If needed, add spironolactone, centrally acting agents, and beta-blockers
CHEP	Start monotherapy with a thiazide diuretic, a beta-blocker, an ACEI in non-Black patients, a long-acting CCB or an ARB in patients <60 y First-line combinations: thiazide diuretic or CCB with an ACEI, ARB, or beta-blocker. Do not combine ACEI and ARB. Caution in combination of nondihydropyridine and a beta-blocker. Single-pill combinations improve control Do not use ACEIs as first-line therapy for uncomplicated hypertension in Black patients. Do not use alpha-blockers as first-line agents for uncomplicated hypertension

[a]As race is a social rather than scientific construct, and purportedly scientific mechanisms to explain the racial differences in outcomes have their roots in biased data, guidelines that suggest different treatments for different races should be considered with caution. Drs. Vyas, Einstein, and Jones offer a thoughtful assessment in *N Engl J Med*. 2020;383:847-882 (https://www.nejm.org/doi/full/10.1056/NEJMms2004740). A more detailed discussion of the role of race in blood pressure guidelines is available from Drs. Williams, Ravenell, Seyedali, Nayef, and Ogedegbe in *Prog Cardiovasc Dis*. 2016;59(3):282–288 (https://www.ncbi.nlm.nih.gov/pubmed/27693861).

Sources

–ACC/AHA; Whelton et al. *JACC*. 2018;71(19):e127-e248.
–JNC8. *JAMA*. 2014;311(5):507-520.
–ESC/EHA: *Eur Heart J*. 2018;39:3021-3104.
–ASH. *J Clin Hypertens*. 2014. doi: 10.1111/jch.12237.
–CHEP. *Can J Cardiol*. 2015;31(5):549-568.

HYPERTENSION TREATMENT—JNC8 2014

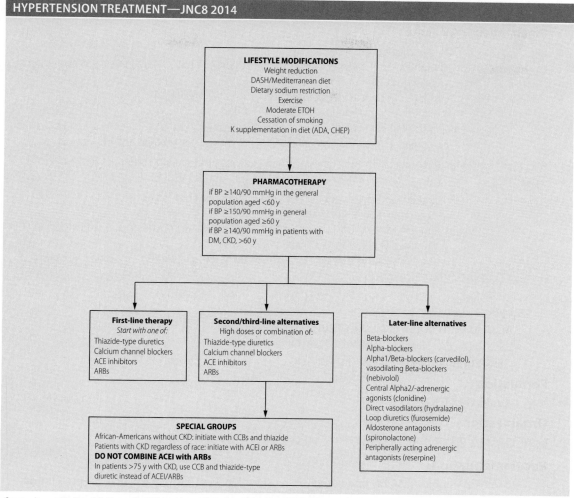

LIFESTYLE MODIFICATIONS
Weight reduction
DASH/Mediterranean diet
Dietary sodium restriction
Exercise
Moderate ETOH
Cessation of smoking
K supplementation in diet (ADA, CHEP)

PHARMACOTHERAPY
if BP ≥140/90 mmHg in the general
population aged <60 y
if BP ≥150/90 mmHg in general
population aged ≥60 y
if BP ≥140/90 mmHg in patients with
DM, CKD, >60 y

First-line therapy
Start with one of:
Thiazide-type diuretics
Calcium channel blockers
ACE inhibitors
ARBs

Second/third-line alternatives
High doses or combination of:
Thiazide-type diuretics
Calcium channel blockers
ACE inhibitors
ARBs

Later-line alternatives
Beta-blockers
Alpha-blockers
Alpha1/Beta-blockers (carvedilol),
vasodilating Beta-blockers
(nebivolol)
Central Alpha2/-adrenergic
agonists (clonidine)
Direct vasodilators (hydralazine)
Loop diuretics (furosemide)
Aldosterone antagonists
(spironolactone)
Peripherally acting adrenergic
antagonists (reserpine)

SPECIAL GROUPS
African-Americans without CKD: initiate with CCBs and thiazide
Patients with CKD regardless of race: initiate with ACEI or ARBs
DO NOT COMBINE ACEI with ARBs
In patients >75 y with CKD, use CCB and thiazide-type
diuretic instead of ACEI/ARBs

Source: James PA, Oparil S, Carter BL. 2014 evidence-based guideline for the management of high blood pressure in adults. Report from the panel members appointed to the Eighth Joint National Committee (JNC8). *JAMA.* 2014;311(5):507-520. doi:10.1001/jama.2013.284427.

Population
–Adults with CAD.

Organizations
▶ ACC/AHA 2017, ESC/ESH 2018, CHEP 2014

Recommendations
–Prioritize medications indicated by CAD.
–Treatment target (ACC/AHA):
  • <130/80 if CAD, prior MI/stroke/TIA/PAD/AAA.
  • <140/90 if chronic stable angina.

GUIDELINES DISCORDANT: CHOICE OF ANTIHYPERTENSIVE AGENT IN CAD	
Organization	**Guidance**
ACC/AHA	Prioritize medications indicated by CAD –Beta-blocker in patients with a history of prior MI. If not tolerated, use nondihydropiridine CCB if no LV dysfunction – ACEI/ARB if prior MI, LV systolic dysfunction, DM, or CKD – A thiazide or thiazide-like diuretic If angina or uncontrolled BP, add nondihydropiridine CCB to beta-blockers. Consider avoiding combination of beta-blocker and CCB—risk of bradyarrhythmias and HF
ESC/ESH	Initial combination should be ACEI/ARB or diuretic plus beta-blocker or CCB
CHEP	Use ACEI first For patients with stable angina, use beta-blockers as initial therapy Avoid combination of ACEI with ARB In high-risk patients, use combination of ACEI and a dihydropyridine CCB rather than an ACEI and a thiazide/thiazide-like diuretic Myocardial ischemia may be exacerbated when DBP ≤60 mmHg—caution in lowering DBP too much (grade D)

Sources
–ACC/AHA; Whelton et al. *JACC.* 2018;71(19):e127-e248.
–ESC/EHA. *Eur Heart J.* 2018;39:3021-3104.
–CHEP. *Can J Cardiol.* 2015;31(5):549-568.

Population
–Adults with CKD.

Organizations
▶ ACC/AHA 2017, ESC/ESH 2018, CHEP 2014, ASH 2014, JNC8 2014

Recommendations
–Use ACE inhibitor (ACEI) or angiotensin receptor blocker (ARB), particularly if proteinuria.
  • Consider starting with ACEI/ARB plus CCB or diuretic as initial therapy. (ESC)
  • In patients over 75 y, use CCB and thiazide-type diuretic instead of ACE/ARB. (JNC8)

GUIDELINES DISCORDANT: BLOOD PRESSURE GOALS IN CKD	
Organization	**Guidance**
ACC/AHA	<130/80
JNC8, CHEP	<140/90
ASH	<140/90—no proteinuria <130/80—proteinuria
ESC/ESH	SBP 130–139

Sources

–ACC/AHA; Whelton et al. *JACC.* 2018;71(19):e127-e248.

–JNC8. *JAMA.* 2014;311(5):507-520. doi:10.1001/jama.2013.284427.

–ESC/EHA. *Eur Heart J.* 2018;39:3021-3104.

–ASH. *J Clin Hypertens.* 2014. doi: 10.1111/jch.12237.

Population

–Adults with HF.

Recommendations

▶ ACC/AHA/ASH 2017, CHEP 2014

–BP target is <130/80 mmHg, but consideration can be given to lowering the BP even further, to <130/80 mmHg. In patients with an elevated DBP who have CAD and HF with evidence of myocardial ischemia, lower the BP slowly. In older hypertensive individuals with wide pulse pressures, lowering SBP may cause very low DBP values (<60 mmHg).

–If stable ischemic heart disease, prioritize medications indicated by CAD/CHF as first drugs: ACEI/ARB, beta-blocker (carvedilol, metoprolol succinate, bisoprolol, or nebivolol), and aldosterone receptor antagonist.

–Use thiazide/thiazide-type diuretic for BP control and to reverse volume overload and associated symptoms. In patients with severe HF (NYHA III or IV), or those with severe renal impairment (eGFR < 30 mL/min), use loop diuretics for volume control (less effective than thiazide/thiazide-type diuretics in lowering BP). Use diuretics together with an ACE/ARB and a beta-blocker.

–Use aldosterone receptor antagonists spironolactone and eplerenone if there is HF (NYHA III or IV) with reduced EF <40%. One or the other may be substituted for a thiazide diuretic in patients requiring a K-sparing agent. If used with an ACEI/ARB in the presence of renal insufficiency, monitor serum K level frequently. Do not use if creatinine level ≥2.5 mg/dL in men or ≥2.0 mg/dL in women, or if serum K level ≥5 mEq/L.

–Add hydralazine plus isosorbide dinitrate to the regimen of diuretic, ACE inhibitor, or ARB, and beta-blocker in African-American patients with NYHA class III or IV HF with reduced ejection fraction.

–Do not use nondihydropyridine CCBs in the treatment of HTN in adults with HFrEF.

–Preserved ejection fraction: consider beta-adrenergic blocking agents, ACEI/ARBs, or CCB as antihypertensives in patients with HF to minimize symptoms of HF.

–Avoid the following drugs in patients with hypertension and HF with reduced ejection fraction:

  • Nondihydropyridine CCBs (such as verapamil and diltiazem).

  • Clonidine.

  • Moxonidine.

  • Hydralazine, without a nitrate.

  • Alpha-adrenergic blockers such as doxazosin (unless all other drugs for the management of hypertension and HF are inadequate to achieve BP control at maximum tolerated doses).

  • Nonsteroidal anti-inflammatory drugs, given their effects on BP, volume status, and renal function.

Source

–ACC/AHA; Whelton et al. *JACC*. 2018;71(19):e127-e248.

Population

–Adults with diabetes.

Recommendations

GUIDELINES DISCORDANT: BLOOD PRESSURE GOALS IN DIABETES	
Organization	**Guidance**
ACC/AHA	<130/80
JNC8	<140/90
ADA	<140/80 <130/80 if younger or "high risk" of cardiovascular disease
CHEP	<130/80
ASH	<140/90 mmHg (without proteinuria) <130/80 mmHg (with proteinuria) or if they are at "high risk" of cardiovascular disease

GUIDELINES DISCORDANT: CHOICE OF ANTIHYPERTENSIVE AGENT IN DIABETES	
Organization	**Guidance**
ACC/AHA	Consider ACEI or ARB if proteinuria
JNC8	Same as non-DM population
ADA	ACEI or ARB: Administer at bedtime
CHEP	Thiazide diuretic or CCB with an ACEI, ARB, or beta-blocker

Sources

–Standards of medical care in diabetes. *Diabetes Care*. 2017;40(suppl 1):S1–S142. (www.care. diabetesjournals.org).

–ACC/AHA; Whelton et al. *JACC*. 2018;71(19):e127-e248.

–JNC8. *JAMA*. 2014;311(5):507-520.

–CHEP. *Can J Cardiol*. 2015;31(5):549-568.

Population

–Adults attempting lifestyle changes for HTN.

Recommendation

IMPACT OF HEALTH BEHAVIOR MANAGEMENT ON BLOOD PRESSURE

Intervention	Systolic BP (mmHg)	Diastolic BP (mmHg)
Diet and weight control	−6.0	−4.8
Reduced salt/sodium intake <2000 mg sodium (Na)[a]	−5.4	−2.8
Reduced alcohol intake (<2 drinks/d)	−3.4	−3.4
DASH diet	−11.4	−5.5
Physical activity (30–40 min 5–7× wk)	−3.1	−1.8
Relaxation therapies	−5.5	−3.5

[a]2000 mg sodium (Na) = 87 mmol sodium (Na) = 5 g of salt (NaCl) ~1 teaspoon of table salt.
Source: Adapted from Canadian Hypertension Education Program (CHEP) Recommendations. 2015. (www.hypertension.ca/en/chep).

LIFESTYLE MODIFICATIONS FOR TREATMENT OF HYPERTENSION

Modification	Recommendation[a]	Approximate SBP Reduction (Range)
Weight reduction	Maintain normal body weight (BMI 18.5–24.9 kg/m^2)	5–20 mmHg per 10-kg weight loss
Adopt DASH eating plan	Consume diet rich in fruits, vegetables, and low-fat dairy products with a reduced content of saturated and total fat	8–14 mmHg
Dietary sodium reduction	Reduce dietary sodium intake to less than 100 mmol/d (2.4 g sodium or 6 g sodium chloride)	2–8 mmHg
Physical activity	Engage in regular aerobic physical activity such as brisk walking (at least 30 min/d, most days of the week)	4–9 mmHg
Moderation of alcohol consumption	Limit consumption to no more than 2 drinks (1 oz or 30 mL ethanol; eg, 24 oz beer, 10 oz wine, or 3 oz 80-proof whiskey) per day in most men and to no more than 1 drink per day in women and lighter-weight persons	2–4 mmHg

DASH, dietary approaches to stop hypertension.
[a]The effects of implementing these modifications are dose- and time-dependent and could be greater for some individuals. DASH diet is effective in lowering SBP in adolescents.
Sources: Couch SC, Saelens BE, Levin L, Dart K, Falciglia G, Daniels SR. The efficacy of a clinic-based behavioral nutrition intervention emphasizing a DASH-type diet for adolescents with elevated blood pressure. *J Pediatr.* 2008;152:494-501. Aronow WS, Fleg JL, Pepine CJ, et al. ACCF/AHA 2011 expert consensus document on hypertension in the elderly: a report of the American College of Cardiology Foundation Task Force on Clinical Expert Consensus documents developed in collaboration with the American Academy of Neurology, American Geriatrics Society, American Society for Preventive Cardiology, American Society of Hypertension, American Society of Nephrology, Association of Black Cardiologists, and European Society of Hypertension. *J Am Coll Cardiol.* 2011:57:2037-2110.

RECOMMENDED MEDICATIONS FOR COMPELLING INDICATIONS

Compelling Indication	Diuretic	BB	ACEI	ARB	CCB	AldoANT
Heart failure	X	X	X	X		X
Post-MI		X	X			X
High coronary disease risk	X	X	X		X	
Diabetes	X		X	X	X	X
Chronic kidney disease[a]			X	X		
Recurrent stroke prevention	X		X			

ACEI, ACE inhibitor; AldoANT, aldosterone antagonist; ARB, angiotensin receptor blocker; BB, beta-blocker; CCB, calcium channel blocker.
Note: Please refer to separate sections of this book to find which medications are considered first line in HTN given the specific comorbidity and why. Each medication has a specific risk/benefit profile.
[a]ALLHAT: Patients with hypertension and reduced GFR: no difference in renal outcomes (development of end-stage renal disease [ESRD] and/or decrement in GFR of ≥50% from baseline) comparing amlodipine, lisinopril, and chlorthalidone (*Arch Intern Med*. 2005;165:936-946). Data do not support preference for CCB, alpha-blockers, or ACEI compared with thiazide diuretics in patients with metabolic syndrome (*Arch Intern Med*. 2008;168:207-217; *J Am Coll Cardiol*. 2011;57:2037-2110; 2012 CHEP Recommendations, http://www.hypertension.ca).

Population
–Adults with refractory hypertension.

Recommendations
–Definition: Failure to reach BP goal (<140/90 mmHg, or 130/80 mmHg in patients with diabetes, heart disease, or chronic kidney disease) using three different antihypertensive drug classes.

–Common causes:
- Nonadherence to drugs/diet.
- Suboptimal therapy/BP measurement (fluid retention, inadequate dosage).
- Diet/drug interactions (caffeine, cocaine, alcohol, nicotine, NSAIDs, steroids, BCP, erythropoietin, natural licorice, herbs).
- Common secondary causes:
  - Obstructive sleep apnea.
  - Diabetes.
  - Chronic kidney disease.
  - Renal artery stenosis.
  - Obesity.
  - Endocrine disorders (primary hyperaldosteronism, hyperthyroidism, hyperparathyroidism, Cushing syndrome), pheochromocytoma.

Therapies
–Exclude nonadherence and incorrect BP measurement.
–Review drug and diet history.
–Screen for secondary causes: History of sleep disorders/daytime sleepiness/tachycardias/BPs in both arms; routine labs: sodium, potassium, creatinine, CBC, ECG, urinalysis, blood glucose,

cholesterol; additional evaluation: aldosterone: renin ratio, renal ultrasound with Doppler flow study, serum or urine catecholamine levels, morning cortisol level.

–Lifestyle therapy: Weight loss (10-kg weight loss results in a 5–20 mmHg decrease in SBP); diet consult for low sodium (2.3 g daily), high fiber, and high potassium (DASH diet results in an 8–14 mmHg decrease in SBP); exercise aerobic training results in a 4–9 mmHg decrease in SBP; and restriction of excess alcohol (1 oz in men and 0.5 oz in women) results in a 2–4 mmHg decrease in SBP.

–Pharmacologic therapy: Consider volume overload.

–Switch from HCTZ to chlorthalidone (especially if GFR < 40 mL/min).

–Switch to loop diuretic if GFR < 30 mL/min (eg, furosemide 40 mg bid).

–Use CCB (amlodipine or nifedipine) + ACE inhibitor or ARB: Consider catecholamine excess.

–Switch to vasodilating beta-blocker (carvedilol, labetalol, nebivolol): Consider aldosterone excess (even with normal serum K+ level).

–Spironolactone or eplerenone.

–Finally, consider hydralazine or minoxidil.

–If already on beta-blocker, clonidine adds little BP benefit.

–Nonpharmacologic therapy: Still under investigation.

–Carotid baroreceptor stimulation (*Hypertension.* 2010;55:1-8): May lower BP 33/22 mmHg.

–Renal artery nerve denervation (SYMPLICITY HTN-3) did not show a significant reduction of SBP in patients with resistant hypertension, 6 mo after the procedure.

Sources

–Bhatt DL, Kandzari DE, O'Neill WW, et al. A controlled trial of renal denervation for resistant hypertension. *N Engl J Med.* 2014;370:1393-1401. Calhoun DA, Jones D, Textor S, et al; American Heart Association Professional Education Committee.

–Resistant hypertension: diagnosis, evaluation, and treatment: a scientific statement from the American Heart Association Professional Education Committee of the Council for High Blood Pressure Research. *Circulation.* 2008;117:e510-e526.

–JNC VII. *Arch Intern Med.* 2003;289:2560-2572.

–European 2007 Guidelines. 2007;28:1462-1536.

–American College of Cardiology/American Heart Association/European Society of Cardiology.

–VA DoD CPG for the Diagnosis and Management of HTN in the Primary Care Setting. https://www.healthquality.va.gov/guidelines/CD/htn/.

Population

–Children and adolescents with hypertension.

Recommendations

–The current definition of HTN in children and adolescents is based on the normative distribution per above; "normal BP" was initially defined as SBP and DBP values <90th percentile (on the basis of age, sex, and height percentiles). See Table 19-8 for age-stratified cutoffs.

–For adolescents, "prehypertension" is BP >120/80 mmHg to <95th percentile or >90th and <95th percentile.

	BP, mmHg			
	Boys		**Girls**	
Age, y	**Systolic**	**DBP**	**Systolic**	**DBP**
1	98	52	98	54
2	100	55	101	58
3	101	58	102	60
4	102	60	103	62
5	103	63	104	64
6	105	66	105	67
7	106	68	106	68
8	107	69	107	69
9	107	70	108	71
10	108	72	109	72
11	110	74	111	74
12	113	75	114	75
≥13	120	80	120	80

TABLE 19-8 SCREENING BP VALUES REQUIRING FURTHER EVALUATION

–Indications for antihypertensive therapy in children and adolescents:
- Symptomatic hypertension.
- Secondary hypertension.
- Hypertensive target organ damage.
- Diabetes (types 1 and 2).
- Persistent hypertension despite nonpharmacologic measures (weight management counseling if overweight; physical activity; diet management).

Sources
–*Pediatrics*. 2011;128(5):S213-S258.
–Kavey RE, Allada V, Daniels SR, et al; American Heart Association Expert Panel on Population and Prevention Science; American Heart Association Council on Cardiovascular Disease in the Young; American Heart Association Council on Epidemiology and Prevention, et al. Cardiovascular risk reduction in high-risk pediatric patients: a scientific statement from the American Heart Association Expert Panel on Population and Prevention Science; the Councils on Cardiovascular Disease in the Young, Epidemiology and Prevention, Nutrition, Physical Activity and Metabolism, High Blood Pressure Research, Cardiovascular Nursing, and the Kidney in Heart Disease; and the Interdisciplinary Working Group on Quality of Care and Outcomes Research: endorsed by the American Academy of Pediatrics. *Circulation*. 2006;114:2710-2738.

PERIPHERAL ARTERIAL DISEASE

Population
  –Adults with lower extremity peripheral arterial disease (PAD).

Organizations
▶ NICE 2020, ACC/AHA 2016

Recommendations
  –In patients with history or physical examination findings suggestive of PAD (most common initial symptom: intermittent claudication), use the resting ankle-brachial index (ABI) to establish the diagnosis.
  –Ensure patient is resting and supine while obtaining systolic blood pressures of brachial arteries, posterior tibialis artery, dorsal pedal artery, and peroneal arteries. If a wave exists, consider using a Doppler probe to determine type of velocity wave form (triphasic, biphasic, or monophasic).
  –Report resting ABI results as abnormal (ABI ≤0.90), borderline (ABI 0.91–0.99), normal (1.00–1.40), or noncompressible (ABI >1.40).
  –Measure toe-brachial index (TBI) to diagnose patients with suspected PAD when the ABI >1.40 (noncompressible).
  –As the ABI in longstanding T2DM may be normal or elevated due to systemic hardening of the arteries, consider imaging if clinically concerned.
  –Use duplex ultrasound of the lower extremities to diagnose anatomic location and severity of stenosis for patients with symptomatic PAD if revascularization is being considered. If nondiagnostic, use MRA. If MRA is contraindicated, use CTA.
  –Counsel patients with PAD and diabetes mellitus about self–foot examination and healthy foot behaviors.
  –Use antiplatelet therapy with aspirin alone (range 75–325 mg/d) or clopidogrel alone (75 mg/d), smoking cessation, a statin, and good glycemic control to reduce MI, stroke, and vascular death in patients with symptomatic PAD.
  –Use cilostazol to improve symptoms and increase walking distance in patients with claudication.
  –Recommend a supervised exercise program for patients with claudication to improve functional status and quality of life and to reduce leg symptoms. A supervised program should involve 120 minutes of supervised exercise a week for at least 3 mo. The exercise should reach a point of maximal reproduced pain.
  –Refer to angioplasty if the exercise program is nonsatisfactory and modifiable risk factors are addressed but nonsatisfactory for symptoms. Endovascular procedures are effective as a revascularization option for patients with lifestyle-limiting claudication and hemodynamically significant aortoiliac occlusive disease.
  –Endovascular procedures establish in-line blood flow to the foot in patients with nonhealing wounds or gangrene.
  –In patients with critical limb ischemia, perform revascularization when possible and construct bypass to the popliteal or infrapopliteal arteries (ie, tibial, pedal) with suitable autogenous vein.

Critical limb ischemia shows diminished circulation, ischemic pain, ulceration, tissue loss, or gangrene. 20% of critical limb ischemia goes onto amputation.

–In patients with acute limb ischemia (ALI), give systemic anticoagulation with heparin immediately unless contraindicated.

–Monitor and treat patients with ALI (eg, fasciotomy) for compartment syndrome after revascularization.

–Perform amputation as the first procedure in patients with a nonsalvageable limb.

Comments

1. Recommend bare metal stents when stenting people with intermittent claudication.
2. Prefer autologous vein bypass when possible for infrainguinal bypass surgery.
3. Prefer bypass surgery over stenting for aortoiliac or femoropopliteal stenosis causing intermittent claudication or critical limb ischemia.
4. Stenting is an option for complete aortoiliac occlusion.

Sources

–*NICE guidelines CG147*. Peripheral arterial disease: diagnosis and management. Updated 11 December 2020.

–2016 AHA/ACC Guideline on the Management of Patients with Lower Extremity Peripheral Artery Disease: executive summary. *Circulation*. 2017;135:e686–e725.

–https://guidelines.gov/summaries/summary/38409

PREOPERATIVE CLEARANCE

Population

–Asymptomatic population without cardiac history.

Organization

▶ ISC1 2019

Recommendations

Preoperative Evaluation

–Do not obtain routine ECG in asymptomatic patients undergoing low-risk[1] surgical procedures.

–Consider ECG in patients with known coronary heart disease, significant arrhythmia, peripheral arterial disease, or other structural heart disease.

–Do NOT routinely perform chest X-rays preoperatively.

–Do NOT routinely test for hemoglobin in healthy, asymptomatic patients. Consider in patients with history of anemia or with prior anticoagulation.

–If known or suspected sleep apnea, communicate with the surgical and anesthesia teams.

–Initiate smoking cessation before elective surgery.

–Delay elective noncardiac surgery at least 60 d after myocardial infarction unless coronary intervention.

[1] ACC/AHA: low risk means combined surgical and patient characteristics that predict risk of a major adverse cardiac event (MACE) of death or MI of <1%.

Perioperative Medications

–If patients have been on beta-blockers, continue, but do not start on the day of surgery to reduce perioperative risk.

–Hold ACEi and ARBs the morning of the surgery (risk for intraoperative hypotension morbidity). No specific recommendation recording calcium channel blockers or diuretic therapies.

–Do not start alpha-2-agonists to prevent cardiac events in noncardiac surgery.

–Continue statins perioperatively.

–If patients require urgent noncardiac surgery in the 4–6 wk after bare metal or drug-eluting stent, continue dual antiplatelets unless relative risk of bleeding exceeds benefit of preventing stent thrombosis.

–If patients on dual antiplatelets for coronary stents require the P2Y12 platelet receptor-inhibitor to be stopped, continue the aspirin if possible and restart the P2Y12 receptor-inhibitor as soon as possible.

Comment

1. ACC Choosing Wisely: Do not obtain stress cardiac imaging or advanced noninvasive imaging as a preoperative assessment in patients scheduled to undergo low-risk noncardiac surgery.

Sources

–http://www.choosingwisely.org/societies/american-college-of-cardiology/
–https://www.icsi.org/guideline/perioperative-guideline/

VALVULAR HEART DISEASE (VHD)

Population

–Adults with mechanical valve or mitral stenosis.

Organizations

▶ AHA/ACC/HRS 2019, ESC 2018, ACCP 2018

Recommendations

–If mechanical valve present, anticoagulate with warfarin titrated to following INR goals:
- Mitral valve: INR 2.5–3.5.
- Aortic valve without increased risk factors for VTE: INR 2.0–3.0.
- Aortic valve with increased risk factors for VTE (AF, prior VTE, LV dysfunction, hypercoagulable state): INR 2.5–3.5. Bridge with heparin or low-molecular-weight heparin for procedures that require warfarin to be held. Do not use direct thrombin inhibitors (dabigatran/edoxaban) or NOACs (rivaroxaban/apixaban).

–NOACs may be used in mild-to-moderate valvular disease. They are also likely acceptable in aortic stenosis (including severe) and >3 mo after mitral valve repair or bioprosthetic valve placement.

Sources

–*JACC.* 2014;64(21):2246-2280. http://www.onlinejacc.org/content/64/21/2246

–*Eur Heart J.* 2016;37:2893-2962.

–*Eur Heart J.* 2018;39(16):1330-1393. https://academic.oup.com/eurheartj/article/39/16/1330/4942493

–*Chest.* 2018;154(4):1121-1201.

–http://www.choosingwisely.org/societies/heart-rhythm-society/

–2016 ESC guidelines for the management of atrial fibrillation developed in collaboration with EACTS.

–2019 AHA/ACC/HRS Focused Update of the 2014 AHA/ACC/HRS. Guideline for the Management of Patients with Atrial Fibrillation.

–Otto CM, Nishimura RA, Bonow RO, et al. 2020 ACC/AHA guideline for the management of patients with valvular heart disease: a report of the American College of Cardiology/American Heart Association Joint Committee on Clinical Practice Guidelines. *Circulation.* 2021;143:e72-e227.

Population

–Adults with valvular heart disease.

–See following sections for specific guidance on aortic stenosis, aortic regurgitation, mitral stenosis, mitral regurgitation, mitral regurgitation as related to infective endocarditis, bicuspid aortic valve.

Organization

▶ ACC/AHA 2020

General Recommendations

–Obtain transthoracic echocardiogram (TTE) with 2D or 3D evaluation of chamber volume. Doppler echo gives noninvasive determination of valve dynamics. Each subtype of VHD has different recommendations of follow-up imaging if TTE is discordant with clinical picture.

–In valvular stenosis, important measurements are maximum velocity across the valve, mean pressure gradient, and valve area.

–In valvular regurgitation, important measurements are regurgitant surface area, volume fraction, and severity grade.

–Patients should be seen at least annually for clinical evaluation. Repeat TTE if there are new symptoms or a change in physical exam.

–Valve replacement replaces a native value disease with a palliated valve disease. If choosing between mechanical and bioprosthetic valves, then patient is choosing between risk of long-term anticoagulation with warfarin versus a risk of reintervention. Therefore, generally older patients receive bioprosthetic valves and younger patients receive mechanical valves.

–If AF develops in first 3 mo after a bioprosthetic valve replacement, use warfarin. After 3 mo with new bioprosthetic valve, if AF develops, can use an NOAC.

–With a mechanical heart valve, the corresponding INR goals for warfarin depend on the location of the valve. Determine the INR at least weekly during initiation and at least monthly when anticoagulation is stable following these goals:

  • Mitral valve: INR 2.5–3.5.
  • Aortic valve without increased risk factors for VTE: INR 2.0–3.0.

- Aortic valve with increased risk factors for VTE (AF, prior VTE, LV dysfunction, hypercoagulable state): INR 2.5–3.5.
  - –Symptoms ongoing after valve replacement may be due to irreversible causes of valve disease such as LV dysfunction, pulmonary HTN, or RV dysfunction. Also may be due to concurrent noncardiac etiologies or other cardiac etiology.
  - –After repair, repeat TTE at 1–3 mo. Then patients should be seen at least annually for clinical evaluation.
  - –**Risk calculator for valve replacement surgery:** https://riskcalc.sts.org/stswebriskcalc/calculate

Population

–Adults with aortic stenosis (AS).

Organization

▶ ACC/AHA 2020

Recommendations

–No medical therapy is available to specifically address AS symptoms or disease progression.

–On TTE, note that velocity and pressure gradients across the valve measured by Doppler may be underestimated if the patient is hypertensive.

–Note that pressure gradients are underestimated if there is LV dysfunction.

–In severe AS with velocity >4.0 m/s, rate of progression is high.

–Exercise treadmill testing is rarely indicated but helpful to evaluate patients who have discordant echo/clinical findings (ie, moderate or severe stenosis in the absence of expected symptoms). Previously undetected symptoms of chest pain, shortness of breath, exertional dizziness, or syncope may be identified to prevent sudden death.

–Guideline-directed medical therapy for HF should be continued in AS.

–Statins prevent atherosclerosis in calcific AS but do not prevent progression of AS hyperdynamics.

–Treat hypertension in the presence of significant AS. HTN doubles the risk for mortality in AS and increases the risk for cardiovascular event in AS. However, abruptly lowering the systolic blood pressure should be avoided so start medication at low dose and increase slowly over months. Resolving the HTN will not stop AS progression.

–Strong indications for aortic valve replacement (AVR):
  - Symptomatic patient (exertional dyspnea or presyncope, HF, angina, syncope).
  - Asymptomatic patients with severe AS and decreased LV function (EF 50%).
  - Asymptomatic patient with severe AS already undergoing another cardiac surgery.

–Percutaneous aortic balloon dilation procedure should be considered a "bridging therapy" to surgical AVR or TAVR/TAVI therapy. However, this procedure is used less frequently in adults given increased availability and success of transcatheter intervention. It is now mostly used in children, adolescents, and young adults.

Population

–Adults with aortic regurgitation (AR).

Organization

▶ ACC/AHA 2020

Recommendations

–Endocarditis is the most common cause of AR. Other causes include aortic dissection, transcatheter procedure, or blunt chest trauma.

–Acute AR may acutely lead to higher LV volumes contributing to low cardiac output and pulmonary congestion.

- Using beta-blockers for associated ascending aortic dissection or aneurysm may increase the transaortic stroke volume, causing a paradoxical increase in systolic blood pressure. Go slowly.
- Do not use beta-blockers in other causes of AR. Cardiac output may suffer without the compensatory tachycardia.

–Cardiac magnetic resonance (CMR) is an alternative form of evaluation if the TTE is nondiagnostic or suboptimal.

–Treat hypertension to keep SBP <140 mmHg with nondihydropyridine calcium channel blocker, ACE inhibitor, or ARB agent.

–Strong indications for AVR:

- Symptomatic (decrease in exercise capacity) with severe AR.
- Asymptomatic with chronic AR and LVEF <55%.
- Going for another cardiac surgery and have severe AR.

Population

–Adults with mitral regurgitation (MR). Includes acute primary, chronic primary, and secondary MR.

Organization

▶ ACC/AHA 2020, 2017

Recommendations

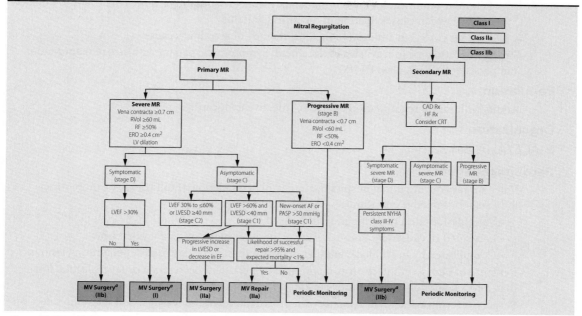

AF, atrial fibrillation; CAD, coronary artery disease; CRT, cardiac resynchronization therapy; EF, ejection fraction; ERO, effective regurgitant orifice; HF, heart failure; LV, left ventricular; LVEF, left ventricular ejection fraction; LVESD, left ventricular end-systolic diameter; MR, mitral regurgitation; MV, mitral valve; NYHA, New York Heart Association; PASP, pulmonary artery systolic pressure; RF, regurgitant fraction; RVol, regurgitant volume; Rx, therapy.
[a]MV repair is preferred over MV replacement when possible.

- Acute primary MR is a rupture of papillary muscles during inferior wall acute STEMI, causing acute hemodynamic decompensation without forward cardiac output and with pulmonary congestion. The vasodilators nitroprusside and nicardipine are good medications while awaiting catheterization because these are easily titrated off in the setting of hypotension due to poor cardiac output.
- Chronic primary MR:
  - Most common cause is mitral valve prolapse.
  - Order of imaging should be TTE to TEE. Use CMR if TTE and TEE are discrepant. If the patient is asymptomatic with severe primary MR, a TTE should be performed every 6–12 mo. TEE is indicated during intraoperative repair.
  - The ideal ejection fraction for the left ventricle is ~70% for adequate leaflet coaptation.

–Secondary MR:
  - Occurs if the left ventricle is too dilated from ischemia or CHF causing awkward positioning of chordae tendineae so there is inadequate leaflet coaptation or if the left atria is too dilated from AF which causes dilation of the mitral annulus
  - Consider CABG in addition to medical therapy of secondary cause.

–Strong indication for mitral valve replacement: Symptomatic patient with severe regurgitation and persistent NYHA class III–IV.

Population

–Adults with mitral regurgitation related to infective endocarditis.

Organization

▶ ACC/AHA 2017

Recommendations

–Valve surgery during initial hospitalization before completion of full course of antibiotics is indicated for infective endocarditis (IE) associated with:
  - Valve dysfunction resulting in symptoms of HF.
  - Left-sided IE caused by *S. aureus*, fungal, or other highly resistant organisms.
  - Complicated by heart block, annular or aortic abscess, or destructive penetrating lesions.

–Evidence of persistent infection as manifested by persistent bacteremia or fevers lasting longer than 5 to 7 d after onset of appropriate antimicrobial therapy.

–Surgery is recommended for patients with prosthetic valve endocarditis and relapsing infection (defined as recurrence of bacteremia after a complete course of appropriate antibiotics and subsequently negative blood cultures) without other identifiable source for portal of infection.

–Complete removal of pacemaker or defibrillator systems, including all leads and the generator, is indicated as part of the early management plan in patients with IE with documented infection of the device or leads.

Population

–Adults with mitral stenosis.

Organization

▶ ACC/AHA 2020

Recommendations

–The majority of mitral stenosis is due to rheumatic heart disease. The time between initial rheumatic illness and MS can be decades. In older people the cause of MS is more often calcific MS. Between age and comorbidities, the prognosis of calcific MS is <50% in 5 y, meaning the indications for intervention are palliative in highly asymptomatic patients.

–Consider transesophageal echocardiogram (TEE) prior to sending the patient for percutaneous mitral balloon commissurotomy (PMBC) to exclude the presence of left atrial thrombus.

–Give warfarin to patients with mitral stenosis and AF, prior embolic event, or intracardiac thrombus. Rheumatic MS patients were excluded from DOAC studies, hence indication for warfarin in Afib.

–Use rate control in Afib and MS to allow optimal diastolic filling time across the stenotic valve. The fibrosis in rheumatic MS may also make it more challenging to rhythm control.

–To increase exercise duration and improve symptoms in younger people, beta-blockers or ivabradine may be beneficial.

–Balloon commissurotomy is indicated in symptomatic patients with severe mitral stenosis (MVA <1.5 cm^2) with no atrial thrombus and no or minimal mitral insufficiency. In rheumatic disease, delay until NYHA III or IV due to slow course of disease.

–Mitral valve replacement is indicated if balloon commissurotomy is contraindicated in a patient with severe symptoms and severe mitral stenosis.

Population

–Adults with bicuspid aortic valve (BAV).

Organization

▶ ACC/AHA 2020

Recommendations

–Aortic aneurysms will affect 20%–40% of adults with BAV. They therefore require lifelong surveillance even in the absence of symptoms.

–Replace the valve if the diameter of the ascending aorta or aortic sinuses is >5.5 cm.

Sources

–Otto CM, Nishimura RA, Bonow RO, et al. 2020 ACC/AHA guideline for the management of patients with valvular heart disease: a report of the American College of Cardiology/American Heart Association Joint Committee on Clinical Practice Guidelines. *Circulation.* 2021;143: e72-e227.

–2017 AHA/ACC focused update of the 2014 AHA/ACC guideline for the management of patients with valvular heart disease: a report of the American College of Cardiology/American Heart Association Task Force on Clinical Practice Guidelines. *Circulation.* 2017;135: e1159–e1195.

Care of the Older Adult

20

DEMENTIA, FEEDING TUBES

Population
- –Patients with advanced dementia.

Organization
▶ American Geriatrics Society 2014

Recommendations
- –Do not use feeding tubes for older adults with advanced dementia.
- –Offer careful hand feeding instead.

Comment
1. Careful hand-feedings and tube-feedings have identical outcomes of death, aspiration pneumonia, functional status, and patient comfort. In addition, tube-feeding is associated with agitation, increased use of physical and chemical restraints, and worsening pressure ulcers.

Source
- –http://americangeriatrics.org/health_care_professionals/clinical_practice/clinical_guidelines_recommendations/2014

DEMENTIA, ALZHEIMER DISEASE

Population
- –Adults.

Organization
▶ NICE 2019, American Geriatric Society 2015

Recommendations
- –Ensure that people with dementia have a designated physician or clinician to coordinate their care.
- –At initial assessment take a history including cognitive, behavioral, psychological symptoms and impact on daily life. Discuss advanced care planning early and ongoing.
- –Donepezil, galantamine, and rivastigmine are options for mild-to-moderate Alzheimer disease.

–Consider memantine for moderate Alzheimer disease in patients who cannot tolerate acetylcholinesterase inhibitors, or in severe Alzheimer disease.

–Offer occupational therapy, group reminiscence therapy, group cognitive stimulation in mild-to-moderate dementia.

–Do not offer ginseng, vitamin E supplements, acupuncture, or herbal formulations to treat dementia. Do not offer cognitive training to treat mild-to-moderate Alzheimer disease or interpersonal therapy to treat cognitive symptoms of mild-to-moderate disease.

–Antipsychotics: Do not use as first line. Only use if acute agitations/hallucinations/delusions are causing severe stress or patient at risk of harm to self or others. Use lowest effective dose and revisit need every 6 wk.

Comments

1. Common adverse effects of acetylcholinesterase inhibitors include diarrhea, nausea, vomiting, muscle cramps, bradycardia, and insomnia.

2. Common adverse effects of memantine are dizziness, headache, constipation, somnolence, and hypertension.

3. Reassess the efficacy of the pharmacological intervention. If the desired clinical effect (eg, stabilization of cognition) is not perceived by 12 wk or so, discontinue the medication. (AGS 2015)

4. Ineffective medications include statins, NSAID, ginkgo, omega-3 fatty acids. (AAFP 2017)

5. Antipsychotics have limited and inconsistent benefit while posing risks including increased fall, strokes, and mortality, oversedation, and cognitive worsening.

Source

–*NICE Guidance: Dementia: Assessment, Management and Support for People Living with Dementia and Their Carers. NICE guideline (NG97); 2019. www.nice.org.uk/guidance/qs184*

DEMENTIA

Population

–Adults with non-Alzheimer dementia.

Organization

▶ NICE 2019

Recommendations

–Offer donepezil or rivastigmine in patients with mild-to-moderate dementia with Lewy bodies. Consider galantamine if donepezil/rivastigmine is not tolerated.

–Consider memantine for patient with Lewy bodies if AChE inhibitors are not tolerated or are contraindicated.

–Only consider AChE inhibitors or memantine for people with vascular dementia if they have suspected comorbid Alzheimer dementia, Parkinson's disease dementia, or dementia with Lewy bodies.

–AChE inhibitors and memantine are not recommended for patients with frontotemporal dementia or cognitive impairment caused by multiple sclerosis.

Source

–NICE Guidance: *Dementia: Assessment, Management and Support for People Living with Dementia and Their Carers.* NICE guideline (NG97); 2019. www.nice.org.uk/guidance/qs184

DELIRIUM, POSTOPERATIVE

Population

–Older adults at risk for or who have postoperative delirium.

Organization

▶ AGS 2021

Recommendations

–Institutions should enact multicomponent nonpharmacologic intervention programs to manage delirium for entire hospitalization.

–Consider regional anesthesia at the time of surgery to improve postoperative pain control and reduce delirium risk.

–Avoid inappropriate medications postoperatively in older adults. Optimize postoperative pain control, preferably with nonopioid pain medication.

–Use antipsychotics at the lowest effective dose and for the shortest duration possible to treat severe agitated delirium.

–Do not newly prescribe prophylactic cholinesterase inhibitors in the perioperative setting to prevent or treat delirium.

–Avoid benzodiazepines for postoperative delirium.

–Avoid pharmacologic therapy for hypoactive delirium.

–Avoid use of physical restraints.

Source

–*J Am Geriatr Soc.* 2015;63(1):124-150.

Comments

1. Inappropriate medications include benzodiazepines, anticholinergics (eg, cyclobenzaprine, paroxetine, tricyclic antidepressants, diphenhydramine), H2-receptor blockers, sedative-hypnotics, and meperidine.

2. Pharmacologic tx of hypoactive delirium has not shown to modify duration or severity of postoperative delirium; do not use antipsychotics in hypoactive delirium unless agitation threatens safety of patient or others.

HIP FRACTURES

Population
–Elderly patients with hip fractures.

Organization
▶ AAOS 2015

Recommendations
–Use preoperative pain control in patients with hip fractures.
–Perform hip fracture surgery within 48 h of admission.
–Do not delay hip fracture surgery for patients on antiplatelet drugs.
–Perform operative fixation for nondisplaced femoral neck fractures.
–Perform unipolar or hemipolar hemiarthroplasty for displaced femoral neck fractures.
–Arrange intensive physical therapy postdischarge to improve functional outcomes.
–Evaluate all patients who have sustained a hip fracture for osteoporosis.

Source
–AAOS. *Management of hip Fractures in the Elderly, Evidence-Based Clinical Practice Guideline.* aaos.org/globalassets/quality-and-practice-resources/hip-fractures-in-the-elderly

PALLIATIVE CARE OF DYING ADULTS

Population
–Dying adults.

Organizations
▶ NICE 2017, NCCN 2020

Recommendations
–Care of the dying patient should be aligned with the patient's goals and wishes and cultural values.
–Give patients and people important to them opportunities to discuss, develop, and review an individualized care plan.
–Symptom management should address physical, emotional, social, and spiritual needs.
–Determine who should be the surrogate decision maker if they cannot make their own decisions.
–Establish if the patient has a preferred care setting.
–Medical management of symptoms:
  • Pain is typically managed with opioids.
  • Breathlessness can be managed with opioids or benzodiazepines +/– oxygen (if on chronic opiates, increase O_2 by 25%). Nonpharmacologic therapies include fans, cooler temperatures, stress management, relaxation therapy, and physical comfort measures.
  • Manage nausea with dopamine antagonists or 5-HT3 antagonists. May add benzodiazepines especially with anxiety component. If vertiginous components, add anticholinergics or

antihistamines. Identify cause of nausea and treat that part of emetic pathway. Haloperidol, metoclopramide, and dexamethasone are options if nausea is refractory.

- Anxiety can be managed with benzodiazepines.
- Reduce or eliminate delirium causing agents such as steroids, anticholinergics, or benzodiazepines. Manage with antipsychotics.
- Manage secretions by reducing fluids (IV or PO), repositioning pt, and using pharmacologic agents such as scopolamine, atropine, or glycopyrrolate.

Comment

1. Recognize and treat opioid-induced neurotoxicity, including myoclonus and hyperalgesia.

Sources

–NICE. 2015 Guideline); *Quality Standard. Care of Dying Adults in the Last Days of Life.* 2017.
–NCCN Guidelines Version 2. 2020 Palliative Care.
–WHO's cancer pain ladder for adults. who.int/cancer/palliative/painladder

PALLIATIVE AND END-OF-LIFE CARE: PAIN MANAGEMENT	
Principles of Analgesic Use	
By the mouth	The oral route is the preferred route for analgesics, including morphine
By the clock	Persistent pain requires round-the-clock treatment to prevent further pain. As-needed (PRN) dosing is irrational and inhumane; it requires patients to experience pain before becoming eligible for relief. Relief is accomplished with long-acting delayed-release preparations (fentanyl patch, slow-release morphine, or oxycodone)
By the WHO ladder	If a maximum dose of medication fails to adequately relieve pain, move up the ladder, not laterally to a different drug in the same efficiency group. Severe pain requires immediate use of an opioid recommended for controlling severe pain, without progressing sequentially through Steps 1 and 2. When using a long-acting opioid, the dose for breakthrough pain should be 10% of the 24-h opioid dose (ie, if a patient is on 100 mg/d of an extended-release morphine preparation, their breakthrough dose is 10 mg of morphine or equivalent every 1–2 h until pain relief is achieved). Refer to appendix "WHO Pain Relief Ladder" in Chapter 33
Individualize treatment	The right dose of an analgesic is the dose that relieves pain with acceptable side effects for a specific patient
Monitor	Monitoring is required to ensure the benefits of treatment are maximized while adverse effects are minimized
Use adjuvant drugs	For example, a nonsteroidal anti-inflammatory drug (NSAID) is often helpful in controlling bone pain. Nonopioid analgesics, such as NSAIDs or acetaminophen, can be used at any step of the ladder. Adjuvant medications also can be used at any step to enhance pain relief or counteract the adverse effects of medications. Neuropathic pain should be treated with gabapentin, duloxetine, nortriptyline, or pregabalin. Moderate- to high-dose dexamethasone is effective as an adjunct to opioids in a pain crisis situation

Source: Adapted from *Pocket Guide to Hospice/Palliative Medicine.*

Endocrine and Metabolic Disorders

21

ADRENAL INCIDENTALOMAS

Population
–Adults.

Organization
▶ AACE 2009

Recommendations
–Evaluate clinically, biochemically, and radiographically for evidence of hypercortisolism, aldosteronism, the presence of pheochromocytoma or a malignant tumor.
–Reevaluate patients who will be managed expectantly at 3–6 mo and then annually for 1–2 y.

Comments
1. A 1-mg overnight dexamethasone suppression test can be used to screen for hypercortisolism.
2. Measure plasma-fractionated metanephrines and normetanephrines to screen for pheochromocytoma.
3. Measure plasma renin activity and aldosterone concentration to assess for primary or secondary aldosteronism.

Source
–https://www.aace.com/files/adrenal-guidelines.pdf

CUSHING'S SYNDROME (CS)

Population
–Pediatric and adult patients with Cushing's syndrome.

Organization
▶ Endocrine Society 2015

Recommendations
–Treatment goals for Cushing's syndrome:
  • Normalize cortisol levels to eliminate the signs and symptoms of CS.
  • Monitor and treat cortisol-dependent comorbidities.

–Recommend vaccinations against influenza, herpes zoster, pneumococcus.

–Recommend perioperative thromboprophylaxis for venous thromboembolism.

–Recommend surgical resection of primary adrenal or ectopic focus underlying CS.

–Assess postoperative serum cortisol levels.

Source

–www.endocrine.org/guidelines-and-clinical-practice/clinical-practice-guidelines/treatment-of-cushing-syndrome

DIABETES MELLITUS (DM), TYPE 1

Population

–Children with Type I DM.

Organizations

▶ ADA 2021, NICE 2020

Recommendations

Evaluation at Diagnosis

– Screen for other autoimmune conditions at time of diagnosis of type 1 DM:
  ○ Celiac disease: IgA tissue transglutaminase antibodies. If negative, rescreen at 2 and 5 y after DM diagnosis.
  ○ Thyroid disease: Check TSH, thyroid peroxidase, and thyroglobulin antibodies; screen q 1-2 y thereafter.
  ○ Pernicious anemia: Check B12 level if anemia or peripheral neuropathy is present. (ADA)

Therapies

– Use intensive insulin therapy with >3 injections daily using either basal and prandial insulin or an insulin pump.

– Instruct patients using multiple insulin injections to self-monitor blood glucose at least 4 times daily.

– Offer Diabetes Self-Management Education and Support (DSMES).

– Offer Medical Nutrition Therapy, preferably with a registered dietician nutritionist.

– Encourage physical activity: 60 min/d of moderate-intensity aerobic activity, 3 d/wk of muscle and bone-strengthening activities.

– Assess psychological and social situation.

– Advise all patients not to smoke.

– Consider statin therapy if age ≥10 y and LDL ≥160 mg/dL, or LDL ≥130 mg/dL and one or more CVD risk factors.

Treatment Goals

– Consider continuous glucose monitoring, as it results in lower HbA1c levels.

GUIDELINES DISCORDANT: GLYCEMIC CONTROL TARGETS	
Organization	**Guidance**
ADA	A1c goal <7% appropriate for most, <6.5% if obtainable without hypoglycemia, or 7%–8% if hypoglycemia unawareness
NICE	Glucose targets are: • 72–126 mg/dL fasting • 72–126 mg/dL before meals • 90–162 mg/dL 90 min after meals • HbA1c ≤6.5%.

Surveillance

GUIDELINES DISCORDANT: SURVEILLANCE TESTING	
Organization	**Guidance**
ADA	Begin screening at age 10, at onset of puberty, or 5 y after diagnosis of type 1 DM, whichever is earlier: • Albuminuria: albumin-to-creatinine ratio (ACR) annually • Retinopathy: fundoscopic exam every 2-4 y • Comprehensive foot exam and monofilament testing annually • Lipid panel near time of diagnosis, at 9–11 y, and q 3 y thereafter – If abnormal, confirm with fasting labs and repeat annually
NICE	Begin screening annually at 12 y of age: • Albuminuria: Urine albumin-to-creatinine ratio (ACR) • Retinopathy: Fundoscopic exam • Comprehensive foot examination and monofilament testing

Sources
–https://diabetesjournals.org/care/article/44/Supplement_1/S180/30606/13-Children-and-Adolescents-Standards-of-Medical
–https://www.nice.org.uk/guidance/ng18

Population
–Adults with Type I DM.

Organizations
▶ ADA 2021, NICE 2020

Recommendations

Evaluation at Diagnosis
– Do *not* routinely confirm diagnosis of type 1 DM by checking C-peptide levels or auto-antibody testing. Consider doing so only if diagnosis is uncertain. (NICE)

- Screen for other autoimmune conditions at time of diagnosis of type 1 DM (ADA):
  - ◦ Celiac disease: IgA tissue transglutaminase antibodies. If negative, rescreen 2 and 5 y after DM diagnosis.
  - ◦ Thyroid dysfunction: Check TSH, thyroid peroxidase, and thyroglobulin antibodies initially; routine screening thereafter.
  - ◦ Pernicious anemia: Check B12 level if anemia or peripheral neuropathy is present.

Therapies
- If using multiple insulin injections, self-monitor blood glucose at least 4 times daily.
- Consider continuous glucose monitoring, as it results in lower HbA1c levels. (ADA)
- Provide all adults with DM 1 a structured education program including carbohydrate counting education, benefits of routine exercise, avoidance of smoking, management of hypoglycemia, and peer support groups.

Treatment Goals
- Measure glycohemoglobin every 3–6 mo. Fructosamine level is an alternative test for anemic patients.

Surveillance
- Surveillance for complications:
  - ◦ Urine albumin-to-creatinine ratio annually.
  - ◦ Dilated fundoscopic exam upon diagnosis and q 2 y after initial assessment.
  - ◦ Monofilament screening for diabetic neuropathy annually.
  - ◦ Comprehensive foot examination at least annually.
- Fasting lipid panel: repeat annually if results are abnormal or every 5 y if results are acceptable (LDL <100 mg/dL).
- TSH annually. (NICE)

GUIDELINES DISCORDANT: INSULIN STRATEGY	
Organization	**Guidance**
ADA	Use intensive insulin therapy with >3 injections daily using either basal and prandial insulin or an insulin pump
NICE	Use basal insulin, preferably insulin detemir BID, or daily glargine if BID detemir isn't acceptable or tolerated
	Use rapid-acting prandial insulin analogs (vs. human or animal insulin) before meals (not after meals)

GUIDELINES DISCORDANT: GLYCEMIC CONTROL TARGETS	
Organization	**Guidance**
ADA	A1c goal <7% appropriate for most, <6.5% if obtainable without hypoglycemia, or 7%–8% if hypoglycemia unawareness

GUIDELINES DISCORDANT: GLYCEMIC CONTROL TARGETS (Continued)	
Organization	**Guidance**
NICE	Glucose targets are: • 90–126 mg/dL fasting • 72–126 mg/dL before meals • 90–162 mg/dL 90 min after meals • HbA1c ≤6.5%

GUIDELINES DISCORDANT: ROLE OF STATINS	
Organization	**Guidance**
ADA	Consider the use of moderate-intensity statin therapy in those with DM1 who have one or more ASCVD risk factors
NICE	Consider statin therapy for all with DM1 Prescribe atorvastatin 20 mg for those that are older than 40 y, have had DM1 > 10 y, have nephropathy, or have other CVD risk factors
ESC 2019[a]	Consider starting a statin in all patients >30 y with T1DM, even if asymptomatic or with normal lipid panel

GUIDELINES DISCORDANT: ROLE OF ASPIRIN	
Organization	**Guidance**
ADA	Consider Aspirin 75–162 mg/d for adults with a 10 y risk of CVD >10% Provide Aspirin 75–162 mg/d if preexisting CVD is present
NICE	Do *not* offer aspirin for primary prevention of CVD to adults with DM1

Sources
–https://diabetesjournals.org/care/issue/44/Supplement_1
–https://nice.org.uk/guidance/ng17
–https://academic.oup.com/eurheartj/article/41/2/255/5556890

DIABETES MELLITUS (DM), TYPE 2

Population
–Nonpregnant adults.
–*Management of adults with comorbid coronary artery disease and hypertension is discussed in Chapter 19: Cardiovascular Diseases.*

Organizations
▶ AACE/ACE 2020, ACP 2017/2018, ADA 2021, ESC 2019, NICE 2020

Recommendations

Lifestyle Interventions

– Weight loss: recommend >5% weight loss if overweight or obese; consider adjunctive weight loss medications approved by FDA. (ADA, AACE, IDF)

– Reduced-calorie meal plan (500–750 kcal/d energy deficit), physical activity (150 min/wk moderate aerobic activity), behavioral intervention. (ADA, AACE, IDF)

– Recommend bariatric surgery for good surgical candidates who meet criteria (see below table).

– Use a multidisciplinary team–based model (including physicians, nurses, dietitians, exercise specialists, dentists, podiatrists, mental health, etc.). Assess barriers to care including food, housing, and financial insecurity as well as literacy and numeracy. Refer to available community resources. (ADA)

– Provide diabetes self-management education and support (DSMES) at appropriate intervals including education about hypoglycemia management and adjustments during illness. (ADA)

– Advise against tobacco use, including e-cigarettes (given evidence of associated deaths), and provide smoking cessation counseling/treatment routinely.

Medication Therapies

– Individualize medication regimens and blood glucose targets (fasting and postprandial) based on patient-specific factors (likely adherence, safety, efficacy, cost, and comorbidities such as cardiac, cerebrovascular, hepatic, and renal disease). (AACE)

– Use metformin as first-line medication.[1] (AACE, ADA, ACP, IDF, NICE)

– Start with metformin monotherapy unless A1c is >9%. (ADA)

– Combination therapy is usually necessary. Choose agents with complementary mechanisms of action, especially in patients with comorbidities (AACE). See Table 21-1 for a more detailed description of various agents available, and Tables 21-2 and 21-3 for further guidance for patients with specific comorbidities.

– Add either a sulfonylurea, a thiazolidinedione (pioglitazone), an SGLT2 inhibitor, or a DPP-4 inhibitor to metformin when a second agent is required, based on discussion of benefits, adverse effects, and cost. (ACP, NICE)

– Considering starting two agents if the HbA1c is 1%–2% or more above target. Combination therapy should be metformin plus sulfonylurea (SU),[2] DPP4 inhibitor, SGLT2 inhibitor,[3] or GLP1 receptor agonist.[4] (IDF)

– Initiate dual therapy if A1c is >1.5% above target; consider early combination therapy (rather than standard stepwise approach) at time of medication initiation to possibly extend time to treatment failure based on VERIFY trial. Individualize medication regimen based on comorbidities, cost, hypoglycemia risk, weight effect, and patient preference. (ADA)

Insulin Therapies

– Consider initiating insulin in the following situations: ongoing catabolic weight loss, symptomatic hyperglycemia, A1c >10% or BG >300 mg/dL. (ADA)

---

[1]Titrate metformin from 500 to 2000 mg/d to minimize GI side effects.
[2]When starting an SU, the patient must learn how to prevent, recognize, and treat hypoglycemia.
[3]SGLT2 inhibitors reduce major cardiovascular events in patients with T2D and are preferred in patients with CVD. Counsel on the increased risk for urinary tract infections.
[4]GLP1 RA can be used if weight loss is a priority and the drug is affordable.

TABLE 21-1 NONINSULIN OPTIONS FOR THE MANAGEMENT OF DIABETES

Agent	Pros	Cons
Metformin	- Mortality Benefit - Low hypoglycemia risk - Weight neutral - Low cost	- Risk of GI upset and lactic acidosis
Sulfonylurea	- Lowers glucose effectively - Low cost	- Weight gain - Moderate hypoglycemia risk
Thiazolidinedione	- Lowers glucose effectively - Low cost	- Weight gain - Risk of edema, heart failure, fractures
DPP-4 inhibitor	- Low hypoglycemia risk - Weight neutral - Rare side effects	- Lowers glucose modestly - Costly
SGLT2 inhibitor	- Low hypoglycemia risk - Causes weight loss	- Lowers glucose modestly - Risk of GU infections, dehydration, fractures - Costly
GLP-1 receptor agonist	- Lowers glucose effectively - Low hypoglycemia risk - Causes weight loss	- Risk of GI upset - Costly

Note: Any of these can be combined except DPP-4 and GLP-1, as their mechanisms of action overlap. Avoid sulfonylureas in patients on insulin therapy because of the hypoglycemia risk.
Source: Adapted from Introduction: Standards of Medical Care in Diabetes. *Diabetes Care.* 2021;44(Suppl 1):S1-S2. doi:10.2337/dc21-Sint

- Start with basal insulin (10 IU/day or 0.1–0.2 IU/kg/d); begin 4 units, 0.1 U/kg or 10% of basal dose, titrate up by 1-2 units or 10-15% weekly; if A1c not controlled add short-acting insulin to other large meals. Can consider adding GLP-1 RA before starting prandial insulin. Can also consider premixed insulin BID instead of prandial insulin.
- If A1c remains above goal, add GLP-1 RA or initiate prandial insulin.
- If initiating prandial insulin, start with 4 units, 0.1 U/kg or 10% of basal dose, titrate up by 1-2 units or 10-15% weekly; if A1c not controlled add short-acting insulin to other large meals.
- As an alternative to prandial insulin, consider changing to premixed insulin before breakfast and dinner.
- Consider starting insulin after addition of second or third oral agent and HbA1c > 7%. (NICE)
  ○ Initial insulin therapy: NPH once or twice daily versus long-acting insulin.
  ○ Consider basal bolus versus pre-mixed biphasic regimen if A1c > 9%.

Treatment Goals
- Glycemic control recommendations [ADA]:
  ○ Pre-prandial glucose: 70–130 mg/dL.
  ○ Postprandial glucose: <180 mg/dL (1–2 h post meals).

TABLE 21-2 RECOMMENDATIONS FOR ADJUNCTIVE DIABETES THERAPIES COMPLEMENTARY TO COMMON COMORBIDITIES

Comorbidity	ADA	ESC
ASCVD	Add an SGLT2 inhibitor or GLP1-RA regardless of A1c unless contraindicated	Prioritize empagliflozin and/or liraglutide (both have mortality benefit and reduce CV events) Then consider canagliflozin, dapagliflozin, semaglutide, and dulaglutide (which reduce CV events)
HF (particularly EF < 45%)	Choose SGLT2 over GLP1-RA	Further considerations in HF: • Preferentially start sacubitril/valsartan instead of ACEI • Use GLP1-RAs and DPP4 inhibitors except saxagliptan if additional agents are needed • Avoid thiazolidinediones • Consider device therapy (ICD, CRT, CRT-D) • Pursue CABG if 2 or 3 vessel CAD • Consider ivabradine in symptomatic patients in sinus rhythm with HR ≥70 and already on max. therapy • Avoid aliskiren
CKD with albuminuria	Use an SGLT2 over GLP1-RA	No recommendation
CKD without albuminuria	Either SGLT2 or GLP1-RA	No recommendation

 ◦ CGM parameters: TIR ("time-in-range") should be used to assess glucose control (associated with risk of microvascular complications) and "time below/above target" should be used to reevaluate treatment regimen.

Prevention of Complications

– Minimize the risks of hypoglycemia, weight gain, and other adverse drug reactions. (AACE)
– Hypoglycemia: Assess for symptomatic/asymptomatic hypoglycemia (BG <70 mg/dL) at each visit. Prescribe IM or intranasal glucagon to patients at high risk of level 2 hypoglycemia (BG <54 mg/dL). Reevaluate treatment regimen and glycemic targets if hypoglycemia unawareness or level 3 hypoglycemia (altered mental/physical functioning requiring assistance). (ADA)
– Control lipids and blood pressure. (AACE)
– Optimize BP alongside glycemic control to prevent progression of diabetic kidney disease.
– All patients with T2DM and HTN > 140/90 should monitor their BP at home. (ADA)
– Recommend ACEI or ARB for patients with hypertension and diabetes with urinary albumin-to-creatinine ratio >30 mg/g creatinine or eGFR <60 mL/min/1.73 m². (ADA, IDF)
 ◦ ACEI/ARB should be started if patient has microalbuminuria without high BP. (IDF)
– Additional therapy with CCB or thiazide diuretic as needed to reach BP goals. (ADA)
– Antiplatelet agents for primary and secondary prevention of CVD are indicated.
– Immunizations: PPSV23 both before and after age 65; influenza annually; 2 or 3 dose hepatitis B series if <60 y, or 3 dose hepatitis B series if ≥60; HPV ≤ 26-y-old, 27–45-y-old if desired; TDAP q10y; Zoster 2 doses ≥ 50. (ADA)

TABLE 21-3 INTERNATIONAL PANEL GUIDELINE ON SELECTING SGLT-2 INHIBITORS OR GLP-1 RECEPTOR AGONISTS

Population	SGLT-2	GLP-1	Comments
Patients with 3 cardiovascular risk factors or fewer	Avoid for most		While there is a small mortality benefit with both agents and small cardiovascular benefit with SGLT-2s, there is a large increase in genital infections (vaginitis, balanitis) with SGLT-2s and severe GI events (pain, nausea, vomiting, diarrhea) with GLP-1s
Patients with >3 cardiovascular risk factors	Consider for most	Avoid for most	The mortality benefit for SGLT-2s becomes more pronounced in higher risk patients
Patients with established cardiovascular or renal disease	Offer one or the other to most		Both agents offer mortality benefit; GLP-1 reduces stroke incidence and SGLT-2s reduce nonfatal MI and heart failure exacerbations in this group
Patients with established cardiovascular and renal disease	Offer to all	Offer as alternative	The benefits seen in patients with cardiovascular or renal disease are more pronounced in those with both, but the mortality benefit is larger with SGLT-2s

Note: A panel reviewed a meta-analysis of benefits and harms from SGLT-2 and GLP-1 agents, incorporated patient focus groups, and assessed practical implications of the recommendations. These recommendations are independent of effect on A1c. Patient-oriented benefits of reducing A1c in type 2 DM are underwhelming, while SGLT-2 and GLP-1 agents have renal- and cardioprotective benefits independent of blood glucose reduction.

Source: BMJ. 2021;373:n1091. https://doi.org/10.1136/bmj.n1091

- Refer patients with any evidence of diabetic retinopathy to ophthalmologist. (ADA, NICE)
- Patients who observe Ramadan should interrupt their fast if SMBG is <70 or >300. High-risk patients are advised not to fast at all.

Surveillance
- Monitor therapy q 3 mo until stable, then at least twice a year. (AACE, ADA)
- Assess for symptomatic/asymptomatic hypoglycemia (BG <70 mg/dL) at each visit. (ADA)
- On follow-up, address interval medical history, medication adherence, side effects including hypoglycemia, lab evaluation, nutrition, psychosocial health, routine health maintenance screening. (AACE, ADA)
- Perform foot examination at every visit for high-risk patients, and annually for lower risk patients. (ADA, IDF, NICE)
- Screen for or check annually:
  ◦ Lipid panel if on statin therapy (otherwise, q 5 y is sufficient). (ADA)
  ◦ Dilated funduscopic exam or retinal photography q1–2 y. (ADA, IDF)
  ◦ Monofilament screening for diabetic neuropathy. (ADA, IDF)

- Screen for peripheral vascular disease by checking foot pulses and/or calculating the ankle/brachial index. (IDF)
- Depression with PHQ-2. (IDF)

GUIDELINES DISCORDANT: WHEN TO REFER TO BARIATRIC SURGERY IN DM2

Organization	Guidance
ADA	BMI ≥40 kg/m² (≥37.5 kg/m² in Asian-Americans), or ≥35 kg/m² without durable weight loss and poor diabetes control with nonsurgical methods
IDF	BMI ≥35 kg/m², or BMI 30–35 kg/m² who have not responded to regular treatment
NICE	Expedited referral for BMI > 35 kg/m², consider referral for BMI 30–34.9 kg/m², or those of Asian descent even with lower BMI than 30 kg/m². All should be receiving concomitant medical therapy

GUIDELINES DISCORDANT: A1C TARGET

Organization	Guidance
ADA	<7%; less (8%) or more stringent (<6.5%) goals may be appropriate for select patients
AACE	6.5%; consider higher targets if older or with comorbidities
ACP	7%–8%; de-intensify therapy if A1c < 6.5% or if life expectancy < 10 y
IDF	<7%; <8% if life expectancy <10 y
NICE	6.5%; higher (7%) if on a drug known to cause hypoglycemia; higher targets on case-by-case basis

GUIDELINES DISCORDANT: LIPID STRATEGY IN DM2

Organization	Guidance
ADA	High-intensity statin therapy if diabetes plus existing ASCVD or 10-y ASCVD risk >20%. Consider addition of ezetimibe or PCSK-9 as well. Moderate-intensity statin therapy if >40 y and no ASCVD or consider if <40 y with ASCVD risk. Add LDL-lowering therapy (ezetimibe or PCSK9 inhibitor) if LDL >70 mg/dL on max statin with existing CVD
ESC	Titrate lipid therapy to CV risk such that LDL <100 for moderate risk, <70 and with ≥50% reduction for high risk, and <55 with ≥50% reduction for very high risk. Consider adding ezetimibe +/− PCSK9 inhibitor if not at goal
IDF	Prescribe a high-intensity statin for patients with: established CVD (secondary prevention) or without CVD who are >40 y with LDL >100 mg/dL (primary prevention)

GUIDELINES DISCORDANT: BP GOALS IN DM2	
Organization	**Guidance**
ADA	Target BP <130/80 mmHg if 10-y ASCVD risk >15% or existing ASCVD, and <140/90 for lower risk patients. Recommend single-agent pharmacotherapy for BP >140/90 and two drug therapy for BP <160/100
ESC	SBP of 120–130 and DBP of 70–80 unless age ≥65 without high risk of cerebrovascular events or diabetic kidney disease, in which case goal is SBP of 130–140
IDF	BP goal is 130–140/80; SBP of 130 is recommended in younger patients and those with CV risk or microvascular disease

GUIDELINES DISCORDANT: ROLE OF ANTIPLATELET THERAPY IN DM2	
Organization	**Guidance**
ADA	ASA 75–162 mg/d if primary prevention of ASCVD if 10-y risk of CAD >10% or for secondary prevention of existing ASCVD. (ADA) Consider ASA 75-162 mg/d plus low dose Rivaroxaban in patients who have stable CAD/PAD and low risk of bleeding
ESC	Start antiplatelet therapy of ASA 81–100 mg daily for primary prevention in high-risk CV patients only, with DAPT for up to 3 y in high-risk patients who tolerate it well for 12 mo; add PPI if high risk for GIB
IDF	Start low-dose aspirin (75–350 mg/d) in patients with T2DM and CVD

Comments

1. Metformin may cause vitamin B12 deficiency; consider periodic monitoring of vitamin B12 levels especially in patients with anemia or neuropathy. Avoid if eGFR <30 mL/min or unstable CHF.
2. Consider GLP1 receptor agonist as first-line injectable medication before insulin.
3. ACEIs or ARBs are first-line antihypertensives. Second-line antihypertensives are dihydropyridine calcium channel blockers, thiazide diuretic if GFR ≥30 mL/min/1.73 m^2 or a loop diuretic if GFR <30 mL/min/1.73 m^2.
4. Metformin, smoking cessation, blood pressure control, and statins consistently improve cardiovascular outcomes.
5. Glycemic control is a staple of care, but controversy exists regarding optimal A1c goals for ambulatory adults. Advocates of tighter control (ie, <7) rely on data from several trials (ACCORD, ADVANCE, UKPDS, VADT) that show improvements in surrogate markers (ie, nerve conduction velocity) but not patient-oriented outcomes (ie, painful neuropathy or mortality) with tighter control. Advocates of more permissive control (ie, <8%) point to potential harm from medication burden and hypoglycemia and the absence of evidence for patient-oriented benefit in tighter control of type 2 DM.

6. The largest trials for glycemic control (such as listed above) do not include SGLT2 inhibitors or GLP-1 receptor agonists, which may provide some cardiovascular benefit apart from glycemic reduction.

7. Continuous glucose monitoring is now recommended for anyone on multiple daily insulin injections, regardless of type of diabetes or age.

8. Self-monitoring of blood glucose levels in patients not on insulin is controversial. There are no agreed upon frequencies within the guidelines (once/d vs. twice/d vs. twice/wk). It is reasonable to consider self-monitoring when making medication changes, diet changes, or alterations in physical activity. It is also reasonable to prescribe self-monitoring in patients on medications with known side-effects of hypoglycemia (such as sulfonylureas).

9. The ODYSSEY OUTCOMES trial demonstrated statistically significant absolute risk reduction in primary endpoints (death from CAD, non-fatal MI, non-fatal ischemic stroke, unstable angina) in patients with T2DM with recent ACS who were treated with combination statin and Alirocumab (PCSK-9). Consider dual therapy in post-ACS patients with T2DM.

10. In patients with ASCVD risk factors with elevated triglycerides (135–499), but controlled LDL cholesterol on a statin, consider treatment with icosapent ethyl.

Sources

–https://www.aace.com/pdfs/diabetes/algorithm-exec-summary.pdf
–https://academic.oup.com/eurheartj/article/41/2/255/5556890
–https://diabetesjournals.org/care/issue/44/Supplement_1
–*Ann Intern Med.* 2017;166:279-290
–*Ann Intern Med.* 2018;168:569-576.
–International Diabetes Federation. *Recommendations for Managing Type 2 Diabetes in Primary Care.* 2017. www.idf.org/managing-type2-diabetes
–https://www.nice.org.uk/guidance/ng28

Population

–Hospitalized adults older than 18 y.

Organizations

▶ AAFP 2017, ADA 2020

Recommendations

–Avoid intensive insulin therapy in hospitalized patients (even in ICU).

–Target blood glucose level of 140–180 mg/dL if insulin therapy is used in hospitalized patients, especially those who are critically ill.

–Either basal insulin or basal plus bolus correctional insulin may be used in the treatment of hospitalized patients; sliding scale regimens are no longer recommended.

–For patients receiving glucocorticoid therapy, consider ordering NPH simultaneously with their steroid to prevent worsening daytime and prandial hyperglycemia. (ADA)

Comment

1. Intensive insulin therapy in SICU/MICU patients does not improve mortality but has a 5-fold increased risk of hypoglycemia.

Sources
–https://www.aafp.org/journalpdfrestricted/afp/2017/1115/p648.pdf
–https://diabetesjournals.org/care/issue/44/Supplement_1

Population
–Children and adolescents with newly diagnosed DM2.

Organizations
▶ AAP 2013, ADA 2021, NICE 2020

Recommendations
–Diet, exercise, and lifestyle modification are recommended for all those diagnosed.
–Offer Diabetes Self-Management Education and Support (DSMES). (ADA)
–Limit nonacademic screen time to <2 h/d.
–Assess psychological and social situation.
–Advise all patients not to smoke.
–Monitor HbA1c every 3 mo.

GUIDELINES DISCORDANT: A1C TARGET	
Organization	**Guidance**
AAP	<7%
ADA	<7%; less (7.5%) or more stringent (<6.5%) goals may be appropriate for select patients
NICE	6.5% or less

GUIDELINES DISCORDANT: PHARMACOLOGIC MANAGEMENT	
Organization	**Guidance**
AAP	Insulin therapy in the following situations: • DKA • HbA1c > 9% • Random glucose > 250 mg/dL Otherwise, metformin therapy is the first-line treatment
ADA	Insulin therapy in the following situations: • DKA • HbA1c > 8.5% • Random glucose > 250 mg/dL Otherwise, metformin therapy is the first-line treatment, with possibility to add liraglutide if not within A1c goal
NICE	Metformin therapy only

Surveillance

– BP measurement at every clinical visit.
  ○ If BP ≥ 95th percentile despite lifestyle management, start ACEI/ARB. (ADA)
– Screening for PCOS at time of diagnosis for adolescent females. (ADA)
– If LDL persistently ≥ 130 after 6 mo of medical nutrition therapy, start statin for goal LDL < 100. (ADA)
– If triglycerides are >400 fasting or >1000 nonfasting, treat with fibrate. (ADA)

GUIDELINES DISCORDANT: SURVEILLANCE TESTING	
Organization	**Guidance**
ADA	Screen annually for: • Albuminuria: Urine albumin-to-creatinine ratio (ACR) • Dyslipidemia with lipid panel • Comprehensive foot examination and monofilament testing • Retinopathy with retinal exam • NAFLD with LFTs • Symptoms of OSA
NICE	Screen annually for: • Albuminuria: Urine albumin-to-creatinine ratio (ACR) • Dyslipidemia with lipid panel • Comprehensive foot examination and monofilament testing • Retinopathy with retinal exam

Sources

–pediatrics.aappublications.org/content/131/2/364.full.pdf
–https://diabetesjournals.org/care/issue/44/Supplement_1
–https://www.nice.org.uk/guidance/ng18

HYPOGONADISM, MALE

Population
–Men with age-related low testosterone.

Organization
▶ ACP 2020

Recommendations
–Discuss risks, benefits, costs, and patient preferences in men with low testosterone and sexual dysfunction who desire to improve sexual function.

–Do not start treatment for goals of improving energy, vitality, physical function, or cognition.

–Reassess in 12 mo and stop treatment if no improvement.

–Consider IM over transdermal therapy, given lower cost with similar risks and efficacy.

Population
–Adult men.

Organizations
▶ Endocrine Society 2018, EAU 2018, AUA 2018

Recommendations
Diagnosis:

– Obtain an AM total testosterone level for men with symptoms and signs of androgen deficiency.[1]

– Consider testing testosterone in men with pituitary masses, obesity, metabolic syndrome, moderate-to-severe COPD, infertility, osteoporosis, HIV, DM type 3, or chronic use of corticosteroids and/or opiates. (EAU)

– Confirm diagnosis with a second AM total testosterone level.

– Diagnose hypogonadism if morning total testosterone level is less than 300 ng/dL on two separate occasions.

– Measure a serum luteinizing hormone (LH) and follicular stimulating hormone (FSH) in all men with testosterone deficiency to distinguish between primary and secondary hypogonadism.

– Measure serum estradiol in testosterone-deficient patients who present with breast symptoms or gynecomastia prior to the commencement of testosterone therapy. (EAU)

– Obtain a dual-energy X-ray absorptiometry (DEXA) scan for all men with severe androgen deficiency.

– Testosterone therapy is indicated for androgen deficiency syndromes (low testosterone with symptoms) unless contraindications exist.[2]

– Obtain a hemoglobin and hematocrit (and PSA in men over 40 y) prior to initiating testosterone therapy and educate patients about the risk of polycythemia. (EAU)

---

[1]Lethargy, easy fatigue, lack of stamina or endurance; reduced libido, decreased spontaneous erections; male infertility; mood changes; gynecomastia, loss of body hair, small testes; osteopenia/osteoporosis.
[2]Breast cancer, prostate cancer, hematocrit >50%, PSA>4 ng/mL, desire for fertility in the near term, MI or CVA within last 6 mo, untreated severe obstructive sleep apnea, severe obstructive urinary symptoms, or uncontrolled heart failure.

- Adjust testosterone therapy dosing to achieve a total testosterone level in the middle tertile of the normal reference range. (AUA)
- Monitor clinical response to therapy, testosterone level, PSA, digital prostate exam, and hematocrit 3, 6, and 12 mo after starting therapy, and annually thereafter. (EAU)
- Consider stopping testosterone therapy after 3–6 mo in patients who normalized total testosterone levels but fail to achieve improvement in clinical signs or symptoms. (AUA)

Comment

1. Testosterone therapy options (goal is a total testosterone level in mid-normal range):
   a. Testosterone enanthate or cypionate: 150–200 mg IM every 2 wk, or 75–100 mg IM weekly.
   b. Testosterone transdermal patch: 4–6 mg daily.
   c. Testosterone 1% gel: 50–100 mg daily.
   d. Testosterone 2% gel: 10–70 mg daily.
   e. Testosterone 2% solution: 60–120 mg (2–4 pumps or twists) applied to the axillae daily.
   f. Testosterone buccal bioadhesive tablets: 30 mg to buccal mucosa q12h.
   g. Testosterone nasal gel: 11 mg (2 pump actuations, 1 actuation per nostril) TID.

Sources

–https://academic.oup.com/jcem/article/103/5/1715/4939465
–https://uroweb.org/guideline/male-hypogonadism/
–http://www.auanet.org/guidelines/testosterone-deficiency-(2018)#x7697

MENOPAUSE

Population

–Menopausal women.

Organizations

▶ AACE 2017, NICE 2015, Endocrine Society 2015

Recommendations

GUIDELINES DISCORDANT: INDICATIONS FOR MENOPAUSAL HORMONE THERAPY	
Organization	**Guidance**
AACE	Severe menopausal symptoms Severe vulvovaginal atrophy Treatment of osteoporosis
NICE	Severe vasomotor symptoms Menopause-related depression Poor libido Urogenital atrophy
Endocrine Society	Severe vasomotor symptoms in women less than 60 y who do not have excess cardiovascular or breast cancer risk

–Duration of therapy should be <5 y. (NICE)

–Cautions with menopausal hormone therapy. (AACE)

- Avoid unopposed estrogen use in women with an intact uterus.
- Micronized progesterone is considered the safer alternative for women needing progesterone.
- Consider transdermal or topical estrogens which may reduce the risk of VTE.
- Use hormonal therapy in the lowest effective dose for the shortest duration possible.
- Custom-compounded bioidentical hormone therapy is *not* recommended.
- Hormone replacement is *not* appropriate for prevention or treatment of dementia, diabetes, or cardiovascular disease (CVD).
- Avoid if at high risk for VTE.

–Contraindications of menopausal hormone therapy (AACE):

- History of breast CA.
- Suspected estrogen-sensitive malignancy.
- Undiagnosed vaginal bleeding.
- Endometrial hyperplasia.
- History of VTE.
- Untreated hypertension.
- Active liver disease.
- Porphyria cutanea tarda.

–Offer vaginal estrogen cream for urogenital atrophy (even if already on systemic estrogen).

–Consider adjuvant testosterone therapy for decreased libido despite HRT. (NICE)

–Offer nonhormonal remedies for women at high risk of CVD or breast cancer. (ES)

- Options include an SSRI, SNRI, gabapentin, or pregabalin.
- Clonidine is an option for women with severe vasomotor symptoms who do not respond to or tolerate nonhormonal modalities.

–For women at moderate risk of CVD, recommend transdermal estradiol and micronized progesterone for severe vasomotor symptoms. (ES)

Comments

1. Use of hormone therapy should always occur after a thorough discussion of the risks, benefits, and alternatives of this treatment with the patient.
2. Risks of HRT:
   a. Venous thromboembolism (VTE): the risk is greater for oral than transdermal preparations.
   b. HRT with estrogen and progesterone may slightly increase risk of breast cancer but declines after stopping HRT.
3. Review benefits of HRT:
   a. Risk of fragility fracture is decreased while taking HRT but this benefit decreases once treatment stops.
4. SSRIs or gabapentin may offer relief of menopausal symptoms for women at high risk from hormone replacement therapy.
   a. Do not use paroxetine or fluoxetine in breast cancer patients as they inhibit the effect of tamoxifen.

Sources
- –www.aace.com/files/position-statements/ep171828ps.pdf
- –https://www.nice.org.uk/guidance/ng23/chapter/Recommendations#managing-short-term-menopausal-symptoms
- –https://www.endocrine.org/guidelines-and-clinical-practice/clinical-practice-guidelines/treatment-of-menopause

OBESITY

Population
–Mature adolescents and adults

Organizations
▶ JCEM 2015, CMAJ 2020

Recommendations

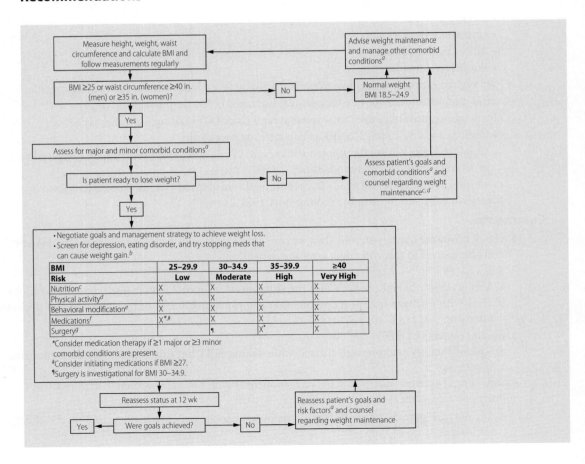

BMI	25–29.9	30–34.9	35–39.9	≥40
Risk	Low	Moderate	High	Very High
Nutrition[c]	X	X	X	X
Physical activity[d]	X	X	X	X
Behavioral modification[e]	X	X	X	X
Medications[f]	X*,#	X	X	X
Surgery[g]		¶	X*	X

*Consider medication therapy if ≥1 major or ≥3 minor comorbid conditions are present.
#Consider initiating medications if BMI ≥27.
¶Surgery is investigational for BMI 30–34.9.

[a]**Minor comorbid conditions:** cigarette smoking; hypertension; LDL cholesterol >130 mg/dL; HDL cholesterol <40 mg/dL (men) or <50 mg/dL (women); glucose intolerance; family history of premature CAD; age ≥65 y (men) or ≥55 y (women).

Major comorbid conditions: waist circumference ≥40 in. (men) or ≥35 in. (women); CAD; peripheral vascular disease; abdominal aortic aneurysm; symptomatic carotid artery disease; type 2 diabetes; and obstructive sleep apnea.

[b]Sulfonylureas; thiazolidinediones; olanzapine, clozapine; risperidone, quetiapine; lithium; paroxetine, citalopram, sertraline; carbamazepine; pregabalin; corticosteroids; megestrol acetate; cyproheptadine; tricyclic antidepressants; monoamine oxidase inhibitors; mirtazapine; valproic acid; and gabapentin.

[c]Encourage a healthy, balanced diet including daily intake of ≥5 servings of fruits/vegetables; 35 g fiber; <30% calories from fat; eliminate takeout, fast foods, soda, and desserts; dietitian consultation for a calorie reduction between 500 and 1000 kcal/kg/d to achieve a 1–2 lb weight reduction per week.

[d]Recommend 30–60 min of moderate activity at least 5 d/wk.

[e]Identify behaviors that may contribute to weight gain (stress, emotional eating, boredom) and use cognitive behavioral counseling, stimulus control, relapse prevention, and goal setting to decrease caloric intake and increase physical activity.

[f]Medications that are FDA approved for weight loss: phentermine; orlistat; lorcaserin phendimetrazine; diethylpropion; and benzphetamine can be used for up to 3 mo as an adjunct for weight loss. Avoid phentermine and diethylpropion in patients with uncontrolled HTN or a history of heart disease.

[g]Bariatric surgery is indicated for patients at high risk for complications. They should be motivated, psychologically stable, have no surgical contraindications, and must accept the operative risk involved.

- –Approach to obesity management (CMAJ):
  - Assess and acknowledge provider bias regarding obesity.
  - Ask permission to discuss obesity with patient in a nonjudgmental way.
  - Assess their story (subjective experiences as well as objective measures such as BMI, height, waist circumference, BP, lipid panel, A1c, LFT measurements).
  - Exercise (30–60 min on most days of the week), with added resistance training.
  - Medical Nutrition Therapy facilitated by registered dietician when possible.
  - Weight loss of 5%–7% in setting of prediabetes, 7%–15% in diagnosed T2DM.
  - Offer multicomponent psychological care in a longitudinal setting.
  - Pharmacotherapy: used when BMI ≥ 30 kg/m², or ≥27 kg/m² with adiposity-related complications, in conjunction with intensive lifestyle changes listed above. Choices for pharmacotherapy include liraglutide 3.0 mg, naltrexone-bupropion combination, orlistat. It is also encouraged to minimize exposure to pharmacotherapy for other medical conditions with the side effect of weight gain.
  - Bariatric surgery considerations: BMI ≥ 40 kg/m², BMI ≥ 35 kg/m² with at least 1 adiposity-related disease, BMI between 30 and 35 kg/m² with presence of poorly controlled T2DM despite maximal medical therapy.
  - Do not offer adjustable gastric banding procedure due to long-term treatment failure and rate of complications.

Comment

1. Bariatric surgery does improve all-cause mortality and comorbidities such as diabetes, hypertension and sleep apnea. (*PLoS Med.* 2020;17(7):e1003206)

Sources

- –*CMAJ.* 2020;192:E875-91. doi: 10.1503/cmaj.191707
- –Adapted from the *ICSI Guideline on the Prevention and Management of Obesity.* https://academic.oup.com/jcem/article/100/2/342/2813109/Pharmacological-Management-of-Obesity-An-Endocrine.

POLYCYSTIC OVARY SYNDROME

Population
  –Women diagnosed with PCOS.

Organization
▶ ACOG 2018

Recommendations
  –Recommend increase in exercise combined with dietary change to reduce diabetes risk and promote weight loss.
  –Prescribe combination low-dose hormonal contraceptives for primary treatment of menstrual disorders.
  –Screen women with PCOS for cardiovascular risk, metabolic syndrome, and type 2 diabetes (fasting glucose followed by 2-h GTT after 75-g glucose load).
  –Consider addition of insulin-sensitizing agent (such as metformin) to decrease androgen levels, improve ovulation rate, improve glucose tolerance, and reduce cardiovascular risk.
  –Prescribe letrozole as first-line therapy for ovulation induction in women with PCOS who desire to conceive.

Comments
  1. Letrozole has shown increased live birth rate compared with clomiphene citrate.
  2. There may be higher pregnancy rates with clomiphene citrate in addition to metformin than with clomiphene alone, particularly in obese women with PCOS.
  3. Second-line intervention for failure of pregnancy with letrozole or clomiphene is exogenous gonadotropins or laparoscopic ovarian surgery.
  4. Women in ethnic groups at higher risk of nonclassical congenital adrenal hyperplasia should be screened with a fasting 17-hydroxyprogesterone level (normal <2–4 ng/mL).
  5. Lower BMI is associated with improved pregnancy rates, decreased hirsutism, and lower risk for metabolic syndrome.
  6. There is no clear primary treatment for hirsutism in PCOS, but the addition of eflornithine to laser treatment is superior to laser alone.

Source
  –https://journals.lww.com/greenjournal/Fulltext/2018/06000/ACOG_Practice_Bulletin_No_194_Polycystic_Ovary.54.aspx

THYROID DISEASE, HYPERTHYROIDISM

Population
  –Adults.

Organizations
▶ NICE 2019, ATA 2016, AACE 2013

Recommendations

–Determine etiology of thyrotoxicosis. If the diagnosis is not apparent, consider obtaining a thyroid receptor antibody level (TRAb) $+/-$ determination of the radioactive iodine uptake (RAIU).

–Use beta-adrenergic blockade in all patients with symptomatic thyrotoxicosis.

–For overt Graves' disease (GD), treat with either radioiodine (RI) therapy, antithyroid drugs (ATDs), or thyroidectomy. Prefer RI unless ATD likely to achieve remission (ie, mild or uncomplicated disease) or patient not an RI/surgery candidate; treat with total thyroidectomy if concern for compression, malignancy, or patient not an RI/surgery candidate.

–For toxic goiter, use RI as first-line if multinodular, then consider total thyroidectomy or ADT; if single nodule, consider RI or hemithyroidectomy.

–For RI therapy:

  • Obtain a pregnancy test within 48 h prior to treatment in any woman with childbearing potential who is to be treated with RAI.

  • Recheck a T4, T3, and TSH level in 4–8 wk after RAI therapy.

  • Assess patients 1–2 mo after ^{131}I therapy with a free T_4 and total triiodothyronine (T_3) level; repeat q 4–6 wk if thyrotoxicosis persists.

  • Consider retreatment with ^{131}I therapy if hyperthyroidism persists 6 mo after ^{131}I treatment.

–For antithyroid drug therapy:

  • When using ADTs for hyperthyroidism, check CBC and liver enzymes prior to starting, and use titration method in young adult vs. either block and replace or titration method in older adults.

  • Methimazole is the preferred antithyroid drug except during the first trimester of pregnancy.

  • Educate patients on the signs and symptoms of agranulocytosis and hepatic injury.

  • Measure TSH receptor antibody level prior to stopping antithyroid drug therapy.

–Thyroidectomy:

  • If near total or total thyroidectomy is chosen as treatment for GD, render patients euthyroid prior to the procedure with ATD pretreatment and beta-adrenergic blockade. Give potassium iodide in the immediate preoperative period.

  • Follow serial calcium or intact PTH levels postoperatively.

  • Start levothyroxine 1.6 μg/kg/d immediately postoperatively.

  • Check a serum TSH level 6–8 wk postoperatively.

  • Wean beta-blockers following thyroidectomy.

–Treat subclinical hyperthyroidism in all individuals ≥65 of age, and in patients with cardiac disease, osteoporosis, or symptoms of hyperthyroidism when the TSH is persistently <0.1 mIU/L. (ATA)

–Treat thyroid storm in the ICU with beta-blockers, antithyroid drugs, inorganic iodide, corticosteroid therapy, volume resuscitation, and aggressive cooling with acetaminophen and cooling blankets. (ATA)

Sources

–https://www.nice.org/uk/guidance/ng145/resources/thyroid-disease-assessment-and-management-pdf-66141781496773

–2016 American Thyroid Association guidelines for diagnosis and management of hyperthyroidism and other causes of thyrotoxicosis. *Thyroid*. 2016;26(10):1343-1421.
–https://www.aace.com/files/hyperguidelinesapril2013.pdf

THYROID DISEASE, HYPOTHYROIDISM

Population
–Nonpregnant adults.

Organizations
▶ NICE 2019, AACE 2012

Recommendations
–Treat with levothyroxine as first-line over natural thyroid extract or liothyronine (no evidence of benefits and long-term outcomes uncertain).
–Start 1.6 µg/kg/d generally, or 25–50 mcg/d with titration if age ≥65 y or history of CVD (higher risk of harm if TSH <10).
–Check antithyroid peroxidase antibodies (TPOAb) in patients with subclinical hypothyroidism or recurrent miscarriages. (AACE)
–Monitor TSH 4–8 wk after starting levothyroxine or adjusting dose, then q 6–12 mo once euthyroid.
–Avoid overtreatment with levothyroxine to minimize risk of cardiovascular, skeletal, or affective disturbances. (AACE)
–Do *not* use levothyroxine to treat obesity or depression in euthyroid patients. (AACE)

GUIDELINES DISCORDANT: WHEN TO INITIATE TREATMENT FOR HYPOTHYROIDISM	
Organization	**Guidance**
NICE	Treat if TSH >10 for 2 tests >3 mo apart If TSH <10, trial 6 mo of treatment and then repeat TSH and up titrate dose if still above reference range or discontinue if symptoms persist and level within reference range
AACE	TSH > 10 mIU/L TSH < 10 mIU/L plus: • Symptomatic • Positive TPO-Ab • History of or at high risk for ASCVD

Sources
–https://www.nice.org/uk/guidance/ng145/resources/thyroid-disease-assessment-and-management-pdf-66141781496773
–https://www.aace.com/files/hypothyroidism_guidelines.pdf

THYROID NODULES

Population
–Nonpregnant adults.

Organization
▶ NICE 2019

Recommendations
–Assess with US if palpable nodule or generalized enlargement, and then proceed with FNA if suspicious by standard grading system (which is based on echogenicity, microcalcifications, border, shape in transverse plane, internal vascularity, and lymphadenopathy).
–If nonmalignant, treat only if airway symptoms or narrowing on imaging; repeat workup if change in symptoms.
–If cystic, treat with aspiration +/− ethanol ablation.
–If noncystic, multinodular, or diffuse goiter, treat with surgery, RIA, or percutaneous thermal ablation.

Source
–https://www.nice.org/uk/guidance/ng145/resources/thyroid-disease-assessment-and-management-pdf-66141781496773

THYROID NODULE FLOW DIAGRAM

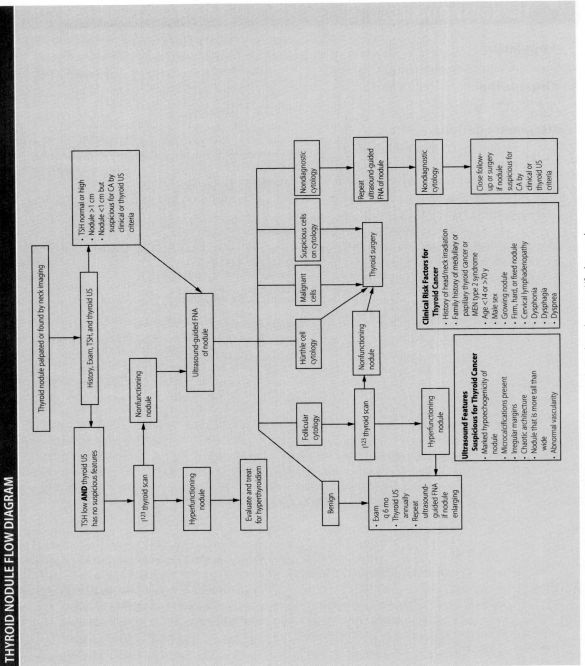

FNA, fine-needle aspiration; MEN, multiple endocrine neoplasia; TSH, thyroid-stimulating hormone; US, ultrasound.

Sources
- –AACE. 2010. https://www.aace.com/files/thyroid-guidelines.pdf
- –ATA. 2015. https://www.ncbi.nlm.nih.gov/pmc/articles/PMC4739132/

TRANSGENDER HEALTH CARE

Population
- –Genderqueer, gender nonconforming, and gender nonbinary people.

Organizations
▶ UCSF 2016, WPATH 2012, Endocrine 2017, ACOG 2021

Recommendations
- –Employ cultural humility. Avoid judgment or editorializing. Use gender pronouns consistent with patients' self-identity. Ask for clarification when uncertain.
- –Diagnose "Gender Dysphoria" when gender identity is incongruent with assignment and there is clinically significant social impairment. Use the term "gender nonconformity" to represent the broader population with incongruent gender identities.
- –Employ informed consent prior to initiating hormone therapy, including effects on fertility; fertility and parenting desires should be discussed early in the process, prior to transition.
- –Offer a multidisciplinary team approach including mental health providers and clinicians to inform and guide treatment modalities, especially for younger patients.
- –Assess for suicide risk. Suicide rates are markedly elevated in this community.

Population
- –Patients transitioning to a female gender expression.

Organizations
▶ UCSF 2016, WPATH 2012, Endocrine 2017, ACOG 2021

Recommendations
- –To develop female secondary sex characteristics, use 17-beta estradiol (typically transdermal patch, oral or sublingual tablet, or injectable). Do not use conjugated equine estrogens because of difficulty. Do not use ethinyl estradiol because of thrombotic risk. Effects include breast development (to Tanner stage 2–3), redistribution of fat, reduction of muscle mass, reduction of body hair, possible arrest/reversal of scalp hair loss, reduced erectile function, and reduced testicular size. There is an increased risk of venous thromboembolism and hypertriglyceridemia, and possibly of hypertension.
- –To suppress male secondary sex characteristics, use antiandrogens such as spironolactone (monitor for hyperkalemia; max dose 200 mg BID). If contraindicated or unable to tolerate, use 5-alpha reductase inhibitors instead. Titrate dose to clinical effect and testosterone levels <55 ng/dL.
- –Screen for breast cancer q2 years if age >50 and 5–10 y of feminizing hormone use. Prostate and testicular cancer risk is reduced by feminizing hormones but not eliminated; individualize screening.

–Hair removal can be achieved through various methods including laser, electrolysis, waxing, plucking, and shaving.

–Consider referral to speech language pathologist if concerns about incongruent voice pitch are present.

–Patients may consider "tucking" (employ tight-fitting underwear to locate the testicles in the inguinal canal and the penis in the perineal region) and "binding" (tight-fitting bras/shirts/wraps/binders) to disguise male anatomical characteristics.

–If considering breast augmentation ("top surgery"), 24 mo of preoperative hormone therapy is recommended, as breast tissue will continue to develop.

–If considering vaginoplasty ("bottom surgery"), requirements include two assessments by a mental health provider, 12 mo of hormone therapy, and 12 mo of living in a gender role congruent with gender identity.

Population

–Patients transitioning to a male gender expression.

Organizations

▶ UCSF 2016, WPATH 2012, Endocrine 2017, ACOG 2021

Recommendations

–To develop male secondary sex characteristics, give testosterone (oral, IM, SQ, or transdermal) and titrate to bioavailable level >72 ng/dL. Effects include development of facial hair, voice changes, fat redistribution, increase in muscle mass, increase in body hair, hairline recession, increase in libido, clitoral growth, vaginal dryness, and cessation of menses. There is an increased risk of polycythemia and possibly of hyperlipidemia.

–In patients receiving testosterone therapy, monitor testosterone levels and hematocrit every 3 mo for the first year, then every 6–12 mo thereafter.

–Discuss contraceptive options, as hormone therapy does not reliably cause infertility and testosterone is teratogenic.

–Discontinue testosterone prior to pregnancy if possible, or immediately upon discovery of pregnancy; consider that pregnancy may worsen feelings of dysphoria.

–Screen for breast and cervical cancer according to current guidelines for cis-gendered women. Do not routinely screen for endometrial cancer but explore the possibility if unexplained vaginal bleeding.

–Evaluation of abnormal uterine bleeding should follow the same guidelines as for cis-gendered women.

–Patients may consider "packing" (use of a penile prosthesis) to provide a male physical appearance.

–If considering mastectomy ("top surgery"), an assessment by a mental health provider is required.

–If considering gonadectomy or hysterectomy ("bottom surgery"), 12 mo of preoperative hormone therapy are required.

–If considering phalloplasty or metoidioplasty, requirements include two assessments by a mental health provider, 12 mo of hormone therapy, and 12 mo of living in a gender role congruent with gender identity.

Population

–Gender nonconforming children and adolescents.

Organizations

▶ UCSF 2016, WPATH 2012, Endocrine 2017

Recommendations

–Suppression of endogenous puberty may represent an opportunity to avoid distressing gender dysphoria and the high rate of suicide that accompanies it.

–Adolescents are candidates for puberty suppression if a long-lasting pattern of gender nonconformity or dysphoria exists, dysphoria emerges or worsens with the onset of puberty, their ability to adhere to treatment is intact, and the adolescent and their parents/guardians have consented to the treatment.

–Do not offer hormonal treatment to prepubertal persons.

–If suppression is desired, use GnRH analogues before the patient has reached Tanner stages 2–3 with frequent monitoring of clinical and lab parameters.

Comments

1. Outcomes data is generally lacking for this population, so most guidelines are based on expert opinion from experienced practitioners.

2. Terminology may be fluid and highly individualized. Approach conversations with humility and open-ended questions.

3. Employ a stepwise approach to therapies. Encourage hormone therapy before surgical intervention for most patients. Informed consent is essential, as every therapy will have reversible and irreversible effects.

4. For patients considering surgical options, refer to surgeon comfortable with the treatment of gender dysphoria. While top surgeries are often well-tolerated, bottom surgeries are relatively complex with higher complication rates and significant postprocedure care. Informed consent is essential and should include the various techniques available, realistic expectations of outcomes, and inherent risks and complications.

5. Dosing of hormones, surveillance regimens, and common adverse effects are detailed in the cited guidelines.

Sources

–AACE. 2010. https://www.aace.com/files/thyroid-guidelines.pdf

–*Guidelines for the Primary and Gender-Affirming Care of Transgender and Gender Nonbinary People*, 2nd ed. University of California, San Francisco Center of Excellence for Transgender Health. 2016. http://www.transhealth.ucsf.edu/guidelines

–*Standards of Care for the Health of Transsexual, Transgender, and Gender-Nonconforming People*, 7th ed. World Professional Association for Transgender Health. 2012. http://wpath.org

–Guidelines on Gender-Dysphoric/Gender-Incongruent Persons. *J Clin Endocrinol Metab.* 2017;102(11):3869-3903.

–https://www.acog.org/clinical/clinical-guidance/committee-opinion/articles/2021/03/health-care-for-transgender-and-gender-diverse-individuals

VITAMIN DEFICIENCIES

Population

–All patients with or suspected of having serum cobalamin and folate deficiency.

Organization

▶ BCSH 2014

Recommendations

–Serum cobalamin <200 ng/L is consistent with cobalamin deficiency.

–Patients with normal cobalamin level but high suspicion of cobalamin and/or folate deficiency should have their methylmalonic acid (MMA) and total homocysteine (tHC) levels measured.

–Patients with cobalamin deficiency or unexplained anemia, neuropathy, or glossitis (regardless of cobalamin level) should have an anti-intrinsic factor antibody test to rule out pernicious anemia.

–Initial therapy for cobalamin deficiency is vitamin B_{12} 1 mg IM TIW for 2 wk and then maintenance therapy.

–Maintenance therapy is either 1 mg IM every 3 mo (if no neurologic symptoms) or every 2 mo (if neurologic symptoms) or vitamin B_{12} 2 mg PO daily.

–Serum folate level <7 nmol/L (<3 µg/L) indicates folate deficiency.

–Treatment of folate deficiency is 1–5 mg PO daily for 1–4 mo, or until folate level normalizes.

Comments

1. Do not use antiparietal cell antibody to test for pernicious anemia.

2. Both MMA and tHC will be elevated in cobalamin deficiency; normal MMA and elevated tHC are consistent with folate deficiency.

Source

–onlinelibrary.wiley.com/doi/full/10.1111/bjh.12959

Disorders of the Eye, Ear, Nose, and Throat

22

Population
–Adults with cataracts.

Organization
▶ AAO 2021

Recommendations
–Refer patients with symptomatic cataracts for surgery. Dietary intake and nutritional supplements have minimal effect on the prevention or treatment of cataract.

–Obtain initial history of symptoms, ocular history, systemic history, assessment of visual functional status, and medications currently used.

–Include the following elements in the initial physical exam: The visual acuity with current correction, external examination, ocular alignment and motility, pupil reactivity and function, measurement of intraocular pressure, slit-lamp exam, and dilated examination with ophthalmology.

–Remove cataracts when visual function no longer meets the patient's needs and cataract surgery provides a reasonable likelihood of quality-of-life improvement.

–Remove cataracts when there is evidence of lens-induced disease or when it is necessary to visualize the fundus in an eye that has the potential for sight.

–Avoid surgery under the following circumstances:
  • Tolerable refractive correction provides vision that meets the patient's needs and desires; surgery is not expected to improve visual function, and no other indication for lens removal exists.
  • The patient cannot safely undergo surgery because of coexisting medical or ocular conditions.
  • Appropriate postoperative care cannot be arranged.
  • Patient or patient's surrogate decision-maker is unable to give informed consent for nonemergent surgery.

Comment
1. Routine preoperative medical testing does not appear to measurably increase the safety of the surgery.

Sources
–*American Academy of Ophthalmology Preferred Practice Pattern: Cataract/Anterior Segment Summary Benchmark.* 2021. http://www.aao.org

–American Optometric Association Consensus Panel on Care of the Adult Patient with Cataract. *Optometric Clinical Practice Guideline: Care of the Adult Patient with Cataract.* 2004. http://www.aoa.org

CATARACT IN ADULTS: EVALUATION AND MANAGEMENT ALGORITHM

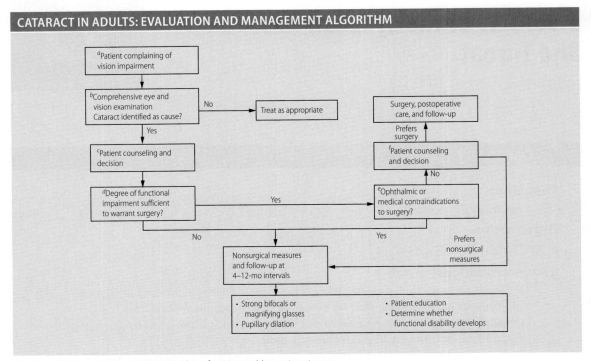

[a]Begin evaluation only when patients complain of a vision problem or impairment.

[b]Essential elements of the comprehensive eye and vision exam:

- Patient history: Consider cataract if acute or gradual onset of vision loss; vision problems under special conditions (eg, low contrast, glare); difficulties performing various visual tasks. Ask about refractive history, previous ocular disease, amblyopia, eye surgery, trauma, general health history, medications, and allergies. It is critical to describe the actual impact of the cataract on the person's function and quality of life. There are several instruments available for assessing functional impairment related to cataract, including VF-14, Activities of Daily Vision Scale, and Visual Activities Questionnaire.
- Ocular examination includes Snellen acuity and refraction; measurement of intraocular pressure; assessment of pupillary function; external exam; slit-lamp exam; and dilated exam of fundus.
- Supplemental testing: May be necessary to assess and document the extent of the functional disability and to determine whether other diseases may limit preoperative or postoperative vision. Most elderly patients presenting with visual problems do not have a cataract that causes functional impairment. Refractive error, macular degeneration, and glaucoma are common alternative etiologies for visual impairment.

[c]Once cataract has been identified as the cause of visual disability, patients should be counseled concerning the nature of the problem, its natural history, and the existence of both surgical and nonsurgical approaches to management. The principal factor that should guide decision making with regard to surgery is the extent to which the cataract impairs the ability to function in daily life. The findings of the physical examination should corroborate that the cataract is the major contributing cause of the functional impairment, and that there is a reasonable expectation that managing the cataract will positively impact the patient's functional activity. Preoperative visual acuity is a poor predictor of postoperative functional improvement: The decision to recommend cataract surgery should not be made solely on the basis of visual acuity.

[d]Patients who complain of mild-to-moderate limitation in activities due to a visual problem, those whose corrected acuities are near 20/40, and those who do not yet wish to undergo surgery may be offered nonsurgical measures for improving visual function. Treatment with nutritional supplements is not recommended. Smoking cessation retards cataract progression. Indications for surgery: Cataract-impaired vision no longer meets the patient's needs; evidence of lens-induced disease (eg, phacomorphic glaucoma, phacolytic glaucoma); necessary to visualize the fundus in an eye that has the potential for sight (eg, diabetic patient at risk of diabetic retinopathy).

CATARACT IN ADULTS: EVALUATION AND MANAGEMENT ALGORITHM

[e]Contraindications to surgery: The patient does not desire surgery; glasses or vision aids provide satisfactory functional vision; surgery will not improve visual function; the patient's quality of life is not compromised; the patient is unable to undergo surgery because of coexisting medical or ocular conditions; a legal consent cannot be obtained; or the patient is unable to obtain adequate postoperative care. Routine preoperative medical testing (12-lead EKG, CBC, measurement of serum electrolytes, BUN, creatinine, and glucose), while commonly performed in patients scheduled to undergo cataract surgery, does not appear to measurably increase the safety of the surgery.

[f]Patients with significant functional and visual impairment due to cataract who have no contraindications to surgery should be counseled regarding the expected risks and benefits of and alternatives to surgery.

Sources: American Academy of Ophthalmology Preferred Practice Pattern: Cataract in the Adult Eye. 2006. http://www.aao.org; American Optometric Association Consensus Panel on Care of the Adult Patient with Cataract. *Optometric Clinical Practice Guideline: Care of the Adult Patient with Cataract.* 2004. http://www.aoa.org.

CERUMEN IMPACTION

Population

–Children and adults.

Organization

▶ AAO-HNS 2017

Recommendations

–Treat cerumen impaction when symptomatic or prevents a needed clinical examination.

–Treat with an appropriate intervention:

- Cerumenolytic agents (water or saline, Cerumenex, addax, Debrox, or dilute solutions of acetic acid, hydrogen peroxide, or sodium bicarbonate).
- Irrigation.
- Manual removal.

Comments

1. Ear candling is not recommended for treatment or prevention of cerumen impaction and has caused harm to patients.
2. Removal of cerumen is not necessary if the patient is asymptomatic and adequate clinical exam is possible.

Source

–https://www.entnet.org//content/clinical-practice-guideline-cerumen-impaction

EPISTAXIS

Population
–Adults and children over age 3.

Organization
▶ AAO-HNS 2020

Recommendations
–Identify the acuity and severity of bleeding to appropriately triage and treat the patient.
- Severe bleeding:
  - Bleeding for greater than 30 min in a 24-h period.
  - History of hospitalization or prior transfusion.
  - Comorbid conditions—uncontrolled HTN, anemia, clotting disorders, etc.

–Perform anterior rhinoscopy to identify a source of bleeding after removal of any blood clot (if present) for patients with nosebleeds.

–Document factors that increase the frequency or severity of bleeding for any patient with a nosebleed, including personal or family history of bleeding disorders, use of anticoagulant or antiplatelet medications, or intranasal drug use.

–First-line interventions:
- Compression: Treat active bleeding with firm sustained compression to the lower third of the nose, with or without the assistance of the patient or caregiver, for 5 min or longer.
- Topical agents (vasoconstrictors).
- Cautery.
- Packing.
- Include patient education and follow-up recommendations for timing of removal.

–Second-line interventions (refractory bleeding):
- Perform, or refer to a clinician who can perform, nasal endoscopy to identify the site of bleeding and guide further management in patients with recurrent nasal bleeding, despite prior treatment with packing or cautery, or with recurrent unilateral nasal bleeding.

–*Invasive treatment options include surgical ligation and/or cautery and endovascular embolization.*

Source
–https://www.entnet.org/quality-practice/quality-products/clinical-practice-guidelines/nosebleed-epistaxis/

HEARING LOSS, SUDDEN

Population
–Adults age 18 y and older.

Organization
▶ AAO-HNS 2019

Recommendations
–Distinguish between sensorineural and conductive hearing loss.

–Diagnose idiopathic sudden sensorineural hearing loss (ISSNHL) when audiometry confirms a 30-dB hearing loss at three consecutive frequencies and no underlying condition can be identified by history and physical.

–Evaluate patients with ISSNHL for retrocochlear pathology by obtaining an MRI of the internal auditory canal, auditory brainstem responses, and an audiology exam.

–Urgent: consider treatment of ISSNHL with incomplete hearing recovery with systemic or intratympanic steroids *within 14 d*. Hyperbaric oxygen therapy is considered only as an adjunct to steroids.

–In patients with ISSNHL, recommend against antivirals, thrombolytics, vasodilators, or antioxidants for treatment and against CT scanning of the head or routine lab testing.

Comments
1. Prompt diagnosis is important.
2. Obtain audiometric testing as soon as possible, and *within 14 d*.
3. Counsel patients with incomplete recovery of hearing about the benefits of hearing aids.

Source
–https://www.entnet.org/quality-practice/quality-products/clinical-practice-guidelines/sudden-hearing-loss-update/

HOARSENESS

Population
–Persons with hoarseness.

Organization
▶ AAO-HNS 2018

Recommendations
–Most, but not all, hoarseness is benign or self-limited; some of the most common causes are URI and vocal overuse.

–Begin assessment with history and physical to identify potential underlying causes and factors.

–If hoarseness fails to resolve or improve within 4 wk, refer for laryngoscopy.

–No need for screening neck imaging (CT or MRI) for chronic hoarseness prior to laryngoscopy.

–Do not routinely use antibiotics or steroids to treat hoarseness.

–Do not use antireflux medications, unless exhibiting signs or symptoms of gastroesophageal reflux disease.

–Encourage or refer to voice therapy for all patients with continued hoarseness and a decreased voice-related quality of life.

–Surgical referral should be given for laryngeal CA, benign laryngeal soft-tissue lesions, or glottis insufficiency.

–Botulinum toxin injections can be beneficial for spasmodic dysphonia.

Comment

1. Nearly one-third of Americans will have hoarseness at some point in their lives.

Source

–https://www.entnet.org//content/clinical-practice-guideline-hoarseness-dysphonia

LARYNGITIS, ACUTE

Population

–Adults.

Organization

▶ Cochrane Database Systematic Reviews 2015

Recommendations

–Insufficient evidence to support the use of antibiotics for acute laryngitis.

–There may be some subjective benefit to erythromycin based on patient-reported symptoms, but cost and negative consequences of use seem to outweigh benefit.

Comment

1. Many methodological flaws in studies evaluated.

Source

–http://www.cochrane.org/CD004783/ARI_antibiotics-to-treat-adults-with-acute-laryngitis

MENIERE'S DISEASE

Population

–Adults, primarily ages 40–60.

Organization

▶ AAO-HNS 2020

Recommendations

–Consider diagnosis in patients presenting with all of the following:
- 2 or more episodes of vertigo.
- Lasting 20 min to 12 h (definite) or up to 24 h (probable).
- Fluctuating or nonfluctuating sensorineural hearing loss, tinnitus, or pressure in the affected ear, when these symptoms are not better accounted for by another disorder.

–Obtain audiogram when assessing for diagnosis of Meniere's.

–Evaluate for vestibular migraine.

–Offer a limited course of vestibular suppressants to patients with Meniere's disease for management of vertigo only during Meniere's disease attacks.

–Do not routinely order vestibular function testing or electrocochleography to establish the diagnosis of Meniere's disease.

–Do not prescribe positive pressure therapy.

–Avoid physical therapy or vestibular therapy for acute vertigo attacks.

–Consider MRI of the internal auditory canal (IAC) and posterior fossa in patients with possible Meniere's disease and audiometrically verified asymmetric sensorineural hearing loss.

–Consider diuretics and/or betahistine for maintenance therapy to reduce symptoms or prevent Meniere's disease attacks.

–Consider intratympanic steroids to patients with active Meniere's disease not responsive to noninvasive treatment.

Source

–https://www.entnet.org/quality-practice/quality-products/clinical-practice-guidelines/menieres-disease/

OTITIS EXTERNA, ACUTE (AOE)

Population

–Children age 2 y or older and adults.

Organization

▶ AAO-HNS 2014

Recommendations

–Do not prescribe systemic antimicrobials as initial therapy for diffuse, uncomplicated acute otitis externa (AOE).

–Use topical antibiotics for initial therapy of AOE.

–In the presence of a perforated tympanic membrane or tympanostomy tubes, prescribe a non-ototoxic topical antibiotic.

Comment

–Recommends reassessment of the diagnosis if the patient fails to respond within 72 h of topical antibiotics.

Source

–https://www.entnet.org//content/clinical-practice-guideline-acute-otitis-externa

OTITIS MEDIA, ACUTE (AOM)

Population
–Children age 3 mo to 18 y.

Organization
▶ AAP 2013

Recommendations
–Make diagnosis with pneumatic otoscopy.
–Use a wait-and-see approach for 48–72 h for children at low risk.[1]
–Provide symptomatic relief with acetaminophen, ibuprofen, and warm compresses to the ear.
–Educate caregivers about prevention of otitis media: encourage breast-feeding, feed child upright if bottle fed, avoid passive smoke exposure, limit exposure to groups of children, careful handwashing prior to handling child, avoid pacifier use >10 mo, ensure immunizations are up to date.
–Amoxicillin is the first-line antibiotic for low-risk children.
–Use alternative medication if failure to respond to initial treatment within 72 h; penicillin allergy; presence of a resistant organism found on culture.
–Refer to an ear, nose, and throat (ENT) specialist for any complications of otitis media including mastoiditis, facial nerve palsy, lateral sinus thrombosis, meningitis, brain abscess, or labyrinthitis.
–Do not require routine rechecks at 10–14 d for children feeling well.
–Management of otitis media with effusion:
  • Educate that effusion will resolve on its own.
  • Do not offer antihistamines or decongestants.
  • Trial antibiotics for 10–14 d prior to referral for tympanostomy tubes.
–Do not routinely prescribe antibiotics in children age 2–12 y with nonsevere AOM when observation is an option.

Comments
1. Amoxicillin is first-line therapy for low-risk children:
    a. 40 mg/kg/d if no antibiotics used in last 3 mo.
    b. 80 mg/kg/d if child is not low risk.
2. Alternative antibiotics:
    a. Amoxicillin-clavulanate.
    b. Cefuroxime axetil.
    c. Ceftriaxone.
    d. Cefprozil.
    e. Loracarbef.

[1]Children older than age 2 y without severe disease (temperature > 102°F [39°C] and moderate-to-severe otalgia), otherwise healthy, do not attend daycare, and have had no prior ear infections within the last month.

  f. Cefdinir.

  g. Cefixime.

  h. Cefpodoxime.

  i. Clarithromycin.

  j. Azithromycin.

  k. Erythromycin.

Sources

 –*Pediatrics*. 2013;131:e964-e999.

 –http://www.choosingwisely.org/societies/american-academy-of-family-physicians/

Population

 –Children 6 mo to 12 y.

Organization

▶ AAP 2013

Recommendations

 –**Diagnosis of AOM**

- Moderate-to-severe bulging of tympanic membrane.
- New-onset otorrhea not due to otitis externa.
- Mild bulging of intensely red tympanic membrane with new otalgia <48 h duration.

 –**Treatment of AOM**

- Analgesics and antipyretics.
- Antibiotic indications:
  - Children <24 mo old with bilateral AOM.
  - No improvement or worsening of symptoms during 48- to 72-h observation period.
  - AOM associated with severe symptoms (extreme fussiness or severe otalgia).
- Observe for 48–72 h in the absence of severe symptoms and fever <102.2°F.

 –Consider tympanostomy tubes for recurrent AOM (3 episodes in 6 mo or 4 episodes in 1 y).

Comments

1. AOM is **not** present in the absence of a middle ear effusion based on pneumatic otoscopy or tympanometry.
2. Amoxicillin is the preferred antibiotics if the child has not received amoxicillin in the last 30 d.
3. Augmentin is the preferred antibiotic if the child has received amoxicillin in the last 30 d.

Source

 –http://www.guidelines.gov/content.aspx?id=43892

PHARYNGITIS, ACUTE

Population
–Children and adults.

Organization
▶ IDSA 2012

Recommendations

APPROACH TO ACUTE PHARYNGITIS

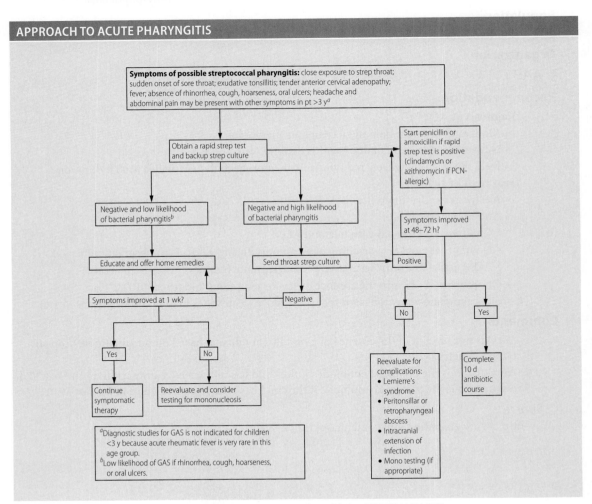

Source: IDSA 2012 guidelines on group A Streptococcus (GAS) pharyngitis. (https://doi.org/10.1093/cid/cis629)

RHINITIS (ALLERGIC)

Population
–Children and adults.

Organizations
▶ ICSI 2011, AAO-HSNF 2015

Recommendations
–Use intranasal steroids when symptoms affect quality of life.
–Use second-generation antihistamines if symptoms of itching or sneezing.
–Perform specific IgE serum or blood allergy testing if no response to treatment, uncertain diagnosis, or specific allergen identity is needed.
–Do not use leukotriene receptor antagonists as primary therapy.

MANAGEMENT OF NONINFECTIOUS RHINITIS

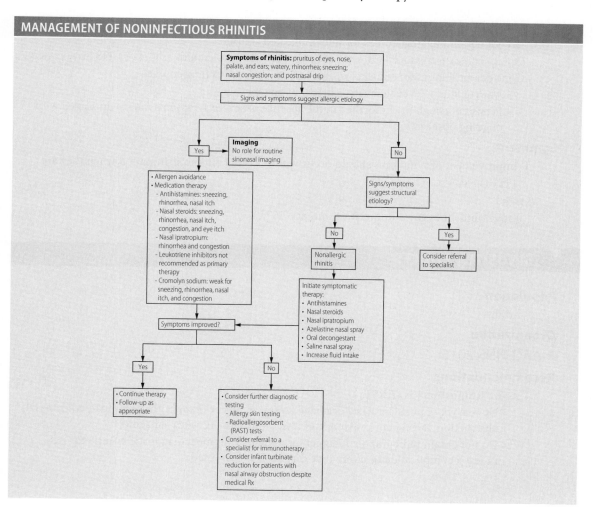

Sources
–ICSI 2011; AAO-HNSF 2015.
–https://www.entnet.org//content/clinical-practice-guideline-allergic-rhinitis

SINUSITIS, PEDIATRICS

Population
–Children.

Organization
▶ AAP 2013

–Presumptively diagnose acute sinusitis if child has acute URI and one of the following:
  • Nasal discharge or persistent cough lasting more than 10 d.
  • Worsening course.
  • Severe onset with fever ≥102.2°F and purulent nasal discharge for at least 3 d.
–Do not obtain imaging studies for uncomplicated sinusitis.
–Obtain contrast-enhanced CT scan of sinuses for any suspicion of orbital or CNS involvement.
–Consider antibiotics for sinusitis with severe onset or worsening course:
  • Amoxicillin +/− clavulanate is first-line therapy.
  • Persistent cough or rhinorrhea in the absence of severe symptoms may be managed with ongoing observation.

Comment
1. Improvement of symptoms should occur within 72 h of antibiotic initiation when they are prescribed.

Source
–https://guidelines.gov/summaries/summary/46939

SINUSITIS, ADULTS

Population
–Adults.

Organization
▶ AAO-HNS 2015

Recommendations
–**Acute Rhinosinusitis (ARS)**
  • Up to 4 wk of purulent nasal drainage (anterior, posterior, or both) accompanied by nasal obstruction, facial pain/pressure/fullness, or both (4–12 wk is subacute).
  • Do not obtain radiographic imaging for patients who meet diagnostic criteria for ARS, unless a complication or alternative diagnosis is suspected.

- **Viral Rhinosinusitis (VRS)**
  - Acute rhinosinusitis that is caused by, or is presumed to be caused by, viral infection. Diagnose viral rhinosinusitis when symptoms or signs of acute rhinosinusitis are present <10 d and the symptoms are not worsening.
- **Symptomatic Relief of VRS**
  - Clinicians may recommend analgesics, topical intranasal steroids, and/or nasal saline irrigation for symptomatic relief of VRS.
- **Differential Diagnosis**
  - Distinguish presumed ABRS from ARS caused by viral upper respiratory infections and noninfectious conditions.
- **Acute Bacterial Rhinosinusitis (ABRS)**
  - Acute rhinosinusitis that is caused by, or is presumed to be caused by, bacterial infection. Diagnose acute bacterial rhinosinusitis when:
    - Symptoms or signs of acute rhinosinusitis fail to improve within 10 d or more beyond the onset of upper respiratory symptoms.
    - Symptoms or signs of acute rhinosinusitis worsen within 10 d after an initial improvement (double worsening).
- **Initial Management**
  - Offer watchful waiting (without antibiotics) or prescribe initial antibiotic therapy for adults with uncomplicated ABRS.
  - Offer watchful waiting only when there is assurance of follow-up such that antibiotic therapy is started if the patient's condition fails to improve by 7 d after ABRS diagnosis or if it worsens at any time.
- **Choice of Antibiotic**
  - If a decision is made to treat ABRS with an antibiotic agent, prescribe amoxicillin with or without clavulanate as first-line therapy for 5–10 d for most adults.
- **Treatment Failure**
  - If the patient's condition worsens or fails to improve with the initial management option by 7 d after diagnosis or worsens during the initial management, reassess the patient to confirm ABRS, exclude other causes of illness, and detect complications.
  - If ABRS is confirmed in the patient initially managed with observation, begin antibiotic therapy.
  - If the patient was initially managed with an antibiotic, change the antibiotic.
- **Symptomatic Relief**
  - Consider recommending analgesics, topical intranasal steroids, and/or nasal saline irrigation for symptomatic relief of ABRS.
- **Chronic Rhinosinusitis (CRS)**
  - Twelve weeks or longer of 2 or more of the following signs and symptoms:
    - Mucopurulent drainage (anterior, posterior, or both).
    - Nasal obstruction (congestion).
    - Facial pain/pressure/fullness.
    - Decreased sense of smell.

- AND inflammation is documented by one or more of the following findings:
  - Purulent (not clear) mucus or edema in the middle meatus or anterior ethmoid region.
  - Polyps in nasal cavity or the middle meatus.
  - Radiographic imaging showing inflammation of the paranasal sinuses.

–**Recurrent Acute Rhinosinusitis**
  - Four or more episodes per year of acute bacterial rhinosinusitis without signs or symptoms of rhinosinusitis between episodes, provided each episode of acute bacterial rhinosinusitis meets diagnostic criteria for ARS.

–**CRS or Recurrent ARS—Diagnosis**
  - Distinguish CRS and recurrent ARS from isolated episodes of ABRS and other causes of sinonasal symptoms.

–**CRS—Objective Confirmation**
  - Confirm a clinical diagnosis of CRS with objective documentation of sinonasal inflammation, which may be accomplished using anterior rhinoscopy, nasal endoscopy, or computed tomography.

–**CRS—Topical Intranasal Therapy**
  - Recommend saline nasal irrigation, topical intranasal corticosteroids, or both for symptom relief of CRS.

–**CRS—Antifungal Therapy**
  - Do not prescribe topical or systemic antifungal therapy for patients with CRS.

Source
  –https://www.entnet.org//content/clinical-practice-guideline-adult-sinusitis

TINNITUS

Population
  –Adults and children.

Organization
▶ AAO-HNS 2014, American Speech-Language-Hearing Association 2018, NICE 2020

Recommendations
  –Obtain a thorough history and exam on patients with tinnitus. Elicit features such as unilateral or pulsatile tinnitus which may suggest more insidious etiology.
  –Refer for a comprehensive audiologic examination for unilateral or persistent tinnitus or any associated hearing impairment.
  –Obtain imaging studies only for unilateral tinnitus, pulsatile tinnitus, asymmetric hearing loss, or focal neurological abnormalities.
  –Refer for a hearing aid for tinnitus with hearing loss.
  –Consider cognitive behavioral therapy or sound therapy for persistent, bothersome tinnitus.
  –Do not offer medical or herbal therapy, including betahistine, or transcranial magnetic stimulation for tinnitus (ASHA: "remain current" in the evidence or lack thereof for these approaches).

Sources

–https://www.entnet.org//content/clinical-practice-guideline-tinnitus
–https://www.asha.org/Practice-Portal/Clinical-Topics/Tinnitus-and-Hyperacusis/
–https://www.nice.org.uk/guidance/ng155

TONSILLECTOMY

Population
–Children.

Organization
▶ AAO-HNS 2019

Recommendations
–Recommends against routine perioperative antibiotics for tonsillectomy.
–Tonsillectomy indicated for:
  • Tonsillar hypertrophy with sleep-disordered breathing.
  • Recurrent throat infections for ≥7 episodes of recurrent throat infection in last year; ≥5 episodes of recurrent throat infection per year in last 2 y; or at least 3 episodes per year for 3 y with documentation in the medical record for each episode of sore throat and ≥1 of the following: temperature >38.3°C (101°F), cervical adenopathy, tonsillar exudate, or positive test for group A beta-hemolytic streptococcus.
–Give post-tonsillectomy pain control, but do not use codeine in children less than age 12.

Source

–https://www.entnet.org/content/clinical-practice-guideline-tonsillectomy-children-update

TYMPANOSTOMY TUBES

Population
–Children 6 mo to 12 y.

Organization
▶ AAO 2013

Recommendations
–Do not insert tympanostomy tubes for children with:
  • A single episode of otitis media with effusion (OME) of <3 mo duration.
  • Recurrent acute otitis media without effusion.
–Obtain a hearing test if OME persists for at least 3 mo or if tympanostomy tube insertion is being considered.
–Offer bilateral tympanostomy tube insertion to children with:
  • Bilateral OME for at least 3 mo **AND** documented hearing impairment.
  • Recurrent acute otitis media with effusions.

- Tympanostomy tube insertion is an option for chronic symptomatic OME associated with balance problems, poor school performance, behavioral problems, or ear discomfort thought to be due to OME.

Comment

1. No need for prophylactic water precautions (avoidance of swimming or water sports or use of earplugs) for children with tympanostomy tubes.

Source

–http://www.guideline.gov/content.aspx?id=46909

VERTIGO, BENIGN PAROXYSMAL POSITIONAL (BPPV)

Population

–Adults.

Organization

▶ AAO-HNS 2017

Recommendations

–Use the Dix–Hallpike maneuver to diagnose posterior semicircular canal BPPV.
–Treat posterior semicircular canal BPPV with a particle repositioning maneuver.
–If the Dix–Hallpike test result is negative, use a supine roll test to diagnose lateral semicircular canal BPPV.
–Offer vestibular repositioning exercises such as the Epley maneuver for the initial treatment of BPPV.
–Observation is an acceptable initial management for patients with BPPV.
–Do not impose postprocedural postural restrictions for posterior canal BPPV.
–Evaluating patients for an underlying peripheral vestibular or central nervous system disorder if they have an initial treatment failure of presumed BPPV.
–Do not routinely obtain radiologic imaging for patients with BPPV.
–Do not routinely order vestibular testing for patients with BPPV.
–Do not routinely use antihistamines or benzodiazepines for patients with BPPV.

Comment

1. BPPV is the most common vestibular disorder in adults, afflicting 2.4% of adults at some point during their lives.
2. A positive Dix-Hallpike test is sufficient to diagnose BPPV, while a negative test is insufficient to rule it out if high pretest probability. (*Otolaryngol Clin North Am.* 2012;45(5):925-940)
3. A demonstration of the Dix-Hallpike maneuver is available here: https://youtu.be/8RYB2QlO1N4
4. A demonstration of the Epley maneuver is available here: https://youtu.be/jBzID5nVQjk

Source

–https://www.entnet.org//content/clinical-practice-guideline-benign-paroxysmal-positional-vertigo-bppv

Gastrointestinal Disorders

23

ABNORMAL LIVER CHEMISTRIES

Organization
▶ American College of Gastroenterology 2017

Recommendations

ALGORITHM FOR EVALUATION OF ASPARTATE AMINOTRANSFERASE (AST) AND/OR ALANINE AMINOTRANSFERASE (ALT) LEVEL

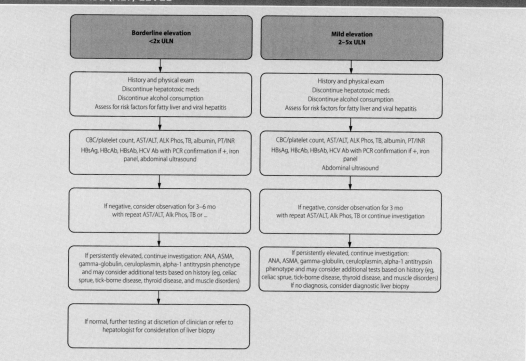

Borderline elevation <2x ULN	Mild elevation 2–5x ULN
History and physical exam Discontinue hepatotoxic meds Discontinue alcohol consumption Assess for risk factors for fatty liver and viral hepatitis	History and physical exam Discontinue hepatotoxic meds Discontinue alcohol consumption Assess for risk factors for fatty liver and viral hepatitis
CBC/platelet count, AST/ALT, ALK Phos, TB, albumin, PT/INR HBsAg, HBcAb, HBsAb, HCV Ab with PCR confirmation if +, iron panel, abdominal ultrasound	CBC/platelet count, AST/ALT, ALK Phos, TB, albumin, PT/INR HBsAg, HBcAb, HBsAb, HCV Ab with PCR confirmation if +, iron panel Abdominal ultrasound
If negative, consider observation for 3–6 mo with repeat AST/ALT, Alk Phos, TB or ...	If negative, consider observation for 3 mo with repeat AST/ALT, Alk Phos, TB or continue investigation
If persistently elevated, continue investigation: ANA, ASMA, gamma-globulin, ceruloplasmin, alpha-1 antitrypsin phenotype and may consider additional tests based on history (eg, celiac sprue, tick-borne disease, thyroid disease, and muscle disorders)	If persistently elevated, continue investigation: ANA, ASMA, gamma-globulin, ceruloplasmin, alpha-1 antitrypsin phenotype and may consider additional tests based on history (eg, celiac sprue, tick-borne disease, thyroid disease, and muscle disorders) If no diagnosis, consider diagnostic liver biopsy
If normal, further testing at discretion of clinician or refer to hepatologist for consideration of liver biopsy	

Source: Reproduced with permission from Kwo PY, Cohen SM, Lim JK. ACG clinical guideline: evaluation of abnormal liver chemistries. *Am J Gastroenterol.* 2017;112(1):18-35.

▶ HCV, hepatitis C virus

ALGORITHM FOR EVALUATION OF ELEVATED SERUM ALKALINE PHOSPHATASE

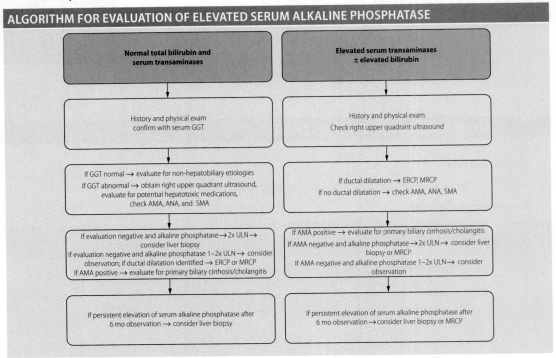

Source: Reproduced with permission from Kwo PY, Cohen SM, Lim JK. ACG clinical guideline: evaluation of abnormal liver chemistries. *Am J Gastroenterol.* 2017;112(1):18-35.

ALGORITHM FOR EVALUTION OF ELEVATED SERUM TOTAL BILIRUBIN

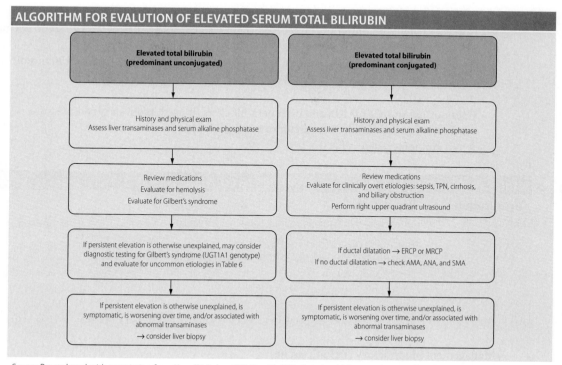

Source: Reproduced with permission from Kwo PY, Cohen SM, Lim JK. ACG clinical guideline: evaluation of abnormal liver chemistries. *Am J Gastroenterol.* 2017;112(1):18-35.

CIRRHOSIS: ASCITES

Population
–Adults with cirrhosis.

Organizations
▶ AASLD 2013, EASL 2018

Recommendations
–Perform diagnostic paracentesis for all patients with new-onset ascites.
–Do not routinely give platelets or fresh frozen plasma (FFP) prior to a paracentesis.
–Ascitic fluid analysis:
  • Cell count with differential.
  • Albumin.
  • Protein.
  • Bedside inoculation of aerobic and anaerobic culture bottles.
–Management of cirrhotic ascites:
  • Alcohol cessation.

- Low sodium diet.[1]
- Control ascites with diuretics. Target maximum weight loss per day of 0.5 kg/d if no edema or 1 kg/d if edema.
- Restrict fluid intake if serum sodium is low (AASLD <125 mmol/L; EASL <130 mmol/L).
- Consider liver transplantation for all patients with cirrhosis and ascites.
- Avoid NSAIDs.
- Cautious use of ACEI, ARB, and even beta-blockers. If used, monitor blood pressure carefully as an independent predictor of survival in patients with cirrhosis.
- Avoid aminoglycosides (EASL).

GUIDELINES DISCORDANT: INITIATING DIURETICS TO CONTROL ASCITES

Organization	Population
AASLD	Give furosemide and spironolactone in a 2:5 ratio
EASL	Start spironolactone at 100 mg/d Increase q3d to max dose of 400 mg/d as tolerated If <2 kg/wk weight loss and patient reaches max dose or develops hyperkalemia, add furosemide, starting at 40 mg/d Increase in 40 mg steps to maximum of 160 mg/d Consider substituting other loop diuretic if furosemide is not effective

–Management of refractory cirrhotic ascites:
- Avoid propranolol.
- Avoid ACEI or ARB.
- Consider oral midodrine, particularly if hypotensive.
- Consider serial therapeutic paracentesis.
- Consider transjugular intrahepatic portosystemic shunt (TIPSS) in carefully selected patients.
- Give albumin for large volume paracentesis (AASLD: give 6–8 g/L of ascitic fluid removed if >5 L; EASL: give 8 g/L ascitic fluid removed and consider even when <5 L).

–Management of spontaneous bacterial peritonitis (SBP):
- Give cefotaxime 2 g IV q8h for 5–7 d. Alternative is ofloxacin 400 mg PO bid.
- For locations with high bacterial resistance use piperacillin/tazobactam or carbapenem (EASL).
- Repeat paracentesis in 48 h to assess for reduction in leukocyte count of >25% (EASL).
- Add albumin 1.5 g/kg/d on day 1 and 1 g/kg/d on day 3 if creatinine >1 mg/dL, BUN >30 mg/dL, or bilirubin >4 mg/dL.

[1]2 g sodium/d is recommended by AASLD. EASL recommends 4.6–6.9 g/d which is equivalent to a no salt-added and no processed food diet.

- Consider diagnosis of secondary bacterial peritonitis and obtain CT scan of abdomen and early surgery if high neutrophil count in ascitic fluid, multiple cultured organisms, or high ascitic protein count (EASL).

–SBP prophylaxis:
- Give cefotaxime or oral norfloxacin for 7 d to anyone with cirrhosis admitted for upper gastrointestinal bleed (regardless of the presence of ascites).
- Give long-term oral trimethoprim-sulfamethoxazole or norfloxacin to any patient with a history of SBP. EASL: stop prophylaxis if long-term improvement with disappearance of ascites.
- Consider SBP prophylaxis if ascitic fluid protein <1.5 g/dL in association with creatinine >1.2 mg/dL or sodium <130 mmol/L or bilirubin >3 mg/dL.
- Consider liver transplant after first episode of SBP due to poor long-term survival (EASL).
- Only use proton pump inhibitors (PPIs) in those with clear indication due to possible increased risk for SBP (EASL).

–Hepatorenal syndrome options for treatment:
- Midodrine + SQ Octreotide + albumin.
- Norepinephrine infusion + albumin.
- Consider terlipressin over the use of norepinephrine since norepinephrine requires a central line with possible ICU admission. Use albumin 20% in doses of 20–40 g/d (EASL).
- Treat to bring the serum creatinine to within 0.3 mg/dL of baseline. If hepatorenal syndrome recurs after treatment, repeat the course. Consider renal replacement therapy in severe illness.
- Refer for liver transplantation.

–Hepatic hydrothorax:
- Do not place chest tube.
- Restrict dietary sodium and give diuretics. EASL: perform therapeutic thoracentesis if dyspnea.
- Consider TIPS for refractory cases.

–Avoid percutaneous gastrostomy tube placement in patients with ascites.

Sources
–AASLD. 2013. https://www.aasld.org/sites/default/files/guideline_documents/ AASLDPracticeGuidelineAsciteDuetoCirrhosisUpdate2012Edition4_.pdf
–EASL. 2018. https://doi.org/10.1016/j.jhep.2018.03.024

CIRRHOSIS: OTHER COMPLICATIONS

Population
–Adults with cirrhosis.

Organization
▶ EASL 2018

Recommendations

–Portal hypertensive gastropathy and intestinopathy (PHG):
- Use nonselective beta-blockers, iron supplementation, and/or blood transfusion as first-line therapy for chronic hemorrhage from PHG.
- Consider TIPS for transfusion-dependent patients.
- Acute PHG bleeding can be treated similarly to variceal bleeding, but there is limited data on efficacy of treatment.

–Renal impairment:
- Categorize renal disease as CKD, AKD, or AKI.
- Remove diuretics, NSBB, and nephrotoxic drugs immediately when impairment suspected.
- Replace fluid losses as needed.
- For AKI stage >1A (based on KDIGO criteria), or from infection-induced AKI, give 20% albumin at 1 g/kg for 2 d. Maximum dose of 100 g/d.
- In patients with AKI and tense ascites, perform paracentesis and replace albumin regardless of the volume removed.

–Acute-on-chronic liver failure:
- Acute-on-chronic liver failure has no particular therapy.
- Seek precipitating factors and treat.
- Expedite consideration for liver transplant.
- Suggest withdrawal of ongoing intensive care support if 4 or more organs are failing after 1 wk of adequate intensive treatment.

–Relative adrenal insufficiency (RAI):
- There is no recommended current treatment for RAI in cirrhosis.

–Cardiopulmonary complications:
- Assess systolic function with cardiac echo with dynamic stress testing (pharmacologic or exercise).
- Diastolic dysfunction may occur as an early sign of cardiomyopathy.
- Evaluate for prolonged QTc and discontinue medications as appropriate.

–Hepatopulmonary syndrome (HPS):
- Assess for HPS in patients with tachypnea, digital clubbing, and/or cyanosis. Screen initially with pulse oximetry, and if SpO2 <96% obtain ABG and further workup as indicated.
- Characterize HPS with contrast (microbubble) echocardiography. Consider transesophageal study to exclude intracardiac shunts.
- Treat patients with HPS and severe hypoxemia with long-term oxygen therapy. It is unclear how this treatment effects survival.
- Liver transplant is the only proven effective treatment for HPS.
- Perform ABG every 6 mo to prioritize liver transplant recipients since severe hypoxemia (PaO2 <45–50 mmHg) predicts increased mortality post–liver transplant.

–Portopulmonary hypertension (PPHT):
- Screen for PPHT with transthoracic echocardiogram and grade as mild, moderate, and severe based on mean pulmonary arterial pressure (mPAP).
- If there is evidence of PPHT, obtain a right heart catheterization.

- Stop beta-blockers and manage varices with endoscopic tools.
- Do not perform TIPS in patients with PPHT.

Comments

1. Confirm diagnosis of cirrhosis with ultrasound or MRI, which is preferred in obesity (Bashir et al. *JACR* 2020;17(5s)).
2. Preferred imaging modality to screen for HCC is ultrasound or MRI with contrast (Bashir et al. *JACR* 2020;17(5s)).

Sources

–AASLD. 2013. https://www.aasld.org/sites/default/files/guideline_documents/ AASLDPracticeGuidelineAsciteDuetoCirrhosisUpdate2012Edition4_.pdf
–EASL. 2018. https://doi.org/10.1016/j.jhep.2018.03.024

BARRETT ESOPHAGUS

Population

–Patients with biopsy diagnosis of Barrett esophagus (metaplastic columnar epithelium in distal esophagus).

Organization

▶ AGA 2011

Recommendations

–Perform endoscopic surveillance in patients with Barrett esophagus at intervals that vary with grade of dysplasia found in the metaplastic epithelium.
–No dysplasia:
  - Endoscopic surveillance (ES) every 3–5 y.
–Low-grade dysplasia: ES every 6–12 mo—consider radiofrequency ablation (RFA)—90% complete eradication of dysplasia.
–High-grade dysplasia: ES every 3 mo if no eradication therapy.
–Eradication therapy: RFA, photodynamic therapy (PDT), or endoscopic mucosal resection (EMR) is preferred over ES in high-grade dysplasia.
  - After complete eradication of intestinal metaplasia, arrange surveillance in 2 y, then every 3 y thereafter.
  - Patients who have not achieved complete eradication require surveillance every 6 mo for 1 y after the last endoscopy, then annually for 2 y, then every 3 y thereafter.
–Long-term use of PPIs:
  - Use long-term PPI in patients with Barrett esophagus, even if asymptomatic.
  - In patients with symptomatic GERD who respond to short-term PPIs, reduce the dose or attempt to stop them.
  - Do not use probiotics in long-term PPI routinely to prevent infection.
  - Do not recommend that long-term PPI users routinely raise their intake of calcium, vitamin B12, or magnesium beyond the Recommended Dietary Allowance.

- Do not routinely screen or monitor long-term PPI users for bone mineral density, serum creatinine, magnesium, or vitamin B12.

Comments

1. In patients with Barrett esophagus without dysplasia, 0.12% develop esophageal cancer per year compared to 0.5% with low-grade dysplasia. Progression from high-grade dysplasia to cancer is 6% per year. (*N Engl J Med.* 2011;365:1375)
2. Forty percent of patients with Barrett esophagus and esophageal cancer have no history of chronic GERD symptoms.
3. Long-term high-dose PPIs or antireflux therapy have been shown to decrease risk of neoplastic progression in patients with Barrett esophagus; however, dose frequency more than once daily is not recommended. (*Clin Gastroenterol Hepatol.* 2013;11:382)
4. Risk of developing cancer is higher among men, older patients (>65 y), and patients with long segments of Barrett mucosa or dysplasia. (*Am J Gastroenterol.* 2011;106:1231) (*Gut.* 2016;65:196)

Sources

–https://www.gastrojournal.org/article/S0016-5085(11)00084-9/fulltext
–https://www.gastrojournal.org/article/S0016-5085(16)35137-X/fulltext
–https://www.gastrojournal.org/article/S0016-5085(17)30091-4/fulltext

CELIAC DISEASE

Population

–Children and adults with celiac disease.

Organization

▶ NICE 2017

Recommendations

–Serological testing for suspected celiac disease:
- Test for total IgA and IgA tissue transglutaminase (tTG).
- Use IgA endomysial antibody test if IgA tTG is weakly positive.

–Other immunoassays regarded as good are the IgA-transglutaminase 2 (TG2) test or IgG-deamidated gliadin peptide (DGP) test.

–Refer individuals with positive serological tests to a GI specialist for endoscopic duodenal biopsy to confirm the diagnosis.

–After diagnosis, monitoring, including antibody tests, is recommended every 3–6 mo in the first year and once a year thereafter in stable patients responding to the gluten-free diet.

–For refractory celiac disease despite strict adherence to gluten-free diet:
- Review certainty of diagnosis.
- Consider coexisting conditions such as irritable bowel syndrome, lactose intolerance, microscopic colitis, or inflammatory bowel disease.

Comments

1. The incidence has been increasing over the last 20 y.
2. The highest incidence of celiac disease seroconversion is between 12 and 36 mo of age.

Source

–https://www.nice.org.uk/guidance/qs134

COLITIS, *CLOSTRIDIUM DIFFICILE*

Population

–Adults and children.

Organization

▶ IDSA SHEA 2017

Recommendations

–Diagnosis of *C. difficile* infection:

- Updated guidelines provide a much clearer algorithm for laboratory testing, though initial step of this algorithm is centered upon each institution's practice.
- In general, Nucleic Acid Amplification Test (NAAT) is preferred to Enzyme Immunoassay (EIA or toxin testing).
- If the institution uses only specimens from patients who are not taking laxatives and have at least 3 or more unformed stools in a 24-h period, then using the NAAT alone is satisfactory.
- Stool toxin test may be used in a multistep algorithm with glutamate dehydrogenase (GDH) to satisfy the recommendation.
- If toxin test is negative, algorithm still recommends follow-up with the NAAT.
- Test for *C. difficile* or its toxins only on diarrheal stool (3 or more unformed stool in 24-h period).
- Avoid testing of stool on asymptomatic patients.
- Repeat testing (within 7 d) during same episode of diarrhea is not recommended.

–Treatment of *C. difficile* infection:

- Discontinue inciting antibiotic agent as soon as possible.
- Avoid antiperistaltic agents.
- New guidelines recommend vancomycin and fidaxomicin, instead of metronidazole, as first-line treatments for *C. difficile*.
- Metronidazole can still be considered as first-line treatment in situations where accessibility to vancomycin and fidaxomicin is limited and in mild-to-moderate disease.
- Initial *C. difficile* infection: vancomycin 125 mg orally 4 times per day or fidaxomicin 200 mg twice daily for 10 d.
- Initial *C. difficile* infection, fulminant[1]: vancomycin 500 mg 4 times per day by mouth or by nasogastric tube. If ileus, consider adding rectal instillation of vancomycin. Intravenously

---

[1]Fulminant *C. difficile* infection, previously referred to as severe, complicated CDI, is characterized by hypotension or shock, ileus, or megacolon.

administer metronidazole (500 mg every 8 h) together with oral or rectal vancomycin, particularly if ileus is present.

- First recurrence, if metronidazole was used for the initial episode: vancomycin 125 mg given 4 times daily for 10 d.
- First recurrence, if standard regimen was used: a prolonged tapered and pulsed vancomycin regimen (eg, 125 mg 4 times per day for 10–14 d, 2 times per day for a week, once per day for a week, and then every 2 or 3 d for 2–8 wk) or fidaxomicin 200 mg twice daily for 10 d.
- Second or subsequent recurrence: prolonged tapered and pulsed vancomycin regimen, or vancomycin 125 mg given 4 times daily for 10 d followed by rifaximin 400 mg 3 times daily for 20 d, or fidaxomicin 200 mg twice daily for 10 d, or fecal microbiota transplantation.

Comments

1. Probiotics such as *Lactobacillus* and *Saccharomyces boulardii* have been associated with some reduction in *C. difficile* recurrence; however, significant results demonstrating efficacy in controlled clinical trials have yet to be seen. Thus, standard utilization of probiotics in the setting of *C. difficile* is not currently supported.
2. Perform hand hygiene before and after contact with patient. Handwashing with soap and water is preferred if there is direct contact.
3. Use disposable patient equipment when possible and ensure that reusable equipment is thoroughly cleaned and disinfected, preferentially with a sporicidal disinfectant.
4. With regard to antibiotic stewardship in order to control increasing rates of *C. difficile*, the guidelines stress attempts to minimize the frequency and duration of high-risk antibiotic therapy and the number of antibiotic agents prescribed.

Source
–https://academic.oup.com/cid/article/66/7/e1/4855916

Population
–Children.

Organization
▶ IDSA SHEA 2017

Recommendations

–Pediatric diagnosis of *C. difficile*:
- Because of the high prevalence of asymptomatic carriage of toxigenic *C. difficile* in infants, do not routinely test for CDI in neonates or infants ≤12 mo of age with diarrhea.
- Colonization rates decrease with increasing age. By 2–3 y of age, approximately 1%–3% of children are asymptomatic carriers of *C. difficile* (a rate similar to that observed in healthy adults).
- In children ≥2 y of age, *C. difficile* testing is recommended for patients with prolonged or worsening diarrhea and risk factors (underlying inflammatory bowel disease, immunocompromising conditions, presence of a gastrostomy or jejunostomy tube) or relevant exposures (contact with the health care system or recent antibiotics).

–Pediatric treatment of *C. difficile*:
- Discontinue inciting antibiotic agent as soon as possible.

- Avoid antiperistaltic agents.
- Either metronidazole or vancomycin is recommended for the treatment of children with an initial episode or first recurrence of nonsevere *C. difficile* infection.
- Initial *C. difficile* infection, nonsevere: metronidazole po for 10 d (7.5 mg/kg/dose tid or qid) or vancomycin po for 10 d (10 mg/kg/dose qid).
- Initial *C. difficile* infection, severe/fulminant: vancomycin po/pr for 10 d (10 mg/kg/dose qid). Consider addition of IV metronidazole for 10 d (10 mg/kg/dose tid).
- First recurrence, nonsevere: metronidazole po for 10 d (7.5 mg/kg/dose tid or qid) or vancomycin po for 10 d (10 mg/kg/dose qid).
- Second or subsequent recurrence: prolonged tapered and pulsed vancomycin regimen,[1] or vancomycin for 10 d (10 mg/kg/dose qid) followed by rifaximin[2] for 20 d, or fecal microbiota transplantation.

Source
–https://academic.oup.com/cid/article/66/7/e1/4855916

Population

–Adult patients with *C. difficile*–associated disease.

Organization

▶ EAST 2014

Recommendations

–If surgery is indicated, recommend a subtotal or total colectomy.
–For severe CDAD, perform surgery prior to the development of shock and need for vasopressors.

Source
–https://www.east.org/education/practice-management-guidelines/clostridium-difficile-associated-disease---timing-and-type-of-surgical-treatment

DIVERTICULAR DISEASE

Population

–Adults with diverticulosis.

Organization

▶ NICE 2020

Recommendations

–Diverticulosis:
  - Recommend high-fiber diet and/or bulk-forming laxatives to reduce constipation.

---

[1]10 mg/kg with max of 125 mg 4 times per day for 10–14 d, then 10 mg/kg with max of 125 mg 2 times per day for a week, then 10 mg/kg with max of 125 mg once per day for a week, and then 10 mg/kg with max of 125 mg every 2 or 3 d for 2–8 wk.
[2]No pediatric dosing for rifaximin given, as it is not approved by the US Food and Drug Administration for use in children.

- Avoid NSAIDs and opioid analgesia if possible.
- Consider antispasmodic for abdominal cramping.

–Acute diverticulitis:
- Offer oral antibiotics if patient is systemically unwell, immunocompromised, or has significant comorbidities.
- Offer IV antibiotics for complicated acute diverticulitis.
- Consider percutaneous drainage or surgery for abscesses >3 cm.
- Offer laparoscopic lavage or surgical resection for diverticular perforation with peritonitis.
- Consider elective resection in patients continuing to have symptoms, such as stricture or fistula, after recovering from acute complicated diverticulitis. There is no recommendation on the timing of surgery.
- Do not use 5-ASA or antibiotics to prevent recurrent acute diverticulitis.

Source
–https://www.nice.org.uk/guidance/ng147

COLORECTAL CANCER FOLLOW-UP CARE

Population
–Adults with nonmetastatic colorectal cancer (Stages II and III).

Organization
▶ American Society of Clinical Oncology Cancer Care Ontario (CCO) 2013

Recommendations
–Highest risk of recurrence during first 4 y after diagnosis; 95% of relapses occur in first 5 y.
–Medical history, physical exam, and CEA testing every 3–6 mo for 5 y. The higher the risk, the more frequent the follow-up.
–Obtain abdominal and chest CT scan annually for 3 y. In highest risk patients (Stage III, >4 nodes+) consider imaging every 4–6 mo.
–Do not use routine PET scan for surveillance.
- If rectal cancer, get pelvic CT annually for 3–5 y.
–Perform surveillance colonoscopy 1 y after initial surgery. If normal, repeat colonoscopy every 5 y. If complete colonoscopy not performed before diagnosis, perform it as soon as the patient recovers from adjuvant therapy.
–Consider recurrence if any new or persistent worsening of symptoms.
–There is insufficient evidence to recommend routine use of FIT or fecal DNA for surveillance after CRC resection.

Comments
1. Stage I colon cancer with very low risk of recurrence. Colonoscopy follow-up every 5 y but CEA and imaging not needed.
2. Colon cancer with >90% to liver as the first site of metastasis. In rectal cancer, 50% of first metastasis is to lung and 50% to liver. (*CA Cancer J Clin.* 2015;65:5)

3. Follow patients found to have resectable metastatic disease (liver, lungs) or local recurrence who are rendered disease free by surgical or radiofrequency ablation (RFA) with frequent surveillance. Ten-year survival is in the 30%–40% range. (*J Clin Oncol.* 2010;28:2300)

4. BRAF mutation prognostic for early relapse and chemotherapy resistance with shortened survival. (*PLoS One.* 2013;8:eb5995)

5. Evaluate patients with CRC younger than 50 y or with significant family history for Lynch syndrome with microsatellite instability and immune histochemistry testing. (*N Engl J Med.* 2009;361:2449)

6. Advise exercise (>150 min/wk), weight loss for high BMI, smoking cessation, and healthy diet—evidence suggests a decrease in disease recurrence.

Sources
–*J Clin Oncol.* 2013;31:4465-4470.
–https://www.ncbi.nlm.nih.gov/pmc/articles/PMC4445789/

CONSTIPATION, IDIOPATHIC

Population
–Children age ≤18 y.

Organization
▶ NICE 2010 (updated 2017)

Recommendations
–Assess all children for fecal impaction.
–If evidence of poor growth, test for celiac disease and hypothyroidism.
–Recommend polyethylene glycol (PEG) as first-line agent for oral disimpaction.
–Add a stimulant laxative if PEG therapy is ineffective after 2 wk.
–Use sodium citrate enemas for disimpaction only if all oral medications have failed.
–Use a maintenance regimen with PEG for several months after a regular bowel pattern has been established.
–Gradually taper maintenance dose over several months as bowel pattern allows.
–Recommend adequate fluid intake.

Comment
1. Minimal fluid intake for age

Age (y)	Volume (mL)
1–3	1300
4–8	1700
9–13	2200
14–18	2500

Source
-https://www.nice.org.uk/guidance/cg99

Population
-Adults.

Organization
▶ AGA 2013

Recommendations
-Digital examination to evaluate resting sphincter tone.
-Discontinue all medications that can cause constipation.
-Assess for hypercalcemia, hypothyroidism.
-Trial of laxatives and fiber:
  • Bisacodyl.
  • Milk of magnesia.
  • Polyethylene glycol.
  • Senna.
-Refractory constipation may require biofeedback or pelvic floor retraining. Severe cases of refractory slow transit constipation may require a total colectomy with ileorectal anastomosis.

Source
-http://www.gastrojournal.org/article/S0016-5085%2812%2901545-4/fulltext

CONSTIPATION, OPIATE INDUCED

Population
-Adults.

Organization
▶ AGA 2019

Recommendations
-Use laxatives as first-line agents.
-For patients with laxative refractory opiate-induced constipation (OIC), use 1 of 3 peripherally acting μ-opioid receptor antagonists (PAMORAs). Avoid these agents in conditions that compromise blood-brain barrier, such as CNS infections, stroke, and traumatic brain injury, to avoid precipitating withdrawal or reversing analgesic effect. Available PAMORAs:
  • Naldemedine (high-quality evidence).
  • Naloxegol (moderate-quality evidence).
  • Methylnatrexone (low-quality evidence).
-Not enough evidence to recommend for or against using lubiprostone (intestinal secretagogue) or prucalopride (selective 5-HT agonist).

Comments

1. Traditional laxatives are divided into 4 categories: osmotic (eg, PEG/lactulose/magnesium citrate), stimulant (eg, bisacodyl/senna/sodium picosulfate), stool softener (eg, docusate), or lubricant (eg, mineral oil).
2. There is limited evidence that routine use of stimulant laxatives for OIC is harmful to the colon despite previous concerns.
3. Fiber has limited effect on OIC, except in patients with fiber-deficient diets.
4. Enemas can sometimes be used as rescue therapy when OIC is refractory to oral treatments.

Source

–https://doi.org/10.1053/j.gastro.2018.07.016

DIARRHEA, ACUTE

Population

–Adults with acute diarrheal illness.

Recommendations

APPROACH TO EMPIRIC THERAPY AND DIAGNOSTIC-DIRECTED MANAGEMENT OF THE ADULT PATIENT WITH ACUTE DIARRHEA (SUSPECT INFECTIOUS ETIOLOGY)

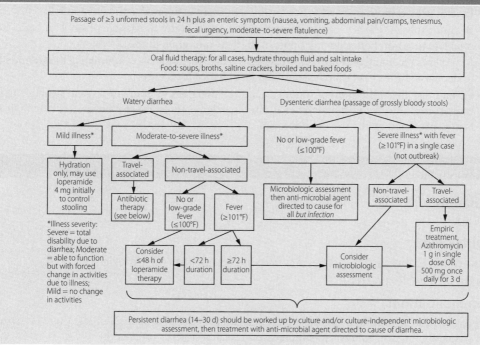

Source: Reproduced with permission from Riddle MS, DuPont HL, Connor BA. ACG clinical guideline: diagnosis, treatment, and prevention of acute diarrheal infections in adults. *Am J Gastroenterol.* 2016;111(5):602-622.

ACUTE DIARRHEA ANTIBIOTIC TREATMENT RECOMMENDATIONS

Antibiotic[a]	Dose	Treatment duration
Levofloxacin	500 mg by mouth	Single dose[b] or 3-d course
Ciprofloxacin	750 mg by mouth or	Single dose[b]
	500 mg by mouth	3-d course
Ofloxacin	400 mg by mouth	Single dose[b] or 3-d course
Azithromycin[c,d]	1000 mg by mouth or	Single dose[b]
	500 mg by mouth	3-d course[d]
Rifaximin[e]	200 mg by mouth 3 times daily	3-d

ETEC, Enterotoxigenic *Escherichia coli*.

[a] Antibiotic regimens may be combined with loperamide, 4 mg first dose, and then 2 mg dose after each loose stool, not to exceed 16 mg in a 24-h period.

[b] If symptoms are not resolved after 24 h, complete a 3-d course of antibiotics.

[c] Use empirically as first line in Southeast Asia and India to cover fluoroquinolone-resistant *Campylobacter* or in other geographical areas if *Campylobacter* or resistant ETEC are suspected.

[d] Preferred regimen for dysentery or febrile diarrhea.

[e] Do not use if clinical suspicion for *Campylobacter, Salmonella, Shigella*, or other causes of invasive diarrhea.

Source: Reproduced with permission from Riddle MS, DuPont HL, Connor BA. ACG clinical guideline: diagnosis, treatment, and prevention of acute diarrheal infections in adults. *Am J Gastroenterol.* 2016;111(5):602-622.

- –Do not use probiotics or prebiotics for the treatment of acute diarrhea in adults.
- –Bismuth subsalicylates can be administered to control rates of passage of stool and may help travelers function better during bouts of mild-to-moderate illness.
- –In patients receiving antibiotics for traveler's diarrhea, administer adjunctive loperamide therapy to decrease duration of diarrhea and increase chance for a cure.
- –Discourage antibiotics for community-acquired diarrhea, as epidemiological studies suggest that most community-acquired diarrhea is viral in origin (norovirus, rotavirus, and adenovirus) and is not shortened by the use of antibiotics.

DYSPEPSIA

Population
- –Adults with dyspepsia.

Organization
▶ American College of Gastroenterology/Canadian Association of Gastroenterology 2017

Recommendations
- –Avoid routine motility studies for patients with functional dyspepsia unless there is a strong suspicion for gastroparesis in which case a motility study is indicated.

WORKUP OF UNDIAGNOSED DYSPEPSIA

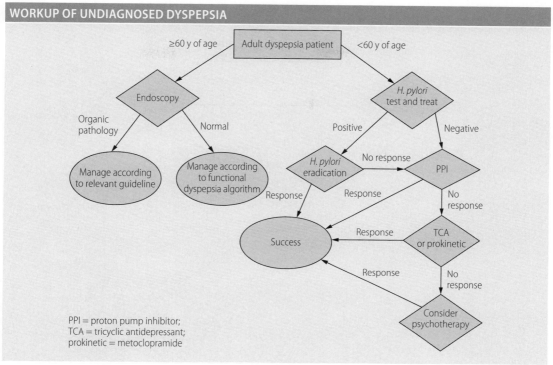

PPI = proton pump inhibitor;
TCA = tricyclic antidepressant;
prokinetic = metoclopramide

Source: Reproduced with permission from Moayyedi P, Lacy BE, Andrews CN, Enns RA, Howden CW, Vakil N. ACG and CAG clinical guideline: management of dyspepsia [published correction appears in Am J Gastroenterol. 2017 Sep;112(9):1484]. *Am J Gastroenterol.* 2017;112(7):988-1013.

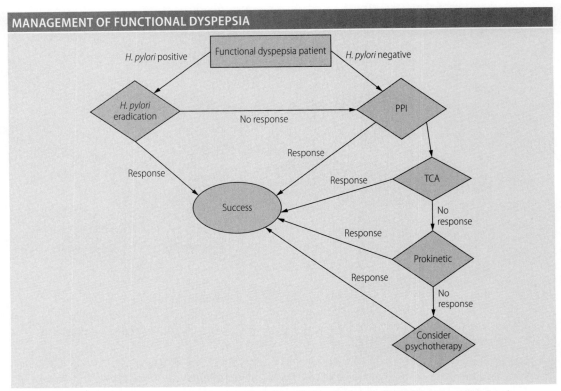

MANAGEMENT OF FUNCTIONAL DYSPEPSIA

Source: Reproduced with permission from Moayyedi P, Lacy BE, Andrews CN, Enns RA, Howden CW, Vakil N. ACG and CAG clinical guideline: management of dyspepsia [published correction appears in Am J Gastroenterol. 2017 Sep;112(9):1484]. *Am J Gastroenterol.* 2017;112(7):988-1013.

Population
–Adults with GERD and dyspepsia.

Organization
▶ NICE 2014

Recommendations
–Recommend smoking cessation and weight reduction.
–Consider discontinuation of offending medications (calcium channel blockers, nitrates, theophylline, bisphosphonates, steroids, and NSAIDs).
–Consider testing for *H. pylori* after a 2-wk washout off PPIs.
–Empiric trial of PPI therapy.
–Consider laparoscopic fundoplication for patients who do not wish to continue with acid suppressive therapy long term.
–Consider specialist referral for:

- Dyspepsia refractory to meds.
- Consideration of surgery.
- Refractory *H. pylori* infection.
- Barrett esophagus.

Source
  –https://www.nice.org.uk/guidance/cg184

GALLSTONES

Population
  –Adults with or suspected of having gallstones.

Organizations
▶ NICE 2014, EASL 2014

Recommendations
  –Diagnosis:
  - Obtain liver function tests and ultrasound if suspected gallstone disease.
  - Suspect acute cholecystitis in a patient with fever, severe pain located in the right upper abdominal quadrant lasting for several hours, and right upper abdominal pain and tenderness on palpation.
  - Consider magnetic resonance cholangiopancreatography (MRCP) if ultrasound has not detected common bile duct stones but the common bile duct is dilated and liver function tests are abnormal.
  –Treatment:
  - Offer cholecystectomy for symptomatic gallstones or acute cholecystitis.
  - Do not offer litholysis using bile acids alone or in combination with extracorporeal shock wave lithotripsy.
  - Offer percutaneous cholecystostomy for acute cholecystitis or gallbladder empyema if surgery is contraindicated.
  - Options for choledocholithiasis:
    ○ Cholecystectomy and intraoperative clearance of CBD stones.
    ○ ERCP prior to cholecystectomy.

Sources
  –https://www.nice.org.uk/guidance/cg188
  –http://www.easl.eu/medias/cpg/Prevention-diagnosis-and-treatment-of-gallstones/English-report.pdf

GASTROINTESTINAL BLEEDING, LOWER

Population
–Adults with suspected lower GI bleeding and coagulopathy.

Organization
▶ ACG 2016

Recommendations
–Consider platelet transfusion to maintain a platelet count of 50,000 in patients with severe bleeding and those requiring endoscopic hemostasis.
–Consider reversal of anticoagulation before endoscopy in patients with an INR > 2.5.

Source
–ACG clinical guideline: management of patients with acute lower gastrointestinal bleeding. *Am J Gastroenterol.* 2016;111:459-474.

ALGORITHM FOR THE MANAGEMENT OF PATIENTS PRESENTING WITH ACUTE LGIB STRATIFIED BY BLEEDING SEVERITY

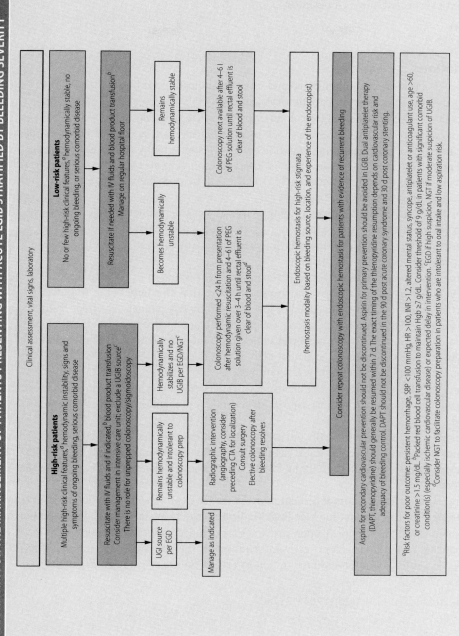

CTA, computed tomographic angiography; DAPT, dual antiplatelet therapy; EGD, esophagogastroduodenoscopy; LGBI, lower gastrointestinal bleeding; NGT, nasogastric tube; PEG, polyethylene glycol; UGIB, upper gastrointestinal bleeding.

Source: Reproduced with permission from Strate LL, Gralnek IM. ACG Clinical guideline: management of patients with acute lower gastrointestinal bleeding [published correction appears in Am J Gastroenterol. 2016 May;111(5):755]. Am J Gastroenterol. 2016;111(4):459–474. doi:10.1038/ajg.2016.41.

Population

–Adults with suspected lower GI bleeding.

Organization

▶ BSG 2019

Recommendations

–Patients with a minor self-limited bleed and no other indication for hospitalization may be discharged home for urgent outpatient investigation.

–Admit patients with major bleed for colonoscopy as soon as possible.

–In patients who are unstable or have a shock index >1 (heart rate/systolic BP) after initial resuscitation or are having ongoing active bleeding, CT angiography is the fastest and least invasive method to localize the site of blood loss. If no source is identified on CT angiography, perform an upper endoscopy immediately as LGIB with hemodynamic instability may indicate an upper gastrointestinal bleed.

–In centers with 24/7 interventional radiology services, consider catheter angiography with the intent to embolize the site of bleeding prior to endoscopic investigation.

–Defer emergency laparotomy unless all effort has been made to localize the bleeding using radiological and endoscopic modalities.

–If transfusion is required, use a restrictive transfusion threshold of 7 g/dL and target of 7–9 g/dL. If history of cardiovascular disease, the threshold is 8 g/dL with a target of 8–10 g/dL.

–Stop warfarin therapy at presentation. For low thrombotic risk patients, consider resuming in 7 d and for high-risk thrombotic patients (ie, prosthetic heart valve in mitral location, atrial fibrillation with prosthetic valve or mitral stenosis, <3 mo after venous thromboembolism) begin low-molecular-weight heparin after 48 h. If unstable from bleeding, reverse with prothrombin complex concentrate and vitamin K.

–If patients with lower GI bleeds take aspirin for primary prophylaxis of cardiovascular events, discontinue it permanently. Restart aspirin for secondary prevention after hemostasis is achieved.

–For patients with coronary stents in situ and on dual antiplatelet therapy, discuss with cardiology but do not stop routinely. For unstable hemorrhage patients, continue aspirin but stop P2Y12 receptor antagonist. Consider restarting P2Y12 receptor antagonist therapy in 5 d after bleeding is controlled.

–Stop direct oral anticoagulants at presentation. Consider treating with inhibitors (idarucizumab or andexanet) for life-threatening bleeding. Medication can be restarted in 7 d after hemorrhage.

–All hospitals should have agreed-upon pathways for management of GI bleeding. Those who admit patients with on-site colonoscopy and endoscopic therapy should have availability 7 d/wk as well as access to 24/7 interventional radiology (either on site or via referral pathway).

Source

–http://dx.doi.org/10.1136/gutjnl-2018-317807

GASTROINTESTINAL BLEEDING, UPPER (UGIB)

Population
–Adults, 16 y or older.

Organizations
▶ NICE 2012 (updated in 2016), EASL 2018

Recommendations
–Recommend a formal risk assessment for patients with a UGIB:
  • Blatchford score at first assessment.
  • Rockall score after endoscopy.
–Avoid platelet transfusions in patients who are not actively bleeding and are hemodynamically stable.
–For UGIB, give FFP if: +
  • Fibrinogen <100 mg/dL.
  • Partial thromboplastin time >1.5× normal.
–Prothrombin complex concentrate (PCC) indicated for UGIB on warfarin.
–Timing of endoscopy:
  • Immediately for unstable patients.
  • Within 24 h for stable patients.
–Management of nonvariceal bleeding:
  • Surgical clips.
  • Thermal coagulation.
  • Epinephrine injection.
  • Fibrin or thrombin glue.
  • Recurrent bleeding can be assessed by repeat endoscopy or by interventional radiology angioembolization.
  • PPIs.
–Management of variceal bleeding:
  • Esophageal variceal band ligation (EASL: within 12 h of admission).
  • Terlipressin or octreotide infusions.
  • Prophylactic third-generation cephalosporin.
  • Transjugular intrahepatic portosystemic shunt for recurrent esophageal variceal bleeding or gastric variceal bleeding.
  • Blood transfusion if necessary (EASL: use restrictive transfusion strategy with threshold of 7 g/dL and target of 7–9 g/dL).
  • Use balloon tamponade only as bridge therapy to definitive treatment and for a maximum of 24 h.
  • Stop beta-blockers and vasodilators and consider using lactulose to prophylaxis for hepatic encephalopathy.
–Prevention and treatment of variceal hemorrhage:

- Primary prophylaxis for varices is indicated for high-risk varices—small varices with red signs, medium or large varices, or small varices in Child-Pugh C patients.
- After banding and stabilization, initiate nonselective beta-blockers used to decrease risk.
- Use propranolol or nadolol. Do not use carvedilol. Use caution in patients with ascites.
- If intolerant to beta-blockers, consider patient for TIPS.

–Gastric varices:
- Use nonselective beta-blockers as primary prevention.
- Give medical therapy for acute gastric variceal hemorrhage as for esophageal variceal hemorrhage. During endoscopy, choose cyanoacrylate as sclerosing agent.
- Consider TIPS or selective embolization thru interventional radiology.

Comments

1. Stop NSAIDs.
2. Alcohol cessation if a factor.
3. Low-dose aspirin can be resumed if needed for secondary prevention of vascular events once hemostasis has been achieved.
4. Use of thienopyridine agents (eg, clopidogrel, ticagrelor, or prasugrel) ongoing only after discussion with appropriate specialist.

Sources

–NICE. 2012. https://www.nice.org.uk/Guidance/cg141
–EASL. 2018. https://doi.org/10.1016/j.jhep.2018.03.024

HELICOBACTER PYLORI INFECTION

Population

–Adults.

Organization

▶ American College of Gastroenterology 2017

Recommendations

–Screen the following patients for *Helicobacter pylori* (*H. pylori*) infection:
- Active peptic ulcer disease (PUD).
- A past history of PUD (unless previous cure of *H. pylori* infection has been documented).
- Low-grade gastric mucosa-associated lymphoid tissue (MALT) lymphoma.
- Undiagnosed dyspepsia.
- Patients who are under the age of 60 y.
- Patients initiating chronic treatment with a nonsteroidal anti-inflammatory drug (NSAID).
- Unexplained iron deficiency anemia.
- Idiopathic thrombocytopenic purpura.
- A history of endoscopic resection of early gastric cancer (EGC).

–Treat all patients who test positive for *H. pylori*.

–Choice of therapy depends on prior antibiotic exposure.

–Consider clarithromycin triple therapy consisting of a PPI, clarithromycin, and amoxicillin or metronidazole for 14 d in regions where *H. pylori* resistance to clarithromycin is known to be <15% and in patients with no previous history of macrolide exposure for any reason.

–Consider bismuth quadruple therapy consisting of a PPI, bismuth, tetracycline, and a nitroimidazole for 10–14 d. Bismuth quadruple therapy is particularly attractive in patients with any previous macrolide exposure or who are allergic to penicillin.

–Consider levofloxacin triple therapy consisting of a PPI, levofloxacin, and amoxicillin for 10–14 d.

–Consider concomitant therapy consisting of a PPI, clarithromycin, amoxicillin, and a nitroimidazole for 10–14 d.

–Whenever *H. pylori* infection is identified and treated, perform testing to prove eradication using a urea breath test, fecal antigen test, or biopsy-based testing at least 4 wk after the completion of antibiotic therapy and after PPI therapy has been withheld for 1–2 wk.

–Bismuth quadruple therapy or levofloxacin salvage regimens are the preferred treatment options if a patient received a first-line treatment containing clarithromycin.

Sources

–ACG clinical guideline: treatment of *Helicobacter pylori* infection. *Am J Gastroenterol.* 2017;112:212-238.

–http://gi.org/guideline/treatment-of-helicobacter-pylori-infection/

Organization

▶ Cochrane Database Systematic Reviews 2013

Recommendation

–Use longer duration therapy for PPI-based *H. pylori* therapy.

Source

–http://www.cochrane.org/CD008337/UPPERGI_ideal-length-of-treatment-for-helicobacter-pylori-h.-pylori-eradication

HEPATITIS B VIRUS (HBV)

Population

–Adults and children with HBV infection.

Organization

▶ AASLD 2016 (with 2018 guidance update)

Recommendations

–Screening, counseling, and prevention:
  • The presence of HBsAg establishes the diagnosis of hepatitis B. Chronic versus acute infection is defined by the presence of HBsAg for at least 6 mo.

- HBV is transmitted by perinatal, percutaneous, sexual exposure and by close person-to-person contact.
- Perinatal transmission is an important cause of chronic infection.
- Recommend HBV immunoglobulin and HBV vaccine to all infants born to HBsAg-positive women.
- Screen high-risk individuals for HBV infection and immunized if seronegative. These include:
  ○ Persons born in regions of high or intermediate HBV endemicity (HBsAg prevalence of >2%).
  ○ US-born persons not vaccinated as an infant whose parents were born in regions with high HBV endemicity (>8%).
  ○ Persons who have ever injected drugs.
  ○ Men who have sex with men.
  ○ Persons needing immunosuppressive therapy, including chemotherapy, immunosuppression related to organ transplantation, and immunosuppression for rheumatologic or gastroenterologic disorders.
  ○ Individuals with elevated ALT or AST of unknown etiology.
  ○ Donors of blood, plasma, organs, tissues, or semen.
  ○ Persons with end-stage renal disease.
  ○ All pregnant women.
  ○ Infants born to HBsAg-positive mothers.
  ○ Persons with chronic liver disease, eg, HCV.
  ○ Persons with HIV.
  ○ Household, needle-sharing, and sexual contacts of HBsAg-positive persons.
  ○ Persons seeking evaluation or treatment for a sexually transmitted disease.
  ○ Health care and public safety workers at risk for occupational exposure to blood or blood-contaminated body fluids.
  ○ Travelers to countries with intermediate or high prevalence of HBV infection.
  ○ Inmates of correctional facilities.
  ○ Unvaccinated persons with diabetes who are aged 19 through 59 y.
–Screen using both HBsAg and anti-HBs:
  - Counsel HBsAg-positive persons regarding prevention of transmission of HBV to others.
  - Other than practicing universal precautions, no special arrangements are indicated for HBV-infected children unless they are prone to biting.
  - Abstinence or only limited use of alcohol is recommended in HBV-infected persons.
–Screen all pregnant women for HBsAg:
  - HBV vaccination is safe in pregnancy. Vaccinate pregnant women who are not immune to or infected with HBV.
  - Treat women who meet standard indications for HBV therapy. Consider treatment for women without standard indications but who have HBV DNA >200,000 IU/mL in the second trimester to prevent mother-to-child transmission.
  - Breastfeeding is not prohibited.

- HBV vaccines have an excellent safety record and are given as a 3-dose series at 0, 1, and 6 mo.
- Vaccinate sexual and household contacts of HBV-infected persons who are negative for HBsAg and anti-HBs.
- Give newborns of HBV-infected mothers at delivery with HBIG and HBV vaccine at delivery and complete the recommended vaccination series. Test infants of HBsAg-positive mothers with postvaccination testing at 9–15 mo of age.

–Diagnosis:
- Diagnostic criteria of chronic hepatitis B:
  ◦ HBsAg present for 6 mo.
  ◦ Subdivided into HBsAg positive and negative. HBV-DNA levels are typically >20,000 IU/mL in HBsAg-positive CHB, and lower values (2000–20,000 IU/mL) are often seen in HBsAg-negative CHB.
  ◦ Normal or elevated ALT and/or AST levels.
  ◦ Liver biopsy results show chronic hepatitis with variable necroinflammation and/or fibrosis.
- Quantitative HBV-DNA testing is essential to guide treatment decisions.
- HBV genotyping can be useful in patients being considered for peg-IFN therapy, otherwise not recommended.
- Testing for viral resistance in treatment-naïve patients is not recommended. Resistance testing can be useful in patients with past treatment experience, those with persistent viremia, or those who experience virological breakthrough during treatment.

–Treatment:
- Recommend antiviral therapy for adults and alanine transaminase (ALT) >2× normal, moderate-to-severe hepatitis on biopsy, compensated cirrhosis or advanced fibrosis, and HBV DNA >20,000 IU/mL; or for reactivation of chronic HBV after chemotherapy or immunosuppression.
- Recommend antiviral therapy in children for ALT >2× normal and HBV DNA >20,000 IU/mL for at least 6 mo.
- Patients who do not meet criteria for treatment require regular monitoring to assess the need for future therapy.
  ◦ Test ALT in HBsAg-positive patients with persistently normal ALT every 3–6 mo.
  ◦ Test patients who are HBsAg positive with HBV DNA levels >20,000 IU/mL and ALT levels less than 2 times the ULN to evaluate histological disease severity with liver biopsy, elastography, or liver fibrosis biomarkers (FIB-4 or FibroTest).
  ◦ Screen all HBsAg-positive patients with cirrhosis with US examination with or without AFP every 6 mo.

Source
–https://www.aasld.org/sites/default/files/HBVGuidance_Terrault_et_al-2018-Hepatology.pdf

HEPATITIS B VIRUS INFECTION—TREATMENT SPECIFICS

Population
–Adults.

Organization
▶ AASLD 2016 (with 2018 guidance update)

Recommendations
–Offer antiviral therapy to adults to decrease the risk of liver-related complications, if:
- Without a liver biopsy to adults with a transient elastography score ≥11 kPa.
- HBV DNA >2000 IU/mL and ALT >30 IU/mL (males) or >19 IU/mL (females).
- Cirrhosis and detectable HBV DNA.

–Initial antiviral options for HBV infection:
- Peginterferon α-2a.
- Entecavir.
- Tenofovir disoproxil.
  - Tenofovir alafenamide fumarate (TAF) has also been approved as a preferred treatment. It has decreased renal and bone toxicity.
  - Test for HIV and baseline Cr before treatment initiation.

–Coinfection with HBV and HCV:
- Test all HBsAg-positive patients for HCV infection.
- HCV treatment is indicated for patients with HCV viremia.
- HBV treatment is determined by HBV-DNA and ALT levels.
- Peginterferon alfa-2a and ribavirin.

Population
–Children and young adults.

Organization
▶ AASLD 2016 (with 2018 guidance update)

Recommendations
–Consider liver biopsy if HBV DNA >2000 IU/mL and ALT >30 IU/mL (males) or >19 IU/mL (females).

–Initial antiviral options:
- Peginterferon α-2a.
- Interferon alpha, nucleos(t)ide analogues (NAs).

Comments
1. Consider a liver biopsy to confirm fibrosis for a transient elastography score 6–10 kPa.
2. Monitor CBC, liver panel, and renal panel at 2, 4, 12, 24, 36, and 48 wk while on interferon therapy.
3. Monitor CBC, liver panel, and renal panel at 4 wk and every 3 mo while on tenofovir therapy.

Population
–Pregnant women.

Organization
▶ AASLD 2016 (with 2018 guidance update)

Recommendations
–The only antivirals studied in pregnant women are lamivudine, telbivudine, and tenofovir disoproxil.

–Of these 3 options, TDF is preferred to minimize the risk of emergence of viral resistance during treatment. Interim studies show high efficacy of TDF in preventing mother-to-child transmission.

–Consider tenofovir disoproxil if HBV DNA >107 IU/mL in the third trimester.

Source
–https://www.aasld.org/sites/default/files/HBVGuidance_Terrault_et_al-2018-Hepatology.pdfc

HEPATITIS C VIRUS (HCV)

Population
–Adults with chronic HCV infection.

Organization
▶ AASLD 2020, AGA 2017, EASL 2020

Recommendations
Evaluation
–If antibody test positive, reflex to an HCV RNA or core antigen confirmation test. In immunocompromised or chronic dialysis patients, use HCV RNA as the first-line test. (EASL)

–If in initial testing anti-HCV antibody is positive but RNA or core antigen are negative, test HCV RNA 12 to 24 wk later to confirm clearance. (EASL)

–Initiate antiviral treatment for all adults with acute or chronic HCV infection, except those with short life expectancy that will not improve with HCV therapy, liver transplant, or other therapies. Few contraindications exist otherwise.

–Consider urgent treatment for patients with significant cirrhosis, extrahepatic manifestations, recurrence after liver transplant, patients at risk for rapid progression because of comorbidities such as HIV or DM, and in individuals at high risk of transmitting HCV.

–Include the following in initial visits:
- History:
  - HCV exposure risk factors and timing of exposure.
  - Symptoms of advanced liver disease such as jaundice, ascites, variceal bleeding, fatigue, pruritus, confusion.
  - Extrahepatic manifestations.
  - Prior HCV treatment.

- Other medical issues: diabetes, CVA, anemia, CKD, HIV, hepatitis B coinfection, depression, solid organ transplant recipient.
  - Family history of cirrhosis, liver cancer, alcohol dependence.
  - Social history of past and current alcohol use, current illicit drug use.
- Labs:
  - HCV RNA quantitative PCR.
  - HCV genotype (unless done previously). Resistance testing is not required prior to first-line treatment.
  - CBC.
  - Serum: Creatinine, sodium, potassium, chloride, albumin, total protein, total bilirubin, ALT, AST, alkaline phosphatase, glucose, protime (INR).
  - Hepatitis A and B immune status.
  - Resistance-associated variant testing in patients with HCV genotype 1a who are using grazoprevir/elbasvir or prior treatment with a direct acting antiviral agent.
  - Hepatic fibrosis severity testing, preferably noninvasively.
  - Hepatic ultrasound.

Treatment

– Use a simple regimen with a single direct antiviral agent (DAA) for treatment-naïve adults without cirrhosis or with compensated cirrhosis. Some regimens treat certain genotypes, and some are pangenotypic. Updated guidelines are available at www.HCVGuidelines.org.
– Conditions requiring a more complex treatment regimen include ESRD, HIV or HBsAg positive, pregnancy, known or suspected HCC, and history of liver transplant.
– Evaluate for drug-drug interactions (www.hep-druginteractions.org) prior to initiating therapy. Interactions exist between certain DAAs and HIV therapies, opiates, lipid-lowering drugs, antipsychotics, antiarrhythmics, antihypertensives, immunosuppressants, antiplatelet agents, anticoagulants, anticonvulsants, PPIs, and others.
– Interferon regimens are the only option for HCV infected or HIV/HCV infected with decompensated cirrhosis.
– There is very limited evidence for treating patients with mixed genotypes (ie, multiple genotypes of HCV infection concurrently). Consider using a pangenotypic regimen and if the optimal regimen or duration is unclear, consult a specialist.
– Treatment monitoring for 8, 12, and 16 wk regimens. (AGA)

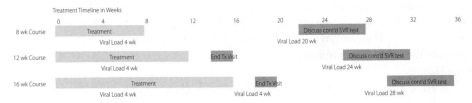

– Vaccinate patients who lack antibodies for hepatitis A and B viruses. If cirrhosis, give pneumococcal vaccine.

–Educate persons with current HCV infection on methods to reduce progression of liver disease (eg, alcohol abstinence) and avoid transmission to others.

–Insufficient evidence to recommend herbal therapy.

–Include the following in subsequent visits:

- For hepatic fibrosis stage 3 or 4:
  ○ EGD evaluation for esophageal varices.
  ○ Alpha fetoprotein.
  ○ Hepatic ultrasound (or, if images inadequate, CT scan of abdomen with contrast).
  ○ Risk reduction/mitigation:
    ▫ Hepatitis A and B vaccinations if not immune.
    ▫ Age-appropriate vaccinations and cancer screening.
    ▫ Counseling on alcohol abstinence.
    ▫ Counseling on transmission/reinfection of HCV.
    ▫ Management of comorbid conditions.
    ▫ Counseling on adherence and consequences of treatment failure if being treated.

–Reassess labs within 12 wk of starting treatment which include: CBC, INR, Hepatic Function Panel (albumin, total and direct bilirubin, ALT/AST, alk phos), renal Function (eGFR). (AGA)

–Refer patients with advanced cirrhosis, multiple treatment failures, coinfection with HIV or hepatitis B to hepatology clinic for proper management. (AGA)

–Declare sustained viral response if RNA or core antigen are undetectable 12–24 wk after the end of treatment.

–Long-term monitoring after successful treatment:

- Fibrosis score 0–2: no further monitoring; counsel on reinfection risk, HIV prevention.
- Fibrosis score 3–4: Ongoing HCC monitoring q6 mo (hepatic ultrasound, AFP levels, LFTs, renal function, INR); yearly visits with hepatology.

Comment

1. High-risk patients are defined as "history of injection drug use, transfusion or organ transplant before 1992, received clotting factors before 1987, history of long-term dialysis, HIV infection, persistently elevated liver enzymes, healthcare and public safety workers after needle sticks, sharps, or mucosal exposure to HCV-positive blood, and children born to HCV-positive women."

Sources

–https://doi.org/10.1002/hep.31060
–https://doi.org/10.1053/j.gastro.2017.03.039
–https://doi.org/10.1016/j.jhep.2020.08.018

Population

–Pregnant adults with HCV infection.

Organization

▶ AASLD 2020, EASL 2020

Recommendations

–Screen all pregnant women for HCV infection at the start of prenatal care.

–Offer treatment to all women with HCV infection prior to becoming pregnant to reduce the risk of vertical transmission.

–Do not treat during pregnancy without a compelling indication and collaboration with obstetric and gastroenterology colleagues.

–Obtain HCV RNA and routine liver function tests at the start of pregnancy to help assess disease severity.

–There is no known way to reduce mother-to-child-transmission risk for HCV-infected women.

–In HCV-infected pregnant women with pruritus or jaundice, evaluate for intrahepatic cholestasis of pregnancy.

–If HCV-infected women with cirrhosis, consult a maternal-fetal medicine (ie, high-risk pregnancy) obstetrician.

–Breastfeeding is not contraindicated in HCV-infected mothers other than when the mother has cracked, damaged, or bleeding nipples or if coinfected with HIV.

–Reassess women with HCV infection after delivery with an HCV-RNA assay to see if they have spontaneously cleared.

Sources
–https://doi.org/10.1002/hep.31060
–https://doi.org/10.1016/j.jhep.2020.08.018

Population
–Adults with acute HCV infection.

Organizations
▶ AASLD 2020, EASL 2020

Recommendations
–Initiate HCV treatment without awaiting spontaneous resolution. Use the same regimens recommended for chronic HCV infection.

–Assess sustained viral response at 12 and 24 wk as late relapses have been reported.

Sources
–https://doi.org/10.1002/hep.31060
–https://doi.org/10.1016/j.jhep.2020.08.018

Population
–Children with HCV infection.

Organizations
▶ AASLD 2020, EASL 2020

Recommendations
Children and adolescents

–Treat patients >3-y-old if a DAA regimen is available for their genotype and age range. Start treatment as soon as possible if the child has cryoglobulinemia, rashes, and glomerulonephritis or advanced fibrosis.

–Avoid interferon-based treatment regimens in children and adolescents.

–Surveil for HCC and varices in children with cirrhosis.

–Therapeutic dose of acetaminophen, steroids, chemotherapy, and organ and bone marrow transplant are not contraindicated in children with chronic hepatitis C.

Perinatal exposure

–Test all children born to HCV-infected women for HCV using an antibody-based test at or after 18 mo of age.

–HCV RNA assay testing can be used in the first year of life but optimal timing is unknown.

–If HCV antibody is positive at 18 mo, test with HCV RNA assay at 3 y of age to confirm chronic HCV infection.

–If a child has HCV, test other siblings born from the same mother.

Counseling parents who have HCV-infected children

–HCV is not transmitted through casual contact, so HCV-infected children do not pose a risk to other children. They can participate in school, sports, athletics, and regular childhood activities without restriction.

–Use universal precautions at school and in the home. Family members should not share toothbrushes, razors, nail clippers, and should use gloves and dilute bleach to clean up blood.

Sources

–https://doi.org/10.1002/hep.31060

–https://doi.org/10.1016/j.jhep.2020.08.018

HEREDITARY HEMOCHROMATOSIS (HH)

Organization

▶ American Association for the Study of Liver Disease (AASLD) 2011

Recommendations

Evaluation:

–Evaluate asymptomatic patients with abnormal iron studies (increased ferritin and iron saturation) for hemochromatosis.

–Evaluate all patients with liver disease for hemochromatosis. (*Ann Intern Med.* 2006;145:209)

–Combine transferrin saturation (TS) and ferritin—if either is abnormal (TS >45% or ferritin >upper limit of normal), the HFE mutation analysis is indicated.

–Screening (iron studies and HFE mutation studies) is recommended for first-degree relatives. (*Ann Intern Med.* 2009;143:522)

–Liver biopsy is recommended for diagnosis and prognosis in patients with phenotypic markers of iron overload who are not C282Y homozygotes or compound heterozygotes (C282Y, H63D).

–Liver biopsy to stage the degree of liver disease in C282Y homozygote or compound heterozygotes if liver enzymes elevated or ferritin >1000 µg/L.

Treatment:

–Therapeutic phlebotomy weekly until ferritin level 50–100 µg/L.

–If C282Y homozygotes with elevated ferritin (but <1000 µg/L), proceed to phlebotomy without liver biopsy.

–If end-organ damage due to iron overload, undergo regular phlebotomy to keep ferritin between 50 and 100 µg/L.

–Avoid vitamin C and iron supplements, but other dietary adjustments not necessary.

–Monitor patients on a regular basis for reaccumulation of iron and undergo maintenance with targeted ferritin levels of 50–100 µg/L.

–Do not use iron chelation with deferoxamine or deferasirox. (*Blood.* 2010;116:317-325) (*Blood.* 2008;111:3373-3376) (*Hepatology.* 2011;54:328-343)

Comments

Problems in hemochromatosis

1. Symptoms besides liver function abnormalities include skin pigmentation, pancreatic dysfunction with diabetes, arthralgias, impotence, and cardiac involvement with ECG changes and heart failure.

2. Other rare mutations causing phenotypic hemochromatosis include transferrin receptor 2 mutation, ferroportin mutation, and H-ferritin mutation.

3. The most devastating complication of hemochromatosis is a 20-fold increase in the risk of hepatocellular carcinoma (HCC). Less than 1% of patients whose ferritin has never been >1000 µg/L develop HCC, while the risk rises considerably in patients with cirrhosis and ferritin level >1000 µg/L. Screen these patients with hepatic ultrasound every 6 mo. Alfa fetoprotein (AFP) is elevated in only 60% of patients with HCC and should not be used as a single screening test. (*Liver Cancer.* 2014;3:31)

4. Patients with hemochromatosis are at increased risk for certain bacterial infections whose virulence is increased in the presence of iron overload. These include *Listeria monocytogenes* (most common in renal dialysis patients), *Yersinia enterocolitica*, and *Vibrio vulniticus* (uncooked seafood is a common source). Infections are made more virulent by iron overload of macrophages impairing their antibacterial activity.

5. Secondary iron overload (most commonly secondary to a transfusion requirement due to blood or bone marrow disease) is best managed by iron chelation beginning when the ferritin rises above 1000 µg/L. In contrast to HH, excess iron is deposited primarily in the reticuloendothelial system, although visceral iron overload does occur over time. (*Blood.* 2014;124:1212)

Source

–Practice guidelines. *Hepatology.* 2011;54:328-343.

INFLAMMATORY BOWEL DISEASE, CROHN'S DISEASE

Population

–Children, young adults, and adults with Crohn's disease.

Organization

▶ ACR 2021

Recommendations

–For initial imaging of suspected Crohn's, choose CT abdomen and pelvis with IV contrast, CT enterography, or MR enterography.

–For imaging in a Crohn's flare, choose CT enterography, MR enterography, and/or CT abdomen and pelvis with IV contrast. Consider using more than one imaging modality to provide complimentary information.

–For surveillance of stable Crohn's, choose MR enterography or CT enterography.

Organization

▶ NICE 2019

Recommendations

–Inducing remission in Crohn's disease.

- Glucocorticoids (prednisolone, methylprednisolone, or IV hydrocortisone) are recommended for first presentation or a single exacerbation in a 12-mo period.
- Consider budesonide or 5-ASA, though less effective, if conventional glucocorticoids are contraindicated or intolerable and if disease is mild-to-moderate.
    - Add azathioprine or mercaptopurine to steroids if steroids cannot be tapered or ≥2 exacerbations in last 12 mo.
    - Assess thiopurine methyltransferase (TPMT) activity before offering azathioprine or mercaptopurine. Do not offer azathioprine or mercaptopurine if TPMT activity is deficient. Consider low-dose thiopurines if TPMT activity is below normal but not deficient.
- Consider adding methotrexate in people who cannot tolerate azathioprine or mercaptopurine, or in whom TPMT activity is deficient.
- Monitor for neutropenia.
- Infliximab or adalimumab is indicated with severe active Crohn's disease refractory to conventional therapy.
    - Given for maximum of 12 mo at a time, or until treatment failure (ie, need for surgery), whichever is shorter.

–Maintaining remission.

- Azathioprine or mercaptopurine as monotherapy in patients achieving remission with steroids.
- Methotrexate (MTX) in patients who need MTX to induce remission or cannot tolerate thiopurines.
- Azathioprine and 3-mo postop metronidazole after complete macroscopic resection. Do not offer biologics or glucocorticosteroids. Do not offer a conventional glucocorticosteroid or budesonide to maintain remission.
- Offer colonoscopic surveillance.

–Surgery: consider when disease is limited to distal ileum and in patients whose disease is refractory to medical therapy or in children/young adults whose growth is impaired.

–Managing strictures: balloon dilation is an option for single stricture that is short, straight, and accessible by colonoscopy.

–Monitor for osteopenia or osteoporosis in children and young adults with risk factors, such as low BMI, pathologic fracture, or repeated glucocorticosteroid use.

Comments

1. Fecal calprotectin is a helpful diagnostic test to differentiate the presence of IBD from irritable bowel syndrome.
2. Avoid NSAIDs as they may exacerbate disease activity.
3. Oral mesalamine has not consistently been demonstrated to be effective for induction of remission and achieving mucosal healing in patients with active Crohn's disease.
4. Consider using natalizumab for induction of symptomatic response and remission in patients with active Crohn's disease, as it is more effective than placebo.
5. Other treatments such as Ustekinumab, novel anti-integrin therapy (with vedolizumab), and diet may be helpful.
6. Surgery is required to treat enteric complications of Crohn's disease; a resection of a segment of diseased intestine is the most common surgery.
7. If a patient has risk factors, it may be helpful to take postoperative prophylaxis with anti-TNF agents.
8. Avoid budesonide or 5-ASA for severe disease.
9. Avoid azathioprine, mercaptopurine, or methotrexate as monotherapy.

Sources
–https://www.nice.org.uk/Guidance/cg152
–Kim et al. Crohn disease. *JACR* 2020;17(5S).

INFLAMMATORY BOWEL DISEASE, ULCERATIVE COLITIS (UC)

Population
–Adults.

Organizations
▶ ACG 2019, AGA 2019/2020

Recommendations

INDUCTION OF REMISSION IN ULCERATIVE COLITIS			
Scenario	ACG	AGA	NICE
Mild proctitis	5-ASA suppositories or enema; rectal corticosteroids if refractory		
Mild, left-sided	Rectal plus oral 5-ASA	Rectal plus oral 5-ASA	Rectal 5-ASA Add oral 5-ASA after 4 wk if refractory
Mild-to-moderate, pancolonic	Oral 5-ASA (low-dose)	Oral 5-ASA (standard-dose, 2–3 g/d) Increase to high-dose (>3 g/d) and add rectal 5-ASA if refractory	Rectal plus high-dose oral 5-ASA Switch to high-dose oral 5-ASA plus oral corticosteroids after 4 wk if refractory

INDUCTION OF REMISSION IN ULCERATIVE COLITIS *(Continued)*

Scenario	ACG	AGA	NICE
Moderate to severe	Anti-TNF monotherapy Consider oral budesonide MMX if anti-TNF is contraindicated Consider infliximab plus azathioprine as alternative to monotherapy Consider vedolizumab or tofacitinib for nonresponders	Use biologics, such as TNF-α inhibitors (eg, infliximab, adalimumab), integrin inhibitor (eg, vedolizumab), JAK inhibitors (eg, tofacitinib), or interleukin inhibitor (eg, ustekinumab). Start with infliximab or vedolizumab in patients naïve to biologics. Use tofacitinib or ustekinumab in nonresponders	
Acute severe	IV methylprednisolone 60 mg/d or hydrocortisone 100 mg 3–4×/d Consider infliximab or cyclosporine in patients not responding to corticosteroids in 3–5 d Test for *C. difficile* and give vancomycin if positive TPN for bowel rest	IV corticosteroids equivalent to 40–60 mg/d of methylprednisolone Use infliximab or cyclosporine in patients not responding to 3–5 d of IV corticosteroids	IV corticosteroids Consider IV cyclosporine after 72 h or if steroids contraindicated If cyclosporine contraindicated, consider infliximab

- Consider oral corticosteroids (eg, budesonide MMX, prednisone) in patients not responding to 5-ASA after 1 mo.

MAINTENANCE OF REMISSION IN ULCERATIVE COLITIS

Scenario	ACG	NICE
Mild proctitis	Rectal 5-ASA	Rectal 5-ASA +/− oral 5-ASA
Mild, left-sided	Oral 5-ASA	Oral 5-ASA, low dose
Mild-to-moderate, pancolonic	Oral 5-ASA	Oral 5-ASA, low dose
Moderate-to-severe	Continue the biologic that induced remission If steroids were used, use thiopurines	
Acute severe	Continue infliximab if it was successful If cyclosporine was used, switch to thiopurine or vedolizumab	Consider oral azathioprine or mercaptopurine

–Colorectal cancer (CRC) prevention:
  - Start colonoscopy screening and surveillance 8 y after diagnosis of UC.
  - If UC and primary sclerosing cholangitis, obtain screening colonoscopy at the time of diagnosis and surveillance annually thereafter.
  - Fecal DNA testing and CT colonography are not recommended due to insufficient evidence.

Comments

1. Addition of 5-ASA to anti-TNF therapy is not recommended if patient failed to respond to 5-ASA prior to switching to biologics.
2. Avoid corticosteroids to maintain remission.
3. Patients with prominent arthritic symptoms may reasonably choose to use sulfasalazine 2–4 g/d if alternatives are cost-prohibitive.
4. Patients who place a higher value on convenience and lower value on effectiveness may use oral rather than rectal administration.
5. Patients who place a higher value on avoiding issues with the mesalamine enemas and do not mind lower effectiveness may use rectal corticosteroid foam preparations.
6. For patients on oral mesalamine once daily, dosing is recommended to increase compliance.
7. There is no good evidence to support the use of probiotics for mild-to-moderate UC. There is limited data showing a benefit of curcumin as adjunctive therapy to 5-ASA in maintaining remission.
8. Oral 5-ASA monotherapy can be considered in cases where topical monotherapy is indicated if patients decline topical treatment. However, inform patient that oral monotherapy may not be as effective.
9. Consider oral azathioprine or oral mercaptopurine to maintain remission after 2 or more exacerbations in 12 mo that require treatment with systemic corticosteroids or if remission is not maintained by aminosalicylates.
10. Monitor bone health, growth, and pubertal development in children and young adults with chronic active disease or who require frequent steroid therapy.
11. Severity of UC is categorized by the Truelove and Witt's Severity Index in adults and by the Pediatric UC Activity Index in children.

Sources

–https://doi.org/10.14309/ajg.00000000000000152
–https://doi.org/10.1053/j.gastro.2018.12.009
–https://doi.org/10.1053/j.gastro.2020.01.006
–https://www.nice.org.uk/Guidance/cg166

INFLAMMATORY BOWEL DISEASE, ULCERATIVE COLITIS, SURGICAL TREATMENT

Population

–Patients with acute severe UC.

Organization

▶ NICE 2019

Recommendations

−Severe acute ulcerative colitis:
- Colectomy may be indicated for patients with any of the following:
  ◦ Persistent diarrhea >8 bowel movements/d.
  ◦ Fevers.
  ◦ Hemodynamic instability.
  ◦ Toxic megacolon.
  ◦ Low albumin, low Hgb, high platelet, CRP >4.5 mg/dL.

−Consider oral azathioprine or mercaptopurine after an episode of acute severe UC.

Source

−https://www.nice.org.uk/Guidance/cg166

Population

−Patients with UC.

Organization

▶ American Society of Colon and Rectal Surgeons 2014

Recommendations

−Indications for surgery in UC:
- Patients with acute colitis and actual or impending perforation.
- Chronic UC refractory to medical therapy.
- Presence of carcinoma or high-grade dysplasia in colon.
- Development of a colonic stricture.
- Consider a second-line agent or surgery for acute colitis that is worsening after 96 h of first-line medical therapy.

Source

−https://www.fascrs.org/sites/default/files/downloads/publication/practice_parameters_ for_the_ surgical_treatment_of.3.pdf

Comments

1. Procedure of choice for emergency surgery is a total or subtotal colectomy with end ileostomy.
2. Procedure of choice for elective surgery is a total proctocolectomy with ileostomy or ileal pouch-anal anastomosis.
3. Patient with severe diarrhea (>8 stools/d) in absence of *C. difficile* colitis and a C-reactive protein >4.5 mg/dL despite medical therapy for 72 h has an 85% chance of requiring a colectomy.

IRRITABLE BOWEL SYNDROME (IBS)

Population

−Adults with symptoms of IBS.

Organizations

▶ NICE 2015, AGA 2019

Recommendations

–Consider IBS for any adult with any of these symptoms for at least 6 mo.

- Abdominal pain.
- Bloating.
- Change in bowel habit.

–Assess all patients with possible IBS for red flag indicators that argue against IBS.

- Unintentional weight loss.
- Rectal bleeding.
- Anemia.
- Abdominal mass.
- Change in bowel habit to looser and more frequent stools if over 60 y.
- Family history of IBD, colon cancer, or celiac disease.
- Recent travel or immigration from high-risk areas.

–Recommend for all patients with suspected IBS.

- Complete blood count.
- ESR.
- C-reactive protein.
- Antiendomysial antibody and antitissue transglutaminase antibody to rule out celiac disease.
- For suspected diarrhea-predominant IBS, consider:
  ○ Fecal calprotectin/lactoferrin to rule out IBD.
  ○ Stool ova and parasites.
  ○ Giardia antigen or PCR.
  ○ 48-h stool bile acid to rule out bile acid malabsorption.

–Lifestyle recommendations for IBS.

- Eat regular meals.
- Drink at least 8 cups of noncaffeinated beverage daily.
- Limit intake of tea, coffee, and alcohol.
- Reduce intake of "resistant starch."
- Avoid sorbitol, an artificial sweetener, for diarrhea-predominant IBS.

–Pharmacologic therapy for IBS.

- Consider laxatives as needed (except lactulose) for constipation.
- Consider linaclotide for refractory constipation for longer than 12 mo.
- Consider antispasmodic agents as needed for pain.
- Loperamide is the antimotility agent of choice for diarrhea.
- Consider low-dose tricyclics (TCAs) as second-line treatment if antispasmodics or antimotility agents have not helped.
- Consider SSRI therapy if TCAs are ineffective.
- Consider cognitive behavioral therapy or hypnotherapy for IBS refractory to above therapies.

Sources

–https://www.nice.org.uk/guidance/qs114
–https://doi.org/10.1053/j.gastro.2019.07.004

LIVER DISEASE, ALCOHOLIC

Population
  –Adults.

Organizations
  ▶ EASL 2018, AASLD 2020

Recommendations
  –Public health policies to reduce alcoholic liver disease (ALD):
  • Address excess alcohol consumption using pricing-based policies and regulation of availability.
  • Ban advertising or marketing of alcohol.
  • Screen for alcohol use disorder (AUD) in primary care and emergency settings using AUDIT or AUDIT-C.
  • Screen for ALD in high-risk populations.
  –Alcohol use disorder (AUD):
  • Alcohol use disorder (defined by DSM-V criteria) is the preferred term in place of alcoholic, alcohol abuse, alcohol dependence, or risky drinker.
  • Include both psychosocial and behavioral approaches (eg, cognitive-behavioral therapy, motivational enhancement therapy, contingency management, 12-step facilitation, network therapy, and couples/family counseling) as well as pharmacotherapy.
  • In patients without ALD, naltrexone or disulfiram can be considered for AUD. In patients with ALD, these medications can cause liver damage due to hepatic metabolism. Safer treatment options are baclofen and acamprosate. Baclofen has more evidence to show improvement in the rate of total alcohol abstinence.
  • There is limited data to show one treatment modality is superior to another; therefore, an integrated and multidisciplinary management of AUD and ALD is recommended.
  • Evaluate patients with AUD for concurrent psychiatric disorders and other addictions.
  • Use benzodiazepines to treat alcohol withdrawal syndrome (AWS) but for no more than 10–14 d due to potential abuse and/or encephalopathy.
  –Management of alcoholic hepatitis (AH):
  • Suspect AH in patients with recent onset of jaundice and excessive alcohol consumption.
  • Use prognostic scores, such as Maddrey Discriminant Function (MDF) and MELD to identify severe AH (MDF $>= 32$ or MELD > 20) who will likely benefit from corticosteroids.
  • If no contraindications to steroids (ie, uncontrolled infections or UGIB, AKI), give prednisolone 40 mg/d or methylprednisolone 32 mg/d for patients with severe AH to reduce short-term mortality. Medium- and long-term survivals do not change.
  • Addition of IV N-acetylcysteine to prednisolone may improve 30-d survival of patients with severe AH.
  • Use Lille model to assess response after 7 d of treatment. If the patient responds (Lille < 0.45), continue steroids for 28 d total. If no response (Lille $>= 0.45$), stop steroids and consider

referral for liver transplant. Provide nutrition orally to maintain ≥35–40 kcal/kg body weight and 1.2–1.5 g/kg protein per day.

- There is insufficient evidence to support the use of granulocyte-colony stimulating factor and pentoxifylline in AH.

–Alcohol-related fibrosis and cirrhosis:

- Complete abstinence from alcohol is recommended for patients with alcohol-related cirrhosis as it reduces liver-related complications and death.
- Identify and manage cofactors including obesity and insulin resistance, malnutrition, cigarette smoking, iron overload, and viral hepatitis.
- Screening and management of complications from cirrhosis are managed similarly for alcohol-related cirrhosis.

–Liver transplantation:

- Consider liver transplant for patients with decompensated cirrhosis, Child-Pugh C, or MELD-Na 2 > 1.
- Do not use a 6-mo sobriety criterion alone for consideration of liver transplant and instead include degree of liver insufficiency, addiction and psychological profile, and support system.
- Check patients on the liver transplant list regularly for abstinence.
- A multidisciplinary approach evaluating medical and psychological suitability for transplant is mandatory.
- An addiction medicine specialist may reduce relapses in heavy drinking patients.
- Severe relapses (defined as >20 g EtOH/d in women and >30 g/d in men) in the posttransplant period can lead to cirrhosis in as little as 5 y.
- Early liver transplant may be proposed in a minority of patients with severe AH and not responding to treatments.
- Screen all liver transplant candidates for cardiovascular, neurological, psychiatric disorders, and neoplasms before and after liver transplant.
- Target risk factors for cancer, such as cigarette smoking, aggressively. Early reduction in calcineurin inhibitor therapy can be considered to decrease the risk for de novo cancers after liver transplant.

Sources
–https://doi.org/10.1016/j.jhep.2018.03.018
–DOI:10.1002/hep.30866

LIVER DISEASE, NONALCOHOLIC (NAFLD)

Population
–Children and adults.

Organization
▶ AASLD 2017

Recommendations

Adults

–Exclude competing etiologies: significant alcohol consumption, hepatitis C, medications, parenteral nutrition, Wilson's disease, autoimmune liver disease, and severe malnutrition.

–If incidental finding of hepatic steatosis (HS) on imaging:

- If LFTs are normal, assess metabolic risk factors (obesity, diabetes mellitus, dyslipidemia) and other causes of HS (significant alcohol consumption or medications).
- If signs/symptoms attributable to liver disease or abnormal LFTs, evaluate for NAFLD.

–Carry a high index of suspicion for NAFLD or nonalcoholic steatohepatitis (NASH) in type 2 diabetic patients and those with metabolic syndrome. A clinical decision tool such as the NFS or fibrosis-4 index can help identify those at low or high risk for advanced fibrosis. Alternatives are using vibration-controlled transient elastography or MR elastography to assess fibrosis.

–Consider liver biopsy in patients:

- With high ferritin and high iron saturation liver to determine the extent of iron accumulation in the liver.
- At increased risk of steatohepatitis and/or advanced fibrosis.
- All patients with a competing etiology for hepatosteatosis which requires a liver biopsy to exclude.

–Use pharmacological treatment only in those with biopsy-proven NASH and fibrosis.

–Weight loss is first-line therapy. Weight loss of 3%–5% of body weight improves steatosis; weight loss of 7%–10% of body weight is needed to improve liver fibrosis. Consider bariatric surgery in select patients to help with weight loss.

–Do not use metformin or GLP-1 agonists to treat NASH.

–Consider pioglitazone only in patients who have biopsy-proven NASH after risks and benefits have been discussed.

–Vitamin E at 800 IU/d in nondiabetic biopsy-proven NASH patients improves liver histology. Do not use with diabetics, NAFLD without liver biopsy, NASH cirrhosis, or cryptogenic cirrhosis.

–Do not use ursodeoxycholic acid or omega-3 fatty acids to treat NAFLD or NASH.

–NAFLD patients are at high risk for cardiovascular disease and require aggressive lifestyle modifications and pharmacotherapy. NAFLD and NASH do not increase risk of liver injury from statins.

–Screen patients with NASH cirrhosis for esophageal varices and HCC with the same frequency/ modalities used for other types of cirrhosis. Noncirrhotic NASH patients do not require screening.

Children

–Test children with fatty liver disease who are very young or not overweight for fatty acid oxidation defects, lysosomal storage diseases, and peroxisomal disorders in addition to the usual causes found in adults.

–Intensive lifestyle modifications are first-line treatment in children.

–Obtain a liver biopsy before starting pharmacotherapy in children.

–Do not use metformin.

–Vitamin E 800 IU/d in biopsy-proven NASH patients has been shown to improve liver histology. Discuss long-term use of vitamin E prior to starting treatment, as efficacy in children is unknown.

Source
–https://doi.org/10.1002/hep.29367

PANCREATITIS, ACUTE (AP)

Population
–Individuals with acute pancreatitis.

Organizations
▶ ACG 2013, AGA 2018, NICE 2020

Recommendations
–Diagnosis of acute pancreatitis (ACG):
- Includes the presence of 2 of the 3 following criteria:
  - Abdominal pain consistent with the disease.
  - Serum amylase and/or lipase greater than 3 times the upper limit of normal.
  - Characteristic findings from abdominal imaging.
- Recommend a contrast-enhanced CT scan or MRI of the pancreas if the diagnosis is unclear or if symptoms are not improving within 72 h.
- Perform a gallbladder ultrasound in all patients with AP.
- Check serum triglyceride level in all patients without a history of alcohol abuse or gallstones.
- Consider ICU or intermediate-level monitoring for any organ dysfunction.

–Initial management.

GUIDELINES DISCORDANT: FLUIDS IN ACUTE PANCREATITIS	
Organization	**Population**
ACG	Aggressive isotonic fluids at 250–500 mL/h
AGA	Use judicious goal-directed therapy for fluid management for resuscitation

- In mild AP, start oral feedings with clear liquids or low-fat diet immediately if there is no nausea and vomiting and the abdominal pain has resolved.
- In severe AP, use enteral nutrition to prevent infectious complications, starting within 72 h of presentation. Avoid parenteral nutrition unless the enteral route is not available, not tolerated, or not meeting caloric requirements.

GUIDELINES DISCORDANT: ROLE OF ERCP IN PANCREATITIS ASSOCIATED WITH GALLSTONES	
Organization	**Population**
ACG	Obtain ERCP
AGA	Do not obtain urgent ERCP unless cholangitis

- In patients found to have gallstones in the gallbladder, perform a cholecystectomy before discharge to prevent a recurrence of AP.
  ◦ In a patient with necrotizing biliary AP, in order to prevent infection, cholecystectomy is to be deferred until active inflammation subsides and fluid collections resolve or stabilize. (ACG)
- Do not use prophylactic antibiotics for severe necrotizing AP.
- In patients with infected necrosis, use antibiotics known to penetrate pancreatic necrosis, such as carbapenems, quinolones, and metronidazole, to delay or perhaps avoid intervention and decrease morbidity and mortality.
  ◦ In stable patients with infected necrosis, delay surgical, radiologic, and/or endoscopic drainage preferably for more than 4 wk to allow liquefaction of the contents and the development of a fibrous wall around the necrosis (walled-off necrosis).

Comments

1. Nasogastric delivery and nasojejunal delivery of enteral feeding appear comparable in efficacy and safety.
2. In addition to gallstones and alcohol, consider causes including metabolic (hypercalcemia, hyperlipidemia), prescription drugs, microlithiasis, hereditary causes, autoimmune pancreatitis, obstructing tumors, or anatomical anomalies.

Sources
–https://gi.org/guideline/acute-pancreatitis/
–www.nice.org.uk/guidance/ng104
–https://doi.org/10.1053/j.gastro.2018.01.032

PANCREATITIS, CHRONIC (CP)

Population
–Individuals with chronic pancreatitis.

Organization
▶ ACG 2020

Recommendations
–Management of pain:
  - Recommend alcohol and smoking cessation.
  - Offer elective interventional procedures (eg, celiac plexus block) for pain palliation.
  - Offer ERCP and/or EUS with pancreatic drainage for pain related to obstructive CP.
  - Consider surgical approaches if endoscopic interventions are not effective.
  - Consider antioxidants (eg, selenium, methionine, vitamins C, A, and D), which may reduce pain.
  - Consider opiates only after all other therapies are exhausted.
  - There is no data supporting the use of pancreatic enzyme supplements to reduce pain.
  - Total pancreatectomy with islet autotransplantation is reserved for refractory pain despite all measures.

–Management of exocrine pancreatic insufficiency (EPI):
- Recommend pancreatic enzyme replacement therapy (PERT) to reduce complications of malnutrition.
- Measure zinc, magnesium, and fat-soluble vitamin levels, and bone density at baseline and periodically.

Source
  –https://doi.org/10.14309/ajg.0000000000000535

PARACENTESIS

Population
  –Adults with ascites.

Organization
▶ AASLD 2012

Recommendations
  –Perform diagnostic abdominal paracentesis in inpatients and outpatients with clinically apparent new-onset ascites.
  –Include ascitic fluid cell count and differential, ascitic fluid total protein, and serum-ascites albumin gradient in initial lab assessment of ascites.
  –Do not routinely administer FFP prior to a paracentesis.

Source
  –https://www.aasld.org/sites/default/files/guideline_documents/
  AASLDPracticeGuidelineAsciteDuetoCirrhosisUpdate2012Edition4_.pdf

ULCERS, STRESS

Organization
▶ SHM 2013

Recommendation
  –Do not prescribe medications for stress ulcer prophylaxis to medical inpatients unless they are at high risk for GI complications.

Source
  –https://www.shmabstracts.com/abstract/evaluation-of-stress-ulcer-prophylaxis-for-patients-with-coagulopathy-secondary-to-chronic-liver-disease/

Genitourinary Disorders

24

ABNORMAL UTERINE BLEEDING

Population
–Adult reproductive-aged women.

Organizations
▶ ACOG 2012, NICE 2018

Recommendations
–Classify bleeding using the PALM (structural) & COEIN (nonstructural) acronyms:
- Polyp.
- Adenomyosis.
- Leiomyoma.
- Malignancy and hyperplasia.
- Coagulopathy.
- Ovulatory dysfunction.
- Endometrial.
- Iatrogenic.
- Not yet classified.

–History: age of menarche, bleeding patterns, severity of bleeding, pain, medical/surgical history, medications, s/sx bleeding disorder, impact on quality of life.

–Physical: pelvic exam including external, bimanual, and speculum exam including Pap if needed.

–Labs: pregnancy test, CBC, TSH, chlamydia, and perhaps a coagulation panel and/or von Willebrand's testing.

–Order transvaginal ultrasound if abnormal physical examination or if symptoms persist despite treatment.

–Perform endometrial biopsy in all patients older than 45 y and patients younger than 45 y with history of unopposed estrogen exposure (including obesity, PCOS), failed medical management, and persistent bleeding. Do not obtain ultrasound measurement of endometrial thickness to rule out malignancy.

–Levonorgestrel IUD is first-line therapy for women with no identified pathology, fibroids <3 cm, or suspected adenomyosis. (NICE)

–If levonorgestrel not used, consider trial of therapies in patients without risk of endometrial hyperplasia, neoplasia, or structural abnormalities (ie, adolescents). Consider NSAIDs, progestins, combination oral contraceptives, or tranexamic acid.

−Structural anatomical causes such as fibroids >3 cm or polyps may require procedural intervention such as endometrial ablation, myomectomy, uterine artery embolization, or hysterectomy.

Sources
−*Obstet Gynecol.* 2012;120(1):197-206.
−www.nice.org.uk/guidance/ng88

BENIGN PROSTATIC HYPERPLASIA (BPH)

Population
−Adult men age >45 with lower urinary tract symptoms (LUTS) from prostatic enlargement.

Organizations
▶ AUA 2010, 2019

Recommendations
−Do not routinely measure serum creatinine in men with BPH.
−Do not recommend dietary supplements or phytotherapeutic agents for LUTS management.
−Patients with LUTS and no signs of bladder outlet obstruction by flow study should be treated for detrusor overactivity.
  • Alter fluid intake.
  • Behavioral modification.
  • Anticholinergic medications.
−Options for moderate-to-severe LUTS from BPH (AUA symptom index score ≥8).
  • Watchful waiting.
  • Medical therapies.
    ◦ Alpha-blockers.[1]
    ◦ 5-Alpha-reductase inhibitors.[2]
    ◦ Anticholinergic agents.
    ◦ Combination therapy.
  • Transurethral needle ablation.
  • Transurethral microwave thermotherapy.
  • Transurethral laser ablation or enucleation of the prostate.
  • Transurethral incision of the prostate.
  • Transurethral vaporization of the prostate.
  • Transurethral resection of the prostate.
  • Laser resection of the prostate.
  • Photoselective vaporization of the prostate.
  • Prostatectomy.

---

[1] Alfa-blockers: alfuzosin, doxazosin, tamsulosin, and terazosin. All have equal clinical effectiveness.
[2] 5-Alfa-reductase inhibitors: dutasteride and finasteride.

–Surgery is recommended for BPH causing renal insufficiency, refractory retention secondary to BPH, recurrent urinary tract infections (UTIs), bladder stones, gross hematuria, refractory LUTS, and/or those unwilling to use other therapies.

Comments

1. Combination therapy with alpha-blocker and 5-alpha-reductase inhibitor is effective for moderate-to-severe LUTS with significant prostate enlargement.
2. Men with planned cataract surgery should have cataract surgery before initiating alpha-blockers.
3. 5-Alpha-reductase inhibitors should not be used for men with LUTS from BPH without prostate enlargement.
4. Anticholinergic agents are appropriate for LUTS that are primarily irritative symptoms, and if patient does not have an elevated post-void residual (>250 mL).
5. The choice of surgical method should be based on the patient's presentation, anatomy, surgeon's experience, and patient's preference.

Sources

–http://www.guidelines.gov/content.aspx?id=25635&search=aua+2010+bph
–https://www.auanet.org/guidelines/benign-prostatic-hyperplasia-(bph)-guideline

CERVICAL CANCER AND ABNORMAL PAP

Population

–Women with abnormal cervical cancer screening studies.

Organization

▶ ASCCP 2019

Recommendations

–Manage abnormal results by assessing risk of CIN3 or higher grade lesion.
–If immediate CIN3+ risk is >4%, intervene.
- 60%–100%: Expedited treatment.[1]
- 25%–59%: Expedited treatment or colposcopy.
- 4%–24%: Colposcopy.

–If immediate CIN3+ risk <4%, choose surveillance interval based on 5-y CIN3+ risk.
- >0.55%: Return in 1 y.
- 0.15%–0.54%: Return in 3 y.
- <0.15%: Return in 5 y for routine screening interval.

–Follow-up intervals or treatment pathways are determined by Pap and HPV results as well as recent history (Tables 24-1 and 24-2).
–When performing colposcopy, obtain 2–4 targeted biopsies of acetowhite lesions.
–Obtain endocervical sample if unable to visualize entire lesion or squamocolumnar junction.

[1]Expedited treatment: start therapy without obtaining colposcopic biopsy.

TABLE 24-1   RESPONSES TO ABNORMAL SCREENING RESULTS, PATIENTS AGE 25–65 WITHOUT PRIOR ANOMALIES[a]

Pap	HPV	Most Recent	Next Step
NILM[b]	Neg	None, HPV−, or Cotest−	Return 5 y
NILM	Pos or 16−/18+	None, HPV−, or Cotest−	Return 1 y
NILM	16+	HPV− or Cotest−	Return 1 y
NILM	16+	None	Colposcopy
LSIL[c]	Neg	Cotest−	Return 3 y
LSIL	Neg	None or HPV−	Return 1 y
LSIL	16−/18+	None, HPV−, or Cotest−	Return 1 y
LSIL	16+	None, HPV−, or Cotest−	Colposcopy
LSIL	Pos	None	Colposcopy
LSIL	Pos	HPV− or Cotest−	Return 1 y
High grade	16+ or 16−/18+	HPV− or Cotest−	Colposcopy
HSIL[d]+	Neg	HPV− or Cotest−	Colposcopy
HSIL+	Pos	HPV− or Cotest−	Treat[e] or Colposcopy
HSIL+	Neg, Pos, or 16−/18+	None	Treat or Colposcopy
HSIL+	16+	None	Treat
ASC-US[f]	Neg	None, HPV−, or Cotest−	Return 3 y
ASC-US	16+	None, HPV−, or Cotest−	Colposcopy
ASC-US	Pos	None	Colposcopy
ASC-US	Pos	HPV− or Cotest−	Return 1 y
ASC-US	16−/18+	None, HPV−, or Cotest−	Return 1 y
ASC-H[g]	Neg	None, HPV−, or Cotest−	Return 1 y
ASC-H	Pos or 16+	None	Treatment or Colposcopy
ASC-H	Pos	HPV− or Cotest−	Colposcopy
ASC-H	16−/18+	None	Colposcopy
AGC[h]	Neg	None, HPV−, or Cotest−	Return 1 y
AGC	Pos, 16+ or 16−/18+	None	Treatment or Colposcopy
AGC	Pos	HPV− or Cotest−	Colposcopy

[a]Abnormal screening results at https://cervixca.nlm.nih.gov/RiskTables/, accessed 9/10/2020.
[b]Negative for intraepithelial lesion or malignancy.
[c]Low-grade squamous intraepithelial lesion.
[d]High-grade squamous intraepithelial lesion.
[e]"Treat" refers to expedited treatment, proceeding to therapy without first obtaining a colposcopic biopsy.
[f]Atypical squamous cells of undetermined significance.
[g]Atypical squamous cells cannot exclude high-grade squamous intraepithelial lesion.
[h]Atypical glandular cells.

TABLE 24-2 RESPONSES TO ABNORMAL SCREENING RESULTS, PATIENTS AGE 25–65 WITH PRIOR ANOMALIES[a]

Pap	HPV	Most Recent	Prior 2	Next Step
NILM	Neg	HPV−/ASC-US		Return 5 y
NILM	Neg	NPV−/LSIL		Return 3 y
NILM	Neg	Cotest−	HPV+/NILM	Return 3 y
NILM	Neg	HPV+/NILM		Return 1 y
NILM	Pos	HPV− or Cotest−	HPV+/NILM	Return 1 y
NILM	Pos	HPV−/ASCUS or HPV−/LSIL		Return 1 y
NILM	16−/18+	HPV+/NILM		Return 1 y
NILM	Pos or 16+	HPV+/NILM		Colposcopy
LSIL	Neg	HPV−/ASC-US, HPV−/LSIL or HPV+/NILM		Return 1 y
LSIL	Pos	HPV−/ASC-US		Return 1 y
LSIL	Pos	HPV−/ASC-US, HPV−/LSIL or HPV+/NILM		Colposcopy
LSIL	16−/18+	HPV+/NILM		Return 1 y
LSIL	16+	HPV+/NILM		Colposcopy
High grade	Pos	HPV− or Cotest−	HPV+/NILM	Colposcopy
High grade	16−/18+ or 16+	HPV+/NILM		Treat or colposcopy
HSIL+	Neg	HPV−/LSIL		Return 5 y
HSIL+	Neg	HPV−/ASC-US		Colposcopy
HSIL+	Neg	HPV+/NILM		Treat or colposcopy
HSIL+	Pos	HPV−/ASC-US, HPV−/LSIL, or HPV+/NILM		Treat or colposcopy
ASC-US	Neg	HPV−/ASC-US, HPV−/LSIL, or HPV+/NILM		Return 1 y
ASC-US	Pos	HPV−/ASC-US		Return 1 y
ASC-US	Pos, 16−/18+, or 16+	HPV−/LSIL or HPV+NILM		Colposcopy
ASC-US, LSIL	Pos	HPV− or Cotest−	HPV+/NILM	Return 1 y
ASC-H	Neg	HPV−/LSIL		Return 5 y
ASC-H	Neg	HPV−/ASC-US		Colposcopy
ASC-H	Pos	HPV−/ASC-US or HPV+/NILM		Colposcopy

TABLE 24-2   RESPONSES TO ABNORMAL SCREENING RESULTS, PATIENTS AGE 25–65 WITH PRIOR ANOMALIES[a] **(Continued)**

Pap	HPV	Most Recent	Prior 2	Next Step
ASC-H	Pos	HPV−/LSIL		Treat or colposcopy
AGC	Neg	HPV−/ASC-US or HPV−/LSIL		Return 5 y
AGC	Neg	HPV+/NILM		Colposcopy
AGC	Pos	HPV−/ASC-US or HPV−/LSIL		Return 5 y
AGC	Pos	HPV+/NILM		Treat or colposcopy

[a]Surveillance following results not requiring immediate colposcopic referral, https://cervixca.nlm.nih.gov/RiskTables/ accessed 9/10/2020.

–If low-risk (cytology <LSIL, no HPV 16/18, and no anomalies on colposcopy), do not obtain random nontargeted biopsies.

–If colposcopy with biopsy shows CIN1 or less, return in 1 y for Pap. Subsequent intervals described in Table 24-3.

–If colposcopy with biopsy shows CIN2, CIN3, AIS, or cancer, proceed to treatment.

Sources

–*J Low Genit Tract Dis.* 2020;24:102-131. https://pubmed.ncbi.nlm.nih.gov/32243307/

–*J Low Genit Tract Dis.* 2017;21:230-234. https://pubmed.ncbi.nlm.nih.gov/28953111/

CHRONIC PELVIC PAIN

Population

–Women with chronic pelvic pain.

Organization

▶ ACOG 2020

Recommendations

–Include in the initial evaluation a thorough history and physical exam. Focus the history on chronology, triggers, treatments of pain, prior medical, surgical, and obstetric history, and psychosocial factors. Focus examination on abdominal and pelvic neuromusculoskeletal system. Palpate the lower back, sacroiliac joints, pubic symphysis, abdomen, and genitalia.

–Beyond the reproductive system, consider interstitial cystitis, irritable bowel syndrome, diverticulitis, and comorbid mood disorders.

–Consider referral to pelvic floor physical therapy, sex therapy, and/or cognitive behavioral therapy when there is pelvic pain with dyspareunia.

TABLE 24-3 MANAGEMENT OF RETURN CYTOLOGY AND HPV AFTER CIN <2 COLPOSCOPY[a]

Initial Abnormality	Prior Post-colpo Result	Current Pap	Current HPV	Next Step
Low grade	None or HPV−	ALL	Neg	Return 3 y
Low grade	HPV− ×2	ALL	Neg	Return 5 y
Low grade	None	ASC-US/LSIL	Neg or Pos	Return 1 y
Low grade	Cotest−	ASC-US/LSIL	Neg	Return 3 y
Low grade	Cotest−	ASC-US/LSIL	Pos	Return 1 y
Low grade	HPV−/ASC-US/LSIL	ASC-US/LSIL	Neg	Return 1 y
Low grade	None or Cotest−	High grade	Neg or Pos	Colposcopy
Low grade	None or Cotest− or HPV−/ ASC-US/LSIL	NILM	Neg	Return 3 y
Low grade	None or Cotest−	NILM	Pos	Return 1 y
Low grade	Cotest− ×2	NILM	Neg	Return 5 y
High grade		ALL	Neg	Return 1 y
High grade	HPV− (×1 or ×2)	ALL	Neg	Return 3 y
High grade		ASC-US/LSIL	Neg	Return 1 y
High grade		ASC-US/LSIL	Pos	Colposcopy
High grade	Cotest−	ASC-US/LSIL	Neg	Return 3 y
High grade	Cotest−	ASC-US/LSIL	Pos	Return 1 y
High grade		High grade	Neg	Colposcopy
High grade		High grade	Pos	Treat or colposcopy
High grade		NILM	Neg	Return 3 y
High grade		NILM	Pos	Colposcopy
High grade	Cotest− (×1 or ×2)	NILM	Neg	Return 3 y
High grade	Cotest−	NILM	Pos	Return 1 y

[a]Surveillance visit following colposcopy/biopsy finding less than CIN-2 (no treatment), https://cervixca.nlm.nih.gov/RiskTables/ accessed 9/10/2020.

– Prescribe serotonin-norepinephrine reuptake inhibitors (ie, duloxetine) if there is a neuropathic component to pain.
– Avoid opioid therapies.
– Consider referral to pain specialists.
– Consider acupuncture and yoga for pain relief.
– Do not routinely refer for laparoscopic lysis of abdominal adhesions.

Source
– *Obstet Gynecol.* 2020;135(3):e98-109.

ERECTILE DYSFUNCTION (ED)

Population
–Adult men.

Organizations
▶ EAU 2018, Endocrine Society 2018, AUA 2018

Recommendations
–Perform a medical and psychosexual history on all patients.

–Perform a focused physical examination to assess CV status, neurologic status, prostate disease, penile abnormalities, and signs of hypogonadism.

–Recommend exercise and decreased BMI.

–Check a fasting glucose, lipid profile, and morning fasting total testosterone levels.

–Refer for psychosexual therapy if psychogenic ED.

–Offer testosterone therapy for androgen deficiency (at least 2 testosterone levels below the normal limit) with associated signs and symptoms if no contraindications are present.[1]

–Routine screening of asymptomatic men for hypogonadism is not recommended. (Endocrine Society 2018)

–Selective phosphodiesterase 5 (PDE5) inhibitors are first-line therapy for idiopathic ED.

–If PDE5 fails, consider intercavernosal injections or penile prosthesis.

Comments
1. Selective PDE5 inhibitors:
   a. Sildenafil (100 mg, half-life 2–4 h).
   b. Tadalafil (20 mg, half-life 18 h).
   c. Vardenafil (20 mg, half-life 4 h).
   d. Avanafil (200 mg, half-life 6–17 h).
2. Avoid nitrates and use alpha-blockers with caution when prescribing a selective PDE5 inhibitor.

Sources
–*J Clin Endocrinol Metab.* 2018;103(5):1-30.

–https://uroweb.org/guideline/male-sexual-dysfunction/

–https://www.auanet.org/guidelines/erectile-dysfunction-(ed)-guideline

---

[1]Prostate CA, breast CA, signs of prostatism, men who intend fertility in short term, PSA >4 ng/mL or >3 ng/mL and high-risk, or comorbidities that would be a contraindication.

HEMATURIA

Population

–Adults with microscopic hematuria.

Organization

▶ AUA 2020

Recommendations

–Define microscopic hematuria as >3 RBC per high-power field on microscopic examination of a properly collected specimen.

–Do not rely on hematuria as defined by a positive dipstick alone.

–Use patient risk to guide further work. Higher risk factors for urothelial disease include smoking, prior pelvic radiation therapy, prior cyclophosphamide therapy, occupational exposures to benzene dyes or aromatic amines, family history of urothelial cancer or Lynch syndrome, or chronic indwelling foreign body in the urinary tract.

–Offer lower risk patients watchful waiting and repeat testing in 6 mo. Refer those with recurrent microscopic hematuria for cystoscopy and renal ultrasound imaging.

–Refer intermediate risk patients for cystoscopy and renal ultrasound imaging.

–Refer higher risk patients for cystoscopy and multiphasic CT urography including urothelial imaging.

Source

–Barocas DA, Boorjian SA, Alvarez RD et al. Microhematuria: AUA/SUFU guideline. *J Urol.* 2020;204:778.

ALGORITHM FOR THE DIAGNOSIS AND MANAGEMENT OF INCIDENTALLY DISCOVERED MICROSCOPIC HEMATURIA

American College of Radiology (ACR) Appropriateness Criteria for Hematuria

Clinical Situation	Imaging Modality
Microhematuria. No risk factors, or history of recent vigorous exercise, or presence of infection, or viral illness, or present or recent menstruation. Initial imaging	CT abd/pelvis w/o IV contrast (May be appropriate)
Microhematuria. Patients with risk factors, without any of the following: history of recent vigorous exercise, or presence of infection or viral illness, or present or recent menstruation, or renal parenchymal disease. Initial imaging	CT urogram with and without IV contrast (Usually appropriate) MR urogram with and without IV contrast CT abd/pelvis with and without IV contrast CT abd/pelvis with IV contrast US kidneys and bladder (May be appropriate)
Microhematuria. Pregnant patient. Initial imaging	US kidneys and bladder (Usually appropriate) MRU without IV contrast (May be appropriate)

ALGORITHM FOR THE DIAGNOSIS AND MANAGEMENT OF INCIDENTALLY DISCOVERED MICROSCOPIC HEMATURIA

American College of Radiology (ACR) Appropriateness Criteria for Hematuria

Clinical Situation	Imaging Modality
Gross hematuria. Initial imaging	CT urogram with and without IV contrast MR urogram with and without IV contrast (Usually appropriate) CT abd/pelvis with and without IV contrast (or either alone) MRI abd/pelvis with and without IV contrast US kidneys and bladder (May be appropriate)

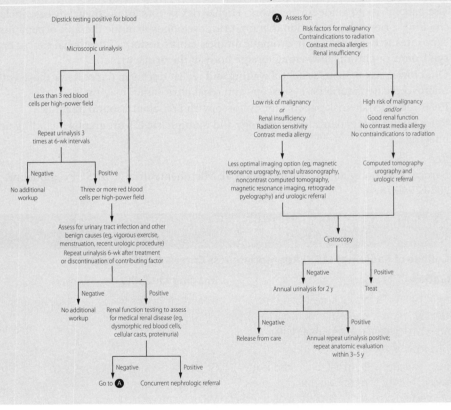

INDWELLING URINARY CATHETERS OR INTERMITTENT CATHETERIZATION

Population
Individuals with indwelling catheter without symptoms of urinary tract infection.

Organization
▶ AUA 2015

Recommendation
–Avoid empiric antibiotics unless the patient has symptoms of a urinary tract infection.

Source
–http://www.choosingwisely.org/clinician-lists/american-urological-association-antimicrobials-indwelling-or-intermittent-bladder-catheterization/

INFERTILITY, MALE

Population
–Adults.

Organization
▶ EAU 2018

Recommendations
–Assessment of male infertility includes:
  • Semen analysis.
–Scrotal ultrasound:
  • If semen analysis is abnormal, check FSH, LH, and testosterone levels.
–Refer patients with abnormal screens to a specialist in male infertility for potential treatments that may include clomiphene citrate, tamoxifen, human chorionic gonadotropin (hCG), dopamine agonists, or surgical treatments depending on the underlying etiology.

Comment
1. Infertility is defined as the inability of a sexually active couple not using contraception to conceive in 1 y.

Source
–https://uroweb.org/guideline/male-infertility/#4

OVARIAN CANCER FOLLOW-UP CARE

Population
–Women treated for ovarian cancer with complete response (Stages I–IV).

Organization
▶ NCCN 2020

Recommendation
–**Follow-up plan:**
  - Office visits every 2–4 mo for 2 y, then 3–6 mo for 3 y, then annually after 5 y.
  - Physical exam including pelvic exam and measurement of CA-125 with each visit.
  - Refer for genetic risk evaluation if not previously done.
  - Chest/abdominal/pelvic CT, MRI, PET-CT, or PET as clinically indicated due to symptoms or rising CA-125.

Comments
1. All patients with ovarian cancer should be screened for BRCA1 and 2 mutations. Ten percent of patients with Lynch syndrome will develop ovarian cancer.
2. Around 22,000 new cases of ovarian cancer are reported in the United States, with approximately 14,000 deaths; 5-y survival is related to stage:
   a. Stage I: 92.6% alive at 5 y.
   b. Stage II: 74.8%.
   c. Stage III–IV: 30.2%.
3. Seventy percent of ovarian cancer patient are initially diagnosed at an advanced stage, usually stage III.
4. Relapsed ovarian cancer is rarely curable, but sequential treatments and intraperitoneal chemotherapy have extended survival to 50–60 mo.

Sources
–https://www/nccn.org/professionals/physician_gls/pdf/ovarian/pdf
–https://www.journalofclinicalpathways.com/overview-updated-nccn-guidelines-ovarian-cancer

POLYCYSTIC OVARY SYNDROME

Population
–Adolescent and adult women.

Organization
▶ Endocrine Society 2013

Recommendations
–Diagnosis if 2 of 3 criteria are met:
  - Androgen excess.

- Ovulatory dysfunction.
- Polycystic ovaries.
–Treatment:
  - Hormonal contraceptives for menstrual irregularities, acne, and hirsutism.
  - Exercise and diet for weight management.
  - Clomiphene citrate recommended for infertility.
  - Recommends against the use of metformin, inositols, or thiazolidinediones.

Source
  –http://www.guideline.gov/content.aspx?id=47899

PROSTATE CANCER: ACTIVE SURVEILLANCE (AS) FOR THE MANAGEMENT OF LOCALIZED DISEASE

Population
  –Men with early clinically localized prostate cancer (Stages T_1 and T_2 and Gleason score less than or equal to 7).

Organizations
▶ CCO 2016, ASCO 2017

Recommendations
  –For most patients with low-risk (Gleason score 6 or less) localized prostate cancer with a PSA <10, employ active surveillance (AS).
  –If younger age, high-volume Gleason 6 cancer, patient preference, and/or African-American ethnicity, consider definitive therapy.
  –For patients with limited life expectancy (<5 y) and low-risk cancer, consider watchful waiting rather than active surveillance.
  –Offer active treatment (radical prostatectomy [RP] or radiation therapy [RT]) for most patients with intermediate-risk (Gleason score 7) localized prostate cancer. For select patients with low-volume, intermediate-risk (Gleason score 3 + 4 = 7) localized prostate cancer, consider active surveillance.
  –Active surveillance consists of:
  - PSA test every 3–6 mo.
  - Direct rectal exam at least once a year.
  - At least a 12-core confirmatory transrectal ultrasound-guided biopsy (including anterior-directed cores) within 6–12 mo and then serial biopsy every 2–5 y thereafter or more frequently if clinically warranted. Men with limited life expectancy may transition to watchful waiting and avoid further biopsies.
  –For patients undergoing AS who are reclassified to a high-risk category (Gleason score now 7 or greater and/or significant increase in volume of Gleason 6 tumor consideration) should be given active therapy (RP or RT).

Comments

1. There are other ancillary tests that may make a difference in deciding when definitive therapy is indicated. The multiparametric MRI (mpMRI) and genomic testing of the malignant prostate cancer may reveal larger tumor size or unfavorable mutations that put the patient in a higher risk category which will need definitive therapy.

2. Data at 10-y follow-up from both observational and randomized trials show a very similar survival, although patients on surveillance had an increase in frequency of metastatic disease and clinical progression. (*N Engl J Med.* 2016;375:1415)

3. This approach is especially beneficial to patients older than 65 who have comorbidities and higher risk of complications. Active surveillance also significantly avoids over-treatment and therapy-related morbidity. A recent 10-y follow-up comparing monitoring, surgery, and radiation therapy treatment outcomes resulted in very similar overall survival.

Sources

–ASCO. *J Clin Oncol.* 2016;34:2182-2190.

–*N Engl J Med.* 2016;375:1415.

–*N Engl J Med.* 2014;370:932.

–*Eur Urol.* 2015;67:233.

PROSTATE CANCER FOLLOW-UP CARE

Population

–Prostate cancer survivors.

Organization

▶ ASCO 2015

Recommendations

–**Surveillance for prostate cancer patient recurrence:**

- Measure serum PSA (prostate-specific antigen) every 4–12 mo (depending on recurrence risk) for the first 5 y then recheck annually thereafter.
- Evaluate survivors with elevated or rising PSA levels as soon as possible by their primary treating specialist.
- Perform an annual direct rectal examination.
- Adhere to ASCO screening and early detection guidelines for 2nd cancers (increased risk of bladder and colon cancer after pelvic radiation).

–**Assessment and management of physical and psychosocial effects of PC and treatment:**

- Anemia related to androgen deprivation therapy (ADT).
- Bowel dysfunction and symptoms especially rectal bleeding.
- Cardiovascular and metabolic effects for men receiving ADT—follow USPSTF guidelines for evaluation and screening for cardiovascular risk factors.
- Assess for distress and depression and refer to appropriate specialist.

- Osteoporosis and fracture risk in men on ADT—do baseline DEXA (dual energy X-ray absorptiometry) scan and support with calcium, vitamin D, and bisphosphonates as indicated.
- Sexual dysfunction—phosphodiesterase type 5 inhibitors may help—refer to appropriate specialist.
- Urinary dysfunction (incontinence and leakage)—refer to urology specialist.
- Vasomotor symptoms (hot flushes) in men receiving ADT—selective serotonin or noradrenergic reuptake inhibitors or gabapentin may be helpful. Low-dose progesterone may be helpful in refractory patients.

Comments

General health promotion can be helpful:

1. Counsel survivors to achieve and maintain a healthy weight by limiting consumption of high-caloric food and beverages.
2. Counsel survivors to engage in at least 150 min/wk of physical activity.
3. Improve dietary pattern with more fruits and vegetables and whole grains.
4. Encourage intake of at least 600 IU of vitamin D per day as well as sources of calcium not to exceed 1200 mg/d.
5. Counsel survivors to avoid or limit alcohol consumption to no more than 2 drinks/d.
6. Counsel survivors to avoid tobacco products.

Rising PSA in patients with nonmetastatic PC:

1. A PSA ≥0.2 ng/mL on 2 consecutive tests is reflective of recurrent prostate cancer. These patients are treated with pelvic radiation with improvement in 10-y survival and freedom from recurrence. The earlier radiation is started after a PSA rise, the better the outcome. Patients who have had previous radiation to the prostate occasionally undergo surgery but most are treated with ADT or cryoablation (*JCO.* 2009;27:4300-4305). A recent trial adding ADT to radiation in this setting increased disease-free progression. (*Eur Urol.* 2016;69:802)
2. Routine CT or bone scanning is not indicated but evaluate new symptoms even if PSA is not rising (transformation to small cell carcinoma in 5% of patients).
3. In newly relapsed patients with visceral metastasis and/or more than 4 separate bone lesions, a combination of concurrent androgen deprivation and taxotere chemotherapy is associated with a 15%–20% increased survival at 5 y vs. sequential therapy. (*N Engl J Med.* 2015;373:737) (*Lancet.* 2016;387:1163)

Source

–Prostate cancer survivorship care guidelines. *J Clin Oncol.* 2015;33: 1078-1085.

URINARY INCONTINENCE, OVERACTIVE BLADDER

Population
–Adults.

Organization
▶ American Urologic Association 2019

Recommendations
–Rule out a urinary tract infection.
–Recommend checking a post-void residual to rule out overflow incontinence.
–First-line treatments:
  • Bladder training.
  • Bladder control strategies.
  • Pelvic floor muscle training.
–Second-line treatments:
  • Antimuscarinic meds or β3-adrenoceptor agonists (ie, darifenacin, fesoterodine, oxybutynin, solifenacin, tolterodine, or trospium).
  • Contraindicated with narrow-angle glaucoma or gastroparesis.
–Third-line treatments:
  • Sacral neuromodulation.
  • Peripheral tibial nerve stimulation.
  • Intradetrusor botulinum toxin A.
–Recommend against indwelling urinary catheters.

Source
–http://www.auanet.org/guidelines/overactive-bladder-(oab)-guideline

URINARY INCONTINENCE, STRESS

Population
–Adult women.

Organization
▶ AUA 2017, ACP 2014

Recommendations

AUA SUI ALGORITHM 2017

Female Stress Urinary Incontinence: AUA/SUFU Evaluation and Treatment Algorithm

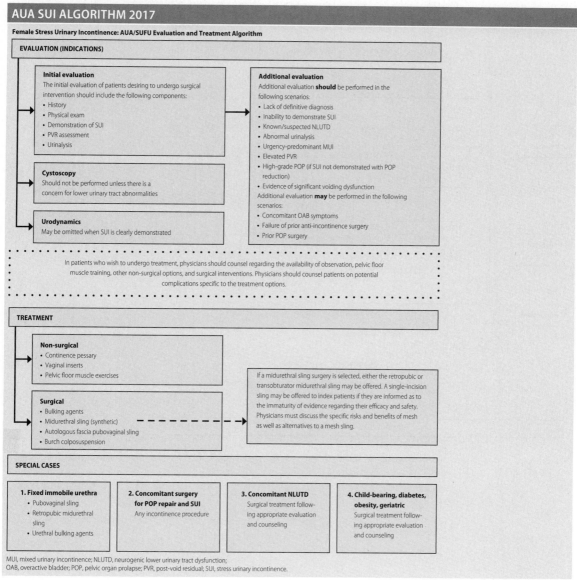

MUI, mixed urinary incontinence; NLUTD, neurogenic lower urinary tract dysfunction;
OAB, overactive bladder; POP, pelvic organ prolapse; PVR, post-void residual; SUI, stress urinary incontinence.

Source: Reproduced with permission from Kobashi KC, Albo ME, Dmochowski RR et al. Surgical treatment of female stress urinary incontinence: AUA/SUFU guideline. *J Urol.* 2017;198:875.

–Refer for pelvic floor muscle training and bladder training.

Source
   –http://www.guideline.gov/content.aspx?id=48543

INITIAL MANAGEMENT OF URINARY INCONTINENCE IN MEN: EAU 2011

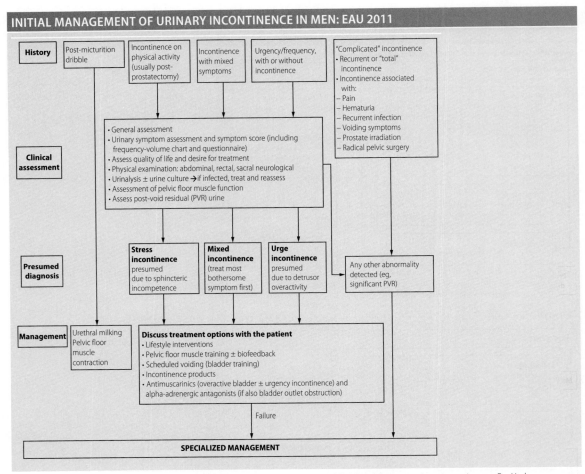

Source: Reproduced with permission from Thüroff JW, Abrams P, Andersson KE, et al. EAU guidelines on urinary incontinence. *Eur Urol.* 2011;59:387-400.

INITIAL MANAGEMENT OF URINARY INCONTINENCE IN MEN: EAU 2011

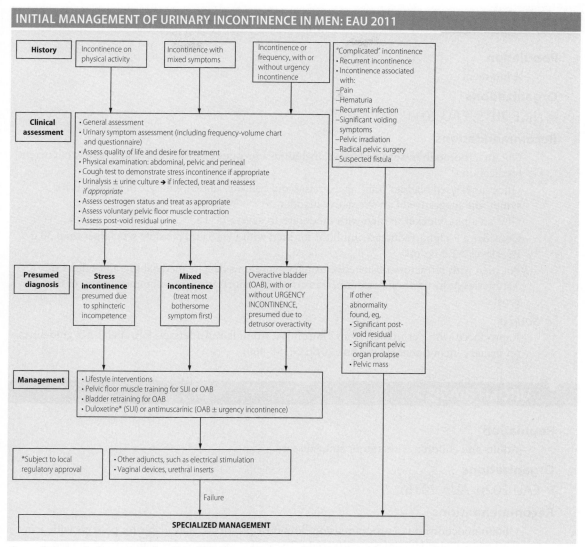

| **History** | Incontinence on physical activity | Incontinence with mixed symptoms | Incontinence or frequency, with or without urgency incontinence | "Complicated" incontinence • Recurrent incontinence • Incontinence associated with: –Pain –Hematuria –Recurrent infection –Significant voiding symptoms –Pelvic irradiation –Radical pelvic surgery –Suspected fistula |

| **Clinical assessment** | • General assessment
• Urinary symptom assessment (including frequency-volume chart and questionnaire)
• Assess quality of life and desire for treatment
• Physical examination: abdominal, pelvic and perineal
• Cough test to demonstrate stress incontinence if appropriate
• Urinalysis ± urine culture ➔ if infected, treat and reassess *if appropriate*
• Assess oestrogen status and treat as appropriate
• Assess voluntary pelvic floor muscle contraction
• Assess post-void residual urine |

| **Presumed diagnosis** | **Stress incontinence** presumed due to sphincteric incompetence | **Mixed incontinence** (treat most bothersome symptom first) | Overactive bladder (OAB), with or without URGENCY INCONTINENCE, presumed due to detrusor overactivity | If other abnormality found, eg, • Significant post-void residual • Significant pelvic organ prolapse • Pelvic mass |

| **Management** | • Lifestyle interventions
• Pelvic floor muscle training for SUI or OAB
• Bladder retraining for OAB
• Duloxetine* (SUI) or antimuscarinic (OAB ± urgency incontinence) |

| *Subject to local regulatory approval | • Other adjuncts, such as electrical stimulation
• Vaginal devices, urethral inserts |

Failure

SPECIALIZED MANAGEMENT

Source: Reproduced with permission from Thüroff JW, Abrams P, Andersson KE, et al. EAU guidelines on urinary incontinence. *Eur Urol.* 2011;59:387-400.

URINARY TRACT SYMPTOMS, LOWER

Population
–Adult men.

Organizations
▶ NICE 2015, EAU 2011

Recommendations
–Obtain a thorough history and exam, including a prostate examination, and a review of current medications.
–Offer supervised bladder training exercises and consider anticholinergic medications for symptoms suggestive of an overactive bladder.
–Give an alpha-blocker to men with moderate-to-severe LUTS.[1]
–Consider a 5-alpha-reductase inhibitor for men with LUTS and prostate size larger than 30 g or PSA level >1.4 ng/mL.
–For men with refractory obstructive urinary symptoms despite medical therapy, offer 1 of 3 surgeries: transurethral resection, transurethral vaporization, or laser enucleation of the prostate.

Source
–Reproduced with permission from Thüroff JW, Abrams P, Andersson KE, et al. EAU guidelines on urinary incontinence. *Eur Urol*. 2011;59:387-400.

UROLITHIASIS

Population
–Adults and children with kidney stone disease.

Organizations
▶ EAU 2020, AUA 2016

Recommendations
–Obtain noncontrast CT urogram using "low-dose protocols" if available for patients with acute flank pain. Consider contrast-enhanced CT scan if stone removal is planned and the renal anatomy needs to be assessed.
–Evaluate renal colic by obtaining:
  • Urinalysis.
  • Serum CBC, creatinine, uric acid, calcium, and albumin +/– intact parathyroid hormone.
  • Stone analysis by X-ray crystallography or infrared spectroscopy.

[1]Alfuzosin, doxazosin, tamsulosin, or terazosin.

–Obtain 24-h urine analysis for complicated calcium stone disease: calcium, oxalate, citrate, creatinine, urate, magnesium, phosphate, sodium, and potassium.

–Renal colic analgesia:

- NSAIDs.
- Opiates.
- Alpha-blockers.

–Treat patients with hypercalciuria with a thiazide diuretic.

–Treat with an alkaline citrate for hypocitraturia, type 1 renal tubular acidosis (RTA), hypercalciuria, and hyperoxaluria.

–Advise adults with a history of urinary stones to drink sufficient water to maintain a urine output >2.5 L/d.

–Consider use of an alpha-receptor blocker to facilitate spontaneous passage of ureteral stones <10 mm.

–Consider active ureteral stone removal for persistent obstruction, failure of spontaneous passage, or the presence of severe, unremitting colic.

- Options include shockwave lithotripsy or ureteroscopy.
- Consider the stone composition before deciding on the method of removal, based on patient history, former stone analysis of the patient, or Hounsfield unit (HU) on unenhanced computed tomography (CT). Stones with density >1000 HU (and with high homogeneity) on noncontrast-enhanced CT are less likely to be disintegrated by shockwave lithotripsy.

–For calcium stones and hypercalciuria:

- Limit sodium intake and consume 1–2 g/d of dietary calcium.
- Thiazide diuretic.

–For calcium oxalate stones:

- If high urinary oxalate, limit intake of oxalate-rich foods and maintain normal calcium consumption.
- If hyperuricosuria, treat with allopurinol.

–For uric acid stones and high urinary uric acid, limit intake of nondairy animal protein.

–For struvite stones refractory to surgical management, consider acetohydroxamic acid therapy.

–For uric acid or cystine stones, consider potassium citrate therapy to raise urinary pH to optimal level.

–Management of sepsis with obstructed kidney:

- Urgent decompression with a ureteral stent or percutaneous nephrostomy tubes.
- Start antibiotics immediately.

Comment

–Patients at high risk for recurrent stone formation:

a. ≥3 stones in 3 y.

b. Infection stones.

c. Urate stones.

d. Children and adolescents with stones.

e. Cystinuria.

f. Primary hyperoxaluria.

    g. Type 1 RTA.
    h. Cystic fibrosis.
    i. Hyperparathyroidism.
    j. Crohn's disease.
    k. Malabsorption syndromes.
    l. Nephrocalcinosis.
    m. Family history of kidney stone disease.
    n. High levels of vitamin D.

Sources
–https://uroweb.org/guideline/urolithiasis/
–http://www.auanet.org/guidelines/kidney-stones-surgical-management-guideline#x14007

Population
–Children with kidney stone disease.

Organization
▶ AUA 2014

Recommendations
–Obtain a complete metabolic workup based on stone analysis.
–Image children with ultrasound or low-dose protocol CT.
–Treat renal pelvic or calyceal stones with diameter >20 mm with percutaneous nephrolithotripsy or shockwave lithotripsy.

Source
–http://www.auanet.org/guidelines/kidney-stones-surgical-management-guideline#x3164

VAGINITIS

Population
–Nonpregnant women.

Organization
▶ ACOG 2020

Recommendations
–Assess with a complete history, physical exam of the vulva and vagina and clinical testing of the discharge.
–See Table 24-4 for a guide to the clinical diagnosis of the most common etiologies.
–Treat bacterial vaginosis with metronidazole (oral or intravaginal) or intravaginal clindamycin.
–Treat trichomoniasis with oral metronidazole
–Avoid treating vaginitis without first performing an examination.

Source
–*Obstet Gynecol.* 2020;135(1)e1-e17.

TABLE 24-4 CLINICAL DIAGNOSIS OF VAGINITIS

Clinical Findings	Normal Discharge	Bacterial Vaginosis	Trichomoniasis	Vulvovaginal Candidiasis
Discharge	White, creamy, or clear	Thin, watery, white-gray; fishy odor	Yellow-green, frothy; odor	Normal or thick, white, curd-like
Other symptoms	None	None	None, or pruritus, irritation, dysuria	Pruritus, burning, dyspareunia, dysuria
Exam	Discharge adherent to walls	Discharge	Discharge; erythema and petechiae of vagina +/− cervix	Discharge; erythema and edema if severe
Microscopy	Mature squams, rare PMNs Mostly lactobacilli	Clue cells (>20%) Positive KOH whiff test No PMNs Decreased/absent lactobacilli; increase cocci and small curved rods	Motile trichomonads Many PMNs Whiff test variable Bacilli and cocci	Branching/budding pseudohyphae (10×), spores (40×) on KOH prep. Rare PMNs Lactobacilli

VULVAR SKIN DISORDERS

Population

–Adult women with inflammatory conditions of the vulva.

Organization

▶ ACOG 2020

Recommendations

–Consider in the differential diagnosis contact dermatitis, lichen simplex chronicus, lichen sclerosus, and lichen planus among other possible etiologies.

–Acute vulvar pruritus: rule out infectious causes (BV, trichomoniasis, candidiasis, molluscum, scabies) using exam and analysis including vaginal pH, saline and KOH preps, amine test, and consider fungal culture or evaluate for noninfectious conditions if the initial analysis is unrevealing.

–Chronic vulvar pruritus: consider dermatoses such as atopic dermatitis, contact dermatitis, lichen simplex chronicus, lichen sclerosus, psoriasis, neoplasia, and other systemic diseases. Biopsy if diagnosis not immediately apparent, if concern for neoplasia, or if diagnosis uncertain after treatment.

- Vulvar pain with pruritus: likely to be either lichen planus or genitourinary syndrome of menopause.
- Vulvar pain without pruritus: evaluate for other etiologies, then consider diagnosis of vulvodynia.
- Treat contact dermatitis with avoidance of offending agents and education about proper vulvar care (avoid irritants, use mild soaps, cleanse vulva with water only, pat dry gently, emollient use, cotton/unscented/fragrance free menstrual pads, adequate lubrication for intercourse). Consider topical corticosteroid (once-twice daily until lesions heal) and oral antipruritics (antihistamines) as needed.
- Treat lichen simplex chronicus with education about vulvar care and a medium- or high-potency corticosteroid.
- Treat lichen sclerosus initially with medium- or high-potency corticosteroid (expert-recommended regimen: clobetasol 0.05% ointment qHS ×4 wk, then alternate nights ×4 wk, then twice weekly ×4 wk). Biopsy if persistent lesions or new growths. Transition to maintenance therapy with twice-weekly medium- or high-potency steroid to improve symptom control, adhesions and scarring, and vulvar cancer.
- Treat lichen planus with high-potency steroid (twice daily initially, then taper). Consider topical calcineurin inhibitors if steroids fail.

Source
- *Obstet Gynecol.* 2020;136(1):e1-e14.

Hematologic Disorders

25

ANEMIA

Population
–Adults and children.

Organization
▶ British Society of Gastroenterology 2011

Recommendation
–Evaluate with complete blood count, including Hb and mean corpuscular volume, reticulocyte count, ferritin level, total iron-binding capacity, and transferrin saturation. Calculate a reticulocyte index and Mentzer index.

Comment
1. Iron deficiency anemia (IDA) and anemia of chronic disease (ACD), sometimes called anemia of inflammation, are the two most common causes of anemia. ACD is often underrecognized, with some hospital-based studies in the United States estimating the prevalence as high as 70%. See Table 25-1 for common causes of anemia.

ANEMIA, CHEMOTHERAPY ASSOCIATED

Population
–Adults with cancer and anemia.

Organization
▶ American Society of Hematology (ASH) 2019

Recommendations
–Offer erythrocyte-stimulating agents (ESAs) if Hb <10 g/dL and curative intent. Consider RBC transfusion as alternative.
–Do not offer ESAs to cancer patients with anemia who are not on chemotherapy who have anemia. Exception: patients with lower risk myelodysplastic syndromes and a serum erythropoietin <500 IU/L.
–In patients with myeloma, non-Hodgkin lymphoma, or chronic lymphocytic leukemia (CLL), observe the response to treatment before considering an ESA.
–Counsel patients on the thromboembolic risks associated with ESAs.

TABLE 25-1	COMMON CAUSES OF ANEMIA					
Cause	MCV	Ferritin Level	RDW	Hb Electrophoresis	Iron/TIBC	Mentzer Index[a]
Iron deficiency anemia (IDA)	Low	<30	High	Normal	<10%	>13
Anemia of chronic disease (ACD)	Normal/Decreased	High	Normal/High	Normal	>15%	>13
IDA + ACD	Normal	<100	High	Normal	<20%	>13
Beta thalassemia	Low	Normal	Normal	↑A_2, F hemoglobin	~20%	<13
Alpha thalassemia	Low	Normal	Normal	Normal	~20%	<13
Hemoglobin E	Low	Normal	Normal	↑HgbE	~20%	<13
B_{12}/Folate deficiency	High	Normal	High	Normal	Normal	<13

[a]Mentzer index = MCV divided by red blood cell number (RBC) in millions.
RDW, red cell distribution of width; TIBC, total iron binding capacity.

−Epoetin beta and alfa, darbepoetin, and biosimilar epoetin alfa have equivalent safety and efficacy.

−Discontinue ESAs if no response within 6–8 wk.

−Consider iron replacement to improve Hb response and reduce RBC transfusions. See "Anemia of Chronic Disease" section for iron store assessment in inflammatory states.

Comment

1. FDA-approved starting dose of epoetin is 150 U/kg 3 times/wk or 40,000 U weekly. For darbepoetin the dose is 2.25 µg/kg weekly or 500 µg every 3 wk subcutaneously.

Source

−*Blood Adv.* 2019;3(8):1197–1210.

ANEMIA, HEMOLYTIC (HA)

Population

−Adults.

Organization

▶ BSH 2016

Recommendations

−Diagnose when there is:
  • Evidence of hemolysis (anemia, jaundice, elevated LDH, decreased haptoglobin, elevated reticulocyte index).
  • A positive direct antiglobulin test.
  • Alternative cause excluded.

−Categorize into primary autoimmune hemolytic anemia (AIHA), secondary AIHA, and drug-induced autoimmune hemolytic anemia (DIIHA).

−Give prednisolone 1 mg/kg/d for primary AIHA or secondary AIHA not responding to other treatments.

−In secondary AIHA, treating the associated condition often improves the AIHA.

−If DIIHA is suspected, stop the offending medication. Improvement usually occurs within 1–2 wk. The addition of steroids is of uncertain benefit though it is frequently used.

−Exclude CMV reactivation and parvovirus B_{12} infection if AIHA is associated with hematologic malignancy.

−If presenting with AIHA during remission of HL, assess for recurrence. If remission is confirmed, treat for primary AIHA.

−Consider azathioprine, danazol, mycophenolate mofetil, and rituximab in AIHA due to systemic lupus erythematosus not responding to steroids.

−In metastatic malignancy, AIHA can respond to disease control or to corticosteroids.

−Use thromboprophylaxis, given association between hemolysis and thrombosis.

−Transfuse for life-threatening anemia with ABO, Rh, and Kell-matched RBCs rather than waiting for full compatibility testing.

−Consider intravenous immunoglobulin (IVIG) as a rescue option in patients with AIHA.

Comments

1. HA is caused by the host's immune system acting against its own red cell antigens.
2. Incidence is 1 per 100,000/y. Approximately half are secondary to an associated disorder. Of these, half are associated with malignancy, a third due to infection, and one-sixth due to collagen vascular disorders.
3. Most cases of AIHA are warm agglutinins, but cold hemagglutinin diseases (CHAD) are also reported.
4. Secondary causes of warm AIHA include neoplasms (CLL, lymphoma, solid organ tumors), infections (hepatitis C, HIV, CMV, VZV, pneumococcal infection, leishmaniosis, tuberculosis), and immune dysregulation (SLE, Sjögren, scleroderma, ulcerative colitis, primary biliary cirrhosis, sarcoidosis, posttransplantation).
5. Secondary causes of cold AIHA include neoplasms (CLL, NHL, solid organ tumors), infections (mycoplasma, viral infections including infectious mononucleosis), autoimmune diseases, and postallogenic hematopoietic stem cell transplant.
6. The most frequent benign associations to AIHA are ovarian teratoma and thymoma. Resection of the tumor consistently resolves the AIHA.
7. Watch out for Evan's syndrome: autoimmune thrombocytopenia plus AIHA, occurring either concurrently or consecutively. Neutropenia is also a common feature. Generally chronic, affects both children and adults. Treatment is largely the same as for AIHA (first line: prednisone 1–2 mg/kg/d; second line: IVIG; third line: cyclosporin, MMF, azathioprine, danazol, rituximab, and splenectomy).

Source
–*Br J. Hematol.* 2016;76(3):395-411.

ANEMIA, IRON DEFICIENCY (IDA)

Population
–Adults.

Organization
▶ British Society of Gastroenterology 2021

Recommendations

Evaluation
–Assess dietary iron intake, malabsorption of iron, menstruation patterns, and blood donation.
–Confirm with iron studies prior to investigation, eg, serum ferritin, transferrin.
–Screen with upper and lower endoscopy for male and postmenopausal female patients unless history of recent significant non-GI blood loss. CT colography is an alternative for assessment of the colon for patient who are not suitable for endoscopy.
–Screen all patients with IDA for celiac disease (CD) and *H. pylori*, but do not defer colonoscopy if the patient is >45 y, has marked anemia, or has a significant family history of colorectal cancer.
–Screen all patients for hematuria and workup accordingly.

–Avoid fecal occult blood testing and rectal exam.

–If the patient has undergone gastrectomy and has IDA, obtain upper and lower endoscopy if >40-y-old.

–If there is no response to iron replacement, perform an iron absorption test: check a baseline iron level and then a second iron level 2–4 h after ingesting a single 325-mg ferrous sulfate tablet with water. An increase in the iron level of at least 100 μg/dL indicates adequate absorption.

–If upper and lower GI tracts are normal, obtain small bowel visualization with capsule endoscopy if the patient has symptoms of small bowel disease and/or continued anemia despite iron replacement. CT or MR enterography can be used if capsule is not available.

–Workup iron deficiency without significant anemia with GI evaluation in postmenopausal women and men >40-y-old.

Treatment

–Do not defer iron replacement while awaiting investigations into IDA unless colonoscopy is imminent.

–Dose ferrous sulfate, fumarate, or gluconate every other day dosing rather than BID dosing. Taking iron 15–30 min before a meal with orange juice or 500 mg of vitamin C may enhance absorption.

–Monitor for response to oral iron in the first 4 wk of treatment then continue for 3 mo.

–Monitor blood count every 6 mo after treatment to evaluate for recurrent IDA.

–If intolerant of iron, noncompliant, or not improving despite oral therapy, give intravenous iron sucrose (dose 200 mg once or twice a week until the calculated iron deficit is administered), ferric carboxymaltose (dose 1000 mg once weekly). Hemoglobin levels can take 8–10 wk to normalize. Reserve transfusion of RBC for cardiovascular instability or persistent symptomatic anemia despite IV iron therapy. See Tables 25-2 and 25-3 for potential complications of blood transfusion.

Comments

1. Symptoms of IDA: weakness, headache, irritability, fatigue, exercise intolerance, and restless leg syndrome. Symptoms may occur without anemia in patients with iron depletion (ferritin <30 ng/mL). As many as 40% of patients with IDA will experience pica (appetite for clay, starch, and paper products) and/or pagophagia (craving for ice) which resolves rapidly with iron repletion.

2. Rarely, in severe prolonged iron deficiency, dysphagia with esophageal webs (Plummer–Vinson syndrome), koilonychias (spoon nails), glossitis with decreased salivary flow, and alopecia can occur.

3. Common causes of occult IDA: aspirin/NSAID use, colonic carcinoma, gastric carcinoma, benign gastric ulcerations, angiodysplasia, and celiac disease. Less common causes include *H. pylori* infection, gastrectomy, esophagitis, hematuria, gastric antral vascular ectasias, and small bowel tumors. Infrequent causes of IDA include *Ancylostoma duodenale* infection, epistaxis, intravascular hemolysis (especially paroxysmal nocturnal hemoglobinuria and microangiopathic hemolytic anemia), pulmonary hemosiderosis, autoimmune gastritis, and congenital IDA (germline mutation in the *TMPRSS6* gene which leads to reduction in iron absorption and mobilization). IDA is also associated with chronic kidney disease (CKD) and CHF and can be multifactorial.

TABLE 25-2   NONINFECTIOUS COMPLICATIONS OF BLOOD TRANSFUSION

Complication	Incidence	Diagnosis	Rx and Outcome
Acute hemolytic transfusion reaction (AHTR)	1:40,000	Serum-free hemoglobin, Coombs	Fluids to keep urine output >1 mL/kg/h, pressors, treat DIC, fatal in $1:1.8 \times 10^6$ RBC exposures
Delayed transfusion reaction (HTR)	1:3000–5000	Timing (10–14 d after tx)–(+) Coombs, ↑ LDH, indirect bilirubin, reticulocyte count—Ab often to Kidd or Rh	Identify responsible antigen, transfuse compatible blood if necessary
Febrile non-HTR	0.1%–1%	Exclude AHTR —↓ risk with leucocyte depletion—starts within 2 h of transfusion	Acetaminophen PO, support and reassurance
Allergic (urticarial)	1%–3%	Urticaria, pruritus but no fever—caused by antibody to donor-plasma proteins	Hold tx—give antihistamines and complete tx when symptoms resolve
Anaphylactic	1:20,000–50,000	Hypotension, bronchospasm, urticaria, anxiety, rule out hemolysis	Epinephrine 1:1000—0.2–0.5 mL. SQ, steroids, antihistamine
Transfusion-related acute lung injury (TRALI)	1:10,000	HLA or neutrophil antibodies in donor blood hypoxia, bilateral lung infiltrates, and fever within 6 h of transfusion	Supportive care—steroids ineffective mortality—10%–20% (most common cause of transfusion-related fatality)

TABLE 25-3   INFECTIOUS COMPLICATIONS OF TRANSFUSION

Transfusion-Transmitted Organism	Risk per Unit of Blood Transfused
HIV	1 in 1,467,000
Hepatitis C	1 in 1,149,000
Hepatitis B	1 in 282,000
West Nile virus	Rare
Cytomegalovirus (CMV)	70%–80% of donors are carriers, leukodepletion ↓ risk but in situation of significant immunosuppression gives CMV-negative blood
Bacterial infection	1 in 3000—5-fold more common in platelet vs. RBC transfusion
Parasitic infection (Babesiosis, malaria, Chagas disease)	Rare

4. 20%–25% of patients will have dose-dependent GI side effects from oral iron including abdominal pain, nausea, constipation, and diarrhea.
5. In new IDA a history of GI or bariatric surgery should not stop an investigation into other causes of IDA.
6. A response of $>/= 10$ g/L rise in Hgb after 2 wk of oral IRT is highly sensitive for a true IDA.
7. IDA is common in young women; usually due to menstrual loss, pregnancy, or dietary insufficiency. Screen for celiac disease and limit other workup unless clinical suggestion for other etiology.
8. IDA in the elderly is common and multifactorial. Weigh risks and benefits of investigations based on comorbidities.

Sources
–https://gut.bmj.com/content/70/11/2030
–*Gut.* 2011;60(10):1309-1316.

ANEMIA OF CHRONIC DISEASE (ACD)

Population
–Adults and children.

Organizations
▶ American Society of Hematology (ASH) 2019, BJH 2011

Recommendations
–Anemia is defined as Hb < 12 g/dL in women, Hb < 13 g/dL in men. Usually, normochromic and normocytic pattern.
–Treat the underlying inflammatory or malignant process.
–Test for concomitant iron deficiency and determine potential responsiveness to iron therapy and long-term iron requirements every 3 mo (every 1–3 mo for people receiving hemodialysis):
  • Percentage of hypochromic cells $>6\%$, reticulocyte hemoglobin content <29 pg, or transferrin saturation $<20\%$, and serum ferritin <100 mg/L are consistent with iron deficiency.
  • The ratio of the serum transferrin receptor (sTFR) to the log of the serum ferritin can also be used to establish the presence of IDA. A ratio <1 makes ACD likely, whereas a ratio >2 suggests that iron stores are deficient, with or without ACD.
–Do not order transferrin saturation or serum ferritin alone to assess iron deficiency in people with ACD or CKD.
–Test as appropriate for kidney and liver function, thyroid function, folic acid, cobalamin (B12), or Vitamin D (negative regulator of hepcidin expression).
–In people with anemia of CKD, treat clinically relevant hyperparathyroidism to improve the management of the anemia.
–In people treated with iron, serum ferritin levels should not rise above 800 mcg/L.
–Treat with transfusion only if patient is clinically unstable or rapid correction of Hb is needed, eg, before surgery.

–Do not initiate ESA therapy in the presence of absolute iron deficiency without also managing the iron deficiency (oral or parenteral).

–Offer treatment with ESAs to patients with ACD/anemia of CKD who are likely to benefit in terms of quality of life and physical function. ESA should not be used if hemoglobin >10 g/dL. The main benefit of ESA is to reduce transfusion need.

–ESA is not to be used in patients with curable malignancies or in patients with cancer not on chemotherapy. Side effects of thrombosis and potentially increased cancer growth should be discussed with the patient.

–Goal Hb is typically 10–12 g/dL for adults, young people, and children 2 y and older, and between 9.5 and 11.5 g/dL for children younger than 2 y of age. Rate of rise goal is typically 1–2 g/dL/mo.

–Avoid blood transfusions in people with anemia of CKD in whom kidney transplant is a treatment option due to antibody formation.

–For patients with anemia of CKD who are iron deficient and not on ESA therapy, consider a trial of oral iron before offering intravenous iron therapy. If intolerant of oral iron or target Hb levels are not reached within 3 mo, offer IV iron therapy. If the patients are receiving hemodialysis, offer IV iron.

–For patients who are iron deficient, receiving ESA therapy, and receiving hemodialysis, offer IV iron.

Comments

1. Frequent causes of ACD include infections (viral, bacterial, parasitic, fungal), malignancies, autoimmune diseases (rheumatoid arthritis, systemic lupus erythematosus, vasculitis, sarcoidosis, inflammatory bowel disease), CKD, and heart failure.
2. IDA frequently occurs concomitantly with ACD.
3. Classically ACD has a mild-to-moderate anemia, normochromic and normocytic, with a low reticulocyte index. Inflammation is typically evident through inflammatory markers such as the white blood cell count, platelet count, C-reactive protein, or erythrocyte sedimentation rate.
4. Routine measurement of erythropoietin is not recommended.
5. Epoetin and darbepoetin are equal in efficacy. FDA-approved starting dose of epoetin is 150 U/kg 3 times/wk or 40,000 U weekly. For darbepoetin the dose is 2.25 µg/kg weekly or 500 µg every 3 wk subcutaneously.
6. When patients stop chemotherapy for any reason, stop ESAs and substitute transfusion therapy according to FDA guidelines.

Source
–*Br J. Hematol* 2011;154(3):289-300.

COBALAMIN (B$_{12}$) AND FOLATE (B$_9$) DEFICIENCY

Population
–Adults ≥19 y of age.

Organization
▶ BJH 2014

Recommendations
–There is no gold standard test for the diagnosis of cobalamin deficiency. Serum cobalamin lacks sensitivity and specificity (a cutoff of 200 ng/L results in a sensitivity of 95% but specificity of 50%).

–Consider cobalamin or folate deficiency when CBC shows oval macrocytes or hyper-segmented neutrophils in the presence of an elevated MCV.

–Cobalamin and folate assays should be assessed concurrently.

–Consider plasma total homocysteine (tHcy) and/or plasma methylmalonic acid (MMA) as supplementary tests if there is clinical suspicion of cobalamin deficiency but intermediate cobalamin level. Both are elevated in cobalamin deficiency. tHcy is a sensitive marker, but MMA is more specific. Holotranscobalamin, the active fraction of plasma cobalamin, may be a suitable assay for assessment of cobalamin status in the future.

–Test all patients with anemia, neuropathy, or glossitis, suspected of having pernicious anemia for anti-intrinsic factor antibodies (IFAB) regardless of cobalamin levels. Do not test for antigastric parietal cell antibodies.

–Test for IFAB in patients with low-serum cobalamin levels in the absence of anemia and who do not have other causes of deficiency. Patients found to have a positive test should have lifelong cobalamin therapy.

–Therapy of cobalamin deficiency is important because neurologic symptoms may be irreversible if treatment is delayed.

–For patients with neurological symptoms, give parenteral cobalamin 1000 mcg IM daily or every other day for 2 wk. Then give 1000 mcg IM q3mo or 1000–2000 mcg PO daily. Oral crystalline cyanocobalamin is as effective as parenteral unless IFAB.

–Retest serum cobalamin levels after 2–4 mo to ensure normalization.

–A serum folate level <7 nmol/L (3 mcg/L) is indicative of folate deficiency. Routine RBC folate testing is not necessary.

–In the presence of strong clinical suspicion of folate deficiency, despite a normal level, an RBC folate assay may be undertaken, having ruled out B$_{12}$ deficiency.

–The dose of folic acid necessary for treatment depends on the cause of the deficiency. Folic acid 0.8 mg PO daily is typically sufficient; however, 5 mg daily is necessary in hemolytic states and patients on hemodialysis.

Comments
1. The interpretation of cobalamin testing should be considered in relation to the clinical circumstances. Falsely low-serum cobalamin levels may be seen in the presence of folate deficiency.

Moreover, neurological symptoms due to cobalamin deficiency can occur in the presence of a normal MCV.

2. The most frequently cited causes of cobalamin deficiency include *H. pylori*, *Giardia lamblia*, fish tapeworm, pernicious anemia, gastric resection, celiac disease, tropical sprue, Crohn disease, low dietary intake (ie, Vegan diet), metformin use, and achlorhydria due to atrophic gastritis or proton pump inhibitors.

3. The incidence of B_{12} deficiency in the elderly (>70-y-old) is 5%–10%.

4. Pernicious anemia (the most common cause of B_{12} deficiency) is an autoimmune illness with antibodies to gastric parietal cells and intrinsic factor resulting in gastric atrophy and malabsorption of food-derived B_{12}. It is associated with Hashimoto disease, type 1 diabetes, vitiligo, and hypoadrenalism.

5. Independent of the etiology of B_{12} deficiency, oral B_{12} (1000–2000 mg) daily will correct lower B_{12} levels due to intrinsic-factor independent absorption.

6. Causes of low folic acid levels include poor diet (lack of legumes and green leafy vegetables), goat's milk (as opposed to cow's milk in children), alcoholism, pregnancy, increased RBC turnover (thalassemia, hemolytic anemias, sickle cell anemia), and hemodialysis.

7. Patients with elevated MCV who are folate deficient must have B_{12} deficiency ruled out since treatment with folate in patients with B_{12} deficiency will accelerate peripheral neuropathy.

8. Drugs that can cause folate deficiency and B_{12} deficiency include trimethoprim, pyrimethamine, methotrexate, and phenytoin.

9. When treating B_{12} and folate deficiency, the MCV may decrease due to acquired iron deficiency as iron is incorporated into red cell precursors in response to B_{12} and/or folate therapy.

Source
−*Br J Haematol.* 2014;166(4):496-513.

DEEP VEIN THROMBOSIS (DVT) AND PULMONARY EMBOLISM (PE)

Population
–Adults.

Organizations
▶ ESC 2019, ACCP 2016, ACP 2015, ASH 2018

Recommendations
–Use a validated tool to diagnose PE that considers clinical probability.
- For suspected initial DVT, use Wells Score for DVT (Table 25-4) to determine pretest probability and therefore diagnostic algorithm (Figs. 25-1–25-3).
- If D-dimer or US can't be obtained within 4 h, consider interim therapeutic anticoagulation while awaiting results.

–Collect baseline blood tests before starting anticoagulation (CBC, renal and hepatic function, PT, APPT), but do not delay starting anticoagulation while awaiting results.
- For suspected recurrent lower extremity DVT, use the diagnostic algorithm in Fig. 25-4.

TABLE 25-4 WELLS SCORE FOR DVT	
Symptoms	**Points**
Malignancy, treatment, or palliation within 6 mo	+1
Bedridden recently >3 d or major surgery within 4 wk	+1
Calf swelling >3 cm compared to the other leg	+1
Collateral superficial veins present	+1
Entire leg swollen	+1
Localized tenderness along the deep venous system	+1
Pitting edema, confined to symptomatic leg	+1
Paralysis, paresis, or recent plaster immobilization of the lower extremity	+1
Previously documented DVT	+1
Alternative diagnosis to DVT as likely or more likely	−2

Low—0 (3% risk of DVT), Moderate—1 or 2 (20% risk of DVT), High—3 or greater (75% risk of DVT).
Source: Goldhaber SZ, Bounameaux H. Pulmonary embolism and deep vein thrombosis. *Lancet.* 2012;379:1835.

Fig. 25-1 Diagnostic algorithm for suspected low pretest probability initial lower extremity deep vein thrombosis (DVT).

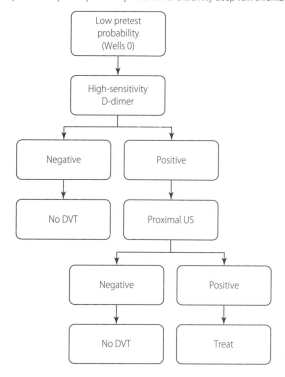

Fig. 25-2 Diagnostic algorithm for suspected moderate pretest probability initial lower extremity deep vein thrombosis (DVT).

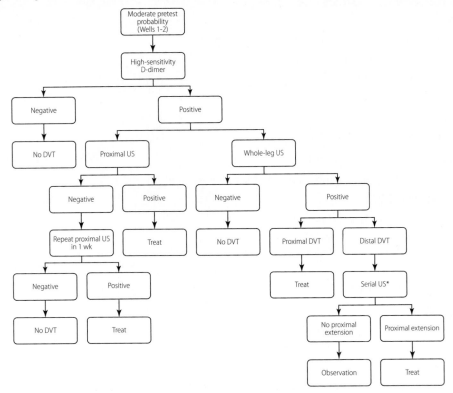

*Treat distal DVT only if patient is at high risk for proximal extension or severely symptomatic.

- For suspected pulmonary embolism, use Wells Score for PE (Table 25-5) or Revised Geneva Score for PE, creatinine clearance, and age-adjusted D-dimer to guide diagnostic strategy.
- Start anticoagulation while initiating workup if PE is suspected.
- Use D-dimer in outpatient settings, or where the probability of PE is low, to reduce unnecessary imaging.
- Use pretest probability to determine further testing (ASH):
  - If low or intermediate PTP of PE ($\leq$5% up to 20%), order D-dimer in an attempt to exclude the diagnosis. If D-dimer positive, order VQ scan or CT pulmonary angiography.
  - If high PTP of PE ($\geq$50%), order CT pulmonary angiography as the initial test, or VQ scan if not feasible.
  - If low PTP of DVT ($\leq$10%), order D-dimer in an attempt to exclude the diagnosis. If D-dimer is positive, order ultrasound.

Fig. 25-3 Diagnostic algorithm for suspected high pretest probability initial lower extremity deep vein thrombosis (DVT).

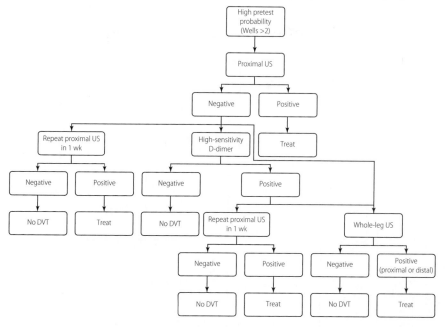

In patients with extensive unexplained leg swelling, if there is no DVT on proximal CUS or whole-leg US and D-dimer testing has not been performed or is positive, the iliac veins should be imaged to exclude isolated iliac DVT.

- If intermediate or high PTP of PE (25% up to ≥50%), order ultrasound of the legs. If initial ultrasound is negative in high-risk patient, follow up with serial ultrasounds.

–If Pulmonary Embolism Rule-out Criteria score is negative, consider foregoing additional testing for PE. (ASH)

–CT Pulmonary Angiogram (CTPA) is the definitive diagnostic study for PE.

–VQ scan can rule out PE if normal and can confirm PE if "high probability."

–In patients with isolated distal DVT consider repeat US once weekly ×2 wk over anticoagulation if no severe symptoms or risk for extension. If found to have extension to distal veins, suggest anticoagulation; if extension to proximal veins, recommend anticoagulation.

–In patients with subsegmental PE without proximal DVT of lower extremity, recommend clinical surveillance over anticoagulation if low risk for recurrent VTE.

–In patients with cerebral vein/venous sinus thrombosis, recommend anticoagulation for at least 3 mo.

–In acute DVT, anticoagulation is recommended over interventional techniques. (In high-risk PE, admit for unfractionated heparin and consider catheter-directed thrombolysis or embolectomy; Fig. 25-6.)

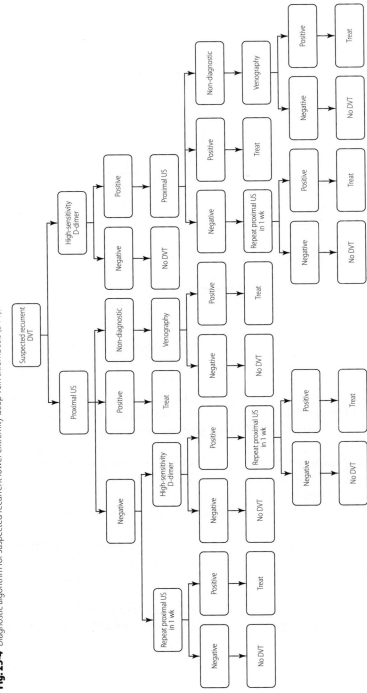

Fig. 25-4 Diagnostic algorithm for suspected recurrent lower extremity deep vein thrombosis (DVT).

TABLE 25-5 WELLS SCORE FOR PE	
Symptoms	**Points**
Clinical signs and symptoms of DVT	+3
PE is #1 diagnosis OR equally likely	+3
Heart rate >100	+1.5
Immobilization at least 3 d OR surgery in the previous 4 wk	+1.5
Previous, objectively diagnosed PE or DVT	+1.5
Hemoptysis	+1
Malignancy, treatment, or palliation within 6 mo	+1

Low—less than 2 (2%–3% risk of PE), Moderate—2–6 (20%–30% risk of PE), High—6 or greater (>70% risk of PE).
Source: Goldhaber SZ, Bounameaux H. Pulmonary embolism and deep vein thrombosis. *Lancet.* 2012;379:1835.

Fig. 25-5 Diagnostic algorithm for suspected pulmonary embolism.

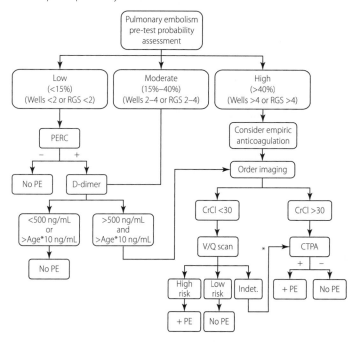

*Consider empiric treatment for PE after risk/benefit analysis.

Fig. 25-6 Treatment algorithm for confirmed pulmonary embolism.

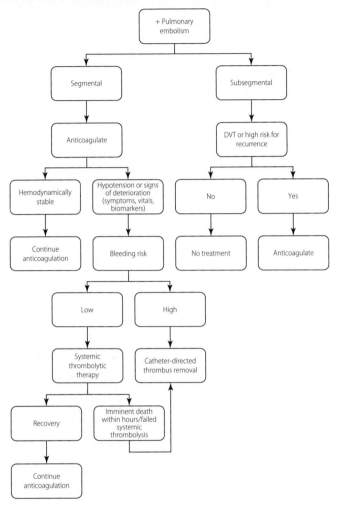

- If low-risk PE (age <80, no cancer, no COPD, HR <110, SBP >100, O2 sat ≥90%, no RV dysfunction, adequate social support, and access to medical care), may discharge home from ER on oral anticoagulation (Table 25-6).
- Offer apixaban or rivaroxaban as first line if no contraindications; if not an option, offer LMWH ×5 d followed by dabigatran or edoxaban or LMWH with VKA ×5 d or until INR is at least 2 × 2 readings then VKA alone.
- Consider regular monitoring for therapeutic levels in patients <50 kg or >120 kg to ensure effectiveness.

TABLE 25-6   RECOMMENDED ANTICOAGULANT SELECTION AND DURATION OF ANTICOAGULATION BASED ON RISK FACTORS AND LOCATION OF DVT

Limb	Prox vs. Dist	Provoked	Cancer	Bleeding Risk	Anticoagulants	Duration
Upper	Prox	Yes	Yes		No specific recommendations	Indefinite
			No		No specific recommendations	3 mo
		No	No	High	No specific recommendations	3 mo
				Low	No specific recommendations	Indefinite
	Dist[a]	Yes	Yes		No specific recommendations	Indefinite
			No		No specific recommendations	3 mo
		No	No	High	No specific recommendations	3 mo
				Low	No specific recommendations	Indefinite
Lower	Prox	Yes	Yes		LMWH over VKA, direct thrombin, or Xa inhibitors	Indefinite
			No		Dabigatran, rivaroxaban, apixaban, or edoxaban over VKA	3 mo
		No	No	High	Dabigatran, rivaroxaban, apixaban, or edoxaban over VKA	3 mo
				Low	Dabigatran, rivaroxaban, apixaban, or edoxaban over VKA	Indefinite
	Dist[a]	Yes	Yes		LMWH over VKA, direct thrombin, or Xa inhibitors	Indefinite
			No		Dabigatran, rivaroxaban, apixaban, or edoxaban over VKA	3 mo
		No	No	High	Dabigatran, rivaroxaban, apixaban, or edoxaban over VKA	3 mo
				Low	Dabigatran, rivaroxaban, apixaban, or edoxaban over VKA	Indefinite

VKA, vitamin K antagonist.

[a]In general, treatment of isolated distal upper or lower extremity DVT is not recommended unless there are severe symptoms or a high risk for or evidence of proximal extension on ultrasound.

–If oral therapy, use DOAC rather than VKA if able (ie, no severe renal impairment, CrCl >15 mL/min), pregnancy/breastfeeding, antiphospholipid syndrome, etc.). If VKA is necessary, bridge with parenteral anticoagulant until INR is 2–3 (Table 25-7).

–Consider IVC filter only if absolute contraindication to anticoagulation or if recurrent PE despite anticoagulation.

TABLE 25-7 RECOMMENDED ANTICOAGULANT SELECTION AND DURATION OF ANTICOAGULATION FOR PULMONARY EMBOLISM BASED ON RISK FACTORS AND LOCATION OF PULMONARY EMBOLISM

Location	Provoked	Cancer	Bleeding Risk	Anticoagulants	Duration
Segmental	Yes	Yes		LMWH over VKA, direct thrombin, or Xa inhibitors	Indefinite
		No		Dabigatran, rivaroxaban, apixaban, or edoxaban over VKA	3 mo
	No	No	High	Dabigatran, rivaroxaban, apixaban, or edoxaban over VKA	3 mo
			Low	Dabigatran, rivaroxaban, apixaban, or edoxaban over VKA therapy	Indefinite
Subsegmental[a]	Yes	Yes		LMWH over VKA, direct thrombin, or Xa inhibitors	Indefinite
		No		Dabigatran, rivaroxaban, apixaban, or edoxaban over VKA	3 mo
	No	No	High	Dabigatran, rivaroxaban, apixaban, or edoxaban over VKA	3 mo
			Low	Dabigatran, rivaroxaban, apixaban, or edoxaban over VKA	Indefinite

VKA, vitamin K antagonist.
[a]In general, treatment of a subsegmental PE is not recommended unless there is a concomitant DVT or high risk for recurrence.

–Remove IVC filter when anticoagulants are no longer contraindicated and have been established.
–ESC: Duration of therapy: ≥3 mo (see Table 25-8).
  • If major reversible/transient risk factor, stop anticoagulation after 3 mo.
  • If recurrent VTE without major reversible/transient risk factor, continue indefinitely.
  • If first VTE and minor or persistent risk factor, consider extending anticoagulation indefinitely.
  • If first VTE without identifiable risk factor, consider extending beyond 3 mo versus discontinuing at 3 mo.
–If extending therapy (in the absence of cancer), consider reducing DOAC dose after 6 mo (apixaban 2.5 mg BID or rivaroxaban 10 mg daily). (ESC 2019)
–If extended therapy indicated but oral anticoagulants are not tolerated or declined, use aspirin or sulodexide instead. (ESC 2019)
–Aspirin 75 mg or 150 mg daily recommended.
–ACCP: Duration based on location (Figure 5).
–If pregnancy, use LMWH at weight-based dose using weight from early pregnancy. Do not use DOACs.

TABLE 25-8 NEW ORAL ANTICOAGULANTS[a] AND WARFARIN

Agent	Target	Dosing	Monitoring	Half-life	Time to Peak Plasma Concentration	Specific Reversible Agent
Warfarin	Vitamin K epoxide	Once daily	INR–adjusted	40 h	72–96 h	Vitamin K[b]
						PCC
Dabigatran	Thrombin	Fixed—once or twice daily	None	14–17 h	2 h	Idarucizumab[c]
Rivaroxaban	Factor Xa	Fixed—once or twice daily	None	5–9 h (50-y-old)	2.5–4 h	Andexxa[c]
				9–13 h (elderly)		
Apixaban	Factor Xa	Fixed twice daily	None	8–15 h	3 h	None[c]
Edoxaban	Factor Xa	Give once daily	None	10–14 h	1–2 h	None[c]

[a]Do not use new oral anticoagulants in patients with mechanical valves. Warfarin is superior.
[b]If significant bleed on warfarin, give vitamin K, and 4-factor prothrombin complex concentrate (PCC/K–centra) or recombinant FVIIa if not controlled.
[c]If significant bleed, aggressively treat source of bleed; consider 4-factor PCC, recombinant FVIIa or Andexxa.

Comments

1. Iodinated contrast agents for CTPA are safe at least to a creatinine clearance of 30, if not lower. (*Ann Emerg Med.* 2018;71(1):44-53)

2. Knee-high GCS (graduated compression stockings) with 30–40 mmHg pressure at ankles for 2 y will reduce postthrombotic syndrome risk by 50%.

3. In patients with acute lower extremity DVT, suggest against using compression stockings to prevent PTS (*Chest.* 2021;160(6):e545-e608). Can consider use for management of leg symptoms after DVT. (*NICE.* 2020;NG158:1-47)

4. Risk factors for warfarin bleeding—age >65 y, history of stroke, history of GI bleed, and recent comorbidity (MI, Hct <30, creatinine >1.5, diabetes). If all 4 factors are present, there is 40% risk of significant bleed in 12 mo; 0.4% of patients on warfarin die of bleeding yearly. (*Chest.* 2016;149:315) (*Am J Med.* 2011;124:111)

5. Calf and iliofemoral thrombosis have increased incidence of false-negative compression ultrasound—recommend CT or MR venogram or venography for suspected iliofemoral thrombosis, and for calf thrombosis, follow-up compression ultrasound (CUS) in 5–7 d is acceptable.

6. Consider high thrombophilic risk in patients with recurrent VTE or patients with first unprovoked VTE who have the following characteristics:
   a. Age <50-y-old.
   b. Family history of VTE.
   c. Unusual site of thrombosis.
   d. Massive venous thrombosis.

7. In unprovoked VTE 3% of patients are found to have associated malignancy, with another 10% diagnosed with cancer over the next 2 y. (*N Engl J Med.* 1998;338:1169) (*Ann Intern Med.* 2008;149:323) (*N Engl J Med.* 2015;373:697)

8. In patients with the antiphospholipid antibody syndrome and a new venous thrombosis, transition to warfarin is superior to using the new oral anticoagulants with adjusted target INR of 2.5. (*Am J Hematol.* 2014;89:1017) (*Chest.* 2021;160(6):e545-e608).

9. The presence of a permanent IVC filter does not mandate continuous anticoagulation unless documented recurrent clot problems.

10. Asymptomatic PE (found incidentally on chest CT) should be treated with same protocol as symptomatic PE.

11. In patients with superficial thrombosis of lower extremity with risk of progression, consider anticoagulation with fondaparinux 2.5 mg daily (or rivaroxaban 10 mg daily as alternative) for 45 d.

12. If anticoagulation treatment fails, increase the dose of change to anticoagulant with different mechanisms of action (after evaluating for adherence and other sources of hypercoagulability).

13. Consider catheter-directed thrombolytic therapy for symptomatic iliofemoral DVT with symptoms <14 d, good functional status, life expectancy >/= 1 y, and low bleeding risk.

Sources

–*Chest.* 2021;160(6):e545-e608.
–*NICE.* 2020;NG158:1-47).
–*J Thromb Hemost.* 2018:16(9);1891-1894. https://doi.org/10.1111/jth.14219
–*Blood Adv.* 2018:2(22);3226.

–*Blood Adv.* 2018:2(22);3257.
–*CHEST* 2016;149(2):315-352.
–*Blood.* 2015;125:1877.

Population

–Adults with cancer and VTE.

Organizations

▶ NICE 2020, ACCP 2021, ESC 2019, International Society on Thrombosis and Hemostasis 2018

Recommendations

GUIDELINES DISCORDANT: MANAGEMENT OF VTE IN PATIENTS WITH ACTIVE CANCER	
Organization	**Guidance**
NICE	–If active cancer, treat for 3 to 6 mo, consider stopping if provoked or HAS-BLED >/= 4 and can't be modified vs. Continuing indefinitely if unprovoked and low bleeding risk
ACCP	If active cancer, use oral Xa inhibitor (apixaban, edoxaban, or rivaroxaban) over LMWH (apixaban or LMWH may be preferred option in luminal GI malignancies)
ESC	If active cancer, use LMWH, but consider edoxaban or rivaroxaban as alternatives if cancer is not gastrointestinal. Treat for at least 6 mo, but consider extending indefinitely or until cure
International Society on Thrombosis and Hemostasis	Employ shared decision making, as overall data is lacking. Consider edoxaban or rivaroxaban as first-line therapy for patients with acute VTE, low bleeding risk, and no drug–drug interactions. Otherwise use low-molecular-weight heparins to treat acute VTE in cancer

Sources
–*Chest.* 2021;160(6):e545-e608.
–*NICE.* 2020;NG158:1-47.
–https://doi.org/10.1111/jth.14219
–*Eur Heart J.* 2020:41;543-603.

HEPARIN-INDUCED THROMBOCYTOPENIA (HIT)

Population

–Adults.

Organization

▶ American Society of Hematology 2018

Recommendations

–Diagnosis: if platelets drop 30%–50%, suspect HIT and use 4T scoring model (see Table 25-9) to assess likelihood of HIT.
  - If intermediate-to-high probability, treat for HIT and send immunologic (enzyme-linked immunosorbent assay [ELISA]) and functional testing (platelet serotonin release assay).
  - Do not test for or empirically treat for HIT in patients with a low-probability 4T score.
–If elevated 4T score, stop heparin and start nonheparin anticoagulation (argatroban, bivalirudin, danaparoid, fondaparinux, or a direct oral anticoagulant [DOAC]) until HIT immunoassay returns negative or platelets are >150,000/mcL.
–Avoid platelet transfusion unless life-threatening bleeding.
–Screen for bilateral lower extremity DVT with ultrasound. Consider screening for upper extremity DVT if upper extremity central venous catheter.

Comments

1. The median platelet count in HIT is 60,000 and seldom falls below 20,000.
2. The development of HIT is not related to the degree of exposure to heparin. A single flush of an IV line or 1 dose of prophylactic heparin can trigger the HIT syndrome. If HIT is not recognized, further administration of heparin will lead to significant increased risk of clot, morbidity, and mortality. (*N Engl J Med*. 2006;355:809-817) (*JAMA*. 2004;164:361-369)
3. The 4T scoring system is most accurate in the low-risk subset, with a negative predictive value of 0.998. (*Blood*. 2012;120:4160-4167)

Source

–*Blood Adv*. 2018;2(22):3360-3392.

IMMUNE THROMBOCYTOPENIA (ITP)

Population

–Adults.

Organization

▶ American Society of Hematology (ASH) 2019

Recommendations

–Diagnosis of exclusion. There is no reliable diagnostic test (including antiplatelet antibody studies). Test for hepatitis C and HIV, and other underlying illnesses suggested by exam.

TABLE 25-9   DIAGNOSTIC TOOL FOR DIAGNOSIS OF HIT

4 Ts	2 Points	1 Point	0 Point
Thrombocytopenia	• Fall in platelet count >50% and nadir of ≥20,000 **AND** • No surgery in preceding 3 d	• >50% fall in platelets but with surgery in preceding 3 d • 30%–50% platelet fall with nadir 10–19,000	• <30% fall in platelets • Any platelet fall with nadir <10,000
Timing of platelet fall	• 5–10 d after start of heparin • Platelet fall <5 d with heparin exposure within past 30 d	• Platelet fall after day 10 • Platelet fall <5 d with heparin exposure in past 100 d	• Platelet fall ≤day 4 without exposure to heparin in last 100 d
Thrombosis or other sequelae	• Confirmed new venous or arterial thrombosis • Skin necrosis at heparin injection sites • Anaphylactoid reaction to IV heparin	• Progressive or recurrent thrombosis while on heparin • Erythematous skin reaction at heparin injection sites	• Thrombosis suspected
Other causes of thrombocytopenia	• No alternative cause of platelet drop evident	• At least 1 other possible cause of drop in platelet count	• Definite or highly likely cause present • Sepsis • Chemotherapy within 20 d • DIC • Drug-induced ITP • Posttransfusion purposes

High probability: 6–8 points; intermediate probability: 4–5 points; low probability: ≤3 points.

–Risk factors:
- Drug induced (trimethoprim-sulfa, rifampin, carbamazepine, vancomycin, quinine derivatives, and many more).
- Systemic lupus/Sjögren syndrome, and other rheumatologic diseases.
- Infections—hepatitis C, HIV, cytomegalovirus (CMV), *H. pylori*, Epstein–Barr virus (EBV), varicella.
- Indolent lymphomas, breast and colon cancer.
- Vaccinations—mostly in children.
- Common variable immunodeficiency—almost exclusively in children.

–Observe if platelet count >30,000 and asymptomatic; do not give steroids except when comorbidities exist, procedures are anticipated, or age > 60-y-old.

–Treat if platelet count <30,000 with or without bleeding.
- Use corticosteroids (prednisone 0.5–2 mg/kg daily with taper) (preferred over observation, even if no bleeding).
- Consider IVIG with corticosteroids when a more rapid rise in platelet count is needed (ie, prior to surgery).
- Second-line therapy: Rituximab.
- If corticosteroids are contraindicated: IVIG or anti-D immune globulin (in patients that are Rh(+) and spleen in place).
- IVIG dose: 1 g/kg as a 1-time dose that may be repeated as necessary. (*Lancet Haematol.* 2016;3:e489) (*Blood.* 2016;127:296) (See Table 25-10.)

–If unresponsive or relapse, consider splenectomy and/or thrombopoietin receptor agonists.

–Treatment of specific forms of secondary ITP (see Table 25-11):
- HCV-associated: Antiviral therapy should be considered in absence of contraindications. Initial therapy in this setting should be IVIG.

TABLE 25-10 FIRST-LINE THERAPY FOR ITP		
Corticosteroids	**RR**	**% With Sustained Response**
Prednisone 0.5–2 mg/kg/d for 2 wk followed by taper	70%–80%	10-y disease-free—13%–15%
Dexamethasone 40 mg daily for 4 d every 2–4 wk for 1–4 cycles	90%	As high as 50% (2–5 y follow-up)
IV anti-D immune globulin	80%	Usually lasts 3–4 wk, but may persist for months in some patients
50–75 μg/kg—warning regarding brisk hemolysis and rare DIC		
IVIG 0.4 g/kg/d × 5 d or 1 g/kg/d for 1–2 d	80%	Transient benefit lasting 2–4 wk

TABLE 25-11 SELECTED SECOND-LINE THERAPY OPTIONS IN ADULT ITP	
TPO Receptor Agonist	**RR**
Eltrombopag 25–75 mg orally daily	70%–80%
Romiplostim 1–10 μg/kg SQ weekly	80%–90%
Immunosuppression	
Azathioprine 1–2 mg/kg	40%
Cyclosporine 5 mg/kg/d for 6 d then 2.5–3 m/kg/d to titrate blood levels of 100–200 mg/mL	50%–60%
Cytoxan 1–2 mg/kg orally or IV (0.3–1 g/m²) for 113 doses every 2–4 wk	30%–60%
Rituximab 375 mg/m² weekly × 4	50%–60% respond—sustained >3–5 y in 10%–15%
Uncertain Mechanism	
Danazol 200 mg 2–4× daily (orally)	~50%
Vinca alkaloid 1–2 mg IV weekly to max of 6 mg	~30% variable

- HIV-associated: start HAART first unless patient has significant bleeding complications. If ITP therapy is required, use corticosteroids, IVIG, anti-D immune globulin, and romiplostim or eltrombopag. Refractory patients should have a splenectomy.
- *H. pylori*–associated: Eradication therapy of newly diagnosed active *H. pylori* infection (stool antigen, urea breath test, endoscopic biopsy) will result in resolution of ITP in 25%–35% of patients.

Comment

1. TTP (thrombotic thrombocytopenic purpura) should always be excluded. Symptoms: ill appearing, low-grade fever, myalgia, chest pain, and altered mental status. Labs: thrombocytopenia and a hemolytic anemia with red cell fragmentation, elevated reticulocyte count, and significant elevation of lactate dehydrogenase. This is a *medical emergency* and should be treated urgently with plasma exchange. See next section for more details.

Sources
–*Blood Adv.* 2019;3(23):3829-3866.
–*Blood.* 2016;128:1547.
–*Blood.* 2011;117:4190-4207.
–*Blood.* 2010;115:168-186.

Population
–Pediatric.

Organization
▶ American Society of Hematology (ASH) 2011

Recommendations

–Do not obtain bone marrow (BM) examination in children and adolescents with typical features of ITP (isolated thrombocytopenia, large, morphologically normal platelets, asymptomatic except for bleeding).

–Initially, observe regardless of platelet count unless moderate-to-severe bleeding.

–If moderate-to-severe bleeding, admit for single dose of IVIG (0.8–1 g/kg) or short-course corticosteroid is first line.

–Consider splenectomy for pediatric patients with chronic or persistent ITP who have significant or persistent bleeding and lack of responsiveness or intolerance to other standard therapies.

–Children with a history of ITP who are unimmunized should receive their scheduled first MMR vaccine. Check titers subsequently and only give further vaccines if immunity is insufficient.

Comments

1. Treatment focuses on severity of bleeding, not platelet cell count. In a study of 505 children with platelets <20,000 and skin bleeding, only 3 patients developed severe bleeding and none had intracranial hemorrhage.
2. Response rate to splenectomy is 70%–80%, but unless a child has severe unresponsive disease, delay the splenectomy for at least 12 mo since 20%–30% will have spontaneous remission.

Sources

–*Pediatr Blood Cancer.* 2009;53:652-654.
–*Blood.* 2010;115:168-186.
–*Blood.* 2013;121:4457-4462.
–*Blood.* 2014;124:3295.

HEMOPHILIA A AND B

Population

–Adults and children.

Organization

▶ NHF 2018

Recommendations

–Hemophilia A is a loss of Factor VIII activity. Hemophilia B is a loss of Factor IX activity. Usually congenital, though can develop acquired hemophilia due to cancer, SLE, or other autoimmune diseases.

–Treat with the corresponding recombinant (r) or plasma-derived (pd) factor concentrates.

–Do not use cryoprecipitate unless there is a risk of loss of life or limb and no FVIII concentrate is available.

–Consider desmopressin (DDAVP, intranasal or parenteral) for patients with mild hemophilia A who have been documented by a DDAVP trial to have a significant rise in fVIII.

–For patients with hemophilia A or B with high titer inhibitors, immune tolerance induction (ITI) is the best option for inhibitor eradication.

–Treatment for patients with hemophilia with inhibitor antibodies include:

- FEIBA (activation prothrombin complex concentration [aPCC]) contains activation factors IIa, VIIa, and Xa and is used to bypass an inhibitor to FVIII or FIX. It is plasma derived.
- NovoSeven RT (recombinant-activated factor VII concentrate) contains activated FVIIa and is used to bypass inhibitors to FVIII or FIX.
- Hemlibra (emicizumab-kxwh) is a bispecific FIXa- and FX-directed monoclonal antibody that bridges FIXa and FX, bypassing the FVIII inhibitor to prevent or treat bleeding in patients with hemophilia A and inhibitors.
- There is a significant risk of thrombosis with the use of these agents. Do not exceed recommended doses.

–Treat patients with acquired hemophilia A with NovoSevenRT or Obizur, a recombinant porcine factor VIII (rpFVIII). Often the human FVIII inhibitor does not cross-react with the porcine FVIII, allowing for cessation of bleeding with Obizur treatment.

–Confirm hepatitis A and B immunity for all patients with hemophilia. Immunize seronegative patients.

Source

–https://www.hemophilia.org/Researchers-Healthcare-Providers/Medical-and-Scientific-Advisory-Council-MASAC/MASAC-Recommendations/Guidelines-for-Emergency-Department-Management-of-Individuals-with-Hemophilia-and-Other-Bleeding-Disorders

NEUTROPENIA WITHOUT FEVER

Population

–Adults.

Organizations

▶ IDSA/ASCO 2018, NIH 2012, ASH 2012

Recommendations

–Neutropenia is defined as an ANC <1500 cells/mm^3.

- Mild: 1500–1000 cells/mm^3.
- Moderate: 1000–500 cells/mm^3.
- Severe: <500 cells/mm^3.

–Most commonly due to chemotherapy, but consider other etiologies including solid malignancies with bone marrow invasion, lymphoproliferative malignancies (eg, natural killer cell lymphomas, hairy cell leukemia, and CLL), radiation therapy, autoimmune etiologies (eg, SLE, rheumatoid arthritis), viral (eg, CMV, EBV, HIV), parasitic (eg, malaria), and genetic (eg, aplastic anemia, paroxysmal nocturnal hemoglobinuria, May-Hegglin anomaly).

–Consider bone marrow biopsy if etiology is not evident.

–Manage chemotherapy-associated neutropenia by dose modification, dose interval delays, and/or prophylaxis with G-CSFs.

–Use antibiotic (fluoroquinolone) and antifungal (oral triazole or parenteral echinocandin) prophylaxis for patients at high risk for febrile neutropenia or profound, protracted neutropenia (defined as ANC <100 for >7 d, eg, most patients with AML/MDS or HSCT treated with myeloablative conditioning regimens).

–If HSV seropositive and undergoing hematopoietic stem cell transplant (HSCT) or leukemia induction therapy, use HSV prophylaxis (eg, acyclovir, valacyclovir).

–Use *Pneumocystis jirovecii* prophylaxis (eg, TMP-SMX, dapsone, aerosolized pentamidine, atovaquone) for patients receiving chemotherapy regimens with >20 mg prednisone equivalents daily for >1 mo or purine analogue usage.

–If high risk of hepatitis B virus reactivation, treat with a nucleoside reverse transcription inhibitor (eg, entecavir or tenofovir).

–Offer yearly influenza vaccination with inactivated vaccine to all patients receiving chemotherapy and all family and household contacts and health care providers.

–Administer Covid-19 vaccination in three doses (not booster dose for 3rd vaccine) and continue precautions due to impaired immune response.

–Use standard precautions (hand hygiene and respiratory hygiene/cough etiquette) to avoid transmission to reduce transmission of pathogens in the health care setting.

–Avoid prolonged contact with environmental airborne fungal spores, ie demolition sites, prolonged gardening/digging, and home renovation.

Comments

1. Risk factors for neutropenia include older age, comorbidities, and a history of multiple cytotoxic chemotherapy regimens.

2. Bone marrow transplantation and chemotherapy for hematologic malignancies are associated with a higher incidence of neutropenia than chemotherapy for solid tumor malignancies.

Sources

–https://www.idsociety.org/covid-19-real-time-learning-network/vaccines/vaccines-information-faq/#

–*J Clin Oncol.* 2018.36:3043-3054.

–*J Clin Oncol.* 2018.36:1443-1453.

–*Clin Adv Hematol Oncol.* 2012;10(12):825-826.

–*Hematol Am Soc Hematol Educ Program.* 2012(1):174-182.

MULTIPLE MYELOMA/MONOCLONAL GAMMOPATHY OF UNDETERMINED SIGNIFICANCE

Population

–Adults.

Organizations

▶ NICE 2016, EMN 2014, EMN 2018, ASCO 2019

Recommendations

–Classic findings of multiple myeloma are CRAB: hyperCalcemia, Renal failure, Anemia, and Bony lesions/pain, in addition to clonal bone marrow plasma cells.

–Serum protein electrophoresis (SPEP) and serum-free light-chain assays confirm the presence of a paraprotein-indicating possible myeloma (MM) or monoclonal gammopathy of undetermined significance (MGUS).

–If SPEP is abnormal, order immunofixation to confirm the presence of a paraprotein-indicating possible myeloma or MGUS.

–Do not use SPEP, immunofixation, serum-free light-chain assay, or urine electrophoresis (UPEP) alone to exclude a diagnosis of myeloma.

–Order whole-body MRI as first-line imaging for all people with a plasma cell disorder suspected to be myeloma.

  • Consider whole-body low-dose CT if whole-body MRI is unsuitable or the patient declines.
  • Only consider skeletal survey if whole-body MRI and low-dose CT are unsuitable or the person declines them.
  • Do not use isotope bone scans to identify myeloma-related bone disease.

–Bone marrow aspirate and trephine biopsy confirm the diagnosis based on plasma cell percentage and flow cytometry morphology.

–New diagnostic criteria for MM are:

  • Involved/uninvolved serum-free light-chain ratio ≥100 and the involved serum-free light-chain level >100 mg/dL.
  • Clonal bone marrow plasma cells ≥60%.
  • Two or more focal lesions on MRI.

–MGUS is differentiated from MM by the absence of end organ damage (ie, hypercalcemia, renal insufficiency, anemia, and bone lesions), decreased amount of serum monoclonal protein (<30 g/L in MGUS), and decreased amount of bone marrow plasma cells (<10% in MGUS).

  • 1% annual risk of progression to other lymphoproliferative disorder.
  • Typically, IgG or IgA MGUS progresses to MM while IgG MGUS progresses to Waldenstrom macroglobulinemia (WM).
  • WM is defined by the presence of an IgM monoclonal gammopathy and ≥10% clonal plasma cells in the bone marrow, as opposed to <10% in IgM MGUS.

–Test for hepatitis B, hepatitis C, and HIV before starting myeloma treatment.

–Smoldering myeloma should be monitored every 3 mo for the first 5 y with CBC, CMP, bone profile, SPEP, serum-free light-chain assay.

  • Do not routinely offer skeletal surveys.

–Any new bone symptoms should receive symptom-directed imaging (MRI, CT FDG PET-CT).

Comments

1. Myeloma is still an incurable disease, although the spectrum of disease is highly variable.
2. MGUS is present in approximately 3.5% of the population over age 50 y.

Sources

–www.nice.org.uk/guidance/ng35

–*Leukemia.* 2018;32(8):1697-1712.
–*Haematologica.* 2015;100(10):1254-1266.
–https://www.asco.org/practice-patients/guidelines/hematologic-malignancies

SICKLE CELL DISEASE

Population
–Adults and children.

Organization
▶ NHLBI 2014

Recommendations

–Give oral penicillin prophylaxis to children <5-y-old and older children who have had splenectomy or invasive pneumococcal infection. Dose (125 mg for age <3 y and 250 mg for age >3 y) twice daily. Consider withholding from children with HbSC diseases and HbS-Beta thalassemia who have not had splenectomy.

–Assure that people of all ages with sickle cell disease (SCD) have been vaccinated against *Streptococcus pneumoniae*. All infants with SCD should receive the complete series of the 13-valent conjugate pneumococcal vaccine series beginning shortly after birth and the 23-valent pneumococcal polysaccharide vaccine at 2 y, with a second dose at age 5 y. Give all other vaccines according to ACIP harmonized vaccine schedule.

–Screen annually for proteinuria beginning at age 10. If positive, perform a first morning void urine albumin-creatinine ratio and if abnormal, consult a renal specialist.

–Evaluate patients with symptoms of dyspnea on exertion for possible pulmonary hypertension.

–Refer all patients to an ophthalmologist for annual dilated eye exam beginning at age 10.

–Screen children with SCD annually with transcranial Doppler beginning at age 2 and continuing until at least age 16. Refer children with conditional (170–199 cm/s) or elevated (>200 cm/s) transcranial Doppler results. Do not screen patients with genotypes other than SCD.

–Ensure every patient with SCD has a reproductive plan. Provide contraceptive counseling to prevent unintended pregnancy and preconception counseling if pregnancy is desired. Progestin-only contraceptives, levonorgestrel IUDs, and barrier methods have no restrictions for use in women with SCD. If the benefits are considered to outweigh the risk, combined hormonal contraceptives (pills, patches, rings) may be used in women with SCD.

–If a partner of a patient with SCA has unknown SCD or thalassemia status, refer the partner for hemoglobinopathy screening.

–Test women with SCD who have been transfused and are anticipating pregnancy for red cell alloantibodies. If she has red cell alloantibodies, test her partner for the corresponding red cell antigens.

–Use an individualized prescribing and monitoring protocol to promote rapid, effective, and safe analgesic management and resolution of vasoocclusive crises (VOC). Use NSAIDs as an adjuvant analgesic in the absence of contraindications as well as adjunctive nonpharmacologic approaches to treat pain such as local heat application and distraction.

- In adults and children with SCD and a VOC, do not administer a blood transfusion unless there are other indications for transfusion.
- In adults and children with SCD and a VOC and an oxygen saturation <95% on room air, administer oxygen.

- Advise that patients seek immediate medical attention for temperatures greater than 101.3°F (38.5°C) due to the risk of severe bacterial infections. Evaluate fevers immediately with a history and physical exam, CBCD, reticulocyte count, blood culture, and urine culture when UTI is suspected.
- In children with SCD and a temperature >101.3 (38.5°C), promptly administer ongoing empiric parenteral antibiotics that provide coverage against *S. pneumoniae* and gram-negative enteric organisms. Subsequent outpatient management using an oral antibiotic is feasible in people who do not appear ill.
- In adults with SCD who have pain that interferes with daily activities and quality of life, treat with hydroxyurea.
- In infants 9 mo of age and older, children, and adolescents with SCD, offer treatment with hydroxyurea regardless of clinical severity to reduce SCD-related complications.
- Discontinue hydroxyurea in females who are pregnant or breastfeeding.
- In people with HbS-Beta thalassemia or HbSC who have recurrent sickle cell–associated pain that interferes with daily activities, consult a sickle cell expert for consideration of hydroxyurea therapy.
- Transfuse RBCs to bring the Hb level to 1 g/dL prior to undergoing a surgical procedure involving general anesthesia.
- Blood transfusion is not indicated for uncomplicated painful crisis, priapism, asymptomatic anemia, recurrent splenic sequestration, and acute kidney injury unless there is multisystem organ failure.
- Chronic transfusion therapy is recommended for a child with TCD >200 cm/s and adults and children with previous clinically overt stroke.
- Monitor for iron overload in chronic transfusion therapy with liver function tests, serum ferritin levels, liver biopsies, and MRIs.
- Administer iron chelation therapy, in consultation with a hematologist, to patients with SCD with documented transfusion-acquired iron overload.

Comments

1. More than 2 million US residents are estimated to be either heterozygous or homozygous for the sickle cell mutation.
2. Those most affected are of African ancestry or self-identified as Black. A minority are Hispanic, southern European, Middle Eastern, or Asian Indian descent.
3. Clinical improvement with hydroxyurea may take 3–6 mo. Watch for thrombocytopenia and neutropenia with hydroxyurea treatment.
4. RBC units that are to be transfused to individuals with SCD should include matching for C, E, and K antigens.

Source

- NHLBI. *Evidence-Based Management of Sickle Cell Disease.* 2014. http://www.nih.gov/guidelines

THROMBOTIC THROMBOCYTOPENIA PURPURA (TTP)

Population
  –Acquired TTP in adults and children.

Organization
  –American Society of Hematology (ASH) 2017, *British Journal of Haematology* 2012

Recommendations
  –Classic pentad (present in only 10% of cases) is microangiopathic hemolytic anemia (MAHA) (jaundice, anemia, schistocytes, low haptoglobin, elevated LDH, increased reticulocyte count), thrombocytopenia (epistaxis, bruising, retinal hemorrhage, hemoptysis), renal impairment (proteinuria, microscopic hematuria), fever (>37.5°C), and neurologic signs (confusion, encephalopathy, coma, headache, paresis, aphasia, dysarthria, visual problems), often with insidious onset.
  - • Revised diagnostic criteria state that TTP must be suspected even with only thrombocytopenia and MAHA.
  - • Up to 35% of patients do not have neurologic symptoms. Renal failure requiring hemodialysis on presentation is more indicative of HUS than in TTP. Median platelet count is 10,000–30,000/mcL at presentation.
  –If TTP is suspected, order ADAMTS-13 activity prior to starting treatment.
  - • Treat empirically. Do not wait for confirmatory tests.
  –Mortality rate of 10%–20% even with appropriate management.
  –Lab tests: ADAMTS-13 assay (activity/antigen and inhibitor/antibody), CBCD, reticulocyte count, peripheral blood smear, haptoglobin, coagulation studies, CMP, cardiac troponins, LDH, urinalysis, Coombs, blood type and antibody screen, TSH, HIV, hepatitis A/B/C viruses, and autoantibodies (ANA/RF/LA/ACLA), stool culture (for pathogenic *E. coli*).
  –Consider CT chest/abdomen pelvis (to look for possible underlying malignancy).
  –Check a pregnancy test in women of childbearing age.
  –Consider EKG or echocardiogram and brain imaging (CT or MRI).
  –TTP is a medical emergency requiring transfer to hospital: 3 units of fresh-frozen plasma should be given while a large-bore catheter is placed for plasma exchange, which should begin within 4–8 h of presentation.
  –Plasma exchange (TPE) should be started with 40 mL/kg body weight plasma volume (PV) exchanges. The volume of exchange can be reduced to 30 mL/kg body weight as clinical conditions and lab studies improve.
  –Continue daily TPE for a minimum of 2 d after platelet count >150,000 and then stopped.
  –Steroids (eg, IV methylprednisolone 10 mg/kg/d × 3 d, then 2.5 mg/kg/d) are often administered, although benefits are uncertain.
  –In patients with neurologic and/or cardiac pathology (associated with increased mortality), rituximab should be used at a dose of 375 mg/m^2 weekly for 4 doses.

Comments

1. TTP results from congenital or autoimmune loss of ADAMTS-13 activity. Loss of ADAMTS-13 prevents cleavage of large high-molecular-weight vWF. vWF binds to platelet receptor GPIB and the resulting complex obstructs the microvasculature leading to red cell fragmentation, thrombocytopenia, and organ ischemia.

2. Differential diagnosis primarily of thrombocytopenia and MAHA includes autoimmune hemolysis/Evans syndrome, disseminated intravascular coagulation (DIC), pregnancy-associated conditions (eg, HELLP, eclampsia, hemolytic uremic syndrome [HUS]), drugs (quinine, simvastatin, interferon, calcineurin inhibitors), malignant hypertension, infections (cytomegalovirus, adenovirus, herpes simplex virus, meningococcus, pneumococcus, fungal), autoimmune diseases (lupus nephritis, acute scleroderma), vasculitis, HUS, malignancy, catastrophic antiphospholipid syndrome.

3. Plasma exchange is not a curative therapy but does protect the patient until antibody levels decline either spontaneously or with use of corticosteroids and rituximab.

4. Precipitating factors: drugs (quinine, ticlopidine, clopidogrel, simvastatin, trimethoprim, interferon, and combined oral contraceptive pills), HIV infection, and pregnancy (usually in the second trimester).

5. HUS clinically resembles TTP, but has a different pathophysiology, and total plasma exchange is of minimal benefit. This illness is commonly caused by bacterial toxins (*Shiga*-like toxin from *E. coli*) or drugs (quinine, gemcitabine, mitomycin C). It is also associated with malignancy and autoimmune disease. In HUS, there is disruption of the endothelium and release of high-molecular-weight vWF that overwhelms the cleaving capacity of ADAMTS-13. An antibody to ADAMTS-13 is not involved. Renal failure dominates the clinical picture and 15%–20% succumb to the disease. (*Br J Haematol.* 2010;148:37) (*N Engl J Med.* 2014;371:654)

Sources
–*Blood* (2017) 129 (21): 2836-2846.
–*Br J Haematol.* 2012;158(3):323-335.

THROMBOPHILIAS

Population
–Adults.

Organizations
▶ NICE 2016, ACOG 2018, Anticoagulation Forum 2016, BSH 2012

Recommendations
–The most common thrombophilias include factor V Leiden (FVL), protein C deficiency (PC), protein S deficiency (PS), antithrombin deficiency (AT), prothrombin gene 20210 A/G mutation (PGM), and antiphospholipid syndrome (APS).
–Do not perform thrombophilia testing at the time of VTE diagnosis or during the first 3 mo of anticoagulation.

- Genotype-based tests (FVL, PGM) and antibody titers (cardiolipin and beta-2 glycoprotein I) can be performed at any point.
- The remaining thrombophilia tests need to be performed 2–4 wk after discontinuation of anticoagulants.

–Only test for thrombophilias when the results will be used to improve or modify management.

- Do not offer thrombophilia testing to patients who are continuing anticoagulation treatment.
- Do not offer thrombophilia testing to patients who have had provoked VTE.
- Consider testing for hereditary thrombophilias or antiphospholipid antibodies in patients who have had unprovoked DVT or PE if it is planned to stop anticoagulation.

–Do not routinely offer thrombophilia testing to first-degree relatives of people with a history of DVT or PE and thrombophilia.

- This includes patients contemplating estrogen use. Even with a negative thrombophilia screen they still have an elevated risk of VTE. Only do so if the test will change your management.
- An exception would be patients who are pregnant or planning to become pregnant as it could change treatment plans.

–A positive thrombophilia evaluation is not a sufficient basis to offer extended anticoagulation following an episode of provoked VTE where the other provoking factor has resolved.

–Testing for APS requires a dual screening testing (eg, DRVVT and aPTT). If either of these is positive, a confirmatory test is performed (eg, high phospholipid concentration, platelet-neutralizing reagent, or LA-insensitive reagent).

- Diagnosis is based on the presence of either vascular thrombosis or pregnancy morbidity plus the presence of lupus anticoagulant, anti-cardiolipin IgG and/or IgM, or anti-beta-2 glycoprotein-I.

–Primary thromboprophylaxis is not recommended for incidentally discovered APS.

–Patients <50-y-old with ischemic stroke should be screened for APS.

- Do not routinely offer APS screening in patients >age 50.
- Antiplatelet therapy is as effective as warfarin for ischemic stroke associated with a single positive APS test result.

–A baseline PT should be ordered when starting warfarin therapy for APS with thrombosis. If this is prolonged, an alternative PT reagent for which the baseline is normal (ie, not affected by lupus anticoagulant) should be used.

–Women with recurrent pregnancy loss (≥3 losses) before 10 wk gestation with normal fetal anatomy/genomics should be screened for APS.

–Always emphasize improvement in modifiable VTE risk factors: obesity, tobacco use, exogenous estrogen use.

Comments

1. Testing for thrombophilias in a patient with unprovoked VTE: the two-step method.
   After 3 mo of anticoagulation, FVL, PGM, cardiolipin, and beta-2 glycoprotein-I antibodies are ordered. If negative, anticoagulation is stopped and 2–4 wk later a D-dimer, lupus

anticoagulant, PC, PS, and AT are ordered. A final decision on anticoagulation can then be made on the basis of results.

2. FVL is the most common inherited thrombophilia, with estimated carrier frequency in the United States in Caucasians 5%, Hispanics 2%, Blacks 1%, Asians 0.5%, and Native Americans 1%.

3. PGM in the United States is present in approximately 4% of Caucasians, 4% in Hispanics, 1% of Blacks, and 0.3% in Native Americans.

4. The prevalence of Protein C (PC) deficiency heterozygosity depends on the cutoff used, but may be as high as 1.5%.

VON WILLEBRAND DISEASE

Population
–Adults and children.

Organizations
▶ ASH 2021, NHF 2018, NHLBI 2007

Recommendations
–Von Willebrand disease is an inherited bleeding disorder due to dysfunctional von Willebrand Factor (VWF).

–Suspect in patients with mucous membrane bleeding, excessive bruising, or bleeding (eg, excessive menstrual bleeding, history of postpartum hemorrhage, excessive bleeding after dental work or a surgical procedure).

–Diagnose based on history and physical examination, CBC, PTT, PT/INR, fibrinogen, PFA-100 (if available), and VWD assays (VWF:Ag, VWF:RCo, and FVIII).

–Treat type 1, 2A, 2M, 2N VWD with DDAVP.[1] If hemostasis is not achieved with DDAVP, use FVIII or recombinant VWF concentrate.

–Treat type 2B and 3 VWD with FVIII concentrate or recombinant VFW concentrate.

–Manage minor bleeding (eg, epistaxis, simple dental extraction, menorrhagia) with DDAVP without laboratory monitoring.

–For patients with cardiovascular disease, give necessary antiplatelet agents or anticoagulation. Desmopressin is generally contraindicated.

–For patients having mucosal procedures, give tranexamic acid alone in patients with mild-to-moderate VWD (VWF activity level $\geq$0.50 IU/mL).

–For patients having minor surgery with mild-to-moderate VWD, antifibrinolytics combined with DDAVP and tranexamic acid are generally effective.

–Refer all major surgeries and bleeding events to hospitals with 24-h laboratory capability, a hematologist, and a surgeon skilled in the management of bleeding disorders. Target FVIII and VWF activity levels $\geq$0.50 IU/mL for >3 d after surgery.

[1]IV DDAVP dosing is 0.3 mcg/kg IV over 30 min. Intranasal dosing of Stimate (1.5 mg/mL DDAVP solution, 0.1-mL puff) is 150 mcg (1 puff) for persons who weigh <50 kg and 300 mcg (2 puffs) for persons weighing 50 kg or more.

–In women who do not desire pregnancy, offer combined oral contraceptives (COC) or the levonorgestrel intrauterine device for menorrhagia in VWD.

–Women with VWD who desire pregnancy should speak with a genetic counselor and a pediatric hematologist.

–Women who desire pregnancy can be treated preferentially with tranexamic acid over DDAVP, antifibrinolytics, or VWF concentrate.

–Women with VWD who are pregnant should achieve VWF/RCo and FVIII levels of at least 50 IU/dL before delivery and maintain that level for at least 3–5 d afterward.

–Women who desire neuraxial anesthesia during labor, target VWF activity level to 0.50–1.5 IU/mL.

–Use tranexamic acid (IV or Oral 25 mg/kg TID for 10–14 d, or longer if blood loss remains heavy) in the postpartum period.

–Do not use cryoprecipitate except in an emergency situation when none of the above-mentioned products are available.

Sources
–*Blood Adv.* 2021;5(1):280-300.
–*Blood Adv.* 2021;5(1):301-325.

Comments

1. The prevalence of protein S deficiency is unknown, but in one case-control study it accounted for 1% of VTEs. Pregnancy, female sex, and estrogen use reduce the levels of protein S. Use of sex-specific reference intervals and testing prior to pregnancy or while not receiving estrogen preparations is preferred.
2. Antithrombin deficiency heterozygosity prevalence is approximately 1 per 2500 people or 0.04%.
3. The presence of hereditary thrombophilia does not affect survival in patients with a history of VTE or the risk of postthrombotic syndrome.
4. Patients with an unprovoked DVT and negative thrombophilia evaluation have the same recurrence rate for VTE as patients with an unprovoked DVT and positive thrombophilia evaluation.
5. Heterozygosity for FVL or PGM does not increase the predicted risk of recurrence to a clinically significant degree after an unprovoked VTE.
6. Family history of thrombosis alone carries an increased risk of thrombosis, even with a negative thrombophilia evaluation.
7. Degree of postthrombotic symptoms, D-dimer levels after a minimum of 3 mo of anticoagulation, and residual vein thrombosis do modify the risk of recurrence in unprovoked VTE.

Sources
–https://www.acog.org/clinical/clinical-guidance/practice-bulletin/articles/2018/07/inherited-thrombophilias-in-pregnancy
–*J Thromb Thrombol.* 2016;41(1):154-164.
–*Br J Hematol.* 2012;159(10):28-38.

Infectious Diseases

26

ASYMPTOMATIC BACTERIURIA (ASB)

Population
–Nonpregnant women.

Organization
▶ IDSA 2019

Recommendations
–Do not treat asymptomatic bacteriuria with antibiotics.
–Do not screen pediatric patients for asymptomatic bacteriuria.
–Only screen pregnant women and patients undergoing urologic procedures.
–Treat ASB in pregnant patients for 4–7 d.

Comments
1. Delirium in older patients is often caused by urinary tract infections. However, in the absence of overt urinary symptoms or signs of systemic infection, empiric treatment of bacteriuria doesn't improve patient-oriented outcomes. (*JAMA Intern Med.* 2019;179(11):1519-1527)

Source
–https://doi.org/10.1093/cid/ciy1121

COMMON COLD

Population
–Healthy adults (those without chronic lung disease or immunocompromising conditions).

Organization
▶ Annals of Internal Medicine 2016

Recommendation
–Do not prescribe antibiotics for the common cold.

Comment
1. Harm from antibiotics outweighs benefits, as all causes of common cold are viral.
2. Evidence-based therapies for cold symptoms include the following:
   a. Ipratropium (4 puffs QID) for cough.

b. NSAIDs for headache, earache, muscle, and joint pains.

c. Acetaminophen for rhinorrhea.

d. Decongestants, with or without antihistamines, for congestion.

e. Zinc (80–92 mg/d within 3 d of symptom onset) to reduce duration.

f. Honey, in children.

3. Nasal saline, oral fluid intake, nasal oxymetazoline, and many herbal therapies lack quality evidence of efficacy.

4. Therapies proven to be no more effective than placebo include antibiotics, antivirals, antihistamines, cough suppressants and expectorants, nasal steroids, steam, Vitamins D and E, and echinacea.

Sources
–http://annals.org/aim/fullarticle/2481815/appropriate-antibiotic-use-acute-respiratory-tract-infection-adults-advice-high

–*Am Fam Physician.* 2019 Sep 1;100(5):281-289.

CORONAVIRUS DISEASE 2019 (COVID-19)

The CDC maintains updated guidelines at https://www.covid19treatmentguidelines.nih.gov/

Organizations
▶ CDC 2022, WHO 2021

Recommendations
–Offer symptomatic management including antipyretics, analgesics, and antitussives.

–Consider educating about breathing exercises.

–Monoclonal antibody therapy: If at risk for progression to severe disease, offer monoclonal antibody therapy. See Tables 26-1 and 26-2 for risk tiers and comorbid conditions that elevate risk.

- CDC: use one of the following, listed in order of preference: ritonavir-boosted nirmatrelvir, sotrovimab, remdesivir, molnupiravir.
- WHO: use casiriimab, imdevimab, or sotrovimab.

–Corticosteroids:

- Do not use for patients not requiring hospitalization or supplemental oxygen.
- If discharged from hospital without supplemental oxygen, stop steroids.
- If discharged from hospital with supplemental oxygen, insufficient evidence exists to guide decision.

–If discharged from ED on oxygen because hospital capacity is limited, give dexamethasone 6 mg PO daily for duration of oxygen use, up to maximum of 10 d.

–Do not use chloroquine, hydroxychloroquine, HIV protease inhibitors, or antibiotic therapy in the absence of other indications.

–Do not use anticoagulants or antiplatelet therapy in outpatients in the absence of other indications.

–Do not stop ACE inhibitors, statin therapy, NSAIDs, or corticosteroids being used for comorbid conditions.

TABLE 26-1 CDC PATIENT RISK GROUPS FOR PRIORITIZING COVID THERAPY

Tier	Risk Groups
1	• Immunocompromised individuals who are not expected to mount an adequate immune response to COVID-19 vaccination or SARS-CoV-2 infection due to their underlying conditions, regardless of their vaccine status • Unvaccinated individuals who are at the highest risk of severe disease (anyone aged ≥75 y or anyone aged ≥65 y with additional risk factors)
2	• Unvaccinated individuals who are at risk of severe disease and who are not included in Tier 1 (anyone aged ≥65 y or anyone aged <65 y with clinical risk factors)
3	• Vaccinated individuals who are at high risk of severe disease (anyone aged ≥75 y or anyone aged ≥65 y with clinical risk factors) • Vaccinated individuals who have not received a COVID-19 vaccine booster dose are likely to be at higher risk for severe disease; patients who have not received a booster dose and who are within this tier should be prioritized for treatment
4	• Vaccinated individuals who are at risk of severe disease (anyone aged ≥65 y or anyone aged <65 with clinical risk factors) • Vaccinated individuals who have not received a COVID-19 vaccine booster dose are likely to be at higher risk for severe disease; patients who have not received a booster dose and who are within this tier should be prioritized for treatment.

Source: https://www.covid19treatmentguidelines.nih.gov/. Accessed 26 February, 2022.

COMPARISON OF RECOMMENDATIONS FOR VARIOUS THERAPIES IN NONSEVERE DISEASE, IN THE NON-HOSPITAL SETTING

	CDC	WHO
Ivermectin	Insufficient evidence to recommend for or against	Do not use except in clinical trials
Convalescent plasma	Insufficient evidence in non-hospitalized patients or in patients with impaired immunity. Do not use in hospitalized patients	Do not use
Supplements (vitamin C, vitamin D, zinc)	Insufficient evidence	Not assessed in guideline
JAK inhibitors (baricitinib, ruxolitinib, tofacitinib)	Do not use	Do not use

Sources
  –https://www.covid19treatmentguidelines.nih.gov/. Accessed 26 February, 2022.
  –*BMJ* 2020;370:m3379.

TABLE 26-2 MEDICAL CONDITIONS THAT INCREASE RISK OF PROGRESSION TO SEVERE COVID

Higher Risk	Suggestion of Higher Risk or Mixed Evidence

– Cancer
– Cerebrovascular disease
– Chronic kidney disease
– Chronic lung diseases limited to:
  • Interstitial lung disease
  • Pulmonary embolism
  • Pulmonary hypertension
  • Bronchiectasis
  • COPD
– Chronic liver diseases limited to:
  • Cirrhosis
  • Nonalcoholic fatty liver disease
  • Alcoholic liver disease
  • Autoimmune hepatitis
– Cystic fibrosis
– Diabetes mellitus, type 1 and type 2
– Disabilities:
  • ADHD
  • Cerebral palsy
  • Congenital malformations
  • Limitations with self-care or activities of daily living
  • Intellectual and developmental disabilities
  • Learning disabilities
  • Spinal cord injuries
– Heart conditions (heart failure, coronary artery disease, or cardiomyopathies)
– HIV
– Mental health disorders limited to:
  • Mood disorders, including depression
  • Schizophrenia spectrum disorders
– Neurologic conditions limited to dementia
– Obesity (BMI ≥ 30 kg/m^2)
– Primary immunodeficiencies
– Pregnancy and recent pregnancy
– Physical inactivity
– Smoking, current and former
– Solid organ or hematopoietic cell transplantation
– Tuberculosis
– Use of corticosteroids or other immunosuppressive medications
	– Children with certain underlying conditions
	– Overweight (BMI ≥ 25 kg/m^2, but < 30 kg/m^2)
	– Sickle cell disease
	– Substance use disorders
	– Thalassemia
	– Alpha 1 antitrypsin deficiency
	– Asthma
	– Bronchopulmonary dysplasia
	– Hepatitis B
	– Hepatitis C
	– Hypertension

Source: https://www.cdc.gov/coronavirus/2019-ncov/hcp/clinical-care/underlyingconditions.html. Accessed 26 February, 2022.

CORONAVIRUS DISEASE 2019 (COVID-19), LONG

Population
–Adults with persistent symptoms 4–12 wk after COVID-19 infection.

Organization
▶ NICE 20221

Recommendations
–Aggressively evaluate for life-threatening causes of concerning symptoms including hypoxia, exertional hypoxia, signs of severe lung disease, or cardiac chest pain.
–Consider labs including CBC, CMP, CRP, ferritin, BNP, A1c, and TSH as directed by symptoms.
–Consider an exercise tolerance test such as the 1-min sit to stand test. If postural symptoms, assess with a 3-min or 10-min active stand test.
–Consider a chest X-ray 12 wk after COVID diagnosis if there are ongoing respiratory symptoms.
–Provide sources of advice and support, including information about common symptoms.
–Insufficient evidence to recommend vitamins and supplements.
–Advise a gradual, phased return to work or school.
–Develop a personalized rehabilitation plan attending to physical, psychological, and psychiatric symptoms.

Source
–https://www.nice.org.uk/guidance/ng188/

COCCIDIOIDOMYCOSIS (VALLEY FEVER)

Population
–Adults.

Organization
▶ IDSA 2016

Recommendations
–Test for coccidioidomycosis in patients presenting with pneumonia in endemic regions (southwest United States).
–Do not start treatment for mild infection.
–Do not treat asymptomatic chronic cavitary coccidioidal pneumonia.
–Use fluconazole as first-line therapy, 400–1200 mg PO daily, including during pregnancy. Check renal function prior to initiating therapy.
–Refer to infection disease specialist for extrapulmonary, disseminated coccidioidomycosis.

Source
–https://academic.oup.com/cid/article/63/6/e112/2389093

DIABETIC FOOT INFECTIONS, OUTPATIENT MANAGEMENT

Population
–Adults older than 18 y with diabetic foot problems.

Organizations
▶ IDF 2017, IWGDF 2019, NICE 2019

Recommendations
–Assess arterial perfusion and need for revascularization.
–Debride callus if necrotic tissue to fully visualize wound, measure depth and extent.
–Check C-reactive protein, erythrocyte sedimentation rate.
–Assess glycemic control.
–Obtain cultures: tissue or bone specimen preferred; deep swab only after debriding wound.
–Obtain X-ray of all new diabetic foot infections. Obtain MRI if osteomyelitis suspected and plain film is not diagnostic.
–Offload diabetic foot ulcers.
–Request surgical consult for deep abscesses, compartment syndrome, and necrotizing soft tissue infection.
–Choose antibiotic based on suspected pathogen and severity.
–Treat clinically infected wounds with antibiotics:
  • 1–2 wk for mild-to-moderate infections, with empiric antibiotics that cover gram-positive organisms.
  • 3 wk for more serious skin and soft tissue infections, with empiric antibiotics that cover gram-positive, gram-negative, and anaerobic bacteria.
  • 6 wk for osteomyelitis.
  • Severe infection: hospital evaluation for parenteral antibiotics and surgical debridement.

Comments
1. A deep space infection may have deceptively few superficial signs.
2. The diabetic foot care team should include:
   a. Diabetologist.
   b. Surgeon with expertise managing DM foot problems.
   c. DM nurse specialist.
   d. Podiatrist.
   e. Tissue viability nurse.
   f. Biomechanic and orthotic specialist.
3. Do not treat diabetic foot ulcers with:
   a. Electrical stimulation therapy, autologous platelet-rich plasma gel, regenerative wound matrices, and dalteparin.
   b. Growth factors.
   c. Hyperbaric oxygen therapy.

Sources

–https://www.idf.org/e-library/guidelines/119-idf-clinical-practice-recommendations-on-diabetic-foot-2017.html
–https://onlinelibrary.wiley.com/doi/full/10.1002/dmrr.3280
–https://www.nice.org.uk/guidance/ng19

HUMAN IMMUNODEFICIENCY VIRUS (HIV)

Population

–HIV-infected adults and children.

Organizations

▶ IDSA 2018, USPSTF 2019

Recommendations

–Obtain a comprehensive present and past medical history, physical examination, medication/social/family history, and review of systems, including HIV-related information upon initiation of care.
–Educate patient on high-risk behaviors to minimize risk of HIV transmission.
–Assess for the presence of depression, substance abuse, or domestic violence.
–Baseline labs upon initiation of care: HIV serostatus; CD4 count; quantitative HIV RNA by PCR (viral load); HIV genotyping; CBCD, chemistry panel, G6PD testing; fasting lipid profile; HLA B5701 test (if abacavir will be used); tropism testing (if the use of a CCR5 antagonist is being considered); urinalysis; Pap smear in women.[1]
–Screening labs: *M. tuberculosis* testing (PPD or interferon-γ release assay); toxoplasma antibodies; Hepatitis B panel, HCV antibodies; VDRL; urine NAAT for gonorrhea; and urine NAAT for chlamydia (except in men age <25 y); anti-CMV IgG in lower risk groups (populations other than men who have sex with men or IV drug users), trichomoniasis in all women, *Chlamydia trachomatis* in all women ≤25 y of age.
–Monitoring labs:
  • CD4 counts and HIV viral load every 3–4 mo.
  • STD screening and TB screening tests should be repeated periodically depending on symptoms and signs, behavioral risk, and possible exposures.
  • Fasting glucose and lipid panel 4–6 wk after initiation of therapy.
–Vaccination for pneumococcal infection, influenza, varicella, hepatitis A, HPV, and HBV according to standard immunization charts.
–All HIV-infected women of childbearing age should be asked about their plans and desires regarding pregnancy upon initiation of care and routinely thereafter.

---

[1]CBCD, complete blood count with differential; G6PD, glucose-6-phosphate dehydrogenase; HLA, human leukocyte antigen; NAAT, nucleic acid amplification test; PCR, polymerase chain reaction; PPD, purified protein derivative; VDRL, Venereal Disease Research Laboratory.

–Pap smear with HPV or reflex to HPV based on age in women every 6 mo and annually thereafter if results are normal. For ASC-US Pap result, if reflex HPV testing is negative, a repeat Pap test in 6–12 mo or repeat co-testing in 12 mo is recommended. For any result ≥ASC-US on repeat cytology, referral to colposcopy is recommended.

–Perform individualized assessment of risk for breast cancer and inform them of the potential benefits and risks of screening mammography for women ages 40–49 y. Perform mammogram annually for age >50 y.

–Hormone replacement therapy is not recommended.

Comments

1. Screen for anogenital human papilloma virus (HPV) with anal Pap testing for men who have sex with men, women with abnormal cervical Pap smear results, and persons with a history of genital warts.
2. Test for serum testosterone level in men complaining of fatigue, ED, or decreased libido.
3. Chest X-ray should be obtained in persons with pulmonary symptoms or who have a positive PPD test result.
4. Screen for STI via mode of intercourse, ie, anal, vaginal, or oral swab for gonorrhea and chlamydia.

Sources

–Aberg JA, Gallant JE, Ghanem KG, Emmanuel P, Zingman BS, Horberg MA. Primary care guidelines for the management of persons infected with HIV: 2013 update by the HIV Medicine Association of the Infectious Diseases Society of America. *Clin Infect Dis*. 2014;58(1):e1-e34, http://academic.oup.com/cid/article/58/1/e1/374007#74163693

–https://www.idsociety.org/globalassets/idsa/practice-guidelines/guidelines-for-prevention-and-treatment-of-opportunistic-infections-in-hiv-infected-adults-and-adolescents.pdf

–https://www.cdc.gov/std/gonorrhea/stdfact-gonorrhea.htm

HUMAN IMMUNODEFICIENCY VIRUS (HIV), ANTIRETROVIRAL THERAPY (ART) IN PEDIATRICS

Population

–HIV-infected children.

Organizations

▶ HHS 2018, IDSA 2019

Recommendations

–Test for maternal HIV in the third trimester, in addition to upon diagnosis of pregnancy.

–ART is recommended for all children, regardless of symptoms or CD4 count.

–HIV genotypic resistance testing is recommended:
- At the time of diagnosis.
- Prior to initiation of therapy.
- For all treatment-naïve children.

–Evaluate for possible side effects and evaluate response to therapy in all children 1–2 wk after initiation of ART or changing ART regimen.

–Recommend laboratory testing for toxicity and viral load response at 2–4 wk after treatment initiation.

–Check absolute CD4 T lymphocyte (CD4) cell count and plasma HIV RNA (viral load) and evaluate therapy adherence, effectiveness, and toxicities every 3–4 mo. CD4 count can be monitored every 6–12 mo in children who are adherent to therapy and have had CD4 counts well above threshold for opportunistic infections, sustained viral suppression, and stable clinical status for 2–3 y.

Comment

1. Specific ART recommendations are beyond the scope of this book.

Sources

–Panel on Antiretroviral Therapy and Medical Management of Children Living with HIV. *Guidelines for the Use of Antiretroviral Agents in Pediatric HIV Infection.*

–http://aidsinfo.nih.gov/contentfiles/lvguidelines/pediatricguidelines.pdf

HUMAN IMMUNODEFICIENCY VIRUS, ANTIRETROVIRAL USE IN ADULTS

Population

–Adults and adolescents.

Organization

▶ HHS 2019

Recommendations

–Start antiretroviral therapy (ART) as soon as feasibly possible.

–Start ART within first 2 wk after initiation of treatment for most opportunistic infections:

- Within 4–6 wk after starting antifungals for cryptococcal meningitis.
- Within 2–8 wk after starting TB treatment in pts with CD4 >50.
- Start immediately in pts with HIV and cancer with special attention to drug interactions

–Use one of these antiretroviral regimens for most patients with HIV:

- Bictegravir/tenofovir alafenamide/emtricitabine.
- Dolutegravir + emtricitabine or lamivudine + tenofovir alafenamide or tenofovir disoproxil fumarate.
- Dolutegravir/Lamivudine (except if HIV RNA >500,000 copies/mL, CD4 <200, on active treatment for opportunistic infection, HBV coinfection and not without HIV genotyping so not to be started on the day of diagnosis).
- Raltegravir + emtricitabine or lamivudine + tenofovir alafenamide (TAF) or tenofovir disoproxil fumarate (TDF).
- For pregnant women/women of childbearing age recommend: dolutegravir, raltegravir, atazanavir/ritonavir, darunavir/ ritonavir (dosed twice daily), or efavirenz, PLUS either tenofovir disoproxil fumarate/emtricitabine or tenofovir disoproxil fumarate/lamivudine.

- Pregnant women on ART not recommended during pregnancy should switch to a recommended regimen after review of genotype testing and ART therapy. Selection of a regimen should be individualized.
- Efavirenz is teratogenic.
- Tenofovir should be used cautiously with renal insufficiency.
- Ritonavir-boosted atazanavir and rilpivirine should not be used with high-dose proton pump inhibitors.
- Regimens that include InSTIs have higher rates of weight gain, greater in dolutegravir, bictegravir.
- Patients on rifamycin-based TB treatment should be on ART with 2 nRTIs plus efavirenz (600 mg/d), raltegravir (800 mg BID), or dolutegravir (50 mg BID).

–How and when to switch between ART therapies:

- To simplify regimen in patients with viral suppression, switch from 3-drug to 2-drug regimens to reduce AEs and adherence. Recommended regimens include dolutegravir/rilpivirine, booted PPT/lamivudine, dolutegravir/lamivudine, and long-acting injectable cabotegravir/rilpivirine q4wk.
- Virologic failure (HIV RNA >200 copies/mL on 2 consecutive measurements): NNRTI failure → dolutegravir + 2 nRTIs, InSTI failure → boosted PI + 2 nRTIs, raltegravir or elvitegravir failure → dolutegravir BID + 1 fully active other agent, multiclass (>3) resistance → construct new regimen from new classes of drugs.
- Development of concomitant disease including kidney, liver, cardiovascular, or bone disease, weight gain, cancer, autoimmune disease, or solid organ transplant may require switching regimens.

–Laboratory testing:

- Screen non-HIV-infected high-risk patients every 3 mo as long as risk persists and offer PrEP (tenofovir disoproxil fumarate/emtricitabine daily, double dose on first day for MSM).
- While on PrEP, screen quarterly with combined HIV Ab/Ag, genital and nongenital GC/Ch, syphilis, pregnancy, and screen annually for estimated CrCl and Hep C Ab.
- If high-risk exposure within 72 h screen with rapid HIV antibody test, if negative offer PEP (3-drug ART regimen within first 24–72 h and continued × 28 d) and obtain testing for Cr, hep B sAg, STIs, and HIV Ab/Ag or HIV RNA.
- If positive for HIV, obtain HIV RNA, CD4, reverse transcriptase-prodrug resistance genotype testing, kidney and liver function, lipid levels, CBC, glucose, pregnancy, viral hep A/B/C, TB and STI testing, but do not delay initiation of ART while awaiting results (add serum cryptococcal Ag if CD4 < 100).
- Within 6 wk of starting ART, repeat HIV RNA; if levels have not declined considerably in adherent patient, then perform genotypic resistance testing.
- If viral suppression is considered stable, monitor HIV RNA levels every 3 mo until 1 y of suppression, then monitor every 6 mo.

- If previously achieved suppression and HIV RNA >50, quickly repeat HIV RNA and assess adherence and tolerability.
- Measure CD4 counts every 6 mo until >250 × 1 y then only repeat if ART failure or immunosuppressive condition.

–Recommend coreceptor tropism assay whenever a CCR5 coreceptor antagonist is considered.

–Screen for HLA-B*5701 before starting abacavir.

–Interruption of HAART is recommended for drug toxicity, intercurrent illness, or operations that precludes oral intake.

–Management of a patient with prior antiretroviral exposure is complex and should be managed by an HIV specialist if changing regimens.

Comments

1. This guideline focuses on antiretroviral management in HIV-1-infected individuals.
2. Alternative regimens for specific clinical scenarios or patient characteristics are beyond the scope of this book.
3. Baseline evaluation should include:
   a. Patient's readiness for ART.
   b. Psychosocial assessment.
   c. Substance abuse screening.
   d. Mental illness screening.
   e. HIV risk behavior screening.
   f. Health insurance and coverage status.
   g. Discussion of risk reduction and disclosure to sexual and/or needle-sharing partners.
   h. Initial labs:
      i. CD4 T-cell count.
      ii. HIV-1 antibody testing.
      iii. HIV RNA viral load.
      iv. Genotypic drug-resistance testing.
      v. CBCD, chemistry panel, LFTs, urinalysis.
      vi. Serologies for hepatitis B & C.
      vii. Fasting glucose or A1c and lipid panel.
      viii. Pregnancy test.
      ix. STD screening.

Sources

–http://aidsinfo.nih.gov/guidelines/html/1/adult-and-adolescent-arv-guidelines/0

–Saag MS, Gandhi RT, Hoy JF, et al. Antiretroviral Drugs for Treatment and Prevention of HIV Infection in Adults: 2020 Recommendations of the International Antiviral Society–USA Panel. *JAMA.* 2020;324(16):1651–1669. doi:10.1001/jama.2020.17025

IDENTIFYING RISK OF SERIOUS ILLNESS IN CHILDREN UNDER 5 Y

TRAFFIC LIGHT SYSTEM FOR IDENTIFYING RISK OF SERIOUS ILLNESS IN CHILDREN UNDER 5 Y

Category	Green—Low Risk	Yellow—Intermediate Risk	Red—High Risk
Color of skin, lips, or tongue	Normal color	Pallor	Mottled, ashen, or blue
Activity	• Responds normally to social cues • Smiles • Awakens easily • Strong cry	• Abnormal response to social cues • No smile • Wakes only with prolonged stimulation • Decreased activity	• No response to social cues • Appears toxic • Stuporous • Weak, high-pitched cry

Respiratory	• Normal breathing	• Nasal flaring
		• Tachypnea
		  ○ >50 breaths/min (6–12 mo)
		  ○ >40 breaths/min (>1 y)
		• SpO_2 ≤95%
		• Pulmonary rales
			• Grunting
			• Marked tachypnea
			  ○ >60 breaths/min
			• Moderate-to-severe chest retractions

Circulation	• Normal skin and eyes
	• Moist mucous membranes
		• Tachycardia
		  ○ >160 beats/min (<12 mo)
		  ○ >150 beats/min (12–24 mo)
		  ○ >140 beats/min (2–5 y)
		• Capillary refill ≥3 s
		• Dry mucous membranes
		• Poor feeding
		• Decreased urine output
			• Findings in yellow zone PLUS
			• Reduced skin turgor

Other	• Nontoxic appearance	• Temperature ≥39°C (age 3–6 mo) • Fever ≥5 d • Rigors • Swelling of a limb or joint • Non-weight bearing on one extremity	• Temperature ≥38°C (<3 mo) • Non-blanching rash • Bulging fontanelle • Neck stiffness • Status epilepticus • Focal neurological signs • Focal seizures

Source: Adapted from National Institute for Health and Care Excellence (NICE). *Guideline on Feverish Illness in Children: Assessment and Initial Management in Children Younger than 5 y.* 2013 May (Clinical Guideline no. 160).

INFLUENZA

Population
 –Adults.

Organization
 ▶ CDC 2020

Recommendations
 –Test for concomitant SARS-CoV-2 (COVID-19).
 –Prioritize treatment: start antiviral treatment as soon as possible for any patient with suspected or confirmed influenza if hospitalized; severe, complicated, or progressive illness; or higher risk for influenza complications, while awaiting lab confirmation.
- Lab-confirmed cases of influenza within 48 h of symptom onset.
- Strongly suspected influenza within 48 h of symptom onset.
- Hospitalized patients with severe, complicated, or progressive lab-confirmed influenza or influenza-like illness with high likelihood of complications even if >48 h from symptom onset.
  ◦ Children aged younger than 2 y or adults aged 65 y and older.
  ◦ Persons with chronic pulmonary (including asthma), cardiovascular (except hypertension alone), renal, hepatic, hematological (including sickle cell disease), metabolic (including diabetes mellitus), or neurologic disorders (including disorders of the brain, spinal cord, peripheral nerve, and muscle, such as cerebral palsy, epilepsy [seizure disorders], stroke, intellectual disability, moderate-to-severe developmental delay, muscular dystrophy, or spinal cord injury).
  ◦ Persons with immunosuppression, including that caused by medications or by HIV infection.
  ◦ Women who are pregnant or postpartum (within 2 wk after delivery).
  ◦ Persons aged younger than 19 y who are receiving long-term aspirin therapy.
  ◦ American Indians/Alaska Natives.
  ◦ Persons who are extremely obese (ie, body mass index is equal to or greater than 40).
  ◦ Residents of nursing homes and other chronic care facilities.
 –Antiviral chemoprophylaxis after exposure to a person with influenza is recommended for:
- Prevention of influenza in persons at high risk of influenza complications during the first 2 wk following vaccination.
- Patients at high risk for complications from influenza who have contraindications to the influenza vaccine.
- Patients with severe immune deficiencies or others who might not respond to influenza vaccination, such as persons receiving immunosuppressive medications.
- NOT recommended if more than 48 h have elapsed since first exposure to a person with influenza.

–Antiviral treatment options include oseltamivir, zanamivir, and peramivir.
- Oseltamivir (oral) for influenza A or B:
  - Treatment dose: 75 mg by mouth (PO) twice daily (BID) × 5 d.
  - Chemoprophylaxis dose: 75 mg by mouth (PO) once daily × 7 d following last known exposure.
  - Will need to be renally dosed for patients with decreased GFR.
- Zanamivir (inhaled) for influenza A or B:
  - Treatment dose: 10 mg (two 5-mg inhalations) twice daily × 5 d.
  - Chemoprophylaxis dose: 10 mg (two 5-mg inhalations) once daily × 7 d after last known exposure.
  - Avoid in patients with underlying respiratory disease (eg, asthma, COPD).
- Peramivir (IV) for influenza A or B:
  - Treatment dose: 600 mg IV once for creatinine clearance ≥50 mL/min × 1 dose.
  - 200 mg IV once for creatinine clearance 30–49 mL/min.
  - 100 mg IV once for creatinine clearance 10–29 mL/min.
  - ESRD patients on dialysis should receive a dose after dialysis at a dose adjusted based on creatinine clearance.
  - Not recommended for chemoprophylaxis.
  - Baloxavir (oral):
    - Treatment dose: 40 to <80 kg = 40 mg × 1; ≥ 80 kg = 80 mg.
    - Not recommended for chemoprophylaxis.

Sources
–http://www.cdc.gov/mmwr/preview/mmwrhtml/rr6001a1.htm
–https://www.cdc.gov/flu/professionals/antivirals/summary-clinicians.htm#:~:text=The%20recommended%20treatment%20course%20for,oral%20baloxavir%20for%201%20day

Population
–Children.

Organizations
▶ ACIP 2011, CDC 2020

Recommendations
–Prioritize treatment: start antiviral treatment as soon as possible for any patient with suspected or confirmed influenza if hospitalized; severe, complicated, or progressive illness; or higher risk for influenza complications, while awaiting lab confirmation.
–Treatment indicated if symptom onset within 48 h and:
- Any child hospitalized with presumed influenza or with severe, complicated, or progressive illness attributable to influenza, regardless of influenza immunization status.
- Influenza infection of any severity in children at high risk of complications of influenza infection.
- Children aged <2 y.
–Chemoprophylaxis indicated as above for adults.

–Antiviral treatment options include oseltamivir and zanamivir.
- Oseltamivir for influenza A or B treatment dose (5 d):
  ○ If <1-y-old: 3 mg/kg/dose twice daily.
  ○ If 1 y or older, dose varies by child's weight:
  ○ 15 kg or less, the dose is 30 mg twice a day.
  ○ >15 to 23 kg, the dose is 45 mg twice a day.
  ○ >23 to 40 kg, the dose is 60 mg twice a day.
  ○ >40 kg, the dose is 75 mg twice a day.
- Oseltamivir chemoprophylaxis dose (7 d):
  ○ Not recommended for <3 mo of age.
  ○ If child is 3 mo or older and younger than 1 y: 3 mg/kg/dose once daily.
  ○ If 1 y or older, dose varies by child's weight:
    ▫ 15 kg or less, the dose is 30 mg once a day.
    ▫ >15 to 23 kg, the dose is 45 mg once a day.
    ▫ >23 to 40 kg, the dose is 60 mg once a day.
    ▫ >40 kg, the dose is 75 mg once a day.
- Zanamivir for influenza A or B:
  ○ Treatment dose (7 y or older): 10 mg (two 5-mg inhalations) twice daily × 5 d.
  ○ Chemoprophylaxis dose (5 y or older): 10 mg (two 5-mg inhalations) once daily × 7 d.
  ○ Avoid in patients with underlying respiratory disease (eg, asthma, COPD).
- Peramivir (IV) for influenza A or B: (2–12 y of age).
  ○ Treatment dose: 12 mg/kg/dose infusion over 15 min (max 600 mg).
  ○ Not recommended for chemoprophylaxis.
  ○ Baloxavir (oral) ≥12 y:
  ○ Treatment dose: >40 to <80 kg = 40 mg × 1; ≥80 kg = 80 mg.
  ○ Not recommended for chemoprophylaxis.

Comments

1. Consider an influenza nasal swab for diagnosis during influenza season in:
   a. Persons with acute onset of fever and respiratory illness.
   b. Persons with fever and acute exacerbation of chronic lung disease.
   c. Infants and children with fever of unclear etiology.
   d. Severely ill persons with fever or hypothermia.
2. Rapid influenza antigen tests have 70%–90% sensitivity in children and 40%–60% sensitivity in adults.
3. Direct or indirect fluorescent antibody staining is useful in screening tests.
4. Influenza PCR may be used as a confirmatory test.

Source

–http://www.cdc.gov/mmwr/preview/mmwrhtml/rr6001a1.htm

LYME DISEASE

Population
–Adults and children.

Organizations
▶ AAN 2020, IDSA 2006

Recommendations
–Prevention: wear light-colored clothing covering all skin, tuck pants into socks, and check for ticks after outdoor activity. Bathe within 2 h of exposure. Apply DEET, oil of lemon, PMD, or permethrin.

–Diagnosis:
  • Diagnose clinically if 1 or more lesions consistent with erythema migrans.
  • If lesions are suggestive but of low risk, perform antibody testing on an acute phase sample followed by antibody testing on convalescent phase serum sample if initial testing negative.
  • Use serum antibody testing over CSF PCR or culture sample testing for Lyme neuroborreliosis.
  • Tick can be submitted for speciation at most labs or health department. Do not test the tick for *B. burgdorferi* as it does not predict clinical infection.
  • Do not routinely test for Lyme disease in workup of psychiatric illness, but can be considered in the evaluation of some neurologic disorders.

–Treatment: promptly remove attached tick and mouthparts by mechanical means (ie, tweezer). Do not burn or apply noxious chemicals or petroleum products to coax detachment.

–Prophylaxis dose: if *I. scapularis* tick is attached for ≥36 h, prophylaxis can be started within 72 h of removal, bite was from identified *Ixodes* spp. vector in an area where Lyme is endemic.
  • Treat adults with single dose of doxycycline 200 mg.
  • Treat children ≥8 y with doxycycline 4.4 mg/kg to max 200 mg.

–Early illness:
  • Adults: doxycycline 100 mg PO BID × 10 d (amoxicillin or cefuroxime × 14 d, if doxycycline contraindication). Azithromycin as second-line therapy × 7 d.
  • Children (≥8 y): amoxicillin, cefuroxime axetil.

–Treat pregnant patients similar to other adults, but do not use doxycycline.

–Early neurologic Lyme:
  • Adults: ceftriaxone 2 g IV × 14–21 d.
  • Children: ceftriaxone 50–75 mg/kg/d IV × 14 d.
  • Alternative agents: cefotaxime, IV penicillin or oral doxycycline.

–Lyme carditis: perform ECG only if suggestive symptoms:
  • Adults: ceftriaxone 2 g IV × 14–21 d, transition to PO doxycycline when appropriate to complete course.

–Late Lyme arthritis:
  • Adults: doxycycline 100 mg PO BID × 28 d.

- Consider ceftriaxone IV for 2–4 wk if no or minimal response to initial oral abx course.
- Children: amoxicillin 50 mg/kg/d divided TID (max 500 mg/dose) × 28 d.

Source
–https://www.idsociety.org/practice-guideline/lyme-disease/

RESPIRATORY TRACT INFECTIONS, LOWER (COMMUNITY-ACQUIRED PNEUMONIA) (CAP)

Population
–Adults.

Organizations
▶ ATS 2019, ESCMID 2011, IDSA 2007

Recommendations
Diagnosis:
–Use severity-of-illness score to determine if inpatient treatment is appropriate:
  - CURB-65: confusion, uremia, respiratory rage, low blood pressure, age ≥65.
  - Pneumonia severity index (PSI).
  - 2007 IDSA Severe CA: 1 major or 3 minor:
    ◦ Minor:
      ◽ Resp rate ≥30 breath/min.
      ◽ PaO_2/FiO_2 ratio ≤250.
      ◽ Multilobar infiltrates.
      ◽ Confusion/disorientation.
      ◽ Uremia (BUN ≥20 mg/dL).
      ◽ Leukopenia (WBC ≤4000 cells/μL).
      ◽ Thrombocytopenia (platelet count ≤100,000/μL).
      ◽ Hypothermia (Temp ≤36°C).
      ◽ Hypotension requiring "aggressive fluid resuscitation."
    ◦ Major:
      ◽ Septic shock.
      ◽ Respiratory failure requiring mechanical ventilation.
  Evaluation:
–Obtain chest radiograph or other imaging.
–Sputum evaluation and blood cultures not recommended for outpatients.
–Routine testing for antigens not recommended, ie, pneumococcal or *Legionella*, unless severe illness (former) or community outbreak (latter).
–Test for influenza during endemic time, rapid test preferred.
–Do not use procalcitonin to guide antibiotic initiation.
–Do not routinely order follow-up chest imaging if symptoms are improving.

Treatment:

–Empiric therapy based on local antibiotic resistance patterns:

- Previously healthy, no risk for drug-resistant *Streptococcus pneumoniae*:
  - Amoxicillin 1 g PO TID.
  - Doxycycline 100 mg PO BID.
  - Macrolide (azithromycin, clarithromycin, or erythromycin) only in areas where resistance <25%.
- Comorbidities (chronic heart, lung, liver, or renal disease; diabetes; alcoholism; malignancy; asplenia; immune suppression; antimicrobials in past 3 mo):
  - Combo therapy:
    - Amoxicillin/clavulanate 500 mg/125 mg PO TID or 875 mg/125 mg PO BID or 2000 mg/125 mg PO BID.
    - Cephalosporin (cefpodoxime 200 mg PO BID or cefuroxime 500 mg PO BID).
    - Macrolide (azithromycin 500 mg PO first day, then 250 mg PO daily or clarithromycin 500 BID) or doxycycline 100 mg PO BID.
  - Mono therapy:
    - Respiratory fluoroquinolone (moxifloxacin 400 mg PO daily, gemifloxacin 320 mg PO daily, or levofloxacin 750 mg PO daily).
    - Beta-lactam + macrolide.
    - If high rate of *S. pneumoniae* macrolide-resistance (MIC ≥ 16 µg/mL), then consider alternative agent to a macrolide.

–Duration of antibiotics: 5–7 d.

Comments

1. Consider aspiration pneumonia in patients with pneumonia and dysphagia. Do not add anaerobic coverage unless lung abscess or empyema is suspected.
2. Steroids are not routinely recommended solely for pneumonia.
3. For *S. pneumoniae*:
   a. Erythromycin MIC >0.5 mg/L predicts clinical failure.
   b. Penicillin MIC ≤ 8 mg/L predicts IV penicillin susceptibility.
4. Influenza in patients being treated for CAP: treat with anti-influenza treatment independent of duration of symptoms prior to diagnosis, but not the converse.
5. A C-reactive protein (CRP) <2 mg/dL at presentation with symptoms >24 h makes pneumonia highly unlikely; a CRP >10 mg/dL makes pneumonia likely.
6. Indications for antibiotics in lower respiratory tract infections (LRTIs):
   a. Suspected pneumonia.
   b. Acute exacerbation of COPD with increased dyspnea, sputum volume, and sputum purulence.

Sources

–https://academic.oup.com/cid/article/44/Supplement_2/S27/372079
–http://www.escmid.org/fileadmin/src/media/PDFs/4ESCMID_Library/2Medical _Guidelines/ ESCMID_Guidelines/Woodhead_et_al_CMI_Sep_2011_LRTI_GL_fulltext.pdf
–https://www.atsjournals.org/doi/full/10.1164/rccm.201908-1581ST

Population

–Infants and children.

Organizations

▶ IDSA 2011

Recommendations

–Hospitalize children with respiratory distress or hypoxia (<90%), or if <6 mo age.
–Use rapid viral detection tests. Avoid urinary antigen tests and blood cultures in children being treated as outpatients.
–Avoid chest X-ray unless ill enough to be hospitalized or failed initial antibiotic therapy. Avoid routine follow-up imaging to document improvement.
–As viral etiologies cause the majority of pneumonia-like illness in pre-school-aged children, do not routinely prescribe antibiotics.
–If evidence of bacterial origin, use amoxicillin, as *S. pneumoniae* is the most common etiology.
–If evidence of atypical pathogens, use macrolides. Test for *M. pneumoniae* if results can be available quickly enough to guide therapy.
–If influenza virus is prevalent in the community, start anti-influenza therapy immediately while awaiting diagnostic test results.
–Consider 10-d duration of antibiotics, though shorter durations may be acceptable for milder illness.
–After initiating therapy, follow up in 48–72 h to ensure improvement.

Comment

1. For outpatients, a duration of 5 d of amoxicillin 75–100 mg/kg/d is equivalent to a duration of 10 –d. (*JAMA Pediatr.* 2021;175(5):475–482)

Source

–*Clin Infect Dis.* 2011:53(7):e25-76.

RESPIRATORY TRACT INFECTIONS, UPPER

Population

Patients with URI.

Organization

▶ IDSA 2015

Recommendation

–Do not prescribe antibiotics for upper respiratory tract infections.

Source

–http://www.choosingwisely.org/societies/infectious-diseases-society-of-america/

SEXUALLY TRANSMITTED DISEASES

SEXUALLY TRANSMITTED DISEASES TREATMENT GUIDELINES

Infection	Recommended Treatment	Alternative Treatment
Chancroid	• Azithromycin 1 g PO × 1 • Ceftriaxone 250 mg IM × 1	• Ciprofloxacin 500 mg PO BID for 3 d • Erythromycin base 500 mg PO TID for 7 d
Genital HSV, first episode	• Acyclovir 400 mg PO TID × 7–10 d[a] • Famciclovir 250 mg PO TID × 7–10 d[a] • Valacyclovir 1 g PO BID × 7–10 d[a]	• Acyclovir 200 mg PO 5 times a day for 7–10 d[a]
Genital HSV, suppressive therapy	• Acyclovir 400 mg PO BID • Valacyclovir 500 mg or 1 g PO daily	• Famciclovir 250 mg PO BID
Genital HSV, episodic therapy for recurrent disease	• Acyclovir 800 mg PO TID × 2 d • Acyclovir 800 mg PO BID × 5 d • Acyclovir 800 mg PO TID × 2 d	• Valacyclovir 500 mg PO BID × 3 d • Valacyclovir 1 g PO daily × 5 d • Famciclovir 125 mg PO BID × 5 d • Famciclovir 1000 mg PO BID × 1 d • Famciclovir 500 mg PO × 1 then 250 mg BID × 2 d
Genital HSV, suppressive therapy for HIV-positive patients	• Acyclovir 400–800 mg PO BID–TID • Famciclovir 500 mg PO BID • Valacyclovir 500 mg PO BID	
Genital HSV, episodic therapy for recurrent genital HSV in HIV-positive patients	• Acyclovir 400 mg PO TID × 5–10 d • Famciclovir 500 mg PO BID × 5–10 d • Valacyclovir 1 g PO BID × 5–10 d	
Granuloma inguinale (Donovanosis)	• Azithromycin 1 g orally once per week or 500 mg daily for at least 3 wk and until all lesions have completely healed	• Doxycycline 100 mg PO BID × ≥3 wk • Erythromycin 500 PO QID × 3 wk • Trimethoprim-sulfamethoxazole 160/800 mg PO BID × 3 wk • Continue all regimens until lesions are completely healed.

SEXUALLY TRANSMITTED DISEASES TREATMENT GUIDELINES

Infection	Recommended Treatment	Alternative Treatment
		• Erythromycin base 500 mg PO QID × ≥3 wk • TMP-SMX 1 double-strength (160/800 mg) tablet PO BID × ≥3 wk • Continue all of these treatments until all lesions have completely healed
Lymphogranuloma venereum	• Doxycycline 100 mg PO BID for × 21 d	• Azithromycin 1 gm PO weekly × 3 wk • Erythromycin base 500 mg PO QID × 21 d
Primary and secondary syphilis in adults	• Benzathine penicillin G 2.4 million units IM × 1	• Doxycycline 100 mg PO BID × 14 d • Tetracycline 500 mg PO QID × 14 d • Amoxicillin 3 g + probenecid 500 mg, both PO BID × 14 d
Primary and secondary syphilis in infants and children	• Benzathine penicillin G 50,000 units/kg IM, up to the adult dose of 2.4 million units × 1	
Early latent syphilis in adults	• Benzathine penicillin G 2.4 million units IM × 1	
Early latent syphilis in children	• Benzathine penicillin G 50,000 units/kg IM, up to the adult dose of 2.4 million units × 1	
Late latent syphilis or latent syphilis of unknown duration in adults	• Benzathine penicillin G 2.4 million units IM weekly × 3 doses	• Doxycycline 100 mg PO BID × 4 wk
Late latent syphilis or latent syphilis of unknown duration in children	• Benzathine penicillin G 50,000 units/kg, up to the adult dose of 2.4 million units, IM weekly × 3 doses	
Tertiary syphilis	• Benzathine penicillin G 2.4 million units IM weekly × 3 doses	• Doxycycline 100 mg PO BID × 4 wk
Neurosyphilis	• Aqueous crystalline penicillin G 3–4 million units IV q4h × 10–14 d	• Procaine penicillin 2.4 million units IM daily × 10–14 d PLUS • Probenecid 500 mg PO QID × 10–14 d

SEXUALLY TRANSMITTED DISEASES TREATMENT GUIDELINES (*Continued*)

Infection	Recommended Treatment	Alternative Treatment
Syphilis, pregnant women	• Pregnant women should be treated with the penicillin regimen appropriate for their stage of infection	• No good alternatives. Recommend penicillin allergy test and desensitization if patient has reported penicillin allergy
Congenital syphilis	• Aqueous crystalline penicillin G 50,000 units/kg/dose IV q12h × 7 d; then q8h × 3 more days	• Procaine penicillin G 50,000 units/kg/dose IM daily × 10 d • Benzathine penicillin G 50,000 units/kg/dose IM × 1
Older children with syphilis	• Aqueous crystalline penicillin G 50,000 units/kg IV q4–6h × 10 d	
Nongonococcal urethritis	• Doxycycline 100 mg PO BID × 7 d	• Azithromycin 1 g PO × 1 • Azithromycin 500 mg PO × 1, then 250 mg PO × 4 d.
Recurrent or persistent urethritis	• Metronidazole 2 g PO × 1 • Tinidazole 2 g PO × 1 • Azithromycin 1 g PO × 1	
Cervicitis[b]	• Doxycycline 100 mg PO BID × 7 d	• Azithromycin 1 g PO × 1
Chlamydia infections in adolescents, adults[b]	• Doxycycline 100 mg PO BID × 7 d	• Azithromycin 1 g PO × 1 • Levofloxacin 500 mg PO daily × 7 d
Chlamydia infections in pregnancy[b]	• Azithromycin 1 g PO × 1	• Amoxicillin 500 mg PO TID × 7 d • Erythromycin base 500 mg PO QID × 7 d • Erythromycin ethylsuccinate 800 mg PO QID × 7 d
Ophthalmia neonatorum from *Chlamydia trachomatis*	• Erythromycin base or ethylsuccinate 50 mg/kg/d PO QID × 14 d	
C. trachomatis pneumonia in infants	• Erythromycin base or ethylsuccinate 50 mg/kg/d PO QID × 14 d	
Chlamydia infections in children ≥45 kg	• Erythromycin base or ethylsuccinate 50 mg/kg/d PO QID × 14 d	
Chlamydia infections in children ≥45 kg and age ≥8 y	• Azithromycin 1 g PO × 1	

SEXUALLY TRANSMITTED DISEASES TREATMENT GUIDELINES

Infection	Recommended Treatment	Alternative Treatment
Chlamydia infections in children age≥8 y	• Azithromycin 1 g PO × 1 • Doxycycline 100 mg PO BID × 7 d	
Uncomplicated gonococcal infections of the cervix, urethra, pharynx, or rectum in adults or children ≥45 kg	• Ceftriaxone 500 mg IM × 1 if < 150 kg. If > 150 kg, ceftriaxone 1 g IM × 1. • Empirically treat for chlamydia if not ruled out with testing with doxycycline 100 mg BID × 7 d.	• If cephalosporin allergy: • Gentamycin 240 mg IM × 1 + azithromycin 2 g PO × 1. • If ceftriaxone not available: Cefixime 800 mg PO × 1. • Empirically treat for chlamydia if not ruled out with testing with doxycycline 100 mg BID × 7 d.
Gonococcal conjunctivitis in adults or children ≥45 kg	• Ceftriaxone 1 g IM × 1	
Gonococcal meningitis or endocarditis in adults or children ≥45 kg	• Ceftriaxone 1 g IV q12h • Empirically treat for chlamydia if not ruled out with testing with doxycycline 100 mg BID × 7 d.	
Disseminated gonococcal infection in adults or children ≥45 kg	• Ceftriaxone 1 g IV/IM daily • Empirically treat for chlamydia if not ruled out with testing with doxycycline 100 mg BID × 7 d.	• Cefotaxime 1 g IV q8h • Ceftizoxime 1 g IV q8h
Ophthalmia neonatorum prophylaxis	• Erythromycin (0.5%) ophthalmic ointment in each eye × 1	
Ophthalmia neonatorum caused by gonococcus	• Ceftriaxone 25–50 mg/kg, not to exceed 250 mg, IV/IM × 1	
Prophylactic treatment of infants born to mothers with gonococcal infection	• Ceftriaxone 25–50 mg/kg, not to exceed 250 mg, IV/IM × 1	
Uncomplicated gonococcal infections of the cervix, urethra, pharynx, or rectum in children ≥45 kg	• Ceftriaxone 125 mg IM × 1 if < 150 kg.	
Gonococcal infections with bacteremia or arthritis in children or adults	• Ceftriaxone 50 mg/kg (maximum dose 1 g) IM/IV daily × 7 d	
Bacterial vaginosis	• Metronidazole 500 mg PO BID × 7 d[c] • Metronidazole gel 0.75%, 1 applicator (5 g) IVag daily × 5 d • Clindamycin cream 2%, 1 applicator (5 g) IVag qhs × 7 d[d]	• Tinidazole 2 g PO daily × 3 d • Clindamycin 300 mg PO BID × 7 d • Clindamycin ovules 100 mg IVag qhs × 3 d

SECTION 3: MANAGEMENT

SEXUALLY TRANSMITTED DISEASES TREATMENT GUIDELINES *(Continued)*		
Infection	**Recommended Treatment**	**Alternative Treatment**
Bacterial vaginosis in pregnancy	• Metronidazole 500 mg PO BID × 7 d • Metronidazole 250 mg PO TID × 7 d • Clindamycin 300 mg PO BID × 7 d	
Trichomoniasis	• Women: Metronidazole 500 mg PO BID × 7 d[c] • Men: Metronidazole 2 g PO × 1 d[c]	• Tinidazole 2 g PO × 1 (women & men)
Candida vaginitis	• Butoconazole 2% cream 5 g IVag × 3 d • Clotrimazole 1% cream 5 g IVag × 7–14 d • Clotrimazole 2% cream 5 g IVag × 3 d • Nystatin 100,000-unit vaginal tablet, 1 tablet IVag × 14 d • Miconazole 2% cream 5 g IVag × 7 d • Miconazole 4% cream 5 g IVag × 3 d • Miconazole 100-mg vaginal suppository, 1 suppository IVag × 7 d	• Fluconazole 150-mg PO × 1
	• Miconazole 200-mg vaginal suppository, 1 suppository IVag × 3 d • Miconazole 1200-mg vaginal suppository, 1 suppository IVag × 1 • Tioconazole 6.5% ointment 5 g IVag × 1 • Terconazole 0.4% cream 5 g IVag × 7 d • Terconazole 0.8% cream 5 g IVag × 3 d • Terconazole 80-mg vaginal suppository, 1 suppository IVag × 3 d	
Severe pelvic inflammatory disease	• Cefotetan 2 g IV q12h PLUS • Doxycycline 100 mg PO/IV q12h OR • Cefoxitin 2 g IV q6h	• Ampicillin/sulbactam 3 g IV q6h PLUS • Doxycycline 100 mg PO/IV BID OR • Clindamycin 900 mg IV q8h PLUS • Gentamicin loading dose IV or IM (2 mg/kg of body weight), followed by a maintenance dose (1.5 mg/kg) q8h. Single daily dosing (3–5 mg/kg) can be substituted
Mild-to-moderate pelvic inflammatory disease	• Ceftriaxone 500 mg IM × 1 PLUS • Doxycycline 100 mg PO BID × 1 d PLUS metronidazole 500 mg PO BID × 14 d[c] OR • Cefoxitin 2 g IM × 1 and probenecid 1 g PO × 1 PLUS • Doxycycline 100 mg PO BID × 14 d ± metronidazole 500 mg PO BID × 14 d[c]	

SEXUALLY TRANSMITTED DISEASES TREATMENT GUIDELINES

Infection	Recommended Treatment	Alternative Treatment

Epididymitis	• Ceftriaxone 500 mg IM × 1, if < 150 kg; if > 150 kg, ceftriaxone 1 g IM × 1 PLUS
	• Doxycycline 100 mg PO BID × 10 d
	For men who practice insertive anal sex:
	  • Ceftriaxone 500 mg IM × 1 PLUS
	  • Levofloxacin 500 mg PO daily × 10 d OR
	  • 1. Ofloxacin 300 mg PO BID × 10 d
		• Fluoroquinolone monotherapy can be considered if enteric organism and gonorrhea ruled out
		• Levofloxacin 500 mg PO daily × 10 d
		• Ofloxacin 300 mg PO BID × 10 d

External genital warts	Provider-administered: • Cryotherapy liquid nitrogen or cryoprobe • TCA or BCA 80%–90% • Surgical removal by tangential scissor excision, tangential shave excision, curettage, or electrosurgery	Patient-applied: • Podofilox 0.5% solution or gel • Imiquimod 5% cream • Sinecatechins 15% ointment
Cervical warts	• Cryotherapy with liquid nitrogen • Surgical removal by tangential scissor excision, tangential shave excision, curettage, or electrosurgery • TCA or BCA 80%–90% applied only to warts • Recommend consulting with specialist in management • Biopsy to exclude high-grade SIL must be performed before treatment is initiated	
Vaginal warts	• Cryotherapy with liquid nitrogen • Surgical removal by tangential scissor excision, tangential shave excision, curettage, or electrosurgery • TCA or BCA 80%–90% applied only to warts	
Urethral meatal warts	• Cryotherapy with liquid nitrogen • Surgical removal by tangential scissor excision, tangential shave excision, curettage, or electrosurgery	
Anal warts	• Cryotherapy with liquid nitrogen • Surgical removal by tangential scissor excision, tangential shave excision, curettage, or electrosurgery • TCA or BCA 80%–90% applied only to warts	• Surgical removal by tangential scissor excision, tangential shave excision, curettage, or electrosurgery

SEXUALLY TRANSMITTED DISEASES TREATMENT GUIDELINES *(Continued)*		
Infection	**Recommended Treatment**	**Alternative Treatment**
Proctitis	• Ceftriaxone 500 mg IM × 1, if < 150 kg; if > 150 kg, ceftriaxone 1 g IM × 1 PLUS • Doxycycline 100 mg PO BID × 7 d (extend to 21 d if bloody discharge, ulceration, or positive for rectal chlamydia	
Pediculosis pubis	• Permethrin 1% cream rinse applied to affected areas and washed off after 10 min • Pyrethrins with piperonyl butoxide applied to the affected area and washed off after 10 min	• Malathion 0.5% lotion applied for 8–12 h and then washed off • Ivermectin 250 µg/kg PO, repeated in 2 wk
Scabies	• Permethrin cream (5%) applied to all areas of the body from the neck down and washed off after 8–14 h • Ivermectin 200 µg/kg PO, repeat in 2 wk	• Lindane (1%) 1 oz of lotion (or 30 g of cream) applied in a thin layer to all areas of the body from the neck down and thoroughly washed off after 8 h • Crotamiton 10% apply thin layer

BCA, bichloroacetic acid; BID, twice a day; h, hour(s); HIV, human immunodeficiency virus; HSV, herpes simplex virus; IM, intramuscular; IV, intravenous; IVag, intravaginally; PO, by mouth; q, every; qhs, at bedtime; QID, 4 times a day; SIL, squamous intraepithelial lesion; TCA, trichloroacetic acid; TID, 3 times a day; TMP-SMX, trimethoprim-sulfamethoxazole.

[a]Treatment can be extended if healing is incomplete after 10 d of therapy.
[b]Consider concomitant treatment of gonorrhea.
[c]Avoid alcohol during treatment and for 24 h after treatment is completed.
[d]Clindamycin cream may weaken latex condoms and diaphragms during treatment and for 5 d thereafter.
Source: Adapted from *CDC Guidelines: Sexually Transmitted Infection Guidelines.* 2021. https://www.cdc.gov/std/treatment-guidelines/default.htm. *MMWR Recomm Rep.* 2021;70(4):1–187.

SINUSITIS

Population
–Adults and children.

Organizations
▶ EPOS 2020, CDC 2017, NICE 2017, IDSA 2012

Recommendations
–Advise patients that etiology is usually viral, course self-limited lasting for 2–3 wk
–Treat with decongestants, nasal irrigation, zinc > 75 mg/d within 24 h of symptom onset.
–Consider nasal steroid and systemic steroid, as they have small beneficial effect.
–Avoid vitamin C and homeopathy, herbal medication (BNO1016 and *Pelargonium sidoides* drops) as there is limited evidence, and antihistamines which offer no benefit.

–Avoid antibiotics early in illness.

–Do not obtain sinus radiographs.

–If persistent symptoms (>10 d) or if severe (>3–4 d + fever or purulent discharge) or change in symptoms (eg, "double sickening"), consider no antibiotic or back-up antibiotic and/or nasal corticosteroid (off-label). (NICE 2017)

–If systemic symptoms or high-risk comorbidity or signs of more serious illness, offer antibiotics.

–Antibiotics (CDC 2017):

- Adult >18-y-old.
- Amoxicillin or amoxicillin-clavulanate × 10 d.
- Macrolides not recommended due to resistance.
- PCN allergy: doxycycline or respiratory fluoroquinolone (levofloxacin or moxifloxacin).
- Children ≤18-y-old:
  ○ Amoxicillin or amoxicillin-clavulanate × 10 d.
  ○ Intractable vomiting: ceftriaxone IM × 1, then oral antibiotics.

Sources

–https://epos2020.com/Documents/supplement_29.pdf

–https://academic.oup.com/cid/article/54/8/1041/364141

–https://www.cdc.gov/antibiotic-use/community/for-hcp/outpatient-hcp/adult-treatment-rec.html

–https://www.nice.org.uk/guidance/ng79

–https://www.cdc.gov/mrsa/pdf/flowchart_pstr.pdf

–https://www.sanfordguide.com/products/digital-subscriptions/sanford-guide-to-antimicrobial-therapy-mobile/

SKIN AND SOFT TISSUE INFECTIONS

Population

–Adults and children.

Organization

▶ IDSA 2014

Recommendations

–Impetigo and ecthyma:

- Gram stain pus or exudate.
- Treat with topical mupirocin or retapamulin BID × 5 d.
- Oral therapy: start with dicloxacillin or cephalexin. If MRSA present, doxycycline, clindamycin, or sulfamethoxazole-trimethoprim (SMX-TMP).

–Purulent infections:

- Gram stain recommended.
- Perform incision and drainage.
- Use antibiotics if signs of systemic infection to cover for MRSA.

–MSSA antibiotics:
- Dicloxacillin 500 mg PO TID.
- Cephalexin 500 mg PO QID.

–MRSA antibiotics:
- Trimethoprim/sulfamethoxazole 160/800 PO BID; if BMI >40, 2 tab PO BID (lacks coverage for Group A streptococcus, not recommended in the third trimester of pregnancy, age <2 y).
- Clindamycin 300–450 mg PO BID; if BMI >40, use higher dose.
- Doxycycline or minocycline 100 mg PO BID; not for use in pregnancy, age <8 y, less effective for *Streptococcus* spp.
- Rifampin; many drug interactions.
- Linezolin; consult infectious disease specialist, many severe side effects, may be used in renal dysfunction.

–Recurrent abscesses:
- Rule out pilonidal cyst, hidradenitis suppurativa, or foreign body.
- Drain and culture drainage.
- Treat with antibiotics for 5–10 d directed by culture result.
- Consider 5-d decolonization: intranasal mupirocin BID, daily chlorhexidine bath, and daily decontamination of personal items.
- Evaluate for neutrophil disorders.

–Erysipelas and cellulitis:
- Routine cultures are not recommended.
- Culture blood and local aspirate if history of malignancy on chemotherapy, neutropenia, cell-mediated immunodeficiency, immersion injury, or animal bite.
- Treat with antibiotics to cover streptococci for 5 d.
- Treat underlying conditions, ie, edema.
- If systemic illness, deep infection, severely immunocompromised, or delirium, then treat with intravenous antibiotics.

–Animal bites (dog or cat):
- Treat with amoxicillin-clavulanate for 3–5 d, if immunocompromised, asplenic, advanced liver disease, antecedent edema, moderate-to-severe injury, involve the hands or face or involve periosteum or joint.
- Evaluate for rabies prophylaxis.
- Evaluate tetanus status, if <10 y, give Tdap.
- Do not perform primary closure, except face following copious irrigation and debridement.

Sources

–https://www.idsociety.org/practice-guideline/skin-and-soft-tissue-infections/
–https://www.cdc.gov/mrsa/pdf/flowchart_pstr.pdf
–https://www.sanfordguide.com/products/digital-subscriptions/sanford-guide-to-antimicrobial-therapy-mobile/

SYPHILIS

Population
–Adults, pregnancy, infants, and children.

Organizations
▶ IDSA 2011, CDC 2021

Recommendations
–Diagnosis: Test all persons who have syphilis for HIV, offer PreEP and retest for HIV in 3 mo if primary test is negative.
–Treatment: See treatment section in table.
–Penicillin G 2.4 million units IM is drug of choice for early syphilis.
–Cerebrospinal fluid (CSF) analysis is indicated if:
- Early syphilis infection and neurologic symptoms.
- Late latent syphilis.

–Obtain CSF examination, for patients with early syphilis do not achieve a >4-fold decline in RPR titers within 12 mo.
–Doxycycline is a second-line therapy for early syphilis in penicillin-allergic patients.
–Ceftriaxone is a second-line therapy for neurosyphilis in penicillin-allergic patients.
–Evaluate and treat sexual partners within preceding 90 d.
–If retreatment is necessary, use Penicillin G 2.4 million units IM × 3 wk, unless neurological involvement.

Comments
1. Penicillin (PCN) G is the only treatment in pregnancy. If PCN allergy, pursue desensitization therapy.
2. Avoid doxycycline in pregnancy.
3. Infants and children: Benzathine PCN G 50,000 U/kg IM up to adult dose 2.4 million units. If secondary syphilis is suspected, consult infectious disease specialist.
4. Treat HIV-positive patients with primary or secondary syphilis as HIV-negative persons.

Sources
–http://cid.oxfordjournals.org/content/53/suppl_3/S110.abstract
–https://www.cdc.gov/std/treatment-guidelines/p-and-s-syphilis.htm

TUBERCULOSIS, MYCOBACTERIUM (MTB), DIAGNOSIS

Population
–Adults and children suspected of having MTB: screen those who spent time with TB patients, are from an endemic country, live/work in high-risk setting, are health care workers.

Organizations

▶ IDSA 2017, NICE 2016

Recommendations

–Do not routinely test for TB.

–Screening: Perform interferon-gamma release assay (IGRA) if >5 y with suspected infection, risk for disease progression, concern for latent MTB (LTBI), or history of BCG vaccination.

–Tuberculin skin test (TST) is an alternative if IGRA is not available, costly, or burdensome.

–Suspected active MTB:

• Perform a chest X-ray in all patients with symptoms.

–Obtain 3 early-morning sputum samples for AFB smear and culture.

–TST preferred in patients <5 y.

–Mandatory screening due to law: IGRA preferred to TST. Perform second test, if initial test is positive in asymptomatic individuals. Diagnose infection if tests are positive twice.

Comment

1. Consider sputum for nucleic acid amplification for mycobacterium TB complex if the person has HIV disease, or there is a need for large contact tracing or rapid diagnosis.

Sources

–https://guidelines.gov/summaries/summary/49964

–https://academic.oup.com/cid/article/64/2/111/2811357

TUBERCULOSIS (TB), MANAGEMENT

Population

–Adults suspected of having active TB.

Organizations

▶ ATS/CDC/IDSA 2016, NICE 2016, ATS 2019

Recommendations

–Report suspect to local public health office for case management and contact screening.

–Refer the patient to a clinician with expertise in TB management.

–Isolate patients in negative pressure rooms within the hospital.

–Test for rifampin resistance, especially if at risk for drug resistance.

–Decision to initiate therapy depends on multiple factors. Refer to a clinician with expertise in TB management. See Figure 26-1 for guidance on initiating therapy.

–If initiating treatment, start patients on RIPE therapy: rifampin (RIF), isoniazid (INH), pyrazinamide (PZA), and ethambutol (EMB). All regimens include an intensive initial phase with four drugs followed by a continuation phase with isoniazid and rifampin alone.

–Preferred regimen: RIPE 5 or 7 d/wk × 8 wk then INH+RIF 5 or 7 d/wk × 18 wk. This has greater efficacy and lower risk of resistance than the alternate regimens below.

Figure 26-1. When to initiate antituberculosis medication.

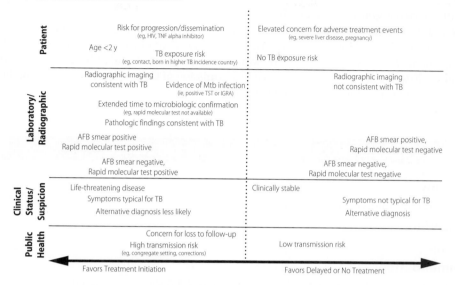

Source: Nahid P, Dorman SE, Alipanah N, et al. Official American Thoracic Society/Centers for Disease Control and Prevention/Infectious Diseases Society of America clinical practice guidelines: treatment of drug-susceptible tuberculosis. *Clin Infect Dis.* 2016;63(7):e147-e195. doi:10.1093/cid/ciw376. Translated and reproduced by permission of Oxford University Press on behalf of the Infectious Diseases Society of America.

–Alternate regimen, if direct observed therapy (DOT) is challenging: RIPE 5 or 7 d/wk × 8 wk then INH+RIF 3 d/wk × 18 wk.

–Alternate regimen, to simplify DOT further: RIPE 3 d/wk × 8 wk then INH+RIF 3d/wk × 18 wk. Use with caution in HIV or cavitary disease, as missed doses can lead to failure/relapse/resistance.

–Simplest acceptable regimen, not for use in HIV, smear positive or cavitary lung disease, or if missed doses are likely: RIPE 7 d/wk × 2 wk, then RIPE 2 d/wk × 6 wk, then INH+RIF 2 d/wk × 18 wk.

–Cavitation on initial CXR with positive cultures at 2 mo of therapy may require extending continuation phase to 31 wk.

–When using INH, give pyridoxine 25–50 mg/d if any risk of neuropathy (pregnancy, breastfeeding, HIV, diabetes, alcohol abuse, malnutrition, chronic renal failure, advanced age).

Comments

1. TB treatment regimens are modified based on TB sensitivities.
2. Consider de-escalation of hospital isolation after 2 wk of therapy if:
   a. Resolution of cough.
   b. Afebrile for a week.
   c. Immunocompetent patient.
   d. No extensive disease by X-ray.
   e. Initial smear grade was 2+ or less.
3. If sputum cultures remain positive after 3 mo of treatment, repeat drug sensitivity testing and assess compliance with regimen.

Sources
–https://www.atsjournals.org/doi/10.1164/rccm.201909-1874ST
–Nahid P, Dorman SE, Alipanah N, et al. Official American Thoracic Society/Centers for Disease Control and Prevention/Infectious Diseases Society of America clinical practice guidelines: treatment of drug-susceptible tuberculosis. *Clin Infect Dis.* 2016;63(7):e147-e195. doi:10.1093/cid/ciw376. Translated and reproduced by permission of Oxford University Press on behalf of the Infectious Diseases Society of America.
–https://guidelines.gov/summaries/summary/49964

TUBERCULOSIS (TB), MANAGEMENT OF LATENT TB

Population
–Adults and children who have latent TB.

Organization
▶ NICE 2016

Recommendations
–High-risk individuals younger than 35 y with latent TB should be offered:
  • 3 mo of rifampin and isoniazid (with pyridoxine).
  • 6 mo of isoniazid (with pyridoxine).
–Offer adults HIV, HBV, and HCV testing before starting treatment for latent TB.
–Offer high-risk individuals between 35 and 65 y latent TB therapy if hepatotoxicity is not a concern.

Comment
1. High-risk patients with latent TB:
   a. HIV-positive.
   b. Younger than 5 y.
   c. Excessive alcohol intake.
   d. Injection drug users.
   e. Solid organ transplant recipients.
   f. Hematologic malignancies.
   g. Undergoing chemotherapy.
   h. Prior jejunoileal bypass.
   i. Diabetes.
   j. Chronic kidney disease.
   k. Prior gastrectomy.
   l. Receiving treatment with antitumor necrosis factor med or other biologic agents.

Source
–https://guidelines.gov/summaries/summary/49964

TUBERCULOSIS (TB), MULTIDRUG-RESISTANT (MDR-TB)

Population

–Patients with suspected or proven drug-resistant TB.

Organization

▶ ATS 2019, WHO 2011

Recommendations

–Perform rapid drug susceptibility testing of isoniazid (INH) and rifampicin at the time of TB diagnosis. If INH resistance is detected, check for fluoroquinolone resistance.
–Use at least 5 drugs during the intensive phase (5–7 mo), followed by 4 drugs during continuation phase (additional 15–21 mo after culture conversion to negative).
–Use sputum smear microscopy and culture to monitor patients with MDR-TB.
–Repeat drug sensitivity testing if cultures remain positive at 3 mo of adherent treatment.
–Add a later-generation fluoroquinolone, bedaquiline, linezolid, clofazimine, and cycloserine. Add ethambutol only if there are no better options for the 5-drug regimen.

Sources

–https://www.atsjournals.org/doi/10.1164/rccm.201909-1874ST
–http://whqlibdoc.who.int/publications/2011/9789241501583_eng.pdf

URINARY TRACT INFECTIONS (UTI)

Population

–Adult women.

Organizations

▶ ACOG 2008, EAU 2010, IDSA 2011, NICE 2018, AUA 2019

Recommendations

–Perform a urinalysis or dipstick testing for symptoms of a UTI: dysuria, urinary frequency, suprapubic pain, or hematuria.
–Send urine culture in men, pregnant women, children, or those with a history of resistant bacteria.
–Use acetaminophen rather than NSAIDs for pain control.
–No evidence for cranberry products or urine alkalization for treatment.
–Duration of antibiotics (consider any previous culture results and sensitivities):
  • Uncomplicated cystitis: 3–7 d (nitrofurantoin requires 5–7 d).
  • Uncomplicated pyelonephritis: 7–10 d.
  • Complicated pyelonephritis or UTI: 3–5 d after control/elimination of complicating factors and defervescence.

–Empiric antibiotics for uncomplicated cystitis[1]:
- Trimethoprim-sulfamethoxazole 800 mg/160 mg BID × 3 d (not recommended if local resistance rate >20%).
- Nitrofurantoin monohydrate 100 mg BID × 5 d.
- Fosfomycin 3 g PO × 1 (second line).
- Beta-lactam antibiotics are alternative agents.[2]

–Empiric antibiotics for complicated UTI or uncomplicated pyelonephritis:
- Fluoroquinolones.
- Ceftriaxone or cefuroxime.
- Aminoglycosides.

–Empiric antibiotics for complicated pyelonephritis:
- Fluoroquinolones.
- Piperacillin-tazobactam.
- Carbapenem.
- Aminoglycosides.

–Consider a fluoroquinolone for symptoms of pyelonephritis or for refractory UTI.

–Special circumstances (NICE 2018):
- Children (age- and weight-specific dosing): cephalexin, amoxicillin-clavulanate (if sensitivities are known).
- Pregnant women: cephalexin 500 mg BID or TID × 7–10 d.
- Men: nitrofurantoin, trimethoprim-sulfamethoxazole, ciprofloxacin, or levofloxacin.

Comments

1. EAU recommends 7 d of antibiotics for men with otherwise uncomplicated cystitis.
2. EAU suggests the following options for antimicrobial prophylaxis of recurrent uncomplicated UTIs in nonpregnant women:
   a. Nitrofurantoin 50 mg PO daily.
   b. TMP-SMX 40/200 mg daily.
3. EAU suggests the following options for antimicrobial prophylaxis of recurrent uncomplicated UTIs in pregnant women:
   a. Cephalexin 125 mg PO daily.
4. Once urine culture and sensitivity results are known, antibiotics can be adjusted to the narrowest spectrum antibiotic.

Sources

–http://www.guidelines.gov/content.aspx?id=12628
–http://www.uroweb.org/gls/pdf/Urological%20Infections%202010.pdf
–http://www.guidelines.gov/content.aspx?id=25652
–http://guidelines.gov/content.aspx?id=12628
–http://cid.oxfordjournals.org/content/52/5/e103.full.pdf+html

[1] TMP-SMX only if regional *Escherichia coli* resistance is
[2] Amoxicillin-clavulanate, cefdinir, cefaclor, or cefpodoxime-proxetil. Cephalexin may be appropriate in certain settings.

–http://nice.org.uk/guidance/ng111

–http://nice.org.uk/guidance/ng109

–https://www.sanfordguide.com/products/digital-subscriptions/sanford-guide-to-antimicrobial-therapy-mobile/

–https://www.auanet.org/guidelines/recurrent-uti

Population

–Febrile children 2–24 mo.

Organizations

▶ AAP 2016, NICE 2019, AAP 2021

Recommendations

–Diagnose a UTI if patient has pyuria, abnormal urinalysis, and ≥50,000 colonies/mL single uropathogenic organism.

–Obtain midstream sample for urine dipstick and culture prior to antibiotics. Bagged specimens can be used for urinalysis, but not for culture. Collect catheterized specimen or suprapubic aspiration for culture only if urinalysis suggests infection.

–Obtain blood cultures if toxic appearing.

–Obtain a renal and bladder ultrasound in all infants 2–24 mo with a febrile UTI.

–Treat febrile UTIs with 7–14 d of antibiotics and tailor antibiotics to culture result.

–Antibiotic prophylaxis is not indicated for a history of febrile UTI.

–A voiding cystourethrogram (VCUG) is indicated if ultrasound reveals hydronephrosis, renal scarring, or other findings of high-grade vesicoureteral reflux, and for recurrent febrile UTIs.

Comments

1. Urine obtained through catheterization has a 95% sensitivity and 99% specificity for UTI.

2. Bag urine cultures have a specificity of approximately 63% with an unacceptably high false-positive rate. Only useful if the cultures are negative.

3. Increased rate of false-positives if the renal ultrasound is performed during acute phase of illness. Consider delaying until illness has defervesced.

Sources

–https://pubmed.ncbi.nlm.nih.gov/34281996/

–http://pediatrics.aappublications.org/content/early/2016/11/24/peds.2016-3026

–http://nice.org.uk/guidance/ng109

–https://www.sanfordguide.com/products/digital-subscriptions/sanford-guide-to-antimicrobial-therapy-mobile/

URINARY TRACT INFECTIONS, PYELONEPHRITIS

Population
–Adults.

Organization
▶ ACP 2021

Recommendations

Diagnosis:

–Urinary symptoms plus fever and costovertebral tenderness.

–Obtain urine culture prior to the initiation of antibiotics.

–Complicated pyelonephritis: obstruction, male sex, immunosuppression, stone disease, anatomic or functional urinary tract abnormality.

Management:

–Hospitalize patients with severe illness, elevated creatinine, severe pain, or who cannot tolerate oral intake.

–Obtain imaging, either ultrasound or CT scan, in patients with severe illness, new renal failure, history of stones, ureteral colic, concern for obstruction (ie, BPH), high urine pH > 7, or failure to respond to therapy.

Treatment:

–Men and women with uncomplicated pyelonephritis: prescribe fluoroquinolone × 5–7 d or trimethoprim-sulfamethoxazole × 14 d.

–Ciprofloxacin 500 mg PO BID × 5 d, or 1000 mg PO daily × 5–7 d or levofloxacin 750 mg PO × 5–7 d.

–Ceftriaxone 1 g IV once with transition to oral therapy for patients who cannot take oral therapy initially.

–Second line:
  • TMP-SMX 160/800 mg PO BID × 14 d.
  • Cefixime 400 mg PO daily.
  • Amoxicillin-clavulanate 875/125 mg PO BID.

–If high risk for resistance, may need inpatient parenteral therapy.

Sources

–Lee, R. Appropriate use of short-course antibiotics in common infections: best practice advice from the American College of Physicians. *Ann Intern Med.* 2021;174(6):822-827.

–https://www.sanfordguide.com/products/digital-subscriptions/sanford-guide-to-antimicrobial-therapy-mobile/

URINARY TRACT INFECTION, RECURRENT

Population
–Adult women.

Organization
▶ AUA 2019

Recommendations
–Obtain results of previous cultures and microbial sensitivity.
–Ensure clean, noncontaminated sample with consideration for catheterized specimen.
–Avoid routine imaging and cystoscopy.
–Do not treat asymptomatic bacteriuria.
–Provide patient-initiated treatment while awaiting culture.
–Prescribe antimicrobial prophylactic antibiotics with caution.
–Recommend cranberry prophylaxis.
–Repeat culture if UTI symptoms persist following antimicrobial therapy.
–Do not perform test of cure if symptoms resolve.
–Prescribe vaginal estrogen in peri- and postmenopausal women.

Source
–https://www.auanet.org/guidelines/recurrent-uti

Disorders of the Musculoskeletal System and Rheumatologic Disorders

27

Population
–Adults with ankylosing spondylitis (AS) or nonradiographic spondyloarthritis.

Organization
▶ ACR/Spondylitis Association of America/Spondyloarthritis Research and Treatment Network 2019

Recommendations
–Treat with scheduled NSAIDs and tumor necrosis factor inhibitor (TNFi) therapy.

–Add slow-acting antirheumatic drugs when TNFi medications are contraindicated. Do not coadminister.

–Do not discontinue/taper tapering biologic with stable disease.

–Use local parenteral corticosteroids for active sacroiliitis, active enthesitis, or peripheral arthritis for symptoms refractory to NSAIDs. Avoid systemic corticosteroid use.

–Refer to an ophthalmologist for concomitant iritis.

–Use TNFi monoclonal antibody therapy for AS with inflammatory bowel disease.

–Refer for a physical therapy program: active and weight-bearing; avoid spine manipulation.

–Do not routinely perform surveillance imaging of spine.

–Screen for fall risk, osteoporosis.

Sources
–Ward MM, Deodhar A, Akl EA, et al. American College of Rheumatology/Spondylitis Association of America/Spondyloarthritis Research and Treatment Network 2015 Recommendations for the treatment of ankylosing spondylitis and nonradiographic axial spondyloarthritis. *Arthritis Rheumatol.* 2016;68(2):282-298.

–rheumatology.org; 2019 Update of the American College of Rheumatology/Spondylitis Association of America/Spondyloarthritis Research and Treatment Network Recommendations for the Treatment of Ankylosing Spondylitis and Nonradiographic Axial Spondyloarthritis.

BACK PAIN, LOW

Population
–Adults.

Organizations
▶ ACP 2020, NICE 2020, ICSI 2018

Recommendations
–Consider various nonpharmacologic treatments for acute or subacute low-back pain including superficial heat, massage, exercise program, acupuncture, and spinal manipulation.
–For chronic low-back pain, start a trial of nonpharmacologic treatments including exercise, multidisciplinary rehabilitation, acupuncture, mindfulness-based stress reduction, tai chi, yoga, biofeedback, cognitive behavioral therapy, or spinal manipulation.
–Consider behavioral health referral for patients with a high disability and/or who experience significant psychological distress from their low-back pain.
–If pharmacologic treatments are needed, offer NSAIDs (topical or oral) or oral acetaminophen or skeletal muscle relaxants in the lowest effective dose for shortest period of time.

Organization	Guidance
GUIDELINES DISCORDANT: ROLE OF OPIATES IN LOW-BACK PAIN	
ACP	Use only if patients have failed all other therapies and only if the potential benefits outweigh the risks of dependency, addiction, overdose, and misuse
NICE	While weak opioids may be helpful in acute phase, do not routinely offer opioids for acute or chronic low-back pain
ICSI	Avoid opioids for acute and subacute low-back pain

–Consider epidural steroid injections as an adjunct for acute and subacute low-back pain with a radicular component. (ICSI)
–Avoid routine imaging (X-ray, CT, MRI) in patients with nonspecific or radicular low-back pain without red flag symptoms.
–Do not offer SSRI, SNRI, tricyclic antidepressants, or anticonvulsants for management of low-back pain. (NICE)
–Do not offer spinal fusion for low-back pain unless part of randomized controlled trial. (NICE)
–Do not offer orthotics such as belts, corsets, foot orthotics for low-back pain. (NICE)

Comments
1. Exercise guided by a physical therapist produces the best long-term results (NNT 7 for pain relief). NSAIDs are also effective (NNT=6) but only when taken. Duloxetine (NNT=10) and opioids (NNT=16) have benefits but also significant side effect profiles. Other interventions don't show consistent long-term benefit. (*Can Fam Physician.* 2021;67(1):e20–e30)
2. When using pharmacologic therapy, consider and counsel the patients on potential side effects.

3. While the guidelines recommend them, muscle relaxants do not improve functional outcomes or pain (*Ann Emerg Med.* 2019;74(4):512-520). If they are used, limit duration to <1 wk.
4. When using opiates, restrict duration to 7 d or less.
5. Topical NSAIDs with or without menthol gel were the most effective first-line therapy.
6. Epidural injections provide a small amount of immediate improvement in both back and leg pain and functional ability, but the benefits were no longer measurable after 2 wk according to a Cochrane review. (*Spine.* 2020;45(21):e1405-e1415)
7. Patients knowingly given placebo report improved pain and function. (*Pain.* 2019;160(12):2891-2897)

Sources

–http://guidelines.gov/summaries/summary/50781/noninvasive-treatments-for-acute-subacute-and-chronic-low-back-pain-a-clinical-practice-guideline-from-the-american-college-of-physicians?q=back+pain

–Qaseem A, Wilt TJ, McLean RM, Forciea MA, Clinical Guidelines Committee of the American College of Physicians. Noninvasive treatments for acute, subacute, and chronic low-back pain: a clinical practice guideline from the American College of Physicians. *Ann Intern Med.* 2017;166(7):514-530.

–Qaseem A, et al.; Clinical Guidelines Committee of the American College of Physicians. Nonpharmacologic and pharmacologic management of acute pain from non-low back, musculoskeletal injuries in adults: a clinical guideline from the American College of Physicians and American Academy of Family Physicians. *Ann Internal Med.* 2020;173(9).

–NICE practice guidelines: Low Back Pain; www.pathways.nice.org.uk/pathways/low-back-pain-and-sciatica/managing-low-back-pain-and-sciatica

–ICSI. *Adult Acute and Subacute Low Back Pain.* March 2018.

LUMBAR DISC HERNIATION

Population
–Adults.

Organization
▶ North American Spine Society 2012

Recommendations
–Offer transforaminal epidural steroid injection for short-term (2–4 wk) pain relief in selected patients.
–Insufficient evidence to recommend for or against the use of IV glucocorticoids, 5-ht receptor inhibitors, gabapentin, amitriptyline, and agmatine sulfate.
–Insufficient evidence to recommend for or against PT/exercise programs as a stand-alone treatment modality, but it is an option for patients with mild-to-moderate symptoms. There is insufficient evidence for traction therapy.
–Consider spinal manipulation as an option for symptomatic relief.
–Do not use TNFα inhibitors.

Source
–North American Spine Society. *Clinical Guidelines for Multidisciplinary Spine Care Diagnosis and Treatment of Lumbar Disc Herniation with Radiculopathy.* 2012.

ROTATOR CUFF TEARS

Population
–Adults.

Organization
▶ AAOS 2019

Recommendations
–Diagnose or stratify patients with suspected rotator cuff tears with a clinical examination. MRI, MRA, and ultrasound are useful adjuncts to clinical exam.
–Small-to-medium tears:
  • Offer physical therapy and/or operative treatment, as both result in significant improvement in patient-reported outcomes.
  • Do not use routine acromioplasty as a concomitant treatment.
–A single injection of corticosteroids with local anesthetic provides short-term improvement in pain and function. Avoid multiple steroid injections, as they may compromise the rotator cuff integrity and affect subsequent repair attempts.
–Limited evidence for the use of hyaluronic acid injections and platelet-rich plasma.
–Encourage early mobilization, as it improves postoperative clinical outcomes.

Source
–AAOS. *Management of Rotator Cuff Injuries Clinical Practice Guideline.* 2019.

BREAST CANCER FOLLOW-UP CARE

Population
–Early-stage women with curable breast cancer.

Organization
▶ American Society of Clinical Oncology (ASCO) 2013

Recommendation
–Careful history and physical examination every 3–6 mo for first 3 y after primary therapy (with or without adjuvant treatment), then every 6–12 mo for next 2 y, and then annually.
–Counsel patients about symptoms of recurrence including new lumps, bone pain, chest pain, dyspnea, abdominal pain, or persistent headaches.
–Counsel all women to perform monthly self-breast examinations.

–Mammography: order first posttreatment mammogram for women treated with breast-conserving therapy no earlier than 6 mo after radiation. Follow with surveillance mammograms every 6–12 mo, preferably annually mammograms are stable.

–Arrange regular pelvic examinations. Tamoxifen can increase risk of uterine cancer, and therefore patients should be advised to report any vaginal bleeding if they are taking tamoxifen.

–Do not routinely perform the following studies for the purpose of breast cancer surveillance:

- CBC and automated chemistry studies.
- Routine chest X-ray.
- Bone scans.
- Liver ultrasound.
- Routine CT scanning.
- Routine FDG-PET scanning.
- Breast MRI (unless patient has BRCA1 or BRCA2 mutation or previous mediastinal radiation at young age).
- Tumor markers including CA27.29, CA15-3, or CEA are not recommended for routine surveillance. (*JAMA*. 1994;27:1587-1592)

Comments

1. Risk of recurrence continues through more than 15 y, especially in woman who are hormone receptor positive. Establish continuity of care with physicians experienced in surveillance of patients and in breast examination. Follow-up by a primary care physician (PCP) leads to the same outcome as specialist follow-up. If the patient desires transfer of care to PCP, 1 y after definitive therapy is appropriate.

2. There is a significant difference in the behavior of hormone receptor (HR)-positive vs. HR-negative disease. HR-negative disease tends to recur earlier (2–3 y) than HR-positive breast cancer (>50% of relapses occur after 5 y). There is also a 3- to 4-fold increase in risk of brain metastasis in HR-negative women vs. HR-positive women.

3. HR-positive patients have a 4-fold increased risk of bone metastasis compared to HR-negative patients in whom metastases to liver, lung, and brain are more common. (*N Engl J Med.* 2007;357:39)

Sources
–*NCCN Guidelines*. 2015;BINV-16:27.
–*J Clin Oncol*. 2013;31:961-965.

GOUT

Population
–Adults with chronic gout.

Organization
▶ ACR 2020

Recommendations

- Primary goal is to minimize inflammation and discomfort for acute gout attacks and prevent future attacks. Future attacks are related to total body uric acid load; thus, urate-lowering therapy (ULT) starts with diet modification followed by pharmacologic interventions targeted to either reducing production or increasing excretion of urate.
- Diet: Limit purine, high-fructose corn syrup, and EtOH intake. Weight loss is beneficial. Do not offer vitamin C supplementation.
- Initiate ULT in the following patients:
  - For patients with frequent gout flares (≥ 2/y).
- For patients with 1 or more tophi.
- For patients with radiographic damage (ie, bony erosions) attributable to gout.
  - Do not initiate ULT for patients experiencing their first flare, unless they have CKD stage ≥ 3, serial serum urate (SU) > 9 mg/dL or urolithiasis.
- Use allopurinol as first-line agent for ULT. Use xanthine oxidase inhibitor over probenecid in CKD stage 3 or greater. Start allopurinol and febuxostat with low dose and titrate up. Do not start pegloticase as first-line therapy.
- Initiate anti-inflammatory prophylaxis concomitantly. Use agents such as colchicine, NSAIDs, or corticosteroids. Continue for 3–6 mo and consider extending as needed if the patient has more flares.
- For patients on ULT, use treat-to-target strategy of ULT dose guided by serial serum urate values with goal < 6 mg/dL.
- For patients where xanthine oxidase inhibitors have failed to achieve serum urate target and have flares or nonresolving tophi, switch to pegloticase. Do not do so if flares are infrequent (<2/y).
- In HTN management, change from hydrochlorothiazide to an alternate antihypertensive. Consider losartan. In HLD, do not add fenofibrate to treatment plan. Continue aspirin if indicated for other diagnoses.

Comments

1. Consider HLA-B*5801 prior to initiating allopurinol for pts of Southeast Asian and African descent. Do not test others.
2. In patients with prior allopurinol allergy, start allopurinol desensitization.
3. In patients with gout on febuxostat therapy with CVD or new CV event, switch to alternative ULT agent.

Source

- 2020 American College of Rheumatology Guideline for the Management of Gout; rhumatology.org/Portals/0/Files/Gout-Guideline-Final-2020.pdf

Population

- Adults experiencing acute gout attack.

Organizations

▶ ACR 2020, ACP 2017

Recommendations

–In acute gout flare, start oral colchicine (low dose), NSAIDs, or glucocorticoids. Topical ice can also be helpful.

–Corticosteroids should be considered first-line therapy in patients without contraindications. Prednisolone 35 mg orally for 5 d. (ACP)

Sources

–2020 American College of Rheumatology Guideline for the Management of Gout; rhumatology. org/Portals/0/Files/Gout-Guideline-Final-2020.pdf

–http://guidelines.gov/summaries/summary/50608/management-of-acute-and-recurrent-gout-a-clinical-practice-guideline-from-the-american-college-of-physicians?q=gout

–Qaseem A, Harris RP, Forciea MA; Clinical Guidelines Committee of the American College of Physicians. Management of acute and recurrent gout: a clinical practice guideline from the American College of Physicians. *Ann Intern Med*. 2017;166(1):58-68.

Population

–Adults with suspected gout.

Organization

▶ American College of Physicians 2017

Recommendation

–Clinicians should use synovial fluid analysis when diagnostic testing is necessary in patients with possible gout.

Sources

–http://guidelines.gov/summaries/summary/50607/diagnosis-of-acute-gout-a-clinical-practice-guideline-from-the-american-college-of-physicians?q=gout

–Qaseem A, McLean RM, Starkey M, Forciea MA; Clinical Guidelines Committee of the American College of Physicians. Diagnosis of acute gout: a clinical practice guideline from the American College of Physicians. *Ann Intern Med*. 2017;166(1):52-57.

HIP FRACTURES

Population

–Elderly patients with hip fractures.

Organization

▶ AAOS 2015

Recommendations

–Use preoperative pain control in patients with hip fractures.

–Perform hip fracture surgery within 48 h of admission.

–Do not delay hip fracture surgery for patients on antiplatelet drugs.

–Perform operative fixation for nondisplaced femoral neck fractures.

–Perform unipolar or hemipolar hemiarthroplasty for displaced femoral neck fractures.

–Arrange intensive physical therapy post-discharge to improve functional outcomes.

–Evaluate all patients who have sustained a hip fracture for osteoporosis.

Source

–AAOS.org: Management of hip Fractures in the Elderly, Evidence-Based Clinical Practice Guideline. aaos.org/globalassets/quality-and-practice-resources/hip-fractures-in-the-elderly

MUSCLE CRAMPS

Population

–Patients with idiopathic muscle cramps.

Organization

▶ AAN 2010

Recommendations

–Consider vitamin B complex, naftidrofuryl, and calcium channel blockers (diltiazem), as they may be effective.

–Data are insufficient on the efficacy of calf stretching in reducing the frequency of muscle cramps.

–AAN recommends that although quinine is likely effective, it should not be used for routine treatment of cramps because of toxicity potential. Reserve quinine derivatives for disabling muscle cramps and monitor dosing carefully. Quinine derivatives are effective in reducing the frequency of muscle cramps, although the magnitude of benefit is smaller than the serious side effects.

Source

–Katzberg HD, Khan AH, So YT. Assessment: symptomatic treatment for muscle cramps (an evidence-based review): report of the Therapeutics and Technology Assessment Subcommittee of the American Academy of Neurology. *Neurology*. 2010;74(8):691-696.

OSTEOARTHRITIS (OA)

Population

–Adults with osteoarthritis.

Organizations

▶ ACR 2019, NICE 2014

Recommendations

–Evaluate ability to perform activities of daily living (ADLs) and teach joint-protection techniques. Provide assistive devices to help perform ADLs including splints for trapeziometacarpal joint OA.

–Strongly recommend exercise and weight loss in overweight and obese patients. Provide information regarding self-efficacy and self-management programs.

–Exercise is a core treatment to include muscle strengthening and general aerobic fitness including aquatic training.

–Refer to physical therapy and/or occupational therapy.

–Consider balance exercises, yoga, tai chi, cognitive behavioral therapy, kinesiotaping, aquatic exercises, medially directed patellar taping.

–Treat pharmacologically with oral NSAIDs, topical NSAIDs, oral acetaminophen, and intra-articular glucocorticoid injections of the knee. Topical capsaicin, acetaminophen, duloxetine, and tramadol are other helpful pharmacologic modalities.

–Consider nonpharmacologic modalities including thermal treatment and radiofrequency ablation for the knee, using canes or braces.

–Consider referral for joint surgery for people with OA and severe joint symptoms refractory to nonsurgical treatments.

–Avoid arthroscopic lavage and debridement unless knee OA with mechanical locking.

Comment

1. Do *not* use the following for OA:
   a. Chondroitin sulfate.
   b. Glucosamine.
   c. Opiates (if possible).
   d. Acupuncture.
   e. Intra-articular hyaluronan.
2. For chronic NSAID use, consider concomitant medical therapy to prevent NSAID-induced ulcers. Avoid long-term PPI use.
3. For knee osteoarthritis, physical therapy produces better long-term outcomes than corticosteroid joint injection, though both provide good short-term effect. (*N Engl J Med.* 2020;382(15):1420-1429)

Sources

–http://www.rheumatology.org/practice/clinical/guidelines/PDFs/ACR_OA_Guidelines_FINAL.pdf

–ACR. *American College of Rheumatology/Arthritis Foundation Guideline for the Management of Osteoarthritis of the hand, Hip, and Knee.* 2019; rheumatology.org/Portals/o/Files/Osteoarthritis-Guideline

–https://guidelines.gov/summaries/summary/47862

Population

–Adults with osteoarthritis of the hip.

Organization

▶ AAOS 2017

Recommendations

–NSAIDs improve short-term pain, function, or both in patients with symptomatic hip OA.

–Avoid glucosamine sulfate for improving function, reducing stiffness, and decreasing pain associated with hip OA.

–Offer intra-articular corticosteroids to improve function and reduce pain in the short-term for symptomatic hip OA.

–Do not offer intra-articular hyaluronic acid to improve function, reducing stiffness, and reducing pain associated with hip OA.

–Recommend physical therapy to improve function and reduce pain in hip OA associated with mild-to-moderate symptoms.

–Recommend postoperative physical therapy to improve early function for those who have undergone total hip arthroplasty.

▼ OSTEOPOROSIS

Population
–Adults at risk for osteoporosis or who have confirmed osteoporosis.

Organizations
▶ ICSI 2011, ACP 2017, AACE 2020

Recommendations
–Evaluate all patients with a low-impact fracture for osteoporosis.

–Advise smoking cessation and alcohol moderation (≤2 drinks/d).

–Advise 1500-mg elemental calcium daily for established osteoporosis, glucocorticoid therapy, or age >65 y.

–Assess for vitamin D deficiency with a 25-hydroxy vitamin D level.
  • Treat vitamin D deficiency if present.

–Advise active lifestyle; weight-bearing exercise, balance training, and resistance exercise.

–Treatment of osteoporosis.
  • Bisphosphonate therapy.
  • Consider estrogen therapy in menopausal women <50 y of age.
  • Consider parathyroid hormone in women with very high risk for fracture.
  • Treat osteoporotic women with pharmacologic therapy for 5 y. Do not monitor bone density during this time.
  • Offer pharmacologic treatment with bisphosphonates to reduce vertebral fracture risk in men with clinically recognized osteoporosis.

–Fall prevention program.
  • Home safety evaluation.
  • Avoid medications that can cause sedation and orthostatic hypotension or affect balance.
  • Assistive walking devices as necessary; physical therapy.

Comments
1. Measure serial heights for all patients and observe for kyphosis.
2. Obtain a lateral vertebral assessment with DXA scan or X-ray if height loss exceeds 4 cm.
3. Repeat DXA bone mineral densitometry no more than every 12–24 mo.

Sources

–https://www.icsi.org/_asset/vnw0c3/Osteo.pdf

–ACP. *Treatment of Low Bone Density or Osteoporosis to Prevent Fractures in Men and Women: A Clinical Practice Guideline Update from the American College of Physicians.* 2017.

Population

–Postmenopausal women.

Organizations

▶ NAMS 2010, AACE 2020, ACOG 2012, ACP 2017

Recommendations

–Recommend maintaining a healthy weight, eating a balanced diet, avoiding excessive alcohol intake, limit caffeine intake, avoiding cigarette smoking, and utilizing measures to avoid falls.

–Recommend supplemental calcium 1200 mg/d and vitamin D_3 1000–4000 international units (IU)/d.

–Recommend an annual check of height and weight and assess for chronic back pain.

–DXA of the hip, femoral neck, and lumbar spine should be measured in women age ≥65 y or postmenopausal women with a risk factor for osteoporosis.[1]

–Recommend repeat DXA testing every 1–2 y for women taking therapy for osteoporosis and every 2–5 y for untreated postmenopausal women.

–Recommend against measurement of biochemical markers of bone turnover.

–Recommend drug therapy for osteoporosis for:

  • Osteoporotic vertebral or hip fracture.

  • DXA with T score ≤ –2.5.

  • DXA with T score ≤ –1 to –2.4 and a 10-y risk of major osteoporotic fracture of ≥20% or hip fracture ≥3% based on FRAX calculator. Available at http://www.shef.ac.uk/FRAX/ or other fracture risk tool.

–Consider the use of hip protectors in women at high risk of falling.

–Avoid menopausal estrogen therapy, estrogen + progesterone therapy, or raloxifene for osteoporosis treatment.

–For patients with significant kyphosis, gait instability, back discomfort, order physical therapy to focus on weight-bearing exercises, back strengthening, balance training.

Comments

1. Options for osteoporosis drug therapy:
   a. Bisphosphonates:
      i. First-line therapy.
      ii. Options include alendronate, ibandronate, risedronate, or zoledronic acid.
      iii. Potential risk for jaw osteonecrosis (uncommon, educate on ONJ risk compared to fracture risk for shared decision-making).

---

[1]Previous fracture after menopause, weight <127 lb, BMI <21 kg/m^2, parent with a history of hip fracture, current smoker, rheumatoid arthritis, or excessive alcohol intake.

      iv. Bisphosphonate holiday may be considered: 5 y if on oral and 3 y if on IV medications; higher risk patients consider 10 y and 6 y; optimal bisphosphonate holiday has not been confirmed.

b. Denosumab: Consider for women at high fracture risk; also potential risk for osteonecrosis.

c. Raloxifene: Second-line agent in younger women with osteoporosis.

d. Teriparatide is an option for high fracture risk or abaloparatide. Therapy should not exceed 24 mo for teraparatide or abaloparatide.

e. Calcitonin:

      i. Third-line therapy for osteoporosis; not recommended for long-term treatment.

      ii. May be used for bone pain from acute vertebral compression fractures.

f. Romosozumab: this anabolic, sclerostin inhibitor has been FDA approved in 2019 for high-risk patients, used for 1 year followed by maintenance pharmacologic agent. Avoid in patients with high-risk cardiovascular or recent MI.

2. Use vitamin D therapy to maintain 25-OH vitamin D level > 30 ng/mL (prefer 30–50 ng/mL).

3. Exercises include weight-bearing exercise plus back and posture exercises.

Sources

–http://www.guidelines.gov/content.aspx?id=15500

–http://www.guidelines.gov/content.aspx?id=38413

–Camacho PM, et al. American Association of Clinical Endocrinologist American College of Endocrinology Clinical Practice Guidelines for the Diagnosis and Treatment of Postmenopausal Osteoporosis. *Endocr Pract*. 2020. AACE 2020.

RHEUMATOID ARTHRITIS (RA), BIOLOGIC DISEASE-MODIFYING ANTIRHEUMATIC DRUGS (DMARDS)

Population

–Adults.

Organization

▶ ACR 2021

Recommendations

–DMARDs (biologics or tofacitinib) and tuberculosis (TB) screening:

• Check a TB skin test or IGRA before initiating these medications.

• Any patient with latent TB needs at least 1 mo treatment prior to the initiation of a biologic or tofacitinib.

–Symptomatic early RA:

• If the disease activity is low, and the patient is naïve to DMARD therapy, use DMARD monotherapy (methotrexate [MTX] preferred) over double or triple therapy.

• If the disease activity is moderate or high, and the patient is naïve to DMARD therapy, use DMARD monotherapy over double or triple therapy.

• If the disease activity remains moderate or high despite DMARD monotherapy (with or without glucocorticoids), use combination DMARDs, a TNFi, or a non-TNF biologic (all with or without MTX).

- If disease flares, add short-term glucocorticoids at the lowest dose and for the shortest duration possible.

−Established RA:

- If disease activity is low and the patient is naïve to DMARD, use DMARD monotherapy (MTX preferred), over TNFi.
- If disease activity is moderate to high and the patient is naïve to DMARD, use DMARD monotherapy (MTX preferred), over tofacitinib and combination DMARD therapy.
- If disease activity remains moderate or high despite DMARD monotherapy, use combination DMARDs, add a TNFi, non-TNF biologic, or tofacitinib (all with or without MTX).

Comments

1. Anti-TNFα agents, abatacept, and rituximab all contraindicated in:
   a. Serious bacterial, fungal, and viral infections, or with latent TB.
   b. Acute viral hepatitis or Child's B or Child's C cirrhosis.
   c. Instances of a lymphoproliferative disorder treated ≤5 y ago; decompensated congestive heart failure (CHF); or any demyelinating disorder.
   d. CBCD, LFTs, and Cr should be monitored every 2–4 wk during the first 3 mo, every 8–12 wk during the next 3–6 mo, and every 12 wk thereafter for patients on leflunomide, MTX, and sulfasalazine. Only baseline levels are recommended for hydroxychloroquine.
   e. Live attenuated vaccines, if indicated, can be given prior to initiating therapy with TNFi biologics or non-TNF biologics. A 2-wk waiting period is recommended before starting biologics. Live attenuated vaccines are not recommended during therapy with biologics.

Source

−ACR. American College of Rheumatology Guideline for the Treatment of Rheumatoid Arthritis. *Arthritis Care Res.* 2021.

POLYMYALGIA RHEUMATICA

Population

−Adults diagnosed with PMR.

Organization

▶ ACR 2015

Recommendations

−Choose glucocorticoid therapy over NSAIDs to treat PMR.
−Initiate glucocorticoids at a minimum dose of 12.5–25 mg prednisone equivalent daily as initial treatment. Avoid doses ≤7.5 mg/d or >30 mg/d.
−Duration of glucocorticoids will be individualized, but a minimum of 12 mo of therapy is assumed. Tapering schedules should be customized based on regular monitoring of disease activity, lab markers, and adverse effects.

–Consider addition of MTX in patients at high risk of relapse, prolonged therapy, or glucocorticoid-related adverse events (due to comorbidities, concomitant medications).

–Avoid TNFα-blocking agents.

–Consider an individualized exercise program targeting maintenance of muscle mass/function and reducing fall risk.

–Avoid the use of Chinese herbal preparations Yanghe and Biqi.

Source

–ACR. Recommendations for the management of polymyalgia rheumatica. *Arthritis Rheumatol.* 2015(67):2569-2580.

SYSTEMIC LUPUS ERYTHEMATOSUS (SLE, LUPUS)

Population

–Adults.

Organization

▶ British Society for Rheumatology (BSR) 2017, EULAR/ACR 2019

Recommendations

–Diagnose lupus in patients with 4 or more of the following symptoms/findings, with at least 1 serological finding and 1 clinical finding, either contemporaneously or sequentially at any time:

- Malar rash.
- Discoid rash.
- Photosensitivity.
- Oral or nasal ulcers.
- Inflammatory arthritis.
- Serositis (ie, pleural effusion, pericardial effusion, pericarditis).
- Renal dysfunction (ie, proteinuria >500 mg/d, cellular casts, lupus nephritis).
- Neurologic dysfunction (ie, severe headache, altered mental status, seizures, psychosis, mononeuritis multiplex, myelitis, peripheral or cranial neuropathy).
- Hematologic dysfunction (ie, hemolytic anemia, WBC < 4000, lymphocytes < 1500, platelets < 100,000).
- Autoimmune dysfunction (ie, positive anti-dsDNA Ab, anti-Sm Ab, lupus anticoagulant test, anticardiolipin or false-positive syphilis FTA; lowered C3/C4).
- Antinuclear antibody (ANA) positivity.

–Mild disease (SLEDAI-2K <6, BILAG C) is characterized by fatigue, malar rash, diffuse alopecia, oral ulcers, arthralgias, myalgias, or platelets 50,000–150,000.

- Acute treatment: Prednisone ≤20 mg daily, hydroxychloroquine ≤6.5 mg/kg/d, MTX 7.5–15 mg/wk, and/or NSAIDs.
- Maintenance treatment: Prednisone ≤7.5 mg/d, hydroxychloroquine 200 mg/d, and/or MTX 10 mg/wk.

–Moderate disease (SLEDAI-2K 6–12, BILAG B) represents potential permanent damage, with fever, rash up to 22% of body surface area, cutaneous vasculitis, alopecia with scalp inflammation, arthritis, pleurisy, pericarditis, hepatitis, or platelets 25,000–50,000.

- Acute treatment: Prednisone ≤0.5 mg/kg/d AND (azathioprine 1.5–2.0 mg/kg/d OR MTX 10–25 mg/wk OR mycophenolate mofetil 2–3 g/d OR cyclosporin ≤2.0 mg/kg/d).
- Maintenance treatment: Prednisone ≤7.5 mg/d AND azathioprine 50–100 mg/d) OR MTX 10 mg/wk OR mycophenolate mofetil 1 g/d OR (cyclosporin 50–100 mg/d AND hydroxychloroquine 200 mg/d).

–Severe disease (SLEDAI-2K >12 or BILAG A) represents organ or life-threatening disease, with rash involving more than 22% of body surface area, myositis, severe pleurisy, and/or pericarditis with effusion, ascites, enteritis, myelopathy, psychosis, acute confusion, optic neuritis, or platelets <25,000.

- Acute treatment: prednisone ≤0.5 mg/kg/d and/or IV methylprednisolone 500 mg × 1–3 OR prednisone ≤0.75–1 mg/kg/d and azathioprine 2–3 mg/kg/d OR mycophenolate mofetil 2–3 g/d OR cyclosporin 2.5 mg/kg/d.
- Maintenance treatment: prednisone 7.5 mg/d AND mycophenolate mofetil 1.0–1.5 g/d OR azathioprine 50–100 mg/d OR cyclosporin 50–100 mg/d and hydroxychloroquine 200 mg/d.

–Consider rituximab and belimumab in patients who do not respond to the regimens above. Consider rituximab especially for patients with severe renal or CNS flare (SLEDAI ≥10). Belimumab is specifically approved for use with antibody positive SLE (anti-dsDNA).

–IVIG and plasmapheresis may be considered in patients with refractory cytopenias, thrombotic thrombocytopenia purpura (TTP), rapid deteriorating acute confusional state, and catastrophic antiphospholipid antibody syndrome.

–Aim to reduce and stop drugs except hydroxychloroquine eventually when in stable remission.

–Test for TPMT (thiopurine S-methyltransferase) activity prior to starting azathioprine:

- Very low levels of TPMT activity are associated with life-threatening bone marrow toxicity.

–Assess blood counts weekly as azathioprine doses are increased.

–Measure serum immunoglobulins prior to starting mycophenolate mofetil, cyclosporin, and rituximab, 3–6 mo later and then annually.

–Screen for chronic infections (tuberculosis, hepatitis B, hepatitis C, HIV, and HPV) prior to starting immunosuppressive therapy.

–Encourage high-SPF UV-A and UV-B sunscreen use for patients with photosensitivity symptoms.

–In patients with stable/low-activity disease, assess the following every 6–12 mo:

- Vital signs, vaccination status, modifiable risk factors (hypertension, hyperlipidemia, diabetes, obesity, tobacco use).
- Blood count, renal function, liver function, vitamin D3, anti-dsDNA titer, C3/C4 level, urinalysis.
- Disease activity using standardized questionnaire (eg, BILAG, SLEDAI, or SLICCC/ACR scores).
- Quality of life using standardized questionnaire (eg, Short-form 36 or LupusQoL).

–In patients with active disease, assess the following every 1–3 mo:
- Blood count, renal function, liver function, creatine, anti-dsDNA titer, C3/C4 level, urinalysis.

–Check anti-Ro and anti-La antibodies prior to pregnancy as these are associated with neonatal lupus/conduction defects.

Comments

1. 5% of the general population will have a positive ANA; 95% of patients with SLE will have a positive ANA.
2. Do not routinely test for ANA or other autoimmune antibodies unless the patient has other signs/symptoms of SLE and a positive result would therefore be diagnostically helpful as non-specific ANA positivity is not uncommon in the general population.
3. Be aware that leukopenia and neutropenia are common in SLE and may therefore be indicative of active disease or a medication side effective.
4. Cyclosporin and tacrolimus may be particularly useful in patients with cytopenias as these medications exhibit this side effect less frequently.
5. Infections, cardiovascular disease, and malignancy are the leading causes of death in patients with SLE.
6. Consider the etiology of an acute flare when treating it. Common causes include medication nonadherence, exposure to sunlight, concurrent or recent infection, hormonal changes, or recent medication changes.
7. CRP is often normal or only mildly elevated in SLE, even with arthritis or serositis. ESR is more sensitive but also not specific.
8. Rising anti-dsDNA antibodies and falling, low complement levels are associated with an acute flare.
9. 40% of patients with SLE, however, don't have positive anti-dsDNA antibodies.
10. ANA, anti-Sm, and anti-RNP antibodies do not fluctuate with disease intensity.

Source

–*Rheumatology*. 2018;57(1):e1-e45. https://doi.org/10.1093/rheumatology/kex286

Neurologic Disorders

28

BELL'S PALSY

Population
–Adults with Bell's palsy.

Organization
▶ AAN 2012

Recommendation
–For patients with recent-onset Bell's palsy (<72 h of symptoms):
- Give steroids (prednisone 1 mg/kg PO daily × 7 d) to increase probability of facial nerve recovery.
- Consider antivirals (eg, acyclovir or valacyclovir) × 7 d.

Comment
1. Antivirals may have a marginal effect on facial nerve recovery when added to steroids, so counsel patients regarding the questionable benefit of antivirals if offered.

Source
–https://n.neurology.org/content/79/22/2209.short

Population
–Adults and children with Bell's palsy.

Organization
▶ AAO 2013

Recommendations
–Do not routinely obtain lab studies, diagnostic imaging, or electrodiagnostic testing for Bell's palsy. Consider Lyme disease (neuroborreliosis) testing in children <15 y.
–Do not routinely obtain diagnostic imaging for straightforward Bell's palsy.
–If presenting within 72 h of symptoms, give steroids with or without antiviral medications to patients 16 y and older.
–Do not use antiviral monotherapy.
–Arrange eye protection for patients with incomplete eye closure.
–Do not use physical therapy or acupuncture for Bell's palsy.

Comment

1. 2019 Cochrane analysis found no benefit from adding antivirals to corticosteroids vs. corticosteroid monotherapy (https://doi.org/ 10.1002/14651858.CD001869.pub9)

Source

—https://pubmed.ncbi.nlm.nih.gov/24189771/

CONCUSSIONS

Population

–Children and young adults.

Organizations

▶ CDC 2016, ACEP 2016, AAN 2013

Recommendations

–Obtain noncontrast CT indicated for loss of consciousness or post-traumatic amnesia. There is no evidence to prefer MRI over CT.

–Use standardized sideline assessment tools to assess athletes with suspected concussions.

–Educate all patients about concussions and post-concussive syndrome. Use tools such as the Acute Concussion Evaluation (ACE) care plan developed by Gioia and Collins to guide follow-up management.

–Immediately remove from play any athlete with a suspected concussion.

–Do not permit an athlete to return to play until he/she has been cleared to play by a licensed health care professional.

Sources

–https://www.cdc.gov/traumaticbraininjury/pdf/tbi_clinicians_factsheet-a.pdf

–https://www.cdc.gov/headsup/pdfs/providers/ACE_care_plan_returning_to_work-a.pdf

–https://www.aan.com/Guidelines/home/GuidelineDetail/582

DELIRIUM

Population

–Adults age ≥18 y in the hospital or in long-term care facilities.

Organization

▶ NICE 2019

Recommendations

–Perform a short Confusion Assessment Method (CAM) screen to confirm the diagnosis of delirium.

–Include the following when managing delirium:
  • Treat the underlying cause.

- Provide frequent reorientation and reassurance to patients and their families.
- Provide cognitively stimulating activities.
- Ensure adequate hydration.
- Provide adequate oxygenation.
- Prevent constipation.
- Ensure early mobilization.
- Provide adequate pain control.
- Provide hearing aids or corrective lenses if sensory impairment is present.
- Promote good sleep hygiene.
  –Avoid Foley catheter.
  –Avoid benzodiazepines.
  –Avoid drugs with anticholinergic side effect profiles.
  - Consider short-term antipsychotic use (<1 wk) for patients who are distressed or considered at risk to themselves or others.
  - Use antipsychotic drugs with caution or not at all for people with conditions such as Parkinson's disease or dementia with Lewy bodies.

Comments

1. Older adults and people with dementia, severe illness, or a hip fracture are more at risk for developing delirium.
2. The prevalence of delirium in people on medical wards in hospital is about 20%–30%, and 10%–50% of people having surgery develop delirium. In long-term care the prevalence is under 20%.
3. Do not use physical restraints for behavioral control in elderly patients with delirium.
4. Delirium can appear both hyperactive and hypoactive, with the above prevalence ensure vigilance when caring for hospitalized, surgical, and long-term care patients..

Sources

–http://www.nice.org.uk/nicemedia/live/13060/49909/49909.pdf
–https://www.hospitalelderlifeprogram.org/uploads/disclaimers/Long_CAM_Training_Manual_10-9-14.pdf
–http://www.choosingwisely.org/societies/american-geriatrics-society/

EPILEPSY

Population

–Children and adults with suspected epilepsy (see "Seizures" section on first-time seizures).

Organization

▶ NICE 2021, ACR 2020

Recommendations

–Educate adults about all aspects of epilepsy.
–Refer to an epilepsy specialist to confirm diagnosis of epilepsy.

–Evaluate epilepsy with the following studies:
- Electroencephalogram (EEG).
- Sleep-deprived EEG if standard EEG is inconclusive.
- Neuroimaging to evaluate for any structural brain abnormalities (see below for appropriate imaging guidance).
- MRI is preferred for children <2 y, adults, refractory seizures, and focal seizures.
- Chemistry panel.
- ECG in adults.
- Urine toxicology screen.

–Imaging may include CT or MRI, typically without contrast, and is typically only necessary if there is a change in semiology or symptoms.
- CT without contrast, MRI without contrast, or MRI with and without contrast is typically appropriate.
- If tumor history, an MRI with contrast or MRI with and without is typically more appropriate.
- For surgical candidates and/or planning, an MRI with contrast, MRI with and without contrast, or FDG-PET/CT brain is usually more appropriate.

–Start antiepileptic drugs (AED) only after the diagnosis of epilepsy is made.

–Do not use valproate in pregnancy. If used in girls and women of childbearing potential, a pregnancy prevention plan must be in place.
- Focal seizures:
  ◦ Carbamazepine.
  ◦ Lamotrigine.
  ◦ Adjunctive AED: levetiracetam, oxcarbazepine, or sodium valproate.
- Generalized tonic–clonic seizures:
  ◦ Sodium valproate.
  ◦ Lamotrigine.
  ◦ Carbamazepine.
  ◦ Oxcarbazepine.
  ◦ Adjunctive AED: levetiracetam or topiramate.
- Absence seizures:
  ◦ Ethosuximide.
  ◦ Sodium valproate.
  ◦ Alternative: lamotrigine.
- Myoclonic seizures:
  ◦ Sodium valproate.
  ◦ Alternatives: levetiracetam or topiramate.

Comment

1. AEDs can decrease the efficacy of combined oral contraceptive pills.

Sources

–http://www.guidelines.gov/content.aspx?id=36082
–https://www.nice.org.uk/guidance/cg137

HEADACHE, MIGRAINE ACUTE TREATMENT

Population

–Adults.

Organization

▶ American Headache Society 2019

Recommendations

–Treat migraines at the first sign of pain.

–For mild-to-moderate attacks, use nonsteroidal anti-inflammatory drugs (NSAIDs), nonopioid analgesics, acetaminophen, or combinations such as aspirin + acetaminophen + caffeine.

–For moderate or severe attacks or milder attacks that fail initial therapy, use triptans or ergotamine derivatives. Antiemetics and IV magnesium (in migraine with aura) are also likely effective.

Source

–*Headache* 2019;59:1-18.

Population

–Children and adolescents.

Organization

▶ AAN 2019

Recommendations

–Diagnostic criteria for pediatric migraine:

• At least 5 headaches over the past year that lasted 2–72 h when untreated.

• Associated with nausea, vomiting, photophobia, or phonophobia.

• 2 of 4 additional features:

○ Pulsatile quality.

○ Unilateral.

○ Worsening with activity or limiting activity.

○ Moderate to severe in intensity.

–Early treatment of migraine (within <1 h of headache onset) improves pain-free rates.

–Offer nonprescription oral analgesics like acetaminophen, ibuprofen, and naproxen.

–Consider triptans, though they are less commonly prescribed in children than in adults.

• Agents FDA-approved for children: almotriptan (age ≥12 y), rizatriptan (age 6–17 y), sumatriptan/naproxen (aged ≥12 y), and zolmitriptan NS (age ≥12 y).

• If incomplete response to triptan, add NSAID (ibuprofen or naproxen).

• Do not prescribe triptans to those with history of ischemic vascular disease or accessory conduction pathway disorders, as the medication can exacerbate these disorders.

• Timing: taking triptan during a typical aura is safe, but it may be more effective if taken at onset of head pain.

–If HA is successfully treated with acute medication but recurs within 24 h, repeat the initial treatment.

–If prominent nausea or vomiting, offer antiemetics.

–Ergots have not been studied in children.

–Consider referral to headache specialist if hemiplegic migraine, migraine with brainstem aura who do not respond to initial treatments.

Sources

–*Neurology* 2019;93:487-499.

HEADACHE, NONMIGRAINE

Population

–Adults.

Organization

▶ ICSI 2011

Recommendations

–The following algorithms detail diagnosis and management pathways for headache disorders in adults.

Source

–Beithon J, Gallenberg M, Johnson K, et al.; Institute for Clinical Systems Improvement. *Diagnosis and Treatment of Headache.* Updated 2011.

HEADACHE DIAGNOSIS ALGORITHM—ICSI 2011

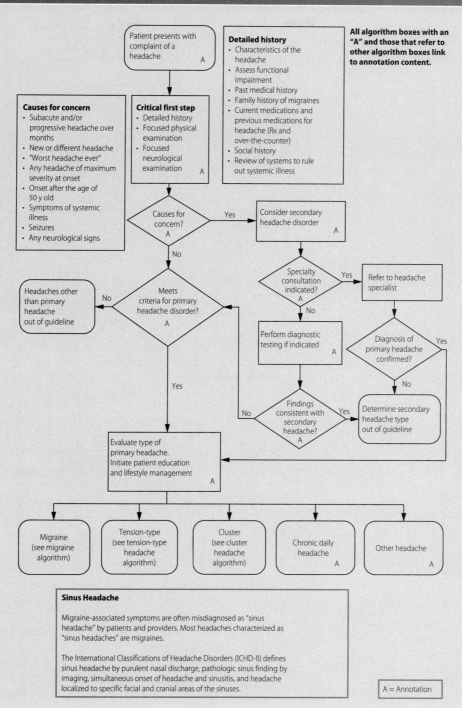

Patient presents with complaint of a headache A

Detailed history
- Characteristics of the headache
- Assess functional impairment
- Past medical history
- Family history of migraines
- Current medications and previous medications for headache (Rx and over-the-counter)
- Social history
- Review of systems to rule out systemic illness

All algorithm boxes with an "A" and those that refer to other algorithm boxes link to annotation content.

Causes for concern
- Subacute and/or progressive headache over months
- New or different headache
- "Worst headache ever"
- Any headache of maximum severity at onset
- Onset after the age of 50 y old
- Symptoms of systemic illness
- Seizures
- Any neurological signs

Critical first step
- Detailed history
- Focused physical examination
- Focused neurological examination A

Causes for concern? A

Yes → Consider secondary headache disorder A

No

Meets criteria for primary headache disorder? A

No → Headaches other than primary headache out of guideline

Specialty consultation indicated? A

Yes → Refer to headache specialist

No

Perform diagnostic testing if indicated A

Diagnosis of primary headache confirmed?

Yes

No → Determine secondary headache type out of guideline

Findings consistent with secondary headache? A

No

Yes → Determine secondary headache type out of guideline

Yes

Evaluate type of primary headache. Initiate patient education and lifestyle management A

- Migraine (see migraine algorithm)
- Tension-type (see tension-type headache algorithm)
- Cluster (see cluster headache algorithm)
- Chronic daily headache A
- Other headache A

Sinus Headache

Migraine-associated symptoms are often misdiagnosed as "sinus headache" by patients and providers. Most headaches characterized as "sinus headaches" are migraines.

The International Classifications of Headache Disorders (ICHD-II) defines sinus headache by purulent nasal discharge, pathologic sinus finding by imaging, simultaneous onset of headache and sinusitis, and headache localized to specific facial and cranial areas of the sinuses.

A = Annotation

TENSION-TYPE HEADACHE ALGORITHM—ICSI 2011

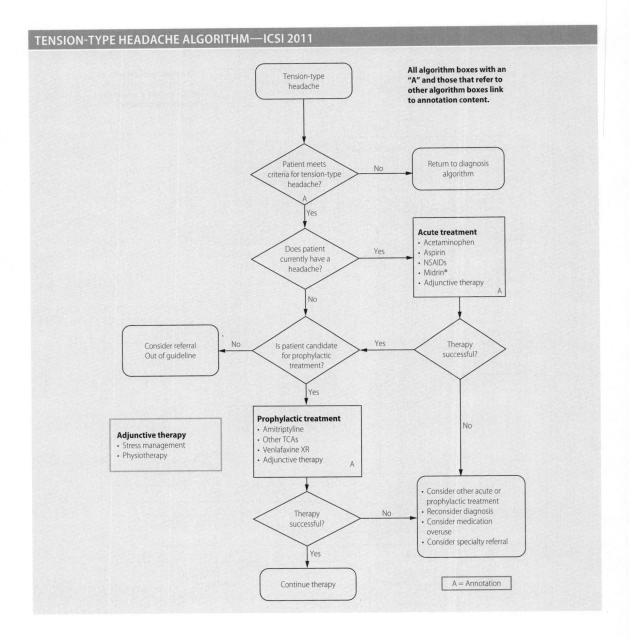

Tension-type headache

All algorithm boxes with an "A" and those that refer to other algorithm boxes link to annotation content.

Patient meets criteria for tension-type headache?
A
No → Return to diagnosis algorithm
Yes

Does patient currently have a headache?
Yes → **Acute treatment**
- Acetaminophen
- Aspirin
- NSAIDs
- Midrin®
- Adjunctive therapy
A
No

Therapy successful?
Yes →

Is patient candidate for prophylactic treatment?
No → Consider referral Out of guideline
Yes
No →

Prophylactic treatment
- Amitriptyline
- Other TCAs
- Venlafaxine XR
- Adjunctive therapy
A

Adjunctive therapy
- Stress management
- Physiotherapy

Therapy successful?
No →
- Consider other acute or prophylactic treatment
- Reconsider diagnosis
- Consider medication overuse
- Consider specialty referral
Yes

Continue therapy

A = Annotation

CLUSTER HEADACHE ALGORITHM—ICSI 2011

All algorithm boxes with an "A" and those that refer to other algorithm boxes link to annotation content.

Cluster headache

Patient meets criteria for cluster headache?
A

No → Return to diagnosis algorithm

Yes

Is patient currently in a cluster cycle?

No →
- Reinforce patient education
- Consider pre-cluster cycle specialty consult

Yes

Acute treatment
- Oxygen
- Sumatriptan SQ
- DHE
- Start prophylactic treatment
A

Bridging treatment
- Corticosteroids
- Ergotamine
- Occipital nerve block
A

Maintenance treatment
- Verapamil (first-line)
- Avoid alcohol consumption during cluster cycle

- Verapamil-high doses
- Steroids and others
- Lithium
- Depakote
- Topiramate
A

A = Annotation

Therapy successful?

No →
- Continue and modify acute treatment
- Continue and modify prophylactic therapy
- Consider referral

Yes

Continue therapy through cycle, then taper

← Yes — Therapy successful? — No → Consider referral/ Out of guideline

HEADACHE, MIGRAINE PROPHYLAXIS

Population
–Adults.

Organization
▶ American Headache Society 2019

Recommendations
–Diagnose migraine using ICHD-3 criteria (Table 28-1).
–Offer prophylaxis if frequent attacks that interfere with regular routines and treatments fail or are overused (ie, used 10+ d/mo).
  • Frequency: offer ppx if 6+ headache days per month, 4+ days per month with some disability, or 3+ days per month with severe disability. May consider for interested patients with lower headache frequency.
–Offer a prevention agent with established efficacy, starting at a low dose and titrate gradually to response or intolerance. Give a trial of at least 8 wk at target dose, and set expectations that a 50% reduction in headache days or a decrease in severity are the goals of therapy. Consider combination therapy if incomplete response. These agents include:
  • Antiepileptics: divalproex sodium, valproate sodium, topiramate.
  • Beta-blockers: metoprolol, propranolol, timolol.
  • Triptans: frovatriptan (only for short-term prevention of menstrual migraine).
  • Onabotulinumtoxin A.

TABLE 28-1 INTERNATIONAL CLASSIFICATION OF HEADACHE DISORDERS CRITERIA FOR MIGRAINE
Episodic
Five attacks with the following criteria, not explained by another condition:
–Duration 4-72 h untreated. –≥ 2 of the following characteristics: unilateral location, pulsating quality, moderate or severe intensity, aggravated by (or causing avoidance of) routine physical activity –Nausea, vomiting, or photophobia and phonophobia
Chronic
≥ 15 d/mo for >3 mo of migraine or tension-type HA H/o at least 5 episodic migraine attacks ≥ 8 d/mo with ≥ 2 of the following characteristics: unilateral location, pulsating quality, moderate or severe intensity, aggravated by (or causing avoidance of) routine physical activity plus duration 4–72 h if migraine with aura or nausea, vomiting or photo/phonophobia if migraine without aura, that patient believes to be a migraine and gets relief from triptan or ergot derivative

–Consider agents with probable effectiveness:
- Antidepressants: amitriptyline, venlafaxine.
- Beta-blockers: atenolol, nadolol.

–If the above are ineffective or if the patient prefers, consider an agent with a single small study of effectiveness: lisinopril, clonidine, guanfacine, carbamazepine, nebivolol, pindolol, cyproheptadine, candesartan.

–Data is insufficient to recommend novel injectable biologic agents for prophylaxis, as they lack long-term safety data and carry uncertain cost-effectiveness.

Source
–*Headache* 2019;59:1-18.

HEADACHE, RADIOLOGY EVALUATION

Population
–Adults.

Organization
▶ ACR 2019

Recommendations
–No imaging:
- Uncomplicated headaches.
- New primary migraine or tension-type headache, with normal neurologic examination.
- In the initial assessment of chronic headache, without new features or neurologic deficit.

–Urgent red flag symptoms require prompt evaluation:
- Signs of systemic illness in the patient with new-onset headache.
- New headache in patients over 50 y of age with symptoms of temporal arteritis.
- Papilledema in an alert patient without focal neurological signs.
- Elderly patient with new headache and subacute cognitive change.

–Emergent red flag symptoms require immediate emergency room evaluation:
- Onset of sudden, severe headache (seconds to a minute to a peak onset of intensity).
- Headache with fever and neck stiffness.
- Papilledema with altered level of consciousness and/or focal neurological signs.

–Consider imaging or specialty consultation if:
- Atypical headaches.
- Changes in headache pattern.
- Unexplained focal signs in the patient with a headache.
- Headache precipitated by exertion, postural change, cough, or valsalva.
- New-onset cluster headache or another trigeminal autonomic cephalgia, hemicrania continua, or new daily persistent headache.

–Neuroimaging recommendations for complicated headache:

- In patients with sudden, severe headache or worst headache of their life, evaluate with CT head without IV contrast for initial imaging.
- In patients with new headache and optic disc edema, evaluate with MRI head without and with IV contrast, MRI head without IV contrast, or CT head without IV contrast for the initial imaging. These procedures are equivalent alternatives.
- In patients with new or progressively worsening headache with one or more of the following "red flags": subacute head trauma, related activity or event (sexual activity, exertion, position), neurological deficit, known or suspected cancer, immunosuppressed or immunocompromised state, age 50 y or older, evaluate with CT head without IV contrast, MRI head without and with IV contrast, or MRI head without IV contrast for the initial imaging. Pregnancy is also considered a "red flag" condition, with separate considerations for radiation and contrast exposure. These procedures are equivalent alternatives.
- In patients with new primary headache of suspected trigeminal autonomic origin, obtain MRI head without and with IV contrast for the initial imaging.
- In patients with chronic headache presenting with new features or increasing frequency, evaluate with MRI head without and with IV contrast or MRI head without IV contrast for the initial imaging. These procedures are equivalent alternatives.

Sources
–https://acsearch.acr.org/docs
–http://www.choosingwisely.org/societies/american-college-of-radiology/

MALIGNANT SPINAL CORD COMPRESSION (MSCC)

Population
–Adults with MSCC.

Organization
▶ Scottish Palliative Care Guidelines 2014, National Collaborating Centre for Cancer—Metastatic Spinal Cord Compression (MSCC) 2012

Recommendations
–Motor deficits are prognostic of ultimate functional outcome.

- In patients presenting with paraplegia >48 h, offer:
  - Radiation for pain control.
  - Surgery only if spine is unstable. The chance for neurological recovery is zero. (*Lancet Oncol.* 2005;6:15)
- In patients presenting with significant or progressing weakness of lower extremities with no previous history of cancer, biopsy for non-neural cancer if accessible.
  - If biopsy is not possible and lymphoma or myeloma unlikely, give dexamethasone 40–100 mg daily and take to surgery to make tissue diagnosis and relieve compression of spinal cord. (*Neurology.* 1989;39:1255. *Lancet Neurol.* 2008;7:459)

- If unstable, the spine should be stabilized. Taper steroids (decrease by ½ every 3 d) and begin radiation in 2–3 wk.
- If tumor is lymphoma or myeloma, consider initiating chemotherapy and high-dose dexamethasone.
- Recovery of lower extremity strength is dependent on degree of paraparesis initially.
- In patients presenting with back pain but mild neurologic symptoms, if no previous cancer:
  - Find site to biopsy, check prostate-specific antigen (PSA), serum protein electrophoresis, beta-2 microglobulin, and alfa-fetoprotein.
  - Begin moderate-dose dexamethasone (16 mg/d) with radiation therapy initially.
  - Surgery reserved for progression of symptoms after starting radiation especially in radio-insensitive cancers (renal cell, sarcoma, melanoma).
  - Recovery of neurologic function in 80%–90% range.
- In patients presenting with back pain but no neurologic symptoms with no previous diagnosis of cancer:
  - Search for site to biopsy (physical exam, PET CT scan, tumor markers) and consult radiation therapy.
  - If myeloma or lymphoma, treat with systemic chemotherapy.
  - Radiation is primary treatment with surgery only on progression.
  - Low dose or no steroids is acceptable.
  - Chance of continued lower extremity strength approaches 100%.

Comments

1. **Clinical considerations:**
   a. MRI with and without gadolinium of the entire spine is mandatory. Thirty percent of patients will have cord compression in more than 1 area.
   b. Twenty percent of patients presenting with MSCC have not had a previous diagnosis of cancer.
   c. Five to eight percent of patients with known cancer will develop MSCC during their course of disease.
   d. Most common tumors associated with MSCC are lung, breast, prostate, myeloma, and lymphoma.
   e. Most common site of MSCC is the thoracic spine (70%) and least common is cervical spine (10%).
   f. Back pain presents in 95% of patients, with average time to MSCC being 6–7 wk. Once motor, sensory, or autonomic dysfunction occur—time to total paraplegia is rapid (hours to days).
   g. Indications for surgery in MSCC include lack of diagnosis, progression on radiation, unstable fracture or bone in spinal canal, and previous radiation to site of MSCC. (*Int J Oncol.* 2011;38:5) (*J Clin Oncol.* 2011;29:3072)
   h. Posterior decompression laminectomy was standard surgery for MSCC, but now resection of tumor with bone reconstruction and stabilization is done most commonly at centers of excellence.
   i. Stereotactic body radiation therapy is being used more commonly with improved results especially in radiation-resistant cancers. (*Cancer.* 2010;116:2258)

Sources
    –*J Palliat Med.* 2015;18:7.
    –*Int J Radiat Oncol Bio/Phys.* 2012;84:312.
    –*Quart J Med.* 2014;107:277-282.
    –*N Engl J Med.* 2017;376:1358.

MULTIPLE SCLEROSIS (MS)

Population
    –Adults.

Organization
▶ AAN 2020

Recommendations
    –Counsel patients with newly diagnosed MS on specific treatment options with disease-modifying therapy (DMT) at a dedicated treatment visit with a clinician who has expertise with DMTs.
    –Ascertain and incorporate patient preferences regarding DMT safety, route of administration, adverse effects, and tolerability. Ongoing dialogue regarding treatment and monitoring for worsening symptoms. Follow up at least annually.
    –Prescribe DMT to patients with a single clinical demyelinating event and two or more brain lesions after discussing risks and benefits with patients for goal to reduce the number of relapses or slow the progression of MS.
    –Prescribe alemtuzumab, fingolimod, or natalizumab for people with highly active MS.
    –DMT can slow or stabilize disease; if disease activity resurfaces, change MS medication.
    –Consider weekly home or outpatient physical therapy (8 wk) as it may improve balance, disability, and gait, but not upper-extremity dexterity.
    –Motor and sensory balance training or motor balance training (3 wk) may improve static and dynamic balance.
    –Consider oral cannabis extract and THC in patients with MS with spasticity and pain (excluding central neuropathic pain).

Sources
    –AAN. *Complementary and Alternative Medicine in Multiple Sclerosis.* 2014; Reaffirmed 2020.
    –AAN. *Comprehensive Systemic Rehabilitation in Multiple Sclerosis.* 2015.
    –AAN. *Practice Guideline: Disease-modifying Therapies for Adults with Multiple Sclerosis.* 2018.

NORMAL PRESSURE HYDROCEPHALUS (NPH)

Population
–Patients with normal pressure hydrocephalus.

Organization
▶ AAN 2015

Recommendations
–Consider shunting for NPH with gait abnormalities.
–A positive response to a therapeutic lumbar puncture increases the chance of success with shunting.
–Patients with impaired cerebral blood flow reactivity to acetazolamide, measured by SPECT, are more likely to respond to shunting.

Source
–https://guidelines.gov/summaries/summary/49957

PAIN, CHRONIC, CANCER RELATED

Population
–Women treated for ovarian cancer with complete response (Stages I–IV).

Organization
▶ ASCO 2016

Recommendations
–Explore multidimensional nature of pain (pain descriptors, distress, impact on function and related physical, psychological, social, and spiritual factors)—explore information about cancer treatment history, comorbid conditions, and psychiatric history, including substance abuse as well as prior treatment for pain.
–Evaluate and monitor for recurrent disease, second cancer, or late-onset treatment effects in patients with new-onset pain (SOR: moderate).
–Prescribe nonopioid analgesics to relieve chronic pain or improve function in cancer survivors. This includes NSAIDs, acetaminophen, and adjuvant analgesics including antidepressants and selected anticonvulsants with evidence of analgesic efficacy (antidepressant duloxetine and anticonvulsants gabapentin and pregabalin) for neuropathic pain.
–Prescribe topical analgesics (NSAIDs, local anesthetics, or compounded creams/gels containing baclofen, amitriptyline, and ketamine).
–Do not use long-term corticosteroids solely to relieve chronic pain.
–Follow specific state regulations that allow access to medical cannabis for patients with chronic pain after consideration of benefits and risk.
–Consider a trial of opioids in carefully selected cancer survivors with chronic pain who do not respond to more conservative management and who continue to experience pain-related

distress or functional impairment. Add nonopioid analgesics and/or adjuvants as clinically necessary. Assess risks of adverse effects of opioids, including persistent common adverse effects (constipation, mental clouding, upper GI symptoms), endocrinopathy (hypogonadism, hyperprolactinemia causing fatigue, infertility, reduced libido), and neurotoxicity (myoclonus, changes in mental status, opioid-induced hyperalgesia, new onset or worsening of sleep apnea syndrome).

Sources
- *J Clin Oncol.* 2016;34:3325-3345.
- *J Pain Symptom Manage.* 2016;51:1070-1090.
- *J Clin Oncol.* 2014;32:1739-1747.
- *JAMA.* 2016;315:1624-1645.
- ASCO. *Management of Chronic Pain in Survivors of Adult Cancers: ASCO Clinical Practice Guideline.* 2016.

PAIN, CHRONIC

Population
- Adults with chronic noncancer pain outside of palliative and end-of-life care.

Organizations
▶ CDC 2016, ICSI 2017

Recommendations
- Use validated tools to assess patient's functional status, pain, and quality of life.

Initial assessment (ICSI):
- Assess for current or prior exposure to opioids and consider checking prescription drug monitoring program data before prescribing opioids.
- Assess for mental health comorbidities in patients with chronic pain.
- Screen all patients with chronic pain for substance use disorders.
- Before initiating opioids for chronic pain, seek a diagnostic cause of the pain and document objective findings on physical exam.

When to initiate or continue opioids for chronic pain (CDC):
- Prefer nonpharmacologic therapy and nonopioid medications for chronic pain.
  Prescribe NSAIDs and acetaminophen for dental pain. (ICSI)
- Use opioid therapy for both pain and function only if the anticipated benefits outweigh the risks.
- Establish treatment goals, including goals for pain and function, before starting opioid therapy for chronic pain. Plan how opioid therapy will be discontinued if benefits do not outweigh the risks.
- Discuss with patients the risks and benefits of opioid therapy before starting opioids and periodically during therapy.
- Incorporate cognitive behavioral therapy or mindfulness-based stress reduction and exercise/physical therapy to pharmacologic therapy in chronic pain patients. (ICSI)

Opioid selection, follow-up, and discontinuation:

–When starting opioid therapy, use immediate-release opioids, and prescribe the lowest effective dose. (CDC)

–Reserve long-acting opioids for patients with opioid tolerance and in whom prescriber is confident of medication adherence. (ICSI)

–Carefully reassess benefits and risks when increasing daily dosage to >50 morphine milligram equivalents.

–Avoid increasing daily dosage to >90–100 morphine milligram equivalents or carefully justify such doses.

–Reassess efficacy within 4 wk of starting opioid therapy for chronic pain and consider discontinuing opioids if benefits do not outweigh risks.

Assessing risk of opioid use:

–Evaluate risks of opioid-related harms.

–Advise patients who are initiating opioids or who have their opioid dose increased not to operate heavy machinery, drive a car, or participate in any activity that may be affected by the sedating effect of opioids.

–Prescribe naloxone emergency kit when patients have an increased risk of opioid overdose especially in patients who are taking ≥50 morphine milligram equivalents per day or concurrently using a benzodiazepine.

–Review prescription drug monitoring program data frequently.

–Obtain periodic urine drug testing to monitor diversion.

–Avoid concurrent opioid and benzodiazepine therapy whenever possible.

–Assess geriatric patients for their fall risk, cognitive impairment, respiratory function, and renal/hepatic impairment prior to initiation of opioids. (ICSI)

–Offer or arrange for medication-assisted treatment for patients with opioid use disorders (eg, buprenorphine or methadone).

Sources

–Dowell D, Haegerich TM, Chou R. CDC guideline for prescribing opioids for chronic pain—United States, 2016. *MMWR Recomm Rep.* 2016;65(1):1-49.

–https://www.cdc.gov/drugoverdose/pdf/guidelines_at-a-glance-a.pdf

–Hooten M, Thorson D, Bianco J, et al. *Pain: Assessment, Non-opioid Treatment Approaches and Opioid Management.* Bloomington, MN: Institute for Clinical Systems Improvement (ICSI); 2016:160.

–https://www.icsi.org/wp-content/uploads/2019/01/Pain.pdf

PAIN, NEUROPATHIC

Population
–Adults with neuropathic pain.

Organization
▶ NICE 2013, 2019

Recommendations
–Offer a choice of amitriptyline, duloxetine, gabapentin, or pregabalin as initial treatment for neuropathic pain (except trigeminal neuralgia).
–Consider tramadol only as acute rescue therapy.
–Offer carbamazepine as initial treatment for trigeminal neuralgia.
–Consider capsaicin cream for localized neuropathic pain.
–Pregabalin and gabapentin carry a risk of dependence and abuse.
–Consider the following agents with expert supervision:
  • Cannabidiol (CBD).
  • Capsaicin patch.
  • Lacosamide.
  • Lamotrigine.
  • Levetiracetam.
  • Morphine.
  • Methadone.
  • Tapentadol.
  • Oxcarbazepine.
  • Topiramate.
  • Tramadol (for long-term use).
  • Venlafaxine.
–Spinal cord stimulation (SCS).

Sources
–http://www.guideline.gov/content.aspx?id=47701
–Neuropathic Pain in Adults: Pharmacological Management in Non-specialist Settings (2013 updated 2019). NICE guideline CG173.

PROCEDURAL SEDATION

Population
–Adults or children.

Organization
▶ ACEP 2014

Recommendations

–Preprocedural fasting is not needed prior to procedural sedation.

–Use continuous capnometry and oximetry to detect hypoventilation.

–A nurse or other qualified individual must be present for continuous monitoring in addition to the procedural operator.

–Safe options for procedural sedation in children and adults include ketamine, propofol, and etomidate.

Comments

1. The combination of ketamine and propofol is also deemed to be safe for procedural sedation in children and adults.

2. Alfentanil can be safely administered to adults for procedural sedation.

Source

–http://www.guideline.gov/content.aspx?id=47772

RESTLESS LEGS SYNDROME AND PERIODIC LIMB MOVEMENT DISORDERS

Population

–Adults.

Organizations

▶ American Academy of Neurology 2016, American Academy of Sleep Medicine 2012

Recommendations

–Nonpharmacologic therapies:
- Avoid or reduce caffeine, nicotine, and EtOH.
- Perform evening stretches, massage, warm or cool baths, light exercise.

–Recommendations for moderate-to-severe restless legs syndrome (RLS).
- Strong evidence for following meds:
  - Pramipexole.
  - Rotigotine.
  - Cabergoline.
  - Gabapentin.
- Moderate evidence for:
  - Ropinirole.
  - Pregabalin.
  - IV ferric carboxymaltose.
- For primary RLS with periodic limb movements of sleep:
  - Ropinirole.

- For primary RLS with concomitant anxiety or depression:
  - Ropinirole.
  - Pramipexole.
  - Gabapentin.
- For RLS and ferritin <75 mcg/mL:
  - Ferrous sulfate with vitamin C.
- For RLS with ESRD on hemodialysis:
  - Vitamin C and E supplementation.
  - Consider adding ropinirole, levodopa, or exercise.

Comments

1. Potential for heart valve damage with pergolide and cabergoline.
2. Insufficient evidence to support any pharmacological treatment for periodic limb movement disorder.

Sources

–Winkelman JW, Armstrong MJ, Allen RP, et al. Practice guideline summary: treatment of restless legs syndrome in adults: report of the Guideline Development, Dissemination, and Implementation Subcommittee of the American Academy of Neurology. *Neurology.* 2016;87(24):2585-2593. http://guidelines.gov/summaries/summary/50689/

–www.guidelines.gov/content.aspx?id=38320

SCIATICA

Population

–People age ≥16 y with suspected sciatica.

Organization

▶ NICE 2016

Recommendations

–Do not routinely offer imaging in a primary care setting to patient with low-back pain with or without sciatica.

–Continue aerobic exercise program.

–Consider spinal manipulation or soft tissue massage as adjunct.

–Consider cognitive behavioral therapy.

–Promote return to work and normal activities.

–Consider NSAIDs and low-dose opioids for acute sciatica.

–Consider epidural steroid injection for acute, severe sciatica.

–Do not prescribe opioids or anticonvulsants for chronic low-back pain with sciatica.

–Consider spinal decompression for people with disabling sciatica for neurological deficits or chronic symptoms refractory to medical management, and spine imaging is consistent with sciatica symptoms.

–Belts, corsets, foot orthotics, rocker sole shoes, spine traction, acupuncture, ultrasound, transcutaneous electrical nerve stimulation (TENS), and interferential therapy have not proven to help patients with sciatica.

Source

–National Guideline Centre. *Low Back Pain and Sciatica in Over 16s: Assessment and Management.* London (UK): National Institute for Health and Care Excellence (NICE); 2016:18.

SEIZURES

Population

–Adults with first unprovoked seizure.

Organizations

▶ AAN 2015, ACR 2020

Recommendations

–Start immediate antiepileptic therapy only if elevated risk of a recurrent seizure. (AAN)
–Obtain initial imaging with a CT without contrast or an MRI without contrast. A CT is typically preferred if seizure is associated with trauma, though an MRI with or with/without may be appropriate. (ACR)
–Risk factors for a recurrent seizure include:
  • Brain injury.
  • Prior stroke.
  • Abnormal EEG with epileptiform activity.
  • Structural abnormality on brain imaging.
  • Nocturnal seizure.

Comment

1. Recurrent seizures occur most frequently in the first 2 y. Over the long term (>3 y), immediate antiepileptic drug (AED) therapy is unlikely to improve the prognosis for sustained seizure remission.

Sources

–https://guidelines.gov/summaries/summary/49218
–https://acsearch.acr.org/docs/69479/Narrative/

Population

–Adults.

Organization

▶ ACEP 2014

Recommendations

–For first generalized convulsive seizure, consider not initiating chronic antiepileptic therapy in the ED.

–Evaluate for a precipitating medical condition.

–Discharge patients home who return to their clinical baseline.

–If known seizure disorder, give antiepileptic therapy in ED orally or by IV.

–For status epilepticus, give benzodiazepines and consider phenytoin, fosphenytoin, valproic acid, and levetiracetam as second-line agents.

Comment

1. For refractory status epilepticus, consider intubation and use of a propofol infusion.

Source

–https://www.acep.org/patient-care/clinical-policies/seizure/

SEIZURES, FEBRILE

Population

–Children age 6 mo to 5 y.

Organization

▶ AAP 2011

Recommendations

–Perform a lumbar puncture if child presents with a fever and seizure and has meningeal signs or a history concerning for meningitis.

–Consider lumbar puncture for children 6–12 mo of age who present with a fever and seizure and are not up to date with their *Haemophilus influenzae* or *Streptococcus pneumoniae* vaccinations.

–Consider lumbar puncture in a child presenting with a fever and a seizure who has been pretreated with antibiotics.

–Do not perform EEG, neuroimaging, or routine labs (basic metabolic panel, calcium, phosphorus, magnesium, glucose, CBC) for a simple febrile seizure.

Comment

1. A febrile seizure is a seizure accompanied by fever ($T \geq 100.4°F$ [38°C]) without CNS infection in a child age 6 mo to 5 y.

Source

–http://pediatrics.aappublications.org/content/127/2/389.full.pdf+html

NATIONAL INSTITUTES OF HEALTH STROKE SCALE SCORE	
1a. Level of consciousness	0 = Alert; keenly responsive
	1 = Not alert, but arousable by minor stimulation
	2 = Not alert; requires repeated stimulation
	3 = Unresponsive or responds only with reflex
1b. Level of consciousness questions: What is the month? What is your age?	0 = Answers two questions correctly
	1 = Answers one question correctly
	2 = Answers neither question correctly

NATIONAL INSTITUTES OF HEALTH STROKE SCALE SCORE *(Continued)*

1c. Level of consciousness commands:
    Open and close your eyes.
    Grip and release your hand.
	0 = Performs both tasks correctly
	1 = Performs one task correctly
	2 = Performs neither task correctly

2. Best gaze	0 = Normal 1 = Partial gaze palsy 2 = Forced deviation
3. Visual	0 = No visual loss 1 = Partial hemianopia 2 = Complete hemianopia 3 = Bilateral hemianopia
4. Facial palsy	0 = Normal symmetric movements 1 = Minor paralysis 2 = Partial paralysis 3 = Complete paralysis of one or both sides

5. Motor arm
    5a. Left arm
    5b. Right arm
	0 = No drift
	1 = Drift
	2 = Some effort against gravity
	3 = No effort against gravity; limb falls
	4 = No movement

6. Motor leg
    6a. Left leg
    6b. Right leg
	0 = No drift
	1 = Drift
	2 = Some effort against gravity
	3 = No effort against gravity
	4 = No movement

7. Limb ataxia	0 = Absent 1 = Present in one limb 2 = Present in two limbs
8. Sensory	0 = Normal; no sensory loss 1 = Mild-to-moderate sensory loss 2 = Severe to total sensory loss
9. Best language	0 = No aphasia; normal 1 = Mild-to-moderate aphasia 2 = Severe aphasia 3 = Mute, global aphasia
10. Dysarthria	0 = Normal 1 = Mild-to-moderate dysarthria 2 = Severe dysarthria
11. Extinction and inattention	0 = No abnormality 1 = Visual, tactile, auditory, spatial, or personal inattention 2 = Profound hemi-inattention or extinction

Total score = 0–42.

STROKE, ACUTE ISCHEMIC

Population
–Adults age 18 y and older presenting to the emergency department with an acute ischemic stroke.

Organization
▶ AHA/ASA 2018

Recommendations

Initial evaluation:

–Obtain noncontrast CT upon arrival to hospital, within 20 min of arrival.

–Obtain CT angiogram with initial imaging for patients who otherwise meet criteria for endovascular treatment (EVT), but do not delay IV alteplase if indicated. Do not delay for a serum creatinine measurement unless history of renal impairment.

–In patients who are potential candidates for mechanical thrombectomy, consider imaging the extracranial carotid and vertebral arteries, in addition to the intracranial circulation for endovascular procedural planning.

–Measure blood glucose and treat hypoglycemia (<60 mg/dL).

–Obtain EKG and baseline troponin (but don't delay IV alteplase).

–Maintain O_2 saturation >94%.

–Identify sources of hyperthermia (>38°C); give antipyretic medications.

–Correct hypotension and hypovolemia.

Thrombolytics:

–For severe/disabling symptoms, give IV alteplase within 3 h from symptom onset, if ischemic stroke. Despite increased risk of hemorrhagic transformation, there is proven clinical benefit for patients with severe stroke symptoms.

–The benefit of IV alteplase between 3 and 4.5 h from symptom onset for patients with very severe stroke symptoms (NIHSS >25) is uncertain. Give IV alteplase in this window for patients ≤80 y of age, without a history of both diabetes mellitus and prior stroke, NIHSS score ≤25, not taking any OACs, and without imaging evidence of ischemic injury involving more than one-third of the MCA territory.

–For mild/nondisabling symptoms, consider IV alteplase up to 4.5 h from symptom onset after discussion of risks and benefits.

–Do not give IV alteplase in the following scenarios:

- Ischemic stroke patients who have an unclear time and/or unwitnessed symptom onset and in whom last known normal (LKN) is >3 or 4.5 h.
- Ischemic stroke patients who awoke with stroke with time LKN >3 or 4.5 h.
- Patients who have had a prior ischemic stroke within 3 mo.
- Recent severe head trauma (within 3 mo).
- Patients who have a history of intracranial hemorrhage.
- Patients with platelets <100,000/mm³, INR >1.7, aPTT >40 s, or PT >15 s (safety and efficacy are unknown). In patients without history of thrombocytopenia, treatment with IV

alteplase can be initiated before availability of platelet count but should be discontinued if platelet count is $<100,000/mm^3$.

- Patients who have received a treatment dose of LMWH within the previous 24 h. The use of IV alteplase in patients taking direct thrombin inhibitors or direct factor Xa inhibitors has not been firmly established but may be harmful.
- In patients with symptoms consistent with infective endocarditis, treatment with IV alteplase should not be administered because of the increased risk of intracranial hemorrhage.

–The following scenarios are not independent contraindications to IV alteplase:

- Age >80.
- Warfarin use with INR ≤1.7.
- ESRD with normal aPTT.
- Seizure.
- Remote h/o GI bleed.
- Recent non-STEMI.

–Special situations:

- Severely elevated BP: lower (to $<185/110$ mmHg) and assess stability before giving IV alteplase.
- Antiplatelet therapy (single or dual): proceed with IV alteplase, as the benefit outweighs the increased risk of symptomatic intracerebral hemorrhage (sICH).
- Major surgery in the prior 14 d: consider IV alteplase but weigh the risk of surgical-site hemorrhage against the anticipated benefits of reduced neurological deficits.
- Concurrent stroke and acute MI: give IV alteplase at the dose appropriate for cerebral ischemia, then pursue percutaneous coronary angioplasty and stenting.
- Current malignancy: safety and efficacy of IV alteplase are not well established. Consider if reasonable (>6 mo) life expectancy and no other contraindications.
- Pregnancy/postpartum: consider when the anticipated benefits of treating moderate or severe stroke outweigh the anticipated increased risks of uterine bleeding.

–Obtain a follow-up CT or MRI scan at 24 h after IV alteplase before starting anticoagulants or antiplatelet agents.

Blood pressure management:

–If otherwise eligible for acute reperfusion therapy but exhibit BP $>185/110$ mmHg, use any of the following to lower blood pressure:

- Labetalol 10–20 mg IV over 1–2 min, may repeat 1 time.
- Nicardipine 5 mg/h IV, titrate up by 2.5 mg/h every 5–15 min, maximum 15 mg/h; when desired BP reached, adjust to maintain proper BP limits.
- Clevidipine 1–2 mg/h IV, titrate by doubling the dose every 2–5 min until desired BP reached; maximum 21 mg/h.
- Other agents including hydralazine and enalaprilat may also be considered.

–If BP is not maintained $\leq185/110$ mmHg, do not administer alteplase.

–Maintain BP $\leq180/105$ mmHg during and after alteplase.

–Monitor BP every 15 min for 2 h from the start of alteplase therapy, then every 30 min for 6 h, and then every hour for 16 h.

–If systolic BP >180–230 mmHg or diastolic BP >105–120 mmHg, use one of the following:
- Labetalol 10 mg IV followed by continuous IV infusion 2–8 mg/min.
- Nicardipine 5 mg/h IV, titrate up to desired effect by 2.5 mg/h every 5–15 min, maximum 15 mg/h.
- Clevidipine 1–2 mg/h IV, titrate by doubling the dose every 2–5 min until desired BP reached; maximum 21 mg/h.
- If BP is not controlled or diastolic BP >140 mmHg, consider IV sodium nitroprusside.

IV Alteplase dosing:

–IV alteplase 0.9 mg/kg, maximum dose 90 mg over 60 min with initial 10% of dose given as bolus over 1 min is recommended for selected patients who may be treated within 4.5 h of ischemic stroke symptom onset or patient LKN.

–Tenecteplase administered as a 0.4-mg/kg single IV bolus has not been proven to be superior or noninferior to alteplase but might be considered as an alternative to alteplase in patients with minor neurological impairment and no major intracranial occlusion.

Mechanical thrombectomy:

–In selected patients with AIS within 6–24 h of LKN who have LVO in the anterior circulation, obtain CTP, DW-MRI, or MRI perfusion to aid in patient selection for mechanical thrombectomy.

–Offer mechanical thrombectomy with a stent retriever for patients with minimal prestroke disability, have a causative occlusion of the internal carotid artery or proximal middle cerebral artery, have an NIHSS score of ≥6, have a reassuring noncontrast head CT (ASPECT score of ≥6), and if they can be treated within 6 h of LKN. No perfusion imaging (CT-P or MR-P) is required in these patients.

–Offer mechanical thrombectomy to selected patients with stroke within 6–16 h of LKN who have large vessel occlusion (LVO) in the anterior circulation and meet other DAWN[1] or DEFUSE 3[2] eligibility criteria.

–Some patients may be eligible for thrombectomy within 16–24 h of LKN per the DAWN eligibility criteria.

Antiplatelet therapy:

–Give aspirin within 24–48 h after onset. For those treated with IV alteplase, delay until 24 h.

–In patients presenting with minor stroke, treat for 21 d with dual-antiplatelet therapy (aspirin and clopidogrel).

Post-ischemic stroke blood pressure management:

–Treat hypertension early only when required by comorbid conditions (eg, concomitant acute coronary event, acute heart failure, aortic dissection, post-thrombolysis, sICH, or preeclampsia/eclampsia). Lowering BP initially by 15% is probably safe.

–Consider lowering BP by 15% in the first 24 h after stroke in patients with BP ≥220/120 mmHg who did not receive IV alteplase or EVT and have no comorbid conditions requiring

[1]*N Engl J Med.* 2018 Jan 4;378(1):11-21. https://pubmed.ncbi.nlm.nih.gov/29129157/
[2]*N Engl J Med.* 2018; 378:708-718. https://pubmed.ncbi.nlm.nih.gov/29364767/

acute antihypertensive treatment, though the benefit of initiating or reinitiating treatment of hypertension within the first 48–72 h is uncertain.

–Start or restart antihypertensive therapy during hospitalization in patients with BP >140/90 mmHg who are neurologically stable.

Stroke rehabilitation:

–Provide rehabilitation to stroke survivors at an intensity commensurate with anticipated benefit and tolerance.

–Provide a formal assessment of ADLs and IADLs, communication abilities, and functional mobility before discharge from acute care hospitalization and incorporate the findings into the care transition and the discharge planning process.

–Perform regular skin assessments with objective scales of risk such as the Braden scale.

–Consider resting ankle splints used at night and during assisted standing for prevention of ankle contracture in the hemiplegic limb.

–Continue regular turning, good skin hygiene, and use of specialized mattresses, wheelchair cushions, and seating until mobility returns.

–Consider resting ankle splints used at night and during assisted standing for prevention of ankle contracture in the hemiplegic limb.

–Use prophylactic-dose subcutaneous heparin (UFH or LMWH) for the duration of the acute and rehabilitation hospital stay or until the stroke survivor regains mobility.

–Remove a Foley catheter within 24 h of hospitalization. Assess urinary retention through bladder scanning or intermittent catheterization.

–Refer individuals discharged to the community to participate in exercise programs with balance training to reduce falls.

–Provide a formal fall prevention program during hospitalization.

–Administer a structured depression inventory such as the Patient Health Questionnaire-2 to routinely screen for poststroke depression.

–Evaluate individuals residing in long-term care facilities for calcium and vitamin D supplementation.

–Assess speech, language, cognitive communication, pragmatics, reading, and writing; identify communicative strengths and weaknesses; and identify helpful compensatory strategies.

–Start enteral diet within 7 d of admission after an acute stroke.

–For patients with dysphagia, consider using nasogastric tubes initially for feeding in the early phase of stroke (starting within the first 7 d) and to place percutaneous gastrostomy tubes in patients with longer anticipated persistent inability to swallow safely (>2–3 wk).

–Consider directing patients and families with stroke to palliative care resources. Caregivers should ascertain and include patient-centered preferences in decision making, especially during prognosis formation and considering interventions or limitations in care.

Source

–Powers WJ, Rabinstein AA, Ackerson T, et al. 2018 Guidelines for the early management of patients with acute ischemic stroke: a guideline for healthcare professionals from the American Heart Association/American Stroke Association [published correction appears in Stroke. 2018 Mar;49(3):e138] [published correction appears in Stroke. 2018 Apr 18]. *Stroke.* 2018;49(3):e46-e110. doi:10.1161/STR.0000000000000158

Population
–Adult stroke patients with comorbidities.

Organization
▶ AHA/ASA 2014, 2018

Recommendations

Atrial fibrillation:
–Start oral anticoagulation within 14 d after the onset of neurological symptoms.

–If high risk for hemorrhagic conversion (ie, large infarct, hemorrhagic transformation on initial imaging, uncontrolled hypertension, or hemorrhage tendency), delay initiation of oral anticoagulation beyond 14 d.

–Choose VKA therapy (Class I; Level of Evidence A), apixaban (Class I; Level of Evidence A), or dabigatran (Class I; Level of Evidence B) for the prevention of recurrent stroke in patients with nonvalvular AF, whether paroxysmal or permanent.

–If unable to take oral anticoagulants, aspirin alone is recommended. Consider the addition of clopidogrel to aspirin therapy.

–The closure of the left atrial appendage with the WATCHMAN device in patients with ischemic stroke or TIA and AF is of uncertain usefulness.

Hypertension:
–Start BP therapy for previously untreated patients with ischemicstroke or TIA who after the first several days have an established SBP ≥140 mmHg or DBP ≥90 mmHg.

–In patients previously treated for HTN, resume BP therapy after the first several days for both prevention of recurrent stroke and other vascular events.

–Goals: <140/90 mmHg; for recent lacunar stroke reasonable SBP target <130 mmHg.

Dyslipidemia:
–Start intensive lipid-lowering therapy for patients with ischemic stroke or TIA presumed to be of atherosclerotic origin and an LDL-C ≥100 mg/dL, regardless of evidence of other clinical ASCVD.

Elevated blood glucose:
–Screen all patients for DM with an HgbA1c.

Obesity:
–Calculate BMI for all patients and start weight-loss management when necessary.

Sleep apnea:
–Consider a sleep study for any patient with history of CVA or TIA on the basis of very high prevalence in this population.

MI and cardiac thrombus:
–Consider VKA therapy (INR: 2–3) for 3 mo in patients with ischemic stroke or TIA in the setting of acute anterior STEMI.

Cardiomyopathy:
–In patients with ischemic stroke or TIA in sinus rhythm who have left atrial or left ventricular thrombus demonstrated by echocardiography or other imaging modality, give anticoagulant therapy with a VKA for ≥3 mo.

Valvular heart disease:

–For patients with ischemic stroke or TIA who have rheumatic mitral valve disease and AF, use long-term VKA therapy with an INR target of 2.5 (range 2.0–3.0).

–For patients with ischemic stroke or TIA and native aortic or nonrheumatic mitral valve disease who do not have AF or another indication for anticoagulation, use antiplatelet therapy.

Prosthetic heart valve:

–For patients with a mechanical aortic valve and a history of ischemic stroke or TIA before its insertion, use VKA therapy with an INR target of 2.5 (range 2.0–3.0).

–For patients with a mechanical mitral valve and a history of ischemic stroke or TIA before its insertion, use VKA therapy with an INR target of 3.0 (range 2.5–3.5).

–For patients with a mechanical mitral or aortic valve who have a history of ischemic stroke or TIA before its insertion and who are at low risk for bleeding, add aspirin 75–100 mg/d to VKA therapy.

–For patients with a bioprosthetic aortic or mitral valve, a history of ischemic stroke or TIA before its insertion, and no other indication for anticoagulation therapy beyond 3–6 mo from the valve placement, use long-term therapy with aspirin 75–100 mg/d rather than long-term anticoagulation.

Aortic arch atheroma:

–For patients with an ischemic stroke or TIA and evidence of aortic arch atheroma, use antiplatelet therapy.

Patent foramen ovale:

–For patients with an ischemic stroke or TIA and a PFO who are not undergoing anticoagulation therapy, use antiplatelet therapy.

–For patients with an ischemic stroke or TIA and both a PFO and a venous source of embolism, anticoagulation is indicated, depending on stroke characteristics. When anticoagulation is contraindicated, an inferior vena cava filter is reasonable.

–For patients with a cryptogenic ischemic stroke or TIA and a PFO without evidence for DVT, available data do not support a benefit for PFO closure.

–In the setting of PFO and DVT, PFO closure by a transcatheter device might be considered, depending on the risk of recurrent DVT.

Patients <30:

–Consider screening for hyperhomocysteinemia among young patients with a recent ischemic stroke or TIA. Most common concern is mutation in *MTHFR* gene. (*Circulation*. 2015;132:e6-e9)

Hypercoagulable states:

–Uncertain utility to screening for thrombophilic states in patients with ischemic stroke or TIA.

–Offer antiplatelet therapy to patients who are found to have abnormal findings on coagulation testing after an initial ischemic stroke or TIA if anticoagulation therapy is not administered.

Sickle cell disease:

–For patients with sickle cell disease and prior ischemic stroke or TIA, use chronic blood transfusions to reduce hemoglobin S to <30% of total hemoglobin.

Pregnancy:

–In the presence of a high-risk condition that would require anticoagulation outside of pregnancy, use one of the following options:

- LMWH twice daily throughout pregnancy, with dose adjusted to achieve the LMWH manufacturer's recommended peak anti-Xa level 4 h after injection, **OR**
- Adjusted-dose UFH throughout pregnancy, administered subcutaneously every 12 h in doses adjusted to keep the mid-interval aPTT at least 2× control or to maintain an anti-Xa heparin level of 0.35–0.70 U/mL, **OR**
- UFH or LMWH (as above) until the 13th wk, followed by substitution of a VKA until close to delivery, when UFH or LMWH is resumed.

–For pregnant women receiving adjusted-dose LMWH therapy for a high-risk condition that would require anticoagulation outside of pregnancy, and when delivery is planned, discontinue LMWH ≥24 h before induction of labor or cesarean section.

–In the presence of a low-risk situation in which antiplatelet therapy would be the treatment recommendation outside of pregnancy, consider UFH or LMWH, or no treatment during the first trimester of pregnancy depending on the clinical situation.

Breast-feeding:

–If anticoagulation required, use warfarin, UFH, or LMWH.

–If antiplatelet therapy required, use low-dose aspirin.

Sources

–Guidelines for the prevention of stroke in patients with stroke and transient ischemic attack: a guideline for healthcare professionals from the American Heart Association/American Stroke Association. *Stroke.* 2014;45.

–http://stroke.ahajournals.org

–2018 Guidelines for the early management of patients with acute ischemic stroke: a guideline for healthcare professionals from the American Heart Association/American Stroke Association. *Stroke.* 2018;49:e46-e99.

SYNCOPE

Population

–Adults presenting with syncope.

Organization

▶ ACC/AHA 2017

Recommendations

–Use the following algorithm to guide additional evaluation and diagnosis for syncope.

Initial Evaluation of Syncope

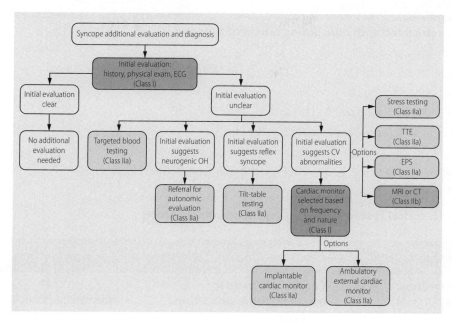

Source: Reprinted with permission Circulation.2017;136:e60-e122 ©2017 American Heart Association, Inc.

HISTORICAL CHARACTERISTICS ASSOCIATED WITH INCREASED PROBABILITY OF CARDIAC AND NONCARDIAC CAUSES OF SYNCOPE

More often associated with cardiac causes of syncope

- Older age (>60 y)
- Male sex
- Presence of known ischemic heart disease, structural heart disease, previous arrhythmias, or reduced ventricular function
- Brief prodrome, such as palpitations, or sudden loss of consciousness without prodrome
- Syncope during exertion
- Syncope in the supine position
- Low number of syncope episodes (1 or 2)
- Abnormal cardiac examination
- Family history of inheritable conditions or premature SCD (<50 y of age)
- Presence of known congenital heart disease

HISTORICAL CHARACTERISTICS ASSOCIATED WITH INCREASED PROBABILITY OF CARDIAC AND NONCARDIAC CAUSES OF SYNCOPE *(Continued)*

More often associated with noncardiac causes of syncope

- Younger age
- No known cardiac disease
- Syncope only in the standing position
- Positional change from supine or sitting to standing
- Presence of prodrome: nausea, vomiting, feeling warmth
- Situational triggers: cough, laugh, micturition, defecation, deglutition
- Frequent recurrence and prolonged history of syncope with similar characteristics

SCD, sudden cardiac death

Historical Features of Cardiac vs. Noncardiac Syncope

EXAMPLE OF SERIOUS MEDICAL CONDITIONS THAT MIGHT WARRANT CONSIDERATION OF FURTHER EVALUTION AND THERAPY IN HOSPITAL SETTING

Cardiac Arrhythmic Conditions	Cardiac or Vascular Nonarrhythmic Conditions	Noncardiac Conditions
• Sustained or symptomatic VT • Symptomatic conduction system disease or Mobitz II or third-degree heart block • Symptomatic bradycardia or sinus pauses not related to neurally mediated syncope • Symptomatic SVT • Pacemaker, ICD malfunction • Inheritable cardiovascular conditions predisposing to arrhythmias	• Cardiac ischemia • Severe aortic stenosis • Cardiac tamponade • HCM • Severe prosthetic valve dysfunction • Pulmonary embolism • Aortic dissection • Acute HF • Moderate-to-severe LV dysfunction	• Severe anemia/gastrointestinal bleeding • Major traumatic injury due to syncope • Persistent vital sign abnormalities

Source: Reproduced with permission from Shen WK, Sheldon RS, Benditt DG, et al. 2017 ACC/AHA/HRS Guideline for the evaluation and management of patients with syncope: executive summary: a report of the American College of Cardiology/American Heart Association Task Force on Clinical Practice Guidelines and the Heart Rhythm Society. *Circulation.* 2017;136(5):e25-e59.

Serious Medical Conditions Associated with Syncope

INDICATIONS FOR HOSPITALIZATION FOR SYNCOPE EVALUATIONS

Source: Reproduced with permission from Shen WK, Sheldon RS, Benditt DG, et al. 2017 ACC/AHA/HRS guideline for the evaluation and management of patients with syncope: executive summary: a report of the american college of cardiology/american heart association task force on clinical practice guidelines and the heart rhythm society. *Circulation*. 2017;136(5):e25-e59.

Recommended Tests for Syncope
–EKG.
–Complete blood count, basic metabolic panel, and other targeted labs based on clinical assessment.
–Echocardiogram if structural heart disease is suspected.
–Stress test if exertional syncope of unclear etiology.
–Continuous telemetry monitoring for patients admitted to hospital.
–Prolonged cardiac monitoring if arrhythmic syncope is suspected.
–Electrophysiologic study if syncope of suspected arrhythmic etiology with negative cardiac monitoring.

Other Interventions for Syncope
–Implantable cardioverter-defibrillator (ICD) implantation for patients with arrhythmogenic right ventricular cardiomyopathy who present with syncope and have a documented sustained ventricular arrhythmia.

Source
–2017 AHA/ACC focused update of the 2014 AHA/ACC guideline for the management of patients with valvular heart disease: a report of the American College of Cardiology/American Heart Association Task Force on clinical practice guidelines. *Circulation*. 2017;135:e1159-e1195.

TRAUMATIC BRAIN INJURY

Population

–Patients with minor head trauma.

Organization

▶ ACEP 2013

Recommendation

–Avoid CT scan of head for minor head trauma in patients who are low risk based on validated decision rules.

Source

–http://www.choosingwisely.org/societies/american-college-of-emergency-physicians/

TREMOR, ESSENTIAL

Population

–Adults.

Organization

▶ AAN 2011

Recommendations

–Treat with propranolol or primidone.
–Alternative treatment options include alprazolam, atenolol, gabapentin, sotalol, or topiramate.
–Do not use levetiracetam, pindolol, trazodone, acetazolamide, or 3,4-diaminopyridine.

Comment

1. Unilateral thalamotomy may be effective for severe refractory essential tremors.

Source

–http://www.neurology.org/content/77/19/1752.full.pdf+html

Prenatal and Obstetric Care

29

ABORTION

Population

–Women with incomplete abortion.

Organization

▶ WHO 2018

Recommendations

–Offer surgical or medical management vs. watchful waiting.
–If patient <13-wk gestation elects medical management, give misoprostol 600 μg orally or 400 μg sublingually. Do not use vaginal misoprostol.
–If patient ≥13-wk gestation elects medical management, give repeated doses of misoprostol 400 μg every 3 h sublingually, vaginally, or buccally.

Population

–Women with intrauterine fetal demise between 14- and 28-wk gestation.

Organization

▶ WHO 2018

Recommendations

–Offer surgical or medical management vs. watchful waiting.
–If patient elects medical management, give 200-mg mifepristone orally; 1–2 d later, give 400-μg misoprostol sublingually or vaginally, and repeat every 4–6 h. If mifepristone is not available or not preferred by the patient, give misoprostol 400 μg every 4–6 h as the initial treatment.

Population

–Women who elect to induce an abortion.

Organization

▶ WHO 2018

Recommendations

–Options include vacuum aspiration (manual or electric), dilation, and evacuation or medical management.

–For medical abortion, give mifepristone 200 mg once as initial dose. At least 24 h later, give misoprostol vaginally, sublingually, or buccally. If <12-wk gestation, use 800 μg. If ≥12-wk gestation, give 400 μg. If mifepristone is not available, use misoprostol as initial dose.

Source
–*Medical Management of Abortion*. Geneva: World Health Organization; 2018. License: CC BY-NC-SA 3.0 IGO.

BREASTFEEDING CHALLENGES

Population
–Women.

Organization
▶ ACOG 2021

Recommendations
–Recommend breastfeeding exclusively for 6 mo with continued breastfeeding as complementary foods are introduced during the infant's first year of life or longer, as mutually desired by the woman and her infant.
–Provide proactive lactation support, including education on hand expression, in anticipation of potential breastfeeding difficulties.
–Manage engorgement expectantly if symptoms are mild and the infant has good latch.
–Perform a focused history and physical exam to distinguish the specific cause of persistent pain while breastfeeding or nipple injury. Treat as indicated.
–Reassure women that their milk supply is adequate if the average feeding frequency is 8–12 times per day, steady weight is gained by day 4 or 5, and 6–8 wet diapers occur on average per day. Counsel on signs of low milk supply or dehydration such as jaundice, insufficient wet or soiled diapers, lethargy, inconsolability, unchanged stool color (not bright yellow by day 5), and a lack of steady infant weight gain.
–Encourage breastfeeding in women who are stable on medication-assisted treatment for opioid use disorders who are not using illicit drugs and who have no other contraindications to breastfeeding.
–Do not use galactagogues as a first-line therapy.

Source
–ACOG. Committee Opinion No 820. Breastfeeding Challenges. 2021.

CONTRACEPTION

Each method column is divided into Initiation (I) and Continuation (C) sub-columns. Values apply to both I and C unless shown separately.

Condition	Sub-Condition	Cu-IUD (I / C)	LNG-IUD (I / C)	Implant (I / C)	DMPA (I / C)	POP (I / C)	CHC (I / C)
Age		Menarche to <20 yrs:2; ≥20 yrs:1	Menarche to <20 yrs:2; ≥20 yrs:1	Menarche to <18 yrs:1; 18-45 yrs:1; >45 yrs:1	Menarche to <18 yrs:2; 18-45 yrs:1; >45 yrs:2	Menarche to <18 yrs:1; 18-45 yrs:1; >45 yrs:1	Menarche to <40 yrs:1; ≥40 yrs:2
Anatomical abnormalities	a) Distorted uterine cavity	4	4				
	b) Other abnormalities	2	2				
Anemias	a) Thalassemia	2	1	1	1	1	1
	b) Sickle cell disease[§]	2	1	1	1	1	2
	c) Iron-deficiency anemia	2	1	1	1	1	1
Benign ovarian tumors	(including cysts)	1	1	1	1	1	1
Breast disease	a) Undiagnosed mass	1	2	2*	2*	2*	2*
	b) Benign breast disease	1	1	1	1	1	1
	c) Family history of cancer	1	1	1	1	1	1
	d) Breast cancer[§]						
	i) Current	1	4	4	4	4	4
	ii) Past and no evidence of current disease for 5 years	1	3	3	3	3	3
Breastfeeding	a) <21 days postpartum			2*	2*	2*	4*
	b) 21 to <30 days postpartum						
	i) With other risk factors for VTE			2*	2*	2*	3*
	ii) Without other risk factors for VTE			2*	2*	2*	3*
	c) 30-42 days postpartum						
	i) With other risk factors for VTE			1*	1*	1*	3*
	ii) Without other risk factors for VTE			1*	1*	1*	2*
	d) >42 days postpartum			1*	1*	1*	2*
Cervical cancer	Awaiting treatment	4 / 2	4 / 2	2	2	1	2
Cervical ectropion		1	1	1	1	1	1
Cervical intraepithelial neoplasia		1	2	2	2	1	2
Cirrhosis	a) Mild (compensated)	1	1	1	1	1	1
	b) Severe[§] (decompensated)	1	3	3	3	3	4
Cystic fibrosis[§]		1*	1*	1*	2*	1*	1*
Deep venous thrombosis (DVT)/Pulmonary embolism (PE)	a) History of DVT/PE, not receiving anticoagulant therapy						
	i) Higher risk for recurrent DVT/PE	1	2	2	2	2	4
	ii) Lower risk for recurrent DVT/PE	1	2	2	2	2	3
	b) Acute DVT/PE	2	2	2	2	2	4
	c) DVT/PE and established anticoagulant therapy for at least 3 months						
	i) Higher risk for recurrent DVT/PE	2	2	2	2	2	4*
	ii) Lower risk for recurrent DVT/PE	2	2	2	2	2	3*
	d) Family history (first-degree relatives)	1	1	1	1	1	2
	e) Major surgery						
	i) With prolonged immobilization	1	2	2	2	2	4
	ii) Without prolonged immobilization	1	1	1	1	1	2
	f) Minor surgery without immobilization	1	1	1	1	1	1
Depressive disorders		1*	1*	1*	1*	1*	1*

Key:

1 No restriction (method can be used)	3 Theoretical or proven risks usually outweigh the advantages
2 Advantages generally outweigh theoretical or proven risks	4 Unacceptable health risk (method not to be used)

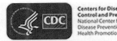

Condition	Sub-Condition	Cu-IUD		LNG-IUD		Implant		DMPA		POP		CHC	
		I	C	I	C	I	C	I	C	I	C	I	C
Diabetes	a) History of gestational disease	1	1	1	1	1	1	1	1	1	1	1	1
	b) Nonvascular disease												
	i) Non-insulin dependent	1	1	2	2	2	2	2	2	2	2	2	2
	ii) Insulin dependent	1	1	2	2	2	2	2	2	2	2	2	2
	c) Nephropathy/retinopathy/neuropathy‡	1	1	2	2	2	2	3	3	2	2	3/4*	3/4*
	d) Other vascular disease or diabetes of >20 years' duration‡	1	1	2	2	2	2	3	3	2	2	3/4*	3/4*
Dysmenorrhea	Severe	2	2	1	1	1	1	1	1	1	1	1	1
Endometrial cancer‡		4	2	4	2	1	1	1	1	1	1	1	1
Endometrial hyperplasia		1	1	1	1	1	1	1	1	1	1	1	1
Endometriosis		2	2	1	1	1	1	1	1	1	1	1	1
Epilepsy‡	(see also Drug Interactions)	1	1	1	1	1*	1*	1*	1*	1*	1*	1*	1*
Gallbladder disease	a) Symptomatic												
	i) Treated by cholecystectomy	1	1	2	2	2	2	2	2	2	2	2	2
	ii) Medically treated	1	1	2	2	2	2	2	2	2	2	3	3
	iii) Current	1	1	2	2	2	2	2	2	2	2	3	3
	b) Asymptomatic	1	1	2	2	2	2	2	2	2	2	2	2
Gestational trophoblastic disease‡	a) Suspected GTD (immediate postevacuation)												
	i) Uterine size first trimester	1*	1*	1*	1*	1*	1*	1*	1*	1*	1*	1*	1*
	ii) Uterine size second trimester	2*	2*	2*	2*	1*	1*	1*	1*	1*	1*	1*	1*
	b) Confirmed GTD												
	i) Undetectable/non-pregnant ß-hCG levels	1*	1*	1*	1*	1*	1*	1*	1*	1*	1*	1*	1*
	ii) Decreasing ß-hCG levels	2*	1*	2*	1*	1*	1*	1*	1*	1*	1*	1*	1*
	iii) Persistently elevated ß-hCG levels or malignant disease, with no evidence or suspicion of intrauterine disease	2*	1*	2*	1*	1*	1*	1*	1*	1*	1*	1*	1*
	iv) Persistently elevated ß-hCG levels or malignant disease, with evidence or suspicion of intrauterine disease	4*	2*	4*	2*	1*	1*	1*	1*	1*	1*	1*	1*
Headaches	a) Nonmigraine (mild or severe)	1	1	1	1	1	1	1	1	1	1	1*	1*
	b) Migraine												
	i) Without aura (includes menstrual migraine)	1	1	1	1	1	1	1	1	1	1	2*	2*
	ii) With aura	1	1	1	1	1	1	1	1	1	1	4*	4*
History of bariatric surgery‡	a) Restrictive procedures	1	1	1	1	1	1	1	1	1	1	1	1
	b) Malabsorptive procedures	1	1	1	1	1	1	1	1	3	3	COCs: 3 P/R: 1	COCs: 3 P/R: 1
History of cholestasis	a) Pregnancy related	1	1	1	1	1	1	1	1	1	1	2	2
	b) Past COC related	1	1	2	2	2	2	2	2	2	2	3	3
History of high blood pressure during pregnancy		1	1	1	1	1	1	1	1	1	1	2	2
History of Pelvic surgery		1	1	1	1	1	1	1	1	1	1	1	1
HIV	a) High risk for HIV	2	2	2	2	1	1	1*	1*	1	1	1	1
	b) HIV infection					1*	1*	1*	1*	1*	1*	1*	1*
	i) Clinically well receiving ARV therapy	1	1	1	1	If on treatment, see Drug Interactions							
	ii) Not clinically well or not receiving ARV therapy‡	2	1	2	1	If on treatment, see Drug Interactions							

Abbreviations: C=continuation of contraceptive method; CHC=combined hormonal contraception (pill, patch, and, ring); COC=combined oral contraceptive; Cu-IUD=copper-containing intrauterine device; DMPA = depot medroxyprogesterone acetate; I=initiation of contraceptive method; LNG-IUD=levonorgestrel-releasing intrauterine device; NA=not applicable; POP=progestin-only pill; P/R=patch/ring ‡ Condition that exposes a woman to increased risk as a result of pregnancy. *Please see the complete guidance for a clarification to this classification: www.cdc.gov/reproductivehealth/unintendedpregnancy/USMEC.htm.

Condition	Sub-Condition	Cu-IUD I	Cu-IUD C	LNG-IUD I	LNG-IUD C	Implant I	Implant C	DMPA I	DMPA C	POP I	POP C	CHC I	CHC C
Hypertension	a) Adequately controlled hypertension	1*	1*	1*	1*	1*	1*	2*	2*	1*	1*	3*	3*
	b) Elevated blood pressure levels (*properly taken measurements*)												
	i) Systolic 140-159 or diastolic 90-99	1*	1*	1*	1*	1*	1*	2*	2*	1*	1*	3*	3*
	ii) Systolic ≥160 or diastolic ≥100[‡]	1*	1*	2*	2*	2*	2*	3*	3*	2*	2*	4*	4*
	c) Vascular disease	1*	1*	2*	2*	2*	2*	3*	3*	2*	2*	4*	4*
Inflammatory bowel disease	(*Ulcerative colitis, Crohn's disease*)	1	1	1	1	1	1	2	2	2	2	2/3*	2/3*
Ischemic heart disease[‡]	Current and history of	1	1	2	3	2	3	3	3	2	3	4	4
Known thrombogenic mutations[‡]		1*	1*	2*	2*	2*	2*	2*	2*	2*	2*	4*	4*
Liver tumors	a) Benign												
	i) Focal nodular hyperplasia	1	1	2	2	2	2	2	2	2	2	2	2
	ii) Hepatocellular adenoma[‡]	1	1	3	3	3	3	3	3	3	3	4	4
	b) Malignant[‡] (hepatoma)	1	1	3	3	3	3	3	3	3	3	4	4
Malaria		1	1	1	1	1	1	1	1	1	1	1	1
Multiple risk factors for atherosclerotic cardiovascular disease	(e.g., older age, smoking, diabetes, hypertension, low HDL, high LDL, or high triglyceride levels)	1	1	2	2	2*	2*	3*	3*	2*	2*	3/4*	3/4*
Multiple sclerosis	a) With prolonged immobility	1	1	1	1	1	1	2	2	1	1	3	3
	b) Without prolonged immobility	1	1	1	1	1	1	2	2	1	1	1	1
Obesity	a) Body mass index (BMI) ≥30 kg/m²	1	1	1	1	1	1	1	1	1	1	2	2
	b) Menarche to <18 years and BMI ≥ 30 kg/m²	1	1	1	1	1	1	2	2	1	1	2	2
Ovarian cancer[‡]		1	1	1	1	1	1	1	1	1	1	1	1
Parity	a) Nulliparous	2	2	2	2	1	1	1	1	1	1	1	1
	b) Parous	1	1	1	1	1	1	1	1	1	1	1	1
Past ectopic pregnancy		1	1	1	1	1	1	1	1	2	2	1	1
Pelvic inflammatory disease	a) Past												
	i) With subsequent pregnancy	1	1	1	1	1	1	1	1	1	1	1	1
	ii) Without subsequent pregnancy	2	2	2	2	1	1	1	1	1	1	1	1
	b) Current	4	2*	4	2*	1	1	1	1	1	1	1	1
Peripartum cardiomyopathy[‡]	a) Normal or mildly impaired cardiac function												
	i) <6 months	2	2	2	2	1	1	1	1	1	1	4	4
	ii) ≥6 months	2	2	2	2	1	1	1	1	1	1	3	3
	b) Moderately or severely impaired cardiac function	2	2	2	2	2	2	2	2	2	2	4	4
Postabortion	a) First trimester	1*	1*	1*	1*	1*	1*	1*	1*	1*	1*	1*	1*
	b) Second trimester	2*	2*	2*	2*	1*	1*	1*	1*	1*	1*	1*	1*
	c) Immediate postseptic abortion	4	4	4	4	1*	1*	1*	1*	1*	1*	1*	1*
Postpartum (*nonbreastfeeding women*)	a) <21 days					1	1	1	1	1	1	4	4
	b) 21 days to 42 days												
	i) With other risk factors for VTE					1	1	1	1	1	1	3*	3*
	ii) Without other risk factors for VTE					1	1	1	1	1	1	2	2
	c) >42 days					1	1	1	1	1	1	1	1
Postpartum (*in breastfeeding or non-breastfeeding women, including cesarean delivery*)	a) <10 minutes after delivery of the placenta												
	i) Breastfeeding	1*	1*	2*	2*								
	ii) Nonbreastfeeding	1*	1*	1*	1*								
	b) 10 minutes after delivery of the placenta to <4 weeks	2*	2*	2*	2*								
	c) ≥4 weeks	1*	1*	1*	1*								
	d) Postpartum sepsis	4	4	4	4								

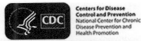

Centers for Disease Control and Prevention
National Center for Chronic Disease Prevention and Health Promotion

Condition	Sub-Condition	Cu-IUD I	Cu-IUD C	LNG-IUD I	LNG-IUD C	Implant I	Implant C	DMPA I	DMPA C	POP I	POP C	CHC I	CHC C
Pregnancy		4*		4*		NA*		NA*		NA*		NA*	
Rheumatoid arthritis	a) On immunosuppressive therapy	2	1	2	1	1		2/3*		1		2	
	b) Not on immunosuppressive therapy	1		1		1		2		1		2	
Schistosomiasis	a) Uncomplicated	1		1		1		1		1		1	
	b) Fibrosis of the liver[‡]	1		1		1		1		1		1	
Sexually transmitted diseases (STDs)	a) Current purulent cervicitis or chlamydial infection or gonococcal infection	4	2*	4	2*	1		1		1		1	
	b) Vaginitis (including trichomonas vaginalis and bacterial vaginosis)	2	2	2	2	1		1		1		1	
	c) Other factors relating to STDs	2*	2	2*	2	1		1		1		1	
Smoking	a) Age <35	1		1		1		1		1		2	
	b) Age ≥35, <15 cigarettes/day	1		1		1		1		1		3	
	c) Age ≥35, ≥15 cigarettes/day	1		1		1		1		1		4	
Solid organ transplantation[‡]	a) Complicated	3	2	3	2	2		2		2		4	
	b) Uncomplicated	2		2		2		2		2		2*	
Stroke[‡]	History of cerebrovascular accident	1		2		2	3	3		2	3	4	
Superficial venous disorders	a) Varicose veins	1		1		1		1		1		1	
	b) Superficial venous thrombosis (acute or history)	1		1		1		1		1		3*	
Systemic lupus erythematosus[‡]	a) Positive (or unknown) antiphospholipid antibodies	1*	1*	3*		3*		3*	3*	3*		4*	
	b) Severe thrombocytopenia	3*	2*	2*		2*		3*	2*	2*		2*	
	c) Immunosuppressive therapy	2*	1*	2*		2*		2*	2*	2*		2*	
	d) None of the above	1*	1*	2*		2*		2*	2*	2*		2*	
Thyroid disorders	Simple goiter/ hyperthyroid/hypothyroid	1		1		1		1		1		1	
Tuberculosis[‡] (see also Drug Interactions)	a) Nonpelvic	1	1	1	1	1*		1*		1*		1*	
	b) Pelvic	4	3	4	3	1*		1*		1*		1*	
Unexplained vaginal bleeding	(suspicious for serious condition) before evaluation	4*	2*	4*	2*	3*		3*		2*		2*	
Uterine fibroids		2		2		1		1		1		1	
Valvular heart disease	a) Uncomplicated	1		1		1		1		1		2	
	b) Complicated[‡]	1		1		1		1		1		4	
Vaginal bleeding patterns	a) Irregular pattern without heavy bleeding	1	1	1		2		2		2		1	
	b) Heavy or prolonged bleeding	2*		1*	2*	2*		2*		2*		1*	
Viral hepatitis	a) Acute or flare	1		1		1		1		1		3/4*	2
	b) Carrier/Chronic	1		1		1		1		1		1	1
Drug Interactions													
Antiretroviral therapy All other ARV's are 1 or 2 for all methods.	Fosamprenavir (FPV)	1/2*	1*	1/2*	1*	2*		2*		2*		3*	
Anticonvulsant therapy	a) Certain anticonvulsants (phenytoin, carbamazepine, barbiturates, primidone, topiramate, oxcarbazepine)	1		1		2*		1*		3*		3*	
	b) Lamotrigine	1		1		1		1		1		3*	
Antimicrobial therapy	a) Broad spectrum antibiotics	1		1		1		1		1		1	
	b) Antifungals	1		1		1		1		1		1	
	c) Antiparasitics	1		1		1		1		1		1	
	d) Rifampin or rifabutin therapy	1		1		2*		1*		3*		3*	
SSRIs		1		1		1		1		1		1	
St. John's wort		1		1		2		1		2		2	

PERCENTAGE OF WOMEN EXPERIENCING AN UNINTENDED PREGNANCY WITHIN THE FIRST YEAR OF TYPICAL USE AND THE FIRST YEAR OF PERFECT USE AND THE PERCENTAGE CONTINUING USE AT THE END OF THE FIRST YEAR: UNITED STATES

% of Women Experiencing an Unintended Pregnancy Within the First Year of Use

Method	Typical Use[a]	Perfect Use[b]	Women Continuing Use at 1 Y[c]
Male sterilization	0.15	0.10	100
Female sterilization	0.5	0.5	100
Nexplanon	0.1	0.1	89
Intrauterine contraceptives			
ParaGard (copper T)	0.8	0.6	78
Mirena/Liletta (LNG)	0.1	0.1	80
Depo-Provera	4	0.2	56
NuvaRing	7	0.3	67
Evra patch	7	0.3	67
Combined pill and Progestin-only pill	7	0.3	67
Diaphragm	17	16	57
Condom			
Female (fc)	21	5	41
Male	13	2	43
Sponge			
Parous women	27	20	
Nulliparous women	14	9	
Withdrawal	20	4	46
Fertility awareness-based methods	15		47
Standard Days method[d]	12	5	
Two-Day method[d]	14	4	
Ovulation method[d]	23	3	
Symptothermal method[d]	2	0.4	
Spermicides[e]	21	16	42
No method[f]	85	85	

Emergency Contraceptive Pills: Treatment with COCs initiated within 120 h after unprotected intercourse reduces the risk of pregnancy by at least 60%–75%.[g] Pregnancy rates are lower if initiated in the first 12 h. Progestin-only EC reduces pregnancy risk by 89%.

Lactational Amenorrhea Method: LAM is a highly effective, temporary method of contraception.[h]

PERCENTAGE OF WOMEN EXPERIENCING AN UNINTENDED PREGNANCY WITHIN THE FIRST YEAR OF TYPICAL USE AND THE FIRST YEAR OF PERFECT USE AND THE PERCENTAGE CONTINUING USE AT THE END OF THE FIRST YEAR: UNITED STATES (*Continued*)

% of Women Experiencing an Unintended Pregnancy Within the First Year of Use

Method	Typical Use[a]	Perfect Use[b]	Women Continuing Use at 1 Y[c]

[a]Among typical couples who initiate use of a method (not necessarily for the first time), the percentage who experience an accidental pregnancy during the first year if they do not stop use for any other reason. Estimates of the probability of pregnancy during the first year of typical use for spermicides, withdrawal, fertility awareness-based methods, the diaphragm, the male condom, the oral contraceptive pill, and Depo-Provera are taken from the 1995 National Survey of Family Growth corrected for underreporting of abortion; see the text for the derivation of estimates for the other methods.

[b]Among couples who initiate use of a method (not necessarily for the first time) and who use it perfectly (both consistently and correctly), the percentage who experience an accidental pregnancy during the first year if they do not stop use for any other reason. See the text for the derivation of the estimate for each method.

[c]Among couples attempting to avoid pregnancy, the percentage who continue to use a method for 1 y.

[d]The Ovulation and Two-Day methods are based on evaluation of cervical mucus. The Standard-Days method avoids intercourse on cycle days 8 through 19. The Symptothermal method is a double-check method based on evaluation of cervical mucus to determine the first fertile day and evaluation of cervical mucus and temperature to determine the last fertile day.

[e]Foams, creams, gels, vaginal suppositories, and vaginal film.

[f]The percentages becoming pregnant in columns (2) and (3) are based on data from populations where contraception is not used and from women who cease using contraception in order to become pregnant. Among such populations, about 89% become pregnant within 1 y. This estimate was lowered slightly (to 85%) to represent the percentage who would become pregnant within 1 y among women now relying on reversible methods of contraception if they abandoned contraception altogether.

[g]ella, Plan B One-Step, and Next Choice are the only dedicated products specifically marketed for emergency contraception. The label for Plan B One-Step (1 dose is 1 white pill) says to take the pill within 72 h after unprotected intercourse. Research has shown that all of the brands listed here are effective when used within 120 h after unprotected sex. The label for Next Choice (1 dose is 1 peach pill) says to take 1 pill within 72 h after unprotected intercourse and another pill 12 h later. Research has shown that both pills can be taken at the same time with no decrease in efficacy or increase in side effects and that they are effective when used within 120 h after unprotected sex. The Food and Drug Administration has in addition declared the following 19 brands of oral contraceptives to be safe and effective for emergency contraception: Ogestrel (1 dose is 2 white pills), Nordette (1 dose is 4 light-orange pills), Cryselle, Levora, Low-Ogestrel, Lo/Ovral, or Quasence (1 dose is 4 white pills), Jolessa, Portia, Seasonale, or Trivora (1 dose is 4 pink pills), Seasonique (1 dose is 4 light-blue-green pills), Enpresse (1 dose is 4 orange pills), Lessina (1 dose is 5 pink pills), Aviane or LoSeasonique (1 dose is 5 orange pills), Lutera or Sronyx (1 dose is 5 white pills), and Lybrel (1 dose is 6 yellow pills).

[h]However, to maintain effective protection against pregnancy, another method of contraception must be used as soon as menstruation resumes, the frequency or duration of breastfeeds is reduced, bottle feeds are introduced, or the baby reaches 6 mo of age.

Source: Zieman M, Hatcher RA, Allen AZ, Haddad L. *Managing Contraception.* 16th ed. 2021. Tiger, GA: Bridging the Gap Foundation.

CONTRACEPTION, EMERGENCY

Population

–Women of childbearing age who had unprotected or inadequately protected sexual intercourse within the last 5 d and who do not desire pregnancy.

Organization

▶ ACOG 2015

Recommendations

–Offer emergency contraception to women who have had unprotected or inadequately protected sexual intercourse and who do not desire pregnancy.

–Offer emergency contraceptive pills or copper IUD to patients who request it up to 5 d after unprotected or inadequately protected sexual intercourse.

–Women should begin using barrier contraceptives to prevent pregnancy after using emergency contraception or abstain from sexual intercourse for 14 d or until her next menses.

Comment

1. Combined progestin-estrogen pills and the copper IUD are not FDA approved for use as emergency contraception but have been shown to be safe and effective and can be used off-label for this indication.

Source

–ACOG Practice Bulletin No. 152. Emergency contraception. *Obstet Gynecol.* 2015;126:e1-e1.

Comments

1. No clinician examination or pregnancy testing is necessary before provision or prescription of emergency contraception.

2. The copper intrauterine device (IUD) is appropriate for use as emergency contraception for women who desire long-acting contraception.

3. Information regarding effective long-term contraceptive methods should be made available whenever a woman requests emergency contraception.

4. Ulipristal acetate is more effective than levonorgestrel-only regimen and maintains its efficacy for up to 5 d.

5. The levonorgestrel-only regimen is more effective than combined hormonal regimen and is associated with less nausea and vomiting compared with the combined estrogen–progestin regimen.

6. Insertion of copper IUD is the most effective method of emergency contraception.

DELAYED UMBILICAL CORD CLAMPING AFTER BIRTH

Population

–Pregnant women.

Organization

▶ ACOG 2020

Recommendations

–Delay umbilical cord clamping for at least 30–60 s in term and preterm infants except when immediate umbilical cord clamping is necessary because of neonatal or maternal indications.

–Do not perform cord milking for extremely preterm infants (<28 wk of gestation).

–There is insufficient evidence to support or refute umbilical cord milking in infants born at 32 wk of gestation or more, including term infants.

Comment

1. A 2019 study of umbilical cord milking was halted early because extremely preterm infants (23–27 wk of gestation) in the cord milking arm more often developed intraventricular hemorrhage compared with similar infants in the delayed cord clamping group.

Source

–ACOG. Committee Opinion No. 814. Delayed Umbilical Cord Clamping After Birth. 2020.

DELIVERY: TRIAL OF LABOR AFTER CESAREAN (TOLAC)

Population

–Pregnant women with a history of 1 previous cesarean delivery with a low-transverse incision.

Organization

▶ ACOG 2019

Recommendations

–Most women with 1 previous cesarean delivery and a low-transverse incision should be counseled about and offered TOLAC.
–In patients who have had a cesarean delivery or major uterine surgery, misoprostol should not be used for cervical ripening.
–Epidural analgesia may be used as a part of TOLAC during labor.

Comment

1. The benefits of a vaginal birth after cesarean (VBAC) include avoiding major abdominal surgery, lower rates of hemorrhage, thromboembolism, infection, and a shorter recovery period. VBAC may also decrease maternal risks associated with cesarean sections, including hysterectomy, bowel/bladder injury, and future abnormal placentation.

Source

–ACOG Practice Bulletin No. 205: Vaginal birth after cesarean delivery. *Obstet Gynecol.* 2019;133(2):e110-e127.

DELIVERY: VAGINAL LACERATIONS

Population

–Women delivering vaginally.

Organization

▶ ACOG 2018

Recommendations

–Insufficient evidence to recommend a specific mode of manual perineal support at delivery:
  • Consider applying warm perineal compresses during pushing to reduce incidence of third-degree and fourth-degree lacerations.

- Consider perineal massage during the second stage of labor to help reduce incidence of third-degree and fourth-degree lacerations.
- Restrictive episiotomy[1] use is recommended over routine episiotomy. A mediolateral episiotomy may be preferred over midline episiotomy.
  –For full-thickness external anal sphincter lacerations, either end-to-end repair or overlap repair is acceptable. There is limited data to support a single dose of antibiotic at the time of anal sphincter repair, though administration is reasonable.

Source
  –ACOG Practice Bulletin No. 198: Prevention and management of obstetric lacerations at vaginal delivery. *Obstet Gynecol.* 2018;132(3):e87-e102.

DIABETES MELLITUS, GESTATIONAL (GDM)

Population
  –Pregnant women.

Organizations
▶ ACOG 2018, SMFM 2018, NICE 2015

Recommendations
  –Treat all women with gestational diabetes with nutrition therapy and exercise.
  –Counsel women with GDM and estimated fetal weight of 4500 g or more regarding the option of scheduled cesarean delivery vs. vaginal trial of labor.
  –Instruct women with GDM to follow fasting and 1-h postprandial glucose levels. Target fasting blood glucose of 95 mg/dL and 1-h postprandial of 140 mg/dL.
  –Start antepartum fetal testing at 32-wk gestational age in women with GDM requiring medication or under poor control and without other comorbidities. Consider starting surveillance earlier if other comorbidities are present.
  –Unless otherwise indicated, do not induce women with well-controlled A1GDM before 39 wk. Expectant management until 40-6/7 wk is appropriate; antepartum fetal testing may not be necessary unless other comorbidities are present.
  –For women with A2GDM, delivery is recommended at 39 0/7 to 39 6/7 weeks of gestation.
  –Screen all women with GDM with a 75-g 2-h GTT 4–12 wk after delivery.

Organization	Guidance
GUIDELINES DISCORDANT: INITIAL PHARMACOTHERAPY IN GESTATIONAL DIABETES	
ACOG	Insulin is preferred (start at 0.7–1.0 U/kg/d); metformin may be a reasonable alternative
NICE (UK), SMFM	Metformin is a reasonable and safe first-line pharmacologic alternative to insulin. If metformin is contraindicated, unacceptable to the woman, or blood glucose levels remain uncontrolled, offer insulin. Glyburide is another alternative oral antihyperglycemic

[1]Restrictive episiotomy denotes episiotomies performed in high-risk cases only, eg, shoulder dystocia, vaginal breech, instrumental deliveries.

Sources
　–ACOG Practice Bulletin No. 190: Gestational Diabetes Mellitus. *Obstet Gynecol.* 2018;131(2):e49-e64.https://www.scribd.com/document/371228843/190-Gestational-Diabetes-Mellitus-Agog
　–NICE. Diabetes in pregnancy: management from preconception to the postnatal period (NG3). 2015.
　–SMFM Statement: Pharmacological treatment of gestational diabetes. *Am J Obstet Gynecol.* 2018;218(5):B2-B4.

EXTERNAL CEPHALIC VERSION

Population
　–Pregnant women near term with breech presentation.

Organization
▶ ACOG 2020

Recommendations
　–Offer external cephalic version (ECV) to all women near term with breech presentations unless there are contraindications.
　–Assess and document fetal presentation starting at 36 0/7 wk of gestation to allow for ECV.

Comments
1. Complications from ECV occur at rates less than 1% and include placental abruption, umbilical cord prolapse, ROM, stillbirth, and fetomaternal hemorrhage.
2. Evidence supports the use of parenteral tocolysis to improve ECV success; adding neuraxial analgesia is reasonable.
3. ECV is approximately 60% successful in achieving a cephalic vaginal birth.

Source
　–ACOG Practice Bulletin No. 221: External Cephalic Version. *Obstet Gynecol.* 2020;135(5):e203-e212.

ECTOPIC PREGNANCY

Population
　–Pregnant women.

Organizations
▶ NICE 2019, ACOG 2017.

Recommendations
　–Evaluation for stable women with an early pregnancy:
　　• Transvaginal ultrasound (TVUS) with a crown-rump length ≥7 mm but no cardiac activity.

- ◦ Repeat ultrasound in 7 d.
- ◦ Quantitative beta-hCG q48h × 2 levels.
- TVUS with gestational sac ≥25 mm and no fetal pole.
  - ◦ Repeat ultrasound in 7 d.
  - ◦ Quantitative beta-hCG q48h × 2 levels.
–Management of ectopic pregnancies.
- Differentiating early intrauterine pregnancy loss from ectopic pregnancy:
  - ◦ Uterine aspiration to identify presence of chorionic villi (indicate intrauterine pregnancy).
  - ◦ If chorionic villi not confirmed, monitor hCG levels:
    - ◻ Take first level 12–24 h after aspiration.
    - ◻ Plateau/increase in hCG suggests incomplete evacuation or nonvisualized ectopic warranting further treatment.
    - ◻ Decrease in hCG suggests failed intrauterine pregnancy; monitor with serial hCG measurements.
- Methotrexate candidates.[1]
  - ◦ No significant pain.
  - ◦ Adnexal mass <3.5 cm.
  - ◦ No cardiac activity on TVUS.
  - ◦ Beta-hCG <5000 IU/L.
  - ◦ Dose is 50 mg/m^2 IM.
- Laparoscopy if:
  - ◦ Unstable patient.
  - ◦ Severe pain.
  - ◦ Adnexal mass ≥3.5 cm.
  - ◦ Cardiac activity seen.
  - ◦ Beta-hCG ≥5000 IU/L.
- Rhogam 250 IU to all Rh-negative women who undergo surgery for an ectopic.

Comments

1. Ectopic pregnancy can present with:
   a. Abdominal or pelvic pain.
   b. Vaginal bleeding.
   c. Amenorrhea.
   d. Breast tenderness.
   e. GI symptoms.
   f. Dizziness.
   g. Urinary symptoms.
   h. Rectal pressure.
   i. Dyschezia.

---

[1]Contraindications to methotrexate use include renal or hepatic disease, bone marrow dysfunction, active gastrointestinal or respiratory disease. Asthma is not a contraindication.

2. Most normal intrauterine pregnancies will show an increase in beta-hCG level by at least 63% in 48 h.

3. Intrauterine pregnancies are usually apparent by TVUS if beta-hCG >1500 IU/L.

Sources
–www.guidelines.gov/content.aspx?id=39274

–NICE. Ectopic pregnancy and miscarriage: diagnosis and initial management (NG126). 2019.

–ACOG Practice Bulletin No. 191: Tubal ectopic pregnancy. *Obstet Gynecol*. 2017. doi: 10.1097/AOG.0000000000002464

FETAL GROWTH RESTRICTION

Population
–Pregnant women.

Organization
▶ ACOG 2021.

Recommendations
–The most frequently used definition is an estimated fetal weight <10th percentile for gestational age.

–Monitor with serial umbilical artery assessments. Umbilical artery Doppler velocimetry used in conjunction with standard fetal surveillance, such as nonstress tests, biophysical profiles, or both, is associated with improved outcomes.

–Offer antenatal corticosteroids if delivery is anticipated before 33 6/7 wk of gestation and between 34 0/7 and 36 6/7 wk of gestation if risk of preterm delivery within 7 d and no previous course of corticosteroids.

–Consider magnesium sulfate for delivery before 32 wk of gestation for fetal and neonatal neuroprotection.

–Do not recommend nutritional and dietary supplemental strategies for the prevention of fetal growth restriction as they are not effective.

Source
–ACOG. Practice Bulletin No 227. Fetal Growth Restriction. 2021.

HUMAN IMMUNODEFICIENCY VIRUS (HIV), PREGNANCY

Population
–Pregnant women.

Organizations
▶ AAFP 2019, USPSTF 2019, ACOG 2018, CDC 2021

Recommendations

–Screen all pregnant women for HIV as early as possible during each pregnancy using an opt-out approach.
–Repeat HIV testing during the third trimester for women known to be at high risk of acquiring HIV.
–Offer rapid HIV screening to women during labor and delivery or during the immediate postpartum period who were not tested earlier in pregnancy or whose HIV is undocumented. If a rapid HIV test result in labor is reactive, antiretroviral prophylaxis should be immediately initiated while awaiting supplemental test results.

Sources

–AAFP. *Clinical Recommendation: HIV Infection, Adolescents and Adults.* 2019.
–USPSTF. *HIV Infection: Screening.* 2019.
–CDC. *Sexually Transmitted Diseases Treatment Guidelines.* 2021.
–ACOG. Practice Bulletin No. 752. Prenatal and perinatal human immunodeficiency virus testing. *Obstet Gynecol.* 2018 Sep;132(3):e138-e142.

Population

–HIV-infected pregnant women.

Organizations

▶ ACOG 2018, IDSA 2020

Recommendations

–Initial prenatal labs should include a quantitative HIV RNA (viral load) level and CD4 cell count with percentage, HIV viral load, and HCV antibody. If HIV RNA is detectable, perform HIV genotypic resistance testing to help guide antepartum therapy.
–Plasma HIV ribonucleic acid (RNA) levels should be monitored at the initial prenatal visit, 2–4 wk after initiating (or changing) cART drug regimens; monthly until RNA levels are undetectable; and then at least every 3 mo during pregnancy.
–Treat with combined antiretroviral therapy (cART) during the antepartum period.
–Women on antiretroviral therapy (ART) that was initiated before pregnancy should continue their current regimen even if the agents are not one of the preferred antiretroviral drugs for use during pregnancy.
–Initiate ART for treatment-naïve women, as early as possible to reduce the risk of transmission at the time of delivery. Delaying ART beyond 28 wk of gestation may not fully suppress HIV RNA by the time of delivery, increasing the risk of perinatal transmission.
–Target sustained maternal viral loads of 1000 copies/mL or less to minimize the risk of perinatal transmission independent of the route of delivery or duration of ruptured membranes before delivery.
–Offer scheduled prelabor cesarean delivery at 38 0/7 wk of gestation if viral loads >1000 copies/mL to reduce the risk of perinatal transmission.
–Screen for hepatitis A virus, tuberculosis, and trichomonas vaginalis in addition to standard prenatal testing.

–Offer primary or booster doses of adult-type tetanus and reduced diphtheria toxoids (Td or TdaP), inactivated influenza vaccine, pneumococcal vaccine, hepatitis A vaccine, and hepatitis B vaccine.

–Counsel women with HIV regarding risk of breast milk transmission of HIV prior to delivery. In the United States, persons with HIV should avoid breastfeeding.

Comments

1. Avoid Methergine for postpartum hemorrhage in women receiving a protease inhibitor or efavirenz.
2. If women do not receive antepartum/intrapartum ART prophylaxis, infants should receive zidovudine for 6 wk.
3. Infants born to HIV-infected women should have an HIV viral load checked at 14 d, at 1–2 mo, and at 4–6 mo.
4. Screening for GDM is generally performed at the usual recommended gestational age of 24–28 wk. However, it is reasonable to perform testing earlier for women on protease inhibitors.

Sources

–ACOG Committee Opinion No. 751: Labor and delivery management of women with HIV infection. *Obstet Gynecol.* 2018;132(3):e131-e137.

–Primary care guidance for persons with HIV: 2020 update by the HIV Medicine Association of the IDSA. *Clin Infect Dis.* 2020; ciaa1391.

GESTATIONAL HYPERTENSION AND PREECLAMPSIA

Population

–Pregnant and postpartum women.

Organization

▶ ACOG 2020

Recommendations

–Initiate low-dose (81 mg/d) aspirin for preeclampsia prophylaxis, between 12 and 28 wk of gestation (ideally before 16 wk of gestation) and continue until delivery in:

- Women with any high-risk factors for preeclampsia (previous pregnancy with preeclampsia, multifetal gestation, renal disease, autoimmune disease, type 1 or type 2 diabetes mellitus, and chronic hypertension).
- Women with more than one of the moderate-risk factors (first pregnancy, maternal age of 35 y or older, a body mass index of more than 30, family history of preeclampsia, sociodemographic characteristics, and personal history factors).

–Antihypertensive treatment should be initiated for acute-onset severe hypertension (SBP ≥160 or DBP ≥110 mmHg) that is confirmed as persistent (15 min or more). Antihypertensive options included hydralazine, labetalol, nifedipine.

–Induce labor at 37 0/7 wk of gestation (or beyond upon diagnosis).

–Proceed toward delivery at 34 0/7 wk of gestation or beyond when gestational hypertension or preeclampsia with severe features is diagnosed.

–Magnesium sulfate should be used for seizure prophylaxis in women with gestational hypertension and preeclampsia with severe features.

–Use nonsteroidal anti-inflammatory medications preferentially over opioid analgesics in postpartum patients, even if on magnesium.

Source

–ACOG. Practice Bulletin No. 222. Gestational Hypertension and Preeclampsia. 2020.

HYPERTENSION, CHRONIC IN PREGNANCY

Population

–Pregnant women with hypertension diagnosed or present before pregnancy or before 20 wk of gestation.

Organization

▶ ACOG 2019

Recommendations

–Obtain baseline evaluation of LFTs, serum creatinine, serum electrolytes, BUN, CBC, spot urine protein/creatinine ratio or 24-h urine for total protein and creatinine. Consider EKG for women with longstanding hypertension ((HTN >4 y duration or age >30 y).

–In cases of diagnostic uncertainty between chronic HTN and superimposed preeclampsia, admit patient for inpatient surveillance with assessment of hematocrit, platelets, creatinine, LFTs, and new-onset proteinuria.

–Initiate low-dose aspirin (81 mg) between 12 and 28 wk of gestation and continue through delivery.

–Initiate antihypertensive medications when SBP >160 mmHg or DBP >110 mmHg.

–For long-term treatment of pregnant women requiring antihypertension medications, use labetalol and nifedipine as first line.

TIMING OF DELIVERY IN PREGNANT PATIENTS WITH CHRONIC HYPERTENSION	
	ACOG Recommended Timing of Delivery (wk of Gestation)
cHTN not requiring medication	≥38+0 to 39+6
cHTN controlled with medication	≥37+0 to 39+0
Severe HTN, difficult to control	34+0 to 36+6

Comments

1. Risks of chronic hypertension in pregnancy include maternal death, stroke, pulmonary edema, renal insufficiency/failure, myocardial infarction, preeclampsia, placental abruption, GDM, postpartum hemorrhage, and cesarean delivery.

2. Risks of chronic hypertension in pregnancy also include stillbirth/perinatal death, growth restriction, preterm birth, and congenital anomalies.

Source
–ACOG Practice Bulletin No. 203: Chronic hypertension in pregnancy. *Obstet Gynecol.* 2019;133(1):e26-e50.

MACROSOMIA

Population
–Pregnant women.

Organization
▶ ACOG 2020.

Recommendations
–Diagnose macrosomia using ultrasound. Prediction of birth weight is imprecise by ultrasonography or clinical measurement. Accuracy of EFW by ultrasound biometry is no better than abdominal palpation.
–Recommend aerobic and strength-conditioning exercise during pregnancy to reduce the risk of macrosomia.
–Optimize maternal glycemic control.
–Discuss risks and benefits of vaginal births and cesarean births based on the degree of suspected macrosomia.
  • Scheduled cesarean birth may be beneficial for newborns with suspected macrosomia with an EFW greater than 5000 g in women without diabetes and an EFW of greater than or equal to 4500 g in women with diabetes.
  • Suspected fetal macrosomia is not an indication for induction of labor before 39 wk of gestation. There is insufficient evidence that benefits of reducing shoulder dystocia risk outweigh harms of early delivery.

Comment
1. Historically macrosomia is defined as >4000 g or 4500 g. No universally accepted definition exists.

Source
–ACOG. Practice Bulletin No 216. Macrosomia. 2020.

POSTPARTUM HEMORRHAGE (PPH)

Population
–Postpartum women.

Organizations
▶ WHO 2012, ACOG 2017, ACR 2020

Recommendations

- Uterotonics for the treatment of PPH:
  - Intravenous oxytocin is the recommended agent.
  - Alternative uterotonics:
    - Misoprostol 800 μg sublingual.
    - Methylergonovine 0.2 mg IM.
    - Carboprost 0.25 mg IM.
- Additional interventions for PPH:
  - Isotonic crystalloid resuscitation.
  - Bimanual uterine massage.
- Therapeutic options for persistent PPH:
  - Tranexamic acid is recommended for persistent PPH refractory to oxytocin.
  - Uterine artery embolization.
  - Balloon tamponade.
- Therapeutic options for a retained placenta:
  - Controlled cord traction with oxytocin 10 IU IM/IV.
  - Manual removal of placenta.
    - Give single dose of first-generation antibiotic for prophylaxis against endometritis.
  - Recommend against methylergonovine, misoprostol, or carboprost (Hemabate) for retained placenta.
- Role of Imaging (ACR):
  - Most of the causes of PPH can be diagnosed clinically, but imaging may play a role in diagnosis.
  - Pelvic ultrasound (transabdominal and transvaginal with Doppler) is the imaging modality of choice for the initial evaluation of PPH.
  - Contrast-enhanced CT of the abdomen and pelvis and CT angiogram of the abdomen and pelvis may be appropriate to determine if active ongoing hemorrhage is present, to localize the bleeding, and to identify the source of bleeding.

Comment

1. Misoprostol 800–1000 μg can also be administered as a rectal suppository for PPH related to uterine atony.

Sources

- ACOG Practice Bulletin No. 183. Postpartum hemorrhage. *Obstet Gynecol.* 2017;130:e168-e186.
- ACR appropriateness criteria postpartum hemorrhage. *J Am Coll Radiol.* 2020;17:S459-S471
- *WHO Recommendations for the Prevention and Treatment of Postpartum Haemorrhage.* Geneva: World Health Organization; 2012. http://www.guidelines.gov/content.aspx?id=39383

PRELABOR RUPTURE OF MEMBRANES

Population
–Pregnant women.

Organizations
▶ ACOG 2020, Cochrane Database of Systematic Reviews 2013, NICE 2021

Recommendations
–Diagnose PROM based on history and physical exam. Per ACOG, digital examinations should be avoided unless patient appears to be in active labor or delivery seems imminent. Sterile speculum exam is preferred.

–In all patients with PROM, initial period of electronic fetal heart monitoring and uterine activity monitoring should be done. Nonreassuring fetal status and clinical chorioamnionitis are indications for delivery.

–<23–24 wk of gestation at risk for imminent delivery:
  • Expectant management or induction of labor.
  • Antibiotics may be considered as early as 20 0/7 wk of gestation.
  • GBS prophylaxis is not recommended before viability.
  • Corticosteroids, tocolysis, and magnesium sulfate are not recommended before viability but may be considered for as early as 23 0/7 wk of gestation.

–24 0/7–33 6/7 wk of gestation at risk for imminent delivery:
  • IV magnesium sulfate treatment for its fetal neuroprotective effect <32 0/7 wk of gestation, if there are no contraindications.
  • Consider trial of expectant management.
  • Antibiotics are recommended to prolong latency if there are no contraindications.
  • Single course of corticosteroids is recommended. Consider at 23 0/7 wk gestation if risk of preterm birth within 7 d.
  • Treat intra-amniotic infection if present (and proceed to delivery).
  • GBS screening and prophylaxis as indicated.

–34 0/7–36 6/7 wk of gestation:
  • Expectant management (NICE) or proceed toward delivery.
  • Consider single-course of corticosteroid. Do not delay delivery for steroids.
  • GBS screening and prophylaxis as indicated. If positive, proceed toward delivery.
  • Treat intra-amniotic infection if present (and proceed toward delivery).

–≥37 0/7 wk of gestation:
  • GBS screening and prophylaxis as indicated.
  • Treat intra-amniotic infection if present.
  • Proceed toward delivery.

–Not enough evidence to show that removal of cerclage after preterm PROM diagnosis has been made. If cerclage remains in place with preterm PROM, prolonged antibiotics prophylaxis beyond 7 d is not recommended.

–Outpatient management of preterm premature rupture of membranes is not recommended.

Comments

1. Twenty-two studies involving over 6800 pregnant women with PROM prior to 37 gestational weeks were analyzed. Routine antibiotics decreased the incidence of chorioamnionitis (RR 0.66), prolonged pregnancy by at least 7 d (RR 0.79), and decreased neonatal infection (RR 0.67), but had no effect on perinatal mortality compared with placebo.
2. Between 34 0/7 and 36 6/7 wk of gestation, NICE recommends expectant management until 37 wk of gestation in the absence of other contraindications. ACOG does not make an explicit recommendation. Either expectant management (with close monitoring) or delivery is reasonable.

Sources

–ACOG Practice Bulletin, No. 217. Prelabor rupture of membranes. *Obstet Gynecol.* 2020;135(3):e80-e97.
–NICE. Inducing labour (NG207). 2021.
–http://www.cochrane.org/CD001058/PREG_antibiotics-for-preterm-rupture-of-membranes

PRETERM LABOR

Population

–Pregnant women.

Organizations

▶ ACOG 2016, Cochrane Database of Systematic Reviews 2013

Recommendations

–Utility of fetal fibronectin testing and/or the cervical length measurement can improve clinical ability to diagnose preterm labor and predict preterm birth in symptomatic women, but the positive predictive value of these tests is poor and should not be used exclusively to direct management in a setting of acute symptoms.
–Single dose of corticosteroids for pregnant women between 24 and 34 gestational weeks or women with ROM or multiple gestations who may deliver within 7 d.
  • Consider single course of corticosteroids at 23-wk gestation for pregnant women who are at risk of delivery within 7 d.
  • Betamethasone or dexamethasone IM are most widely studied corticosteroids.
–Magnesium sulfate for possible preterm delivery prior to 32 wk for neuroprotection.
  • Indomethacin is a potential option for use in conjunction with magnesium sulfate.
–Tocolytic options for up to 48 h. Upper limit for use of tocolytic agents to prevent preterm birth is 34-wk gestation. Do not recommend maintenance therapy.
  • Beta-agonists.
  • Nifedipine.
  • Indomethacin.
–Women with preterm contractions without cervical change, especially if <2 cm, should not be treated with tocolytics.
–No role for antibiotics in preterm labor and intact membranes.
–Bedrest and hydration have not been shown to prevent preterm birth and should not be routinely recommended.

Comments

1. Magnesium sulfate administered prior to 32 wk reduces the severity and risk of cerebral palsy.
2. Cochrane analysis found no difference in the incidence of preterm delivery comparing hydration and bedrest with bedrest alone.

Sources

–ACOG. Practice Bulletin No. 171: Management of preterm labor. *Obstet Gynecol.* 2016;128:e155-e164.
–http://www.cochrane.org/CD003096/PREG_hydration-for-treatment-of-preterm-labour

PREGNANCY, PRETERM LABOR, TOCOLYSIS

Population

–Pregnant women in preterm labor.

Organization

▶ ACOG 2016

Recommendation

–Tocolytic options for up to 48 h. Upper limit for use of tocolytic agents to prevent preterm birth is 34-wk gestation. Do not recommend maintenance therapy.
  • Beta-agonists.
  • Nifedipine.
  • Indomethacin.

Source

–ACOG. Practice Bulletin No. 171: Management of preterm labor. *Obstet Gynecol.* 2016;128:e155-e164.

ROUTINE PRENATAL CARE

COMPILED RECOMMENDATIONS FOR ROUTINE PRENATAL CARE

Preconception visit

1. Measure height, weight, and blood pressure.
2. Assess immunization status for tetanus toxoid, reduced diphtheria toxoid, and acellular pertussis (Tdap); measles–mumps–rubella; hepatitis B; rubella, and varicella. Immunize as indicated. Live vaccines should be administered at least one month prior to pregnancy.
3. Assess all patients for pregnancy risk: substance abuse, domestic violence, sexual abuse, psychiatric disorders, risk factors for preterm labor, exposure to chemicals or infectious agents, hereditary disorders, gestational diabetes, or chronic medical problems. Initiate interventions to optimize maternal, fetal, and pregnancy outcomes.
4. Educate patients about proper nutrition; offer weight reduction strategies for obese patients.
5. With the exception of universal HIV and Hepatitis C screening, screening lab tests should be considered selectively in appropriate high-risk groups.
6. Initiate folic acid 400–800 μg/d; 4 mg/d for a history of a child affected by a neural tube defect.

Initial prenatal visit

1. Confirm pregnancy.
2. Assess medical, surgical, obstetric, psychosocial, and family history, and perform a complete physical examination. Record baseline blood pressure, height, weight, and calculate BMI.
3. Order CBC, blood type (ABO & RhD) and antibody screen, rubella titer, varicella titer, HIV, syphilis screening, Hepatitis B surface antigen, Hepatitis C antibody, urine NAAT for gonorrhea and chlamydia, urinalysis (proteinuria, glucosuria), urine culture. Pap smear if not up to date. Other selective screening tests as indicated.
4. Order an obstetrical ultrasound for dating if any of the following: beyond 16-wk gestational age, unsure of last menstrual period, size/date discrepancy on examination, or for inability to hear fetal heart tones by 12 gestational weeks.
5. Discuss fetal aneuploidy screening and counseling regardless of maternal age.
6. Prenatal testing for sickle cell anemia (African descent), thalassemia (African, Mediterranean, Middle Eastern, Southeast Asians), Canavan disease and Tay-Sachs (Jewish patients), cystic fibrosis (whites and Ashkenazi Jews), and fragile X syndrome (family history of nonspecified mental retardation).
7. Test for tuberculosis in medium- to high-risk patients.[a]
8. Consider a 1-h 50-g glucose tolerance test for certain high-risk groups.[b]
9. Obtain an operative report in all women who have had a prior cesarean section.
10. Psychosocial risk assessment for mood disorders, substance abuse, or domestic violence.

Frequency of visits for uncomplicated pregnancies

1. Every 4 wk until 28 gestational weeks; q2 wk from 28 to 36 wk; weekly >36 wk.
2. Offer a single ultrasound examination at 18- to 20-wk gestation if not indicated earlier (ACOG). Consider offering routine ultrasonography between 11- and 14-wk gestation even if not medically indicated (NICE). There is no evidence to support routine ultrasonography in uncomplicated pregnancies.

Routine checks at follow-up prenatal visits

1. Assess weight, blood pressure, and urine for glucose and protein.
2. Exam: edema, fundal height, and fetal heart tones at all visits; fetal presentation starting at 36 wk.
3. Ask about regular uterine contractions, leakage of fluid, vaginal bleeding, or decreased fetal movement.
4. Discuss labor precautions.

Antepartum lab testing

1. Offer first trimester, second trimester, or combined testing to screen for fetal aneuploidy; invasive diagnostic testing for fetal aneuploidy should be available to all women regardless of maternal age.
   a. First trimester.
   b. Second trimester screening options: amniocentesis at 14 wk; a Quad Marker Screen at 16–18 wk; and/or a screening ultrasound with nuchal translucency assessment.
2. Consider serial transvaginal sonography of the cervix every 2–3 wk to assess cervical length for patients at high risk for preterm delivery starting at 16 wk.
3. No role for routine bacterial vaginosis screening.
4. 1 hour 50-g glucose tolerance test in all women between 24 and 28 wk.
5. Screen for group B beta-hemolytic streptococcus (GBS) colonization between 36- and 38-wk gestation with rectovaginal swab.
6. Recommend weekly amniotic fluid assessments and twice weekly nonstress testing starting at 41 wk.

Prenatal counseling

1. Cessation of smoking, drinking alcohol, or use of any illicit drugs.
2. Avoid cat litter boxes, hot tubs, certain foods (ie, raw fish or unpasteurized cheese).
3. Proper nutrition and expected weight gain: National Academy of Sciences advises weight gain 28–40 lb (prepregnancy BMI <20), 25–35 lb (BMI 20–26), 15–25 lb (BMI 26–29), and 15–20 lb (BMI ≥30).
4. Inquire about domestic violence and depression at initial visit, at 28 wk, and at postpartum visit.
5. Recommend regular mild-to-moderate exercise 3 or more times a week.
6. Avoid high-altitude activities, scuba diving, and contact sports during pregnancy.
7. Benefits of breast-feeding vs. bottle-feeding.
8. Discuss postpartum contraceptive options (including tubal sterilization) during third trimester.
9. Discuss analgesia and anesthesia options and offer prenatal classes at 24 wk.
10. Discuss repeat C-section vs. vaginal birth after cesarean (if applicable).
11. Discuss the option of circumcision if a boy is delivered.
12. Avoid air travel and long train or car trips beyond 36 wk.
13. Discuss the uncertain benefit of kick counting in the prevention of stillbirth. Kick counting may be associated with increased risk of iatrogenic preterm birth, induction of labor, and cesarean birth.

Prenatal interventions

1. Suppressive antiviral medications starting at 36 wk for women with a history of genital herpes.
2. Cesarean delivery is indicated for women who are HIV positive or have active genital herpes and are in labor.
3. For patients who report a history of abuse, offer interventions and resources to increase their safety during and after pregnancy.
4. For patients with severe depression, consider treatment with an SSRI (avoid paroxetine if possible).
5. Rh immune globulin 300 µg IM for all Rh-negative women with negative antibody screens between 26 and 28 wk.
6. Refer for nutrition counseling at 10–12 wk for BMI <20 kg/m^2 or at any time during pregnancy for inadequate weight gain.
7. Start prenatal vitamins with iron and folic acid 400–800 µg/d and 1200 mg elemental calcium/d starting at 4-wk preconception (or as early as possible during pregnancy) and continued until 6-wk postpartum.
8. Give inactivated influenza vaccine IM to all pregnant women during influenza season.
9. Give Tdap vaccine during each pregnancy between 27- and 36-wk gestation.
10. Consider progesterone therapy IM weekly or intravaginally daily to women at high risk for preterm birth.
11. Recommend an external cephalic version at 37 wk for all noncephalic presentations.
12. Offer labor induction to women at 41 wk by good dates.
13. Treat all women with confirmed syphilis with penicillin G during pregnancy.
14. Treat all women with gonorrhea with ceftriaxone; follow treatment with a test of cure.
15. Treat all women with chlamydia with azithromycin; follow treatment with a test of cure. Doxycycline is contraindicated during the second and third trimesters of pregnancy.
16. Treat all GBS-positive women with penicillin G when in labor or with spontaneous rupture of membranes.
17. Offer group prenatal care as an alternative to traditional prenatal care if available and involve partners.
18. Discuss and document preferences about mode of birth early on and confirm toward the end of pregnancy, as preferences may have changed.

Postpartum interventions

1. Treat all infants born to HBV-positive women with hepatitis B immunoglobulin (HBIG) and initiate HBV vaccine series within 12 h of life.
2. All women with a positive tuberculosis skin test and no evidence of active disease should receive a postpartum chest X-ray; treat with isoniazid 300 mg PO daily for 9 mo if chest X-ray is negative.
3. Administer a Tdap booster if tetanus status is unknown or the last Td (tetanus-diphtheria) vaccine was >10 y ago.
4. Administer an MMR vaccine to all rubella nonimmune women.
5. Offer HPV vaccine to all women ≤26 wk who have not been immunized.
6. Initiate contraception.
7. Repeat Pap smear at 6-wk postpartum check.

[a]Post gastrectomy, gastric bypass, immunosuppressed (HIV-positive, diabetes, renal failure, chronic steroid/immunosuppressive therapy, head/neck or hematologic malignancies), silicosis, organ transplant recipients, malabsorptive syndromes, alcoholics, intravenous drug users, close contacts of persons with active pulmonary tuberculosis, medically underserved, low socioeconomic class, residents/employees of long-term care facilities and jails, health care workers, and immigrants from endemic areas.

[b]Overweight (BMI ≥25 kg/m^2) and an additional risk factor: physical inactivity; first-degree relative with DM; high-risk ethnicity (eg, African-American, Latino, Native American, Asian-American, Pacific Islander); history of gestational diabetes mellitus (GDM); prior baby with birthweight >9 lb; unexplained stillbirth or malformed infant; HTN on therapy or with BP ≥140/90 mmHg; HDL cholesterol level <35 mg/dL (0.90 mmol/L) and/or a triglyceride level >250 mg/dL (2.82 mmol/L); polycystic ovary syndrome; history of impaired glucose tolerance or HgbA1c ≥5.7%; acanthosis nigricans; cardiovascular disease; or ≥2+ glucosuria.

Sources:
Adapted from ACOG ICSI Guideline on Routine Prenatal Care, July 2010. http://www.icsi.org/prenatal_care_4/prenatal_care_routine_full_version_2.html;
Am Fam Physician. 2014;89(3):199-208.
USPSTF. *Hepatitis C Virus Infection in Adolescents and Adults: Screening.* 2020.
NICE. Antenatal Care (NG201). 2021.
NICE. Inducing Labour (NG207). 2021.
NICE. Postnatal Care (NG194). 2021.
ACOG. Practice Bulletin No 229. Antepartum Fetal Surveillance. 2021.

AAP AND AFP PERINATAL AND POSTNATAL GUIDELINES

Breast-feeding	Strongly recommends education and counseling to promote breast-feeding.
Hemoglobinopathies	Strongly recommends ordering screening tests for hemoglobinopathies in neonates.
Hyperbilirubinemia	Perform ongoing systematic assessments during the neonatal period for the risk of an infant developing severe hyperbilirubinemia.
Phenylketonuria	Strongly recommends ordering screening tests for phenylketonuria in neonates.
Thyroid function abnormalities	Strongly recommends ordering screening tests for thyroid function abnormalities in neonates.

Sources: Pediatrics. 2004;114:297-316; 2005;115:496-506.

THYROID DISEASE, PREGNANCY AND POSTPARTUM

Population
–Women during and immediately after pregnancy.

Organizations
▶ ATA 2017, ACOG 2020

Recommendations
–Hypothyroidism in pregnancy is defined as:
  - An elevated TSH (>2.5 mIU/L) and a suppressed free thyroxine (FT_4).
  - TSH ≥10 mIU/L (irrespective of FT_4).

–Do not treat subclinical hypothyroidism (TSH 2.5–9.9 mIU/L and a normal FT_4) in pregnancy.

–If hypothyroid treat with levothyroxine, starting with 1–2 mcg/kg or 100 mcg daily. Goal of therapy is to normalize TSH levels (between lower limit of reference range and 2.5 mU/L). Monitor TSH levels every 4 wk when treating thyroid disease in pregnancy.

–Measure a TSH receptor antibody level at 20–24 wk for any history of Graves' disease (GD).

–If a thyroid nodule is found, arrange thyroid ultrasound and TSH testing.

–Patients found to have thyroid cancer during pregnancy would ideally undergo surgery during second trimester.

–Do not treat transient hCG-mediated TSH suppression in early pregnancy with antithyroid drug therapy.

–If hyperthyroid, use propylthiouracil (PTU) or methimazole. Avoid methimazole in the first trimester.

–Treat Graves' disease during pregnancy with the lowest possible dose of antithyroid drug needed to keep the mother's thyroid hormone levels at or slightly above the reference range for total T4 and T3 values in pregnancy (1.5 times above nonpregnant reference ranges in the second and third trimesters), and the TSH below the reference range for pregnancy.

–Pregnancy is a relative contraindication to thyroidectomy and should only be used when medical management has been unsuccessful or ATDs cannot be used.

Comment
1. Surgery for well-differentiated thyroid carcinoma can often be deferred until postpartum period.

Sources
–2016 American Thyroid Association guidelines for diagnosis and management of hyperthyroidism and other causes of thyrotoxicosis. *Thyroid*. 2016;26(10):1343-1421.

–2017 Guidelines of the American Thyroid Association for the diagnosis and management of thyroid disease during pregnancy and the postpartum. *Thyroid*. 2017;27(3):315-390.

–http://thyroidguidelines.net/sites/thyroidguidelines.net/files/file/thy.2011.0087.pdf

–*Obstet Gynecol*. 2020; 135(6):e261-274.

Pulmonary Disorders

30

APNEA, CENTRAL SLEEP (CSAS)

Population
–Adults.

Organization

▶ American Academy of Sleep Medicine 2012

Recommendations
–**Primary CSAS**
- Use positive airway pressure therapy.
- Limited evidence to support the use of acetazolamide for CSAS.
- Consider zolpidem or triazolam if patients are not at high risk for respiratory depression.
–**CSAS related to CHF**
- Nocturnal oxygen therapy.
- Continuous positive airway pressure (CPAP) therapy targeted to normalize the apnea-hypopnea index.
–**CSAS related to ESRD**
- Options for therapy include CPAP, nocturnal oxygen, and bicarbonate buffer use during dialysis.

Source
–http://www.guideline.gov/content.aspx?id=35175

APNEA, OBSTRUCTIVE SLEEP (OSA)

Population
–Adults.

Organization

▶ AASM 2017, 2019

Recommendations
–**Diagnosis**
- Test for OSA in conjunction with a comprehensive sleep evaluation.

- Diagnose OSA when apnea-hypopnea index (AHI) is ≥5 events/h. Severe OSA is AHI ≥ 30 events/h.
- Use a polysomnogram or home sleep apnea testing with a technically adequate device to diagnose OSA in uncomplicated adult patients presenting with signs and symptoms that indicate an increased risk of moderate-to-severe OSA.
- Use a polysomnogram, rather than home sleep apnea testing, to diagnose OSA in patients with significant cardiorespiratory disease, potential respiratory muscle weakness due to neuromuscular condition, awake hypoventilation or suspicion of sleep-related hypoventilation, chronic opioid medication use, and history of stroke or severe insomnia.
- If a single home sleep apnea testing is negative, inconclusive, or technically inadequate, a polysomnogram be performed for the diagnosis or exclusion of OSA.

–**Treatment with positive airway pressure (PAP)**
- Treat OSA with PAP, either CPAP or autoadjusting PAP (APAP).
- Choose CPAP and APAP rather than bi-level PAP (BPAP) because BPAP is more costly and does not prevent obstructive breathing events at low expiratory pressure levels. Patients with a PAP requirement over 20 cm H_2O will require BPAP because of the limitation of settings on CPAP.
- Alternatives to PAP include weight loss, positional therapy, oral appliance therapy, surgical management of anatomical nasal obstruction, or maxillomandibular advancement.
- To improve adherence, choose nasal or intranasal mask interface rather than oronasal or oral, use heated humidification (reduces sleepiness, dry mouth/throat/nose, nasal congestion, hoarseness, headache, epistaxis), and offer educational, behavioral, and other troubleshooting interventions particularly in the setting of PTSD/anxiety.

Comments

1. Excessive daytime sleepiness: PAP, when compared to no treatment, shows significant improvement in sleepiness.
2. Impaired sleep: mixed data that PAP will alleviate this symptom.
3. HTN: PAP therapy causes a clinically significant BP reduction. But, if PAP is burdensome to sleep cycle, patients without sleep symptoms may be treated with standard anti-HTN treatment in lieu of PAP.
4. CV events/mortality: insufficient evidence to recommend PAP as a means to reduce CV events or CV mortality.

Sources

–*J Clin Sleep Med.* 2017;13(3):479-504.
–*J Clin Sleep Med.* 2019;15(2):335-343.
–VA/DoD CPG for the Management of Chronic Insomnia Disorder and Obstructive Sleep Apnea, Version 1.0-2019.

ASTHMA, EXACERBATIONS

Population
–Children >5 y and adults.

Organization
▶ GINA 2020

Recommendations
–**Acute exacerbation**
  - If in the clinic, assess severity of asthma exacerbation while starting SABA and supplemental oxygen as needed.
  - Transfer to acute care facility if altered mentation, silent chest, or signs of severe exacerbation (agitated, accessary muscle use, HR > 120, 90% SatO2 on RA) are observed. Give inhaled SABA, inhaled ipratropium bromide, oxygen, and systemic corticosteroids as soon as possible.
  - Consider alternative causes for the patient's respiratory symptoms. Consider anaphylaxis, foreign body, bronchiectasis, congenital heart disease/cardiac failure, pulmonary embolism, chronic obstructive pulmonary disease (COPD).
  - If in the ED, start treatment with repeated doses of inhaled SABA, early oral corticosteroids, and supplemental oxygen. Titrate oxygen to maintain oxygen saturation 93%–95% in adults, and 94%–98% in children ages 6–12 y.
  - Consider IV magnesium if patient is not responding to initial SABA, ipratropium bromide, oxygen, and systemic steroids.
  - No role for routine antibiotics, chest X-ray (CXR), or blood gases in asthma exacerbation. Use antibiotics only for suspected bacterial infections.

–**Subsequent care**
  - Initiate inhaled corticosteroid (ICS) before hospital discharge or step up ICS treatment for 2–4 wk. Stress daily use.
  - Prescribe 5–7 d course oral corticosteroid for adults and 3–5 d course for children. Follow-up within 2–7 d. Ensure symptoms are well controlled and that the treatment is continued.
  - Use the exacerbation as an opportunity to review the patient's chronic medication regimen, identify misunderstanding, and review the asthma action plan.

Comment
1. Corticosteroids dosing:
   a. For children: prednisolone 1–2 mg/kg/d to max 40 mg/d.
   b. For adults: methylprednisolone 1 mg/kg IV q6h initially for severe exacerbations. Prednisolone 40–50 mg PO for mild-to-moderate.
   c. Magnesium dosing: Magnesium sulfate 2 g IV.
   d. Rapid-acting beta-agonists (SABA) dosing: 4–10 puffs albuterol pMDI with spacer or 2.5–5 mg nebulized every 20 min for 1 h.

Source
–Global Strategy for Asthma Management and Prevention 2020 Update. Global Initiative for Asthma. http://www.ginasthma.org

ASTHMA, STABLE

Population
–Children age >5 y, adolescents, and adults.

Organization
▶ GINA 2020, NICE 2017

Recommendations
–**Basic principles**
  - Diagnose asthma by history: typical symptoms are a combination of shortness of breath, cough, wheezing, and chest tightness; variability over time and in intensity; frequent triggers.
  - Recommend spirometry with bronchodilators to confirm diagnosis, determine the severity of airflow limitation and its reversibility. Repeat spirometry at least every 1–2 y for asthma monitoring. FEV_1 and FEV_1/FVC ratio are reduced in asthma and increase by more than 12% after a bronchodilator challenge.
  - Classify asthma by level of symptom control.
  - Obtain a chest radiograph at the initial visit to exclude alternative diagnoses.
  - Assess for tobacco use and strongly advise smokers to quit.
  - Consider allergy testing for history of atopy, rhinitis, rhinorrhea, and seasonal variation or specific extrinsic triggers.
  - Encourage allergen and environmental or occupational trigger avoidance.
  - Recommend an asthma action plan based on peak expiratory flow (PEF) monitoring for all patients.
  - Educate patients, assist them in self-management, develop goals of treatment, create an asthma action plan, and regularly monitor asthma control.

STEPWISE APPROACH TO ASTHMA MANAGEMENT

Stepwise approach to asthma treatment

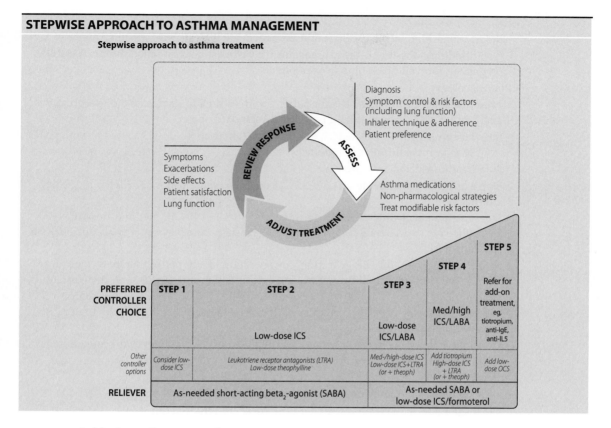

	STEP 1	STEP 2	STEP 3	STEP 4	STEP 5
PREFERRED CONTROLLER CHOICE		Low-dose ICS	Low-dose ICS/LABA	Med/high ICS/LABA	Refer for add-on treatment, eg, tiotropium, anti-IgE, anti-IL5
Other controller options	*Consider low-dose ICS*	*Leukotriene receptor antagonists (LTRA)* *Low-dose theophylline*	*Med-/high-dose ICS* *Low-dose ICS+LTRA* *(or + theoph)*	*Add tiotropium* *High-dose ICS* *+ LTRA* *(or + theoph)*	*Add low-dose OCS*
RELIEVER	As-needed short-acting beta₂-agonist (SABA)		As-needed SABA or low-dose ICS/formoterol		

–**Achieving asthma control**

- Assess: in the last 4 wk, has patient had:
  - Daytime asthma symptoms >2×/wk.
  - Night waking due to asthma.
  - Need for SABA reliever for symptoms >2×/wk.
  - Any activity limitations due to asthma.
- Well-controlled asthma is defined by 0 of the above.
- Partly controlled asthma is 1–2 of the above.
- Uncontrolled asthma is 3–4 of the above.
- Major independent risk factors for exacerbations:
  - Uncontrolled asthma.
  - Frequent asthma exacerbations (>1 in the past year).
  - History of ICU admission or intubation for asthma exacerbation.

- Potentially modifiable risk factors:
  - Medications: high SABA use, lack of ICS, inadequate ICS.
  - Comorbidities: obesity, chronic rhinosinusitis, gastroesophageal reflux disease (GERD), pregnancy, food allergies, blood eosinophilia.
- Pharmacology:
  - Prescribe at least a low-dose ICS for patients with asthma to reduce risk of exacerbations and death. SABA-only treatment is no longer standard of care.
  - Step 1 asthma: PRN low-dose ICS + formoterol (children 6–11: ICS alone prn with SABA +/− ICS for breakthrough symptoms).
  - Step 2 asthma: daily low-dose ICS.
  - Step 3 asthma: daily low-dose ICS + LABA (6–11 y: medium-dose ICS is a reasonable alternative).
  - Step 4 asthma: daily low-dose ICS/formoterol daily and PRN, or medium-dose ICS/LABA daily with SABA PRN (6–11 y: refer to specialty care if symptoms uncontrolled on medium-dose ICS).
  - Step 5 asthma: refer for allergy testing, consideration of adjunctive therapies (high-dose ICS/LABA, tiotropium, azithromycin, anti-IgE, anti-IL5, anti-IL4Rα, oral corticosteroids, etc.).
  - For patients at steps 2+, also prescribe SABA or low-dose ICS + formoterol to use PRN breakthrough symptoms.
  - Consider leukotriene receptor antagonists in place of ICS in patients with concomitant allergic rhinitis or who are intolerant of ICS.
  - For difficult-to-control asthma:
    - Treat potentially aggravating conditions: rhinitis, GERD, nasal polyps.
    - Consider alternative diagnoses: COPD or vocal cord dysfunction.

Source

–Reproduced with permission © 2022 Global Initiative for Asthma. Global Strategy for Asthma Management and Prevention 2020 Update. www.ginasthma.org

BRONCHIOLITIS, ACUTE

Population

–Infants and children.

Organization

▶ NICE 2015

Recommendations

Evaluation

–Consider diagnosis in children under 2 y of age, especially in the first year of life. Incidence peaks between 3 and 6 mo.

–Symptoms typically peak between 3 and 5 d. Cough resolves in 90% of infants within 3 wk.

–Diagnose bronchiolitis if the patient has a coryzal prodrome lasting 1 to 3 d, followed by all of the following:

- Persistent cough.
- Either tachypnea or chest recession (or both).
- Either wheeze or crackles on chest auscultation (or both).

–Other common symptoms include fever (30% of cases, usually <39°C) and poor feeding (typically after 3–5 d of illness).

–Consider a diagnosis of pneumonia if the patient has high fever (>39°C) and/or persistently focal crackles.

–Admit to hospital if any of the following:

- Apnea (observed or reported).
- Persistent room air oxygen saturation <90% (age ≥ 6 wk) or <92% (age < 6 wk or any age with underlying health conditions).
- Inadequate oral fluid intake.
- Persisting severe respiratory distress (ie, grunting, marked chest recession, or respiratory rate > 70 breaths/min).

–When deciding whether to admit a baby or child with bronchiolitis, take account of any known risk factors for more severe bronchiolitis.

–Do not routinely perform blood tests or CXR (changes on X-ray may mimic pneumonia but do not require antibiotics).

Management

–Do not perform chest physiotherapy unless relevant comorbidities (ie, spinal muscular atrophy, severe tracheomalacia).

–Do not use any of the following to treat bronchiolitis in babies or children:

- Antibiotics.
- Hypertonic saline.
- Adrenaline (nebulized).
- Salbutamol.
- Montelukast.
- Ipratropium bromide.
- Systemic or inhaled corticosteroids/a combination of systemic corticosteroids and nebulized adrenaline.

–Give oxygen supplementation to babies and children with bronchiolitis if their oxygen saturation is <90% (age ≥ 6 wk) or <92% (age < 6wk or any age with underlying health conditions).

–Do not routinely perform upper airway suctioning in babies or children with bronchiolitis. Consider upper airway suctioning in babies and children who have respiratory distress or feeding difficulties because of upper airway secretions.

Source
  –https://www.nice.org.uk/guidance/ng9

BRONCHITIS, ACUTE

Population
–Adults age ≥ 18 y.

Organization
▶ CDC 2017

Recommendations
–Avoid CXR if all the following are present:
- Heart rate <100 beats/min.
- Respiratory rate <24 breaths/min.
- Temperature <100.4°F (38°C).
- No exam findings consistent with pneumonia (consolidation, egophony, fremitus).

–Colored sputum does not predict bacterial infection.
–Avoid routine use of antibiotics regardless of duration of cough.
–Treat symptomatically, as necessary:
- Cough suppression (codeine, dextromethorphan).
- Antihistamines (first or second generation).
- Pharyngeal drainage with decongestants (phenylephrine).

Comments
1. Primary clinical goal is to exclude pneumonia.
2. Consider antitussive agents for short-term relief of coughing.
3. Avoid routine beta-2 agonists or mucolytic agents to alleviate cough.

Source
–https://www.cdc.gov/antibiotic-use/community/for-hcp/outpatient-hcp/adult-treatment-rec.html

CHRONIC OBSTRUCTIVE PULMONARY DISEASE, EXACERBATIONS

Population
–Adults.

Organizations
▶ GOLD 2022, ERS/ATS 2017

Recommendations
–Consider alternate diagnoses: PNA, pneumothorax, pleural effusion, pulmonary embolism, pulmonary edema, cardiac arrhythmias.
–Classify and treat according to severity (GOLD):
- Mild: short-acting bronchodilators.
- Moderate: SABA + antibiotics and/or oral glucocorticoids.
- Severe (acute respiratory failure): hospitalization or ER.

CONFLICTING GUIDANCE: THERAPY FOR COPD EXACERBATIONS IN THE AMBULATORY SETTING		
	GOLD	**ERS/ATS**
Corticosteroids	Use glucocorticoids for moderate or severe exacerbations: Prednisone 40 mg PO daily × 5 d or Prednisolone 40 mg PO or IV daily × 5 d	Suggest ≤ 14 d corticosteroid course
Antibiotics	Treat with antibiotics for 5–7 d if exacerbation is associated with sputum color change, increased volume or thicknessChoose an aminopenicillin w/ clavulanic acid, macrolide, or a tetracycline, depending on local bacterial resistance patterns	Suggest administration of antibiotics

- Use noninvasive positive pressure ventilation for moderate-to-severe hypercapnic respiratory failure. Bi-PAP improves survival, and decreases need for intubation, infectious complications, and hospital length of stay in moderate-to-severe COPD exacerbations.
- Use bronchodilators for acute treatment despite lack of high-quality evidence (GOLD). Deliver by nebulizer or metered-dose inhalers. Inhale 1–2 puffs q1h for 2–3 doses and then q2–4h. Do not use continuous nebulizer.
- Do not use methylxanthines due to side-effect profiles.
- **Postexacerbation care:**
  - Before 1 mo, review discharge therapy and inhaler technique. Assess for need for long-term oxygen treatment through a new ABG and SatO2%. Document symptoms via CAT or mMRC and document capacity for ADLs. (GOLD)
  - At 3–4 mo, reassess lung function by spirometry and prognosis (ie, BODE index[1]). (GOLD)
  - Enroll in pulmonary rehabilitation within 3 wk of hospital discharge. (ERS/ATA)

Comments

1. The scope of the ERS/ATS guidelines is much narrower, owing to the lack of conclusive evidence for much of the detail in the GOLD recommendations.
2. Short courses of oral antibiotics and oral corticosteroids are the only evidence-based therapies that improve outcomes in COPD exacerbations. There is insufficient data to guide choice of antibiotic or treatment duration. (*Ann Intern Med.* 2020;172:413-422)

Sources

- Wedzicha JA, Miravitlles M, Hurst JR et al. *Management of COPD Exacerbations: A European Respiratory Society/American Thoracic Society Guideline.* Reproduced with permission of the © ERS 2021: *Eur Respir J.* 2017;49:1600791. doi: 10.1183/13993003.00791-201
- https://goldcopd.org/

[1]*N Engl J Med.* 2004;350:1005-1012. http://www.nejm.org/doi/full/10.1056/NEJMoa021322#t=article

CHRONIC OBSTRUCTIVE PULMONARY DISEASE (COPD), STABLE

REVISED GOLD COPD GRADING AND STAGING

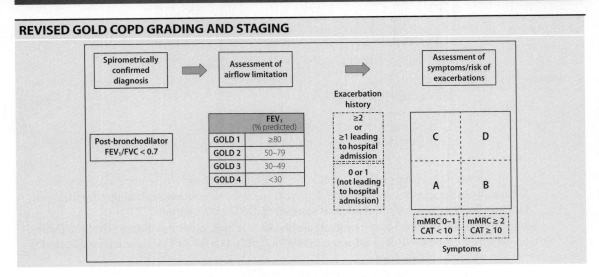

Population

–Adults.

Organizations

▶ GOLD 2020, ATS 2020

Recommendations

–Counsel for smoking cessation. Smoking cessation has the greatest capacity to influence the natural history of COPD.

–Evaluate symptoms using COPD Assessment Tool (CAT) or Modified British Medical Research Council Dyspnea Scale (mMRC). Risk factors for chronic airflow limitation include smoking, alpha-1 antitrypsin deficiency, occupational dust/agent/fume exposure, asthma, factors that affect lung growth. (GOLD)

–GOLD Grading and Staging: assess severity of COPD by GOLD Grades 1–4 based on spirometry and GOLD Stages A–D based on symptoms and exacerbation history. Label is expressed as "GOLD grade _, group _."

GUIDELINES DISCORDANT: STEPWISE MEDICATION APPROACH TO CHRONIC COPD

GOLD	ATS

1. SABA + SAMA PRN.
2. If persistent symptoms, add:
  a. FEV1 > 50% of predicted: either LABA or LAMA
  b. FEV1 < 50% of predicted: either LABA, ICS, or LAMA
3. If persistent symptoms: LAMA+LABA+ICS[a]
	1. LABA + LAMA if dyspnea and exercise intolerance[b]
	2. If persistent symptoms and 1+ exacerbation requiring treatment in the past year: ICS + LABA + LAMA
	3. If a patient on ICS + LABA + LAMA goes a year without an exacerbation, stop the ICS

Other suggestions:
  Phosphodiesterase-4 inhibitors improve lung function and reduce moderate-to-severe exacerbations for patients with severe COPD
  In refractory cases, consider extended course (up to 1 y) azithromycin 250 mg/d
	Other suggestions:
	  −Avoid maintenance oral corticosteroids for frequent severe exacerbations
	  −In patients with severe refractory dyspnea, consider opiates to manage the symptom

[a] Triple therapy ICS/LABA/LAMA is superior in reducing exacerbations compared to ICS/LABA, LABA/LAMA, or LAMA alone (NNT 16). Evidence for mortality benefit is mixed.

[b] The combination improved symptom scores and reduced exacerbations more than monotherapy with LABA or LAMA without additional adverse effects.

GUIDELINES DISCORDANT: ROLE OF EOSINOPHILIA IN PATIENTS ELIGIBLE FOR ICS

Organization	Guidance
GOLD	Use blood eosinophil count to determine if ICS is safe to use. Use caution if eosinophils <300 cells/μL. Eosinophils <100, repeated pneumonia events, or history of mycobacterial infection are contraindications to ICS
ATS	Insufficient evidence to make a statement

- Administer annual influenza vaccination, and pneumococcal vaccination PPSV23 for adults <65 y with FEV1 < 40%; PCV13 for adults in general population age ≥65 y.
- Arrange pulmonary rehabilitation for symptomatic patients with moderate-to-severe COPD (FEV1 < 50% of predicted).
  - Prescribe continuous oxygen therapy for COPD patients with room air hypoxemia (PaO_2 ≤ 55 mmHg or SpO_2 ≤ 88%).
  - Screen COPD patients for osteoporosis and depression.
  - Avoid regular mucolytic therapy.
  - Offer nutritional support for patients with severe COPD with malnutrition.
  - Calculate the BODE index (BMI, airflow obstruction, dyspnea, and exercise capacity on a 6-min walk test) to assess the risk of death in severe COPD.[1]

[1] See http://www.nejm.org/doi/full/10.1056/NEJMoa021322#t=article

Comments

1. Confirm suspected COPD with postbronchodilator spirometry. Perform spirometry in patients with symptoms and/or risk factors.
2. $FEV_1/FVC < 0.7$ confirms the presence of airflow obstruction and COPD.
3. Classification of COPD by spirometry:
   a. Mild COPD = $FEV_1 \geq 80\%$ of predicted.
   b. Moderate COPD = FEV_1 50%–79% of predicted.
   c. Severe COPD = FEV_1 30%–49% of predicted.
   d. Very severe COPD = $FEV_1 < 30\%$ of predicted.
4. Can consider lung volume reduction surgery in patients with severe upper lobe emphysema and low post-pulmonary rehab exercise capacity.
5. Consider roflumilast, a phosphodiesterase-4 inhibitor, to reduce exacerbations for patients with severe chronic bronchitis and frequent exacerbations.

Source

–Global Initiative for Chronic Obstructive Lung Disease: Global Strategy for the Diagnosis, Management and Prevention of Chronic Obstructive Pulmonary Disease 2020 Report. https://goldcopd.org/

–*Am J Respir Crit Care Med.* 2020;201(9):e56-e69.

COMMON MEDICATIONS FOR THE MANAGEMENT OF COPD

Drug	Inhaler (µg/dose)	Nebulizer (mg/mL)	Drug	Inhaler (µg/dose)	Nebulizer (mg/mL)
Short-acting beta₂-agonists			**Combination beta₂-agonist-anticholinergics**		
Albuterol	100–200[M/D]	5	Albuterol-ipratropium	100/20[SMI]	1 vial
Levalbuterol	45–90[M]	0.21, 0.42	**Methylxanthines**		
Long-acting beta₂-agonists			**Aminophylline**	**200–600 mg pill PO**	
Arformoterol		0.0075	Theophylline SR	100–600 mg pill PO	
Formoterol	4.5–12[M/D]	0.01	**Inhaled corticosteroids**		
Indacaterol	75–300[D]		Beclomethasone	50–400[M/D]	0.2–0.4
Salmeterol	25–50[M/D]		Budesonide	100, 200, 400[D]	0.2, 0.25, 0.5
Short-acting anticholinergics			Fluticasone	50–500[M/D]	
Ipratropium bromide	20, 40[M]	0.25–0.5	**Combination beta₂-agonist-corticosteroids**		
Long-acting anticholinergics			Formoterol-budesonide	4.5/160[M]; 9/320[D]	
Aclidinium bromide	322[D]		Formoterol-mometasone	10/200[M] or 10/400[M]	

COMMON MEDICATIONS FOR THE MANAGEMENT OF COPD *(Continued)*					
Drug	**Inhaler (μg/ dose)**	**Nebulizer (mg/mL)**	**Drug**	**Inhaler (μg/ dose)**	**Nebulizer (mg/ mL)**
Tiotropium	18[D], 5[SMI]		Salmeterol-fluticasone	50/100, 50/250, 50/500[D]	
				25/50, 25/125, 25/250[M]	
Phosphodiesterase-4 inhibitors			Vilanterol-fluticasone	25/100[D]	
Roflumilast	500 μg PO daily				

M = metered-dose inhalers.
D = dry powder inhalers.
SMI = soft mist inhalers.
Source: Data from *GOLD Guide to COPD Diagnosis, Management and Prevention.* http://goldcopd.org

COUGH, CHRONIC

Population
–Adults and children >14 y/o with cough >8-wk duration.

Organizations
▶ ACCP 2020, ERS 2020

Recommendations
–Determine the duration of the cough as acute (<3 wk), subacute (3–8 wk), or chronic (>8 wk), as this can guide the differential diagnosis.
–Evaluate for red flag symptoms, occupational/environmental exposures, travel exposures, physical exam, and CXR.
–Consider the common causes of chronic cough with a normal CXR:
  • Smoking.
  • ACE inhibitor use.
  • Upper airway cough syndrome (formerly known as postnasal drip syndrome).
  • Asthma (classic, cough-variant, or nonasthmatic eosinophilic bronchitis).
  • GERD.
  • Nonasthmatic eosinophilic bronchitis.
  • Cough hypersensitivity.
–Oral prednisolone ×1 wk helps in classic asthma in adults, but there's greater efficacy of systemic leukotriene antagonists (Montelukast) in all groups.
–Consider 2–4 wk of ICS (though may not be superior to placebo).
–Avoid using bronchodilators alone as maintenance treatment for cough in asthma.
–Avoid empiric therapy for GERD if no peptic/esophageal symptoms.

–Diagnose "unexplained chronic cough" if lasting >8 wk without an identifiable cause after investigation and supervised therapeutic trials.

–Consider cough hypersensitivity and treat with speech therapy or cough neuromodulators: morphine 5 mg BID has strong evidence, while gabapentin and pregabalin have moderate evidence.

–Do not routinely perform chest CT scans on patients with chronic cough, normal CXR, and normal physical exam.

Population

–Children <14 y with cough >4-wk duration.

Organization

▶ ACCP 2020

Recommendations

–Evaluate cough >4-wk for signs/symptoms such as productive cough, wheezing, recurrent infections, hemoptysis, growth failure, facial pain, dyspnea, chest pain, and digital clubbing.

–Order CXR and spirometry if >6 y.

–"Specific cough" has signs/symptoms and/or spirometry/CXR findings. Indicates underlying disorder like bronchiectasis, retained foreign body or large airway obstruction, aspiration, cardiac anomalies, cystic fibrosis, asthma, TB, and tracheomalacia.

–"Protracted bacterial bronchitis" (PBB) is a chronic wet cough w/o other specific SXS or findings on imaging/spirometry. Prescribe 2–4 wk of antibiotics following local antibiograms.

–"Nonspecific cough" is a dry cough without signs/symptoms and with normal CXR and spirometry:

- Usually postviral cough or acute viral bronchitis.
- Watch, wait, review every 2–4 wk evaluating for specific signs or symptoms.
- Discuss with parents the trial of therapy with ICS (400 µg/d budesonide equivalent). Follow up in 2 wk; if cough resolves, may be asthma.

–Do not recommend OTC medications for symptomatic relief of cough.

Comments

1. Red flag symptoms for cough:
   a. Hemoptysis.
   b. Smoker age >45 with new cough, change in cough, or coexisting voice disturbance.
   c. Adults age 55–80 with a 30 pack-year history or who have quit less than 15 y ago.
   d. Dyspnea, especially at rest or at night.
   e. Hoarseness.
   f. Systemic symptoms: fever, weight loss, peripheral edema with weight gain.
   g. Dysphagia.
   h. Vomiting.
   i. Recurrent pneumonia.
   j. Abnormal physical exam or CXR.

2. The quality of evidence surrounding cough suppressants is poor. None routinely outperform placebo, but placebo improves symptoms in >50% of patients in many studies. Few have serious adverse effects, but antihistamines and dextromethorphan have a higher rate of nonserious adverse effects.[1]

Sources

–Morice AH et al. ERS guidelines on the diagnosis and treatment of chronic cough in adults and children. *Eur Respir J*. 2020;55:1901136.

–CHEST Guideline and Expert Panel Report. Managing chronic cough as a symptom in children and management algorithms. *Chest*. 2020;158(1):P303-P329.

–CHEST Guideline and Expert Panel Report. *Chest*. 2018;153(1):196-209.

Population

–Adults and children >12 y/o with chronic cough due to asthma or nonasthmatic eosinophilic bronchitis (NAEB).

Organization

▶ ACCP 2020

Recommendations

–Use noninvasive measurement of airway inflammation. Eosinophilic airway inflammation is likely to be associated with a more favorable response to ICS.

–Use ICS as first-line therapy.

–If response to ICS is incomplete, step up the ICS dose and consider a therapeutic trial of a leukotriene inhibitor after reconsideration of alternative causes of cough.

–In cough-variant asthma (but not NAEB), consider beta-agonist in combination with ICS.

Comment

1. Evidence is much greater for trial of leukotriene inhibitor in chronic cough due to asthma than NAEB due to the smaller amount of trials for NAEB.

Source

–*CHEST* 2020;158(1):68-96.

OBESITY HYPOVENTILATION SYNDROME

Population

–Patients with BMI > 30, especially in BMI > 40.

Organization

▶ ATS 2019

Recommendations

–Diagnose obesity hypoventilation syndrome (OHS) in the setting of:

[1]*Cochrane Database Syst Rev.* 2014;2014(11). https://www.ncbi.nlm.nih.gov/pmc/articles/PMC7061814/

- BMI > 30 kg/m^2.
- Sleep-disordered breathing (SDB).
- Awake daytime hypercapnia, awake resting PaCO2 > 45 mmHg at sea level.
–In high pretest probability of OHS, screen with PaCO2.
–In low-to-moderate probability of OHS (BMI 30–40 w/SDB), a serum bicarbonate level <27 mmol/L can rule out OHS. If ≥27, screen with a PaCO2.
–Follow up elevated PaCO2 with both a sleep study (polysomnography or respiratory polygraph) and awake ABG.
–Use CPAP, regardless of concomitant OSA.
–If CPAP is inadequate, change to noninvasive ventilation.
–If hospitalized adults are suspected to have OHS w/o prior formal sleep study diagnosis, discharge on noninvasive ventilation and refer to sleep laboratory within 3 mo after hospital discharge due to high-risk short-term mortality w/o therapy.
–Pursue weight-loss interventions that produce sustained 25%–30% weight loss of actual body weight. This is the level of weight loss that may be required to resolve hypoventilation.
–Even multifaceted weight-loss lifestyle programs may not produce these results.
–If patient has no contraindications, evaluate for bariatric surgery.

Comment

1. Of obese patients referred to sleep centers for OSA or SDB, 8%–20% are diagnosed with OHS. 90% of OHS patients have coexistent OSA, 70% of total OHS patients have severe OSA. The other 10% have nonobstructive, sleep-dependent hypoventilation.

Source
–*Am J Resp Crit Care Med.* 2019;200(3):e6-e24.

NON-SMALL-CELL LUNG CANCER (NSCLC) FOLLOW-UP CARE

Population

–Non-small-cell lung cancer patients treated with curative intent.

Organization

▶ American College of Chest Physicians (ACCP) 2013

Recommendation

–**Follow-up program**
- Perform chest CT scan every 6 mo for first 2 y after resection then once a year thereafter out to 10 y (second primary in 10% who survive first lung cancer).
- Avoid routine imaging with PET scanning.
- See patients every 3–4 mo for 2 y then less frequently. Assess health-related quality of life with each visit.
- Avoid surveillance biomarker testing outside of clinical trials.
- Offer smoking cessation interventions, annual influenza vaccine, and every 5 y pneumococcal vaccinations.

- Evaluate any headache or neurologic symptoms with MRI brain with gadolinium, as lung cancer is the most common cancer to have brain metastases.

Comments

1. Cure rates are reflective of stage:
   a. Stage I—65%–70%.
   b. Stage II—40%.
   c. Stage IIIA—25%.
   d. Stage IIIB—18%.
2. Symptoms of local recurrence include increase or change in cough, dyspnea, and chest pain.

Source
   –*JAMA*. 2010;303:1070.

PLEURAL EFFUSION, NEW

Population

–Adults with undiagnosed unilateral pleural effusion.

Organization

▶ BTS 2010

Recommendations

–Use ultrasound or a posteroanterior CXR to detect the presence of a pleural effusion. Consider a lateral decubitus CXR to differentiate pleural liquid from pleural thickening.

–CT scans detect very small effusions (less than 10 mL of fluid). Use CT scan to evaluate undiagnosed exudative pleural effusions prior to complete pleural fluid drainage. Obtain CT scan in the setting of pleural infection which has not responded to initial chest tube drainage.

–Thoracic ultrasound is more sensitive than CT scan to distinguish loculations.

–During thoracentesis, bedside ultrasound guidance improves the likelihood of successful aspiration and reduces risk of organ puncture.

–Perform thoracentesis for any undiagnosed effusions of more than 1 cm from the chest wall on lateral decubitus CXR. Do not perform thoracentesis on bilateral pleural effusions in a setting which is strongly suggestive of a transudative process, unless there are atypical features or a failure to respond to therapy. In patients with advanced cancer, do not perform thoracentesis for small effusions.

–Perform diagnostic thoracentesis for all patients with a pleural effusion in the setting of sepsis or pneumonic illness.

–Send pleural fluid for cell count and differential, Gram stain and culture, protein, lactate dehydrogenase (LDH), and cytology. A minimum of 50–60 mL of pleural fluid should be withdrawn for analysis. Assess pleural fluid pH in nonpurulent effusions when pleural infection is suspected. Check pleural fluid glucose when pleural fluid pH is not available and pleural infection is suspected.

–Involve a chest physician or thoracic surgeon in the care of all patients who require chest tube drainage for pleural infection.

Sources
–BTS *Pleural Disease Guideline.* 2010
–*Thorax.* 2010;65(suppl 2):ii1-76.

PLEURAL EFFUSION, MALIGNANT (MPE)

Population
–Adults with lung cancer or metastatic malignancy to the lung with a malignant pleural effusion.

Organizations
▶ BTS 2010, ACCP 2014

Recommendations
–If MPE suspected, send pleural fluid for cytology (minimum 50 mL; ideally 200 mL to allow for cell block and molecular testing).
–Refer all patients with MPE to pulmonologist and/or thoracic surgery for treatment options.
–Asymptomatic patients require frequent follow-up but no treatment.
–Treat symptomatic patients initially with therapeutic thoracentesis (1000–1500 mL) to relieve symptoms.
–Consider recurrent outpatient therapeutic thoracentesis for patients with expected survival less than 1 mo and/or poor performance status (PS) and/or slow reaccumulation of the pleural effusion (ie, >1 mo).
–Otherwise, pursue definitive intervention after first or second thoracentesis. Choice of therapy depends on projected survival and availability of resources. Individualize management and present to a multidisciplinary Tumor Board for advice. (*JAMA.* 2012;307:2432)
–Treatment options:
  • Indwelling (tunneled) pleural catheter (considered for patients with trapped lung who experience some relief following thoracentesis): for patients who want to avoid hospitalization or discomfort of pleurodesis.
  • Talc pleurodesis (Talc poudrage) via thoracoscopy: consider for patients with longer projected survival and those who don't want an indwelling catheter. Contraindicated for patients with trapped lung.
  • Talc pleurodesis (slurry) via chest tube: consider for patients with longer projected survival or contraindication to thoracoscopy. Contraindicated for patients with trapped lung.
  • Consider chemotherapy as an adjunct treatment option. Patients undergoing first-line systemic therapy for tumors with high response rates (small-cell lung cancer and lymphoma) may avoid definitive treatments.

Comment
1. Indwelling pleural catheter (IPC-pleurex catheter) requires a regular outpatient drainage schedule. Address potential burden for the patient or caregiver. Complications from IPCs are

uncommon. The infection rate is 5%, with more than half the patients responding to antibiotics without removing the catheter. (*Chest.* 2013;144:1597) Other problems with IPCs include pneumothorax (5.9%), cellulitis (3.4%), obstruction/clogging (3.7%), and unspecified catheter malfunction (9.1%). The most common adverse events with talc pleurodesis include fever, pain, and GI symptoms. Less common are cardiac arrhythmia, dyspnea, systemic inflammatory response, empyema, and talc dissemination.

Sources

–https://www.guideline.gov/summaries/summary/49355/management-of-malignant-pleural-effusion
–*Chest.* 2012;142:394
–*Chest.* 2013;143(5):e4555-e4975.
–*J Natl Compr Canc Netw.* 2012;10:975.
–*Thoracic Society Pleural Disease Guideline.* 2010.
–*Thorax.* 2010;65(suppl 2):132.

PNEUMOTHORAX, SPONTANEOUS

Population

–Adults with diagnosis of spontaneous pneumothorax.

Organization

▶ BTS 2010

Recommendations[1]

–Use standard standing CXR for the initial diagnosis; expiratory films are not necessary. CT scan is recommended for uncertain or complex cases.
–Tension pneumothorax is a medical emergency. Suspect in the setting of respiratory distress or hypotension. Treat with oxygen supplementation and needle decompression.
–Symptoms including dyspnea are more important than the size of pneumothorax in determining the management strategy.
–If the patient has pneumothorax size <2 cm and minimal symptoms, consider discharge with outpatient follow-up and return precautions.
–If the patient has significant dyspnea or pneumothorax size >2 cm, recommend needle aspiration with 16–18 G needle. If pneumothorax is then >2 cm and symptoms improved, consider discharge with outpatient follow-up. For pneumothorax <2 cm with minimal symptoms, consider conservative management/observation. If after needle aspiration, the patient is still symptomatic, or size still <2 cm, recommend chest drain size 8–14 Fr and admission.
–Use needle aspiration and small-bore chest drains (<20 Fr) rather than large-bore chest drains for reduced hospitalization and length of stay.

[1]These recommendations do not apply for secondary pneumothorax, or pneumothorax in the setting of underlying lung disease. For these patients, admit at a minimum for observation and oxygen, even if not actively managed.

–If there is a persistent air leak at 48 h, consult with chest physician.

–Smoking cessation counseling is recommended to prevent recurrence.

Comment

1. Ultrasound with attention to pleural interface for lung sliding (sea shore sign on M-mode) is highly sensitive for pneumothorax. While the guidelines are yet to be updated, ultrasound has proven more sensitive than CXR for pneumothorax. (*Acad Emerg Med.* 2010;17(1):11-17) (*Am J Emerg Med.* 2019. https://doi.org/10.1016/j.ajem.2019.02.028)

Sources

–*Thoracic Society Pleural Disease Guideline.* 2010.

–*Thorax.* 2010;65(suppl 2):ii18-31.

–Wilkerson RG, et al. Sensitivity of bedside ultrasound and supine anteroposterior chest radiographs for the identification of pneumothorax after blunt trauma. *Acad Emerg Med.* 2010. PMID: 20078434.

PULMONARY HYPERTENSION

Population

–Adults diagnosed with pulmonary hypertension or with suspected diagnosis.

Organization

▶ ACCP 2019

Recommendations

–Refer all pulmonary arterial hypertension (PAH) patients to a center with expertise in diagnosis before therapy is started.

–Evaluate severity consistently. WHO Functional Classification for PAH has ranking I–IV based on progression of symptoms of dyspnea, fatigue, weakness on exertion and not on exertion. Evolution of symptoms includes lower extremity edema, angina, or syncope which would indicate right heart dysfunction/failure.

–Treat aggressively contributing causes such as sleep apnea and systemic hypertension.

–Arrange a supervised exercise activity.

–Keep patient up-to-date on influenza and pneumococcal PNA immunization schedules.

–Avoid pregnancy and nonessential surgery in PAH. When these do occur, refer to a multidisciplinary PAH center.

–Avoid exposure to high altitude. Supplemental oxygen may be needed to keep O2 Sat >91% in air travel.

–Incorporate palliative care services.

–If acute vasoreactivity testing is positive, start calcium channel blockers unless contraindicated (ie, right heart failure).

–Otherwise, use combination therapy (ambrisentan + tadalafil) or monotherapy (bosentan, macitentan, ambrisentan, riociguat, sildenafil, or tadalafil).

TABLE 30-1 FLEISCHNER SOCIETY 2017 GUIDELINES FOR MANAGEMENT OF INCIDENTALLY DETECTED PULMONARY NODULES IN ADULTS

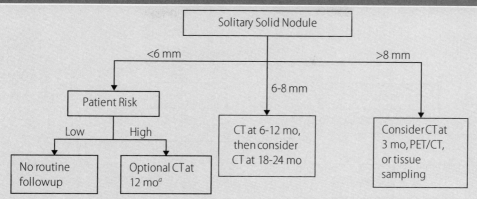

a Certain patients at high risk with suspicious nodule morphology, upper lobe location or both may warrant 12 mo f/u.

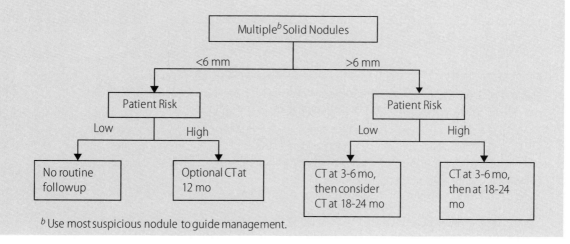

b Use most suspicious nodule to guide management.

TABLE 30-1 FLEISCHNER SOCIETY 2017 GUIDELINES FOR MANAGEMENT OF INCIDENTALLY DETECTED PULMONARY NODULES IN ADULTS *(Continued)*

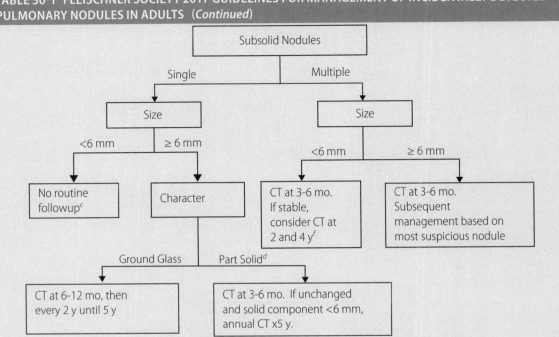

[c] In certain suspicious nodules <6 mm, consider follow-up at 2 and 4 y. If solid component(s) or growth develops, consider resection (recommendations 3A and 4A).

[d] In practice, part-solid nodules cannot be defined as such until [3]6 mm, and nodules <6 mm do not usually require follow-up. Persistent part-solid nodules with solid components [3]6 mm should be considered highly suspicious (recommendations 4A–4C).

[f] Multiple <6 mm pure ground-glass nodules are usually benign, but consider follow-up in selected patients at high risk at 2 and 4 y (recommendation 5A).

Note: These recommendations do not apply to lung cancer screening, patients with immunosuppression, or patients with known primary cancer.

–If rapid disease progression or poor prognosis, initiate parenteral prostanoids such as IV epoprostenol, IV treprostinil, or SC treprostinil. If parenteral prostanoids are not tolerated, the patient can take inhaled prostanoids with oral PDE-5 inhibitors and oral endothelin receptor antagonists. The patient can take up to 3 classes of PAH pharmacotherapy until consideration for lung transplant.

Source
–Chest Guideline and Expert Panel Report Update. Therapy for pulmonary arterial hypertension in adults. *Chest*. 2019;15(3):565-586.

PULMONARY NODULES

Population

–Adults with incidental pulmonary nodules. These guidelines do not apply to immunocompromised patients, patients with cancer, or for lung cancer screening.

Organization

▶ Fleischer Society 2017

Recommendations

–Fleischner Society Guidelines recommend:
  • Categorize nodules by size, solid or subsolid, single or multiple, low or high risk.
–Do not follow up solid nodules 6 mm or less in diameter in low-risk adults >35-y-old, even if multiple nodules are present.
  • Use the Brock model for initial risk assessment of pulmonary nodules larger than 8 mm in patients who have ever smoked.
–Do not follow up diffuse, central, or laminated pattern of calcification or fat.
–Consider a PET-CT scan for patients with a pulmonary nodule and an initial risk of malignancy >5%.
–Suggestions for pulmonary nodules management:
  • Serial CT scans when the malignancy risk is <5%.
  • CT-guided biopsy when the risk of malignancy is 5%–65%.
  • Video-assisted thoracoscopic surgery when the chance of malignancy exceeds 65%.
  • Consider bronchoscopy when a bronchus sign is present on CT scan.

Source

–Table (Fleischner Society 2017 Guidelines for Management of Incidentally Detected Pulmonary Nodules in Adults) MacMahon H, Naidich D P, Goo J M, et al. Guidelines for management of incidental pulmonary nodules detected on CT images: from the Fleischner Society 2017. *Radiology*. 2017;284:228-243.

Renal Disorders

31

Population
—Adults.

Organizations
▶ KDIGO 2021, NKF-KDOQI 2014, NICE 2021, VA/DoD 2019

Recommendations
—Establish CKD stage by eGFR and presence of albuminuria with abnormalities being present for at least 3 mo. Establish etiology. Refer to urology or nephrology if appropriate.[1]
- Etiology: Assign probable cause of CKD based on absence or presence of systemic disease and the location within the kidney of observed or presumed pathologic-anatomic abnormalities.
- GFR category[2]:
  ○ G1: GFR > 90 (mL/min/1.73 m^2).
  ○ G2: GFR 60–89.
  ○ G3a: GFR 45–59.
  ○ G3b: GFR 30–44.
  ○ G4: GFR 15–29.
  ○ G5: GFR < 15.
- Albuminuria category by urine albumin-to-creatinine ratio (ACR):
  ○ A1: ACR < 3 (mg/mmol).
  ○ A2: ACR 3–30.
  ○ A3: ACR > 30.
—Evaluate for chronicity.
- In those with GFR < 60 mL/min/1.73 m^2 (GFR categories G3a–5), evaluate history of prior indicators for kidney disease and prior measurements.

[1]Possible indications for urology consultation: isolated or gross hematuria, renal masses or complex cysts, symptomatic or obstructing nephrolithiasis, hydronephrosis or bladder abnormalities, urinary symptoms.
Possible indications for nephrology consultation: eGFR < 30, decline in eGFR > 5 per year, non-DM with heavy proteinuria or hematuria, unclear cause of CKD, complications of CKD (anemia, acidosis, hyperphosphatemia, hyperparathyroidism, electrolyte abnormalities), DM with heavy proteinuria or hematuria, management of nephrolithiasis, ADPKD.
[2]Use serum creatinine-based eGFR for initial assessment. If eGFR < 60, consider one time serum cystatin C-based eGFR to confirm diagnosis and refine staging of CKD.

- If duration is >3 mo then CKD is confirmed. If not >3 mo CKD is not confirmed or is unclear.
  - —Monitor for CKD progression with annual GFR and ACR. Assess more frequently if higher risk for progression based on GFR and ACR.
  - —Monitor for complications in CKD stage 3a–5 with hemoglobin, electrolytes, calcium, phosphate, intact parathyroid hormone (PTH), 25-OH vitamin D.
  - —Management and prevention of disease progression and complications:
    - Treat the underlying cause of the CKD.
    - Control BP and individualize BP targets based on age, coexisting comorbidities, presence of retinopathy, and tolerance of treatment.

GUIDELINE DISCORDANT: TARGET BLOOD PRESSURE GOAL IN CKD NOT ON HD	
KDIGO 2021	SBP < 120 on standardized in-office measurement
NICE 2020	• If ACR < 70, goal BP <140/<90 • If ACR > 90, goal SBP <130/<80

- Use ACE-I or ARB in CKD and ACR > 70 or CKD with DM and ACR > 30.
- Target a hemoglobin A1c of approximately 7% in people with diabetes and CKD, although HbA1c should be individualized to a range of <6.5% to <8% based on multiple factors. (KDIGO)
- First-line glycemic control for CKD with DM includes metformin[1] and SGLT2[2] inhibitor, with additional therapy added as needed.
- Lower protein intake to 0.8 g/kg/d in adults with diabetes and nondiabetics with GFR categories G4–5.
- Recommend salt intake of <2 g/d in people with CKD.
- Supplement bicarbonate in CKD with metabolic acidosis.
- Give oral iron therapy every other day for Stage 3 or worse CKD with anemia.
- Use erythropoietic-stimulating agents only if hemoglobin <10 g/dL.
- Refer to nephrology for consideration of renal replacement therapy after shared decision-making if 5-y risk of RRT is >5%, if ACR >70, or on >4 antihypertensives. (NICE)
- Recommend immunizations for influenza, Tdap, 13-valent pneumococcal conjugate vaccine, hepatitis B virus, zoster, MMR.

Comments

1. Recommendation for low protein (0.6–0.8 g/kg/d) diet: If offered to CKD stage 3 and 4 patients, it may slow progression to ESRD, but also may be associated with risk of calorie malnutrition; thus, multidisciplinary support is recommended with use (VA/DoD). Alternate committees recommend to not offer low-protein diets (dietary protein intake less than 0.6–0.8 g/kg/d) (NICE).

---

[1]Metformin: Reduce dose once eGFR < 45. Discontinue if eGFR < 30 or HD initiation.
[2]SGLT2-I: Do not start if eGFR < 30. Discontinue with HD initiation.

2. eGFR calculators that incorporate race are based on flawed data and may exacerbate health inequities. Use caution when adjusting eGFR calculations based on race. (*NEJM* 2020; 383(9):874-882)

Sources

—https://www.ajkd.org/article/S0272-6386(14)00491-0/pdf
—KDIGO. Clinical practice guideline for diabetes management in chronic kidney disease. *Kidney Int.* 2020;98:S1-S115.
—KDIGO. Clinical practice guideline for the management of blood pressure in chronic kidney disease. *Kidney Int.* 2021;99:S1-S87.
—NICE. Chronic kidney disease: assessment and management. *NICE Guideline*. 25 August 2021. www.nice.org.uk/guidance/ng203.
—VA/DoD. *VA/DoD Clinical Practice Guideline for the Management of Chronic Kidney Disease*. 2019. https://www.healthquality.va.gov/guidelines/CD/ckd/VADoDCKDCPGProviderSummaryFinal5082142020.pdf

KIDNEY DISEASE, CHRONIC—MINERAL AND BONE DISORDERS (CKD-MBDS)

Population

—Adults and children.

Organization

▶ KDIGO 2017

Recommendations

—Monitor serum calcium, phosphorus, immunoreactive parathyroid hormone (iPTH), and alkaline phosphatase levels:
  • Beginning with Stage G3a CKD (adults).
  • Beginning with Stage G2 CKD (children).
—Measure 25-OH vitamin D levels beginning in stage G3a CKD.
—Treat all vitamin D deficiency with vitamin D supplementation with standard recommended dosing. Decisions to treat should be based on trends of vitamin D levels, not a single level.
—In Stages G3–5 CKD, consider a bone biopsy before bisphosphonate therapy if a dynamic bone disease is a possibility.
—In Stages G3–5 CKD, aim to normalize calcium and phosphorus levels.
—In Stage G5 CKD, seek to maintain a PTH level of approximately 2–9 times the upper normal limit for the assay.

Comment

1. Options for oral phosphate binders:
   a. Calcium acetate.
   b. Calcium carbonate.
   c. Calcium citrate.

   d. Sevelamer carbonate.

   e. Lanthanum carbonate.

Source

   —https://kdigo.org/wp-content/uploads/2017/02/KDIGO_CKD_MBD_Guideline_r6.pdf

KIDNEY INJURY, ACUTE (AKI)

Population

   —Children and adults.

Organization

▶ NICE 2013, 2019

Recommendations

   —Perform a urinalysis in all patients with AKI. Consider checking urine electrolytes (ie, urine sodium, urine creatine, urine urea, and urine osmolarity) to calculate a FENa or FEUrea.

   —Do not routinely obtain a renal ultrasound when the cause of the AKI has been identified.

   —Detect AKI with any of the following criteria:

   • Rise in serum creatinine ≥0.3 mg/dL in 48 h.

   • 50% or more rise in creatinine in last 7 d.

   • Urine output <0.5 mL/kg/h.

   —Refer for renal replacement therapy the patients with any of the following refractory to medical management:

   • Hyperkalemia.

   • Metabolic acidosis.

   • Uremia.

   • Fluid overload.

Sources

   —https://doi.org/10.1016/0002-9343(84)90368-1

   —https://www.nice.org.uk/guidance/ng148

RENAL CANCER (RCC) FOLLOW-UP CARE

Organization

▶ NCCN 2016

Recommendations

   —**Follow-up after a partial or radical nephrectomy**

   • History and physical (H&P) every 6 mo for 2 y then annually up to 5 y after surgery.

   • Comprehensive metabolic panel or other blood tests as indicated every 6 mo for 2 y then annually until 5 y.

- Baseline abdominal CT, MRI, or US within 3–9 mo of surgery. If initial scan-negative abdominal imaging may be considered annually for 3 y based on overall risk factors.
- **Follow-up after radical nephrectomy**
  - H&P every 3–6 mo for 3 y then annually up to 5 y after radical nephrectomy, then as clinically indicated.
  - Comprehensive metabolic panel, LDH, and C-reactive protein every 6 mo for 2 y then annually up to 5 y.
  - Baseline abdominal CT or MRI within 3–6 mo then CT, MRI, or US every 3–6 mo for 3 y then annually up to 5 y.
  - Chest imaging—baseline chest CT within 3–6 mo.
  - Pelvic, brain, or spinal imaging as clinically indicated. Nuclear bone scan as clinically indicated.

Comments

1. **RCC staging**
   a. Stage I—Tumor <7 cm N0M0.
   b. Stage II—Tumor >7 cm limited to kidney N0M0.
   c. Stage III—Any tumor size with regional node metastasis.
   d. Stage IV—T4 (spread beyond Gerota's fascia—any T, any N, M [-systemic metastases]).
2. Features of high risk for relapse: Stage III, size of tumor, high grade (Fuhrman 3 or 4), coagulative tumor necrosis (5 times increase in risk of death). (*Br J Urol.* 2009;103:165)

Source
—*J Clin Oncol.* 2014; j32:4059.

RENAL MASSES, SMALL

Population
—Adults with small renal masses (SRM < 4 cm).

Organization
▶ ASCO 2017

Recommendations
—Based on tumor-specific findings and competing risks of mortality, all patients with an SRM (<4 cm in size) should be considered for renal tumor biopsy (RTB) when the results may alter management (strength of recommendation: strong).
—Active surveillance should be an initial management option for patients who have significant comorbidities and limited life expectancy (end-stage renal disease, SRM < 1 cm, life expectancy < 5 y).
—Partial nephrectomy (PN) for SRM is the standard treatment that should be offered to all patients for whom an intervention is indicated and who possess a tumor that is amenable to this approach (recommendation: strong).

—Percutaneous thermal ablation should be considered an option for patients who possess tumors such that complete ablation will be achieved. A biopsy should be obtained before or at the time of ablation (recommendation: moderate).

—Radical nephrectomy for SRM should be reserved only for patients who possess a tumor of significant complexity that is not amenable to PN or where PN may result in unacceptable morbidity even when performed at centers of excellence. Referral to experienced surgeon and a center with experience should be considered (recommendation: strong).

—Referral to a nephrologist should be considered if CKD (GFR < 45 mL/min) or progressive CKD develops after treatment, especially if associated with proteinuria (recommendation: moderate).

Comments

1. SRMs are commonly discovered incidentally during diagnostic evaluation for other medical conditions. A significant number of SRMs are benign. As the size increases (especially >4 cm), the likelihood of malignancy increases. Imaging with MRI, CT scans, and ultrasound cannot make an absolute diagnosis of malignancy, necessitating a core biopsy if possible. About 10%–15% of patients will have a nondiagnostic biopsy and must be followed closely and rebiopsied if the mass is growing. Radiofrequency ablation (RFA) is commonly used to ablate small cancers but should have a biopsy done first to document malignancy.

2. Decision regarding therapy in patients with significant comorbidities is difficult. The Charleston Comorbidity Index (CCI) is a tool that can predict 1-y mortality. In patients with a short life expectancy, surveillance and supportive care is the best approach for this population. Partial nephrectomy is the treatment of choice for SRM that are amenable to nephron-sparing surgery. Radical nephrectomy in the past has been the procedure of choice in managing small RCC. Today partial nephrectomy is preferred and radical nephrectomy now is the treatment of choice in <30% of patients with SRM.

Sources

—*J Clin Oncol.* 2017;35:668-680
—*N Engl J Med.* 2010;362:624.
—*Eur Urol.* 2016;69:116.
—*JAMA.* 2015;150:664.
—*Eur Urol.* 2015;67.

Disorders of the Skin

32

ACNE

Population
—Adolescents or young adults.

Organizations
▶ AAD 2016, NICE 2021

Recommendations

TREATMENT OPTIONS FOR ACNE		
Acne	**First-Line Treatment**	**Alternative Treatment**
Mild	—Benzoyl peroxide (BP) —Topical retinoid —Topical combination (BP + antibiotic or retinoid + BP or all three)	—Add topical retinoid or BP —Consider alternate retinoid —Consider topical dapsone
Moderate	—Topical combination (BP + antibiotic or retinoid + BP or all three) —Oral antibiotic + topical retinoid + BP —Oral antibiotic +topical retinoid + BP + topical antibiotic	—Alternate combo therapy —Change oral abx —Add combo oral contraceptive or oral spironolactone (females) —Consider oral tretinoin
Severe	—Oral antibiotic + Topical combination (BP + antibiotic or retinoid + BP or all three) —Oral isotretinoin	—Change oral abx —Add combo oral contraceptive or oral spironolactone (females) —Consider oral tretinoin

—**Oral Abx:** prefer **doxycycline** or **minocycline** over **tetracycline**. Don't use in pregnant women or children <8 y of age; instead consider erythromycin or azithromycin.

—Use topical dapsone 5% gel postinflammatory dyspigmentation.

—Consider oral contraceptives (OCDs) for inflammatory acne in females.

—Consider spironolactone in females.

—If adrenal hyperandrogenism, consider low-dose oral corticosteroids.

—Data is limited for pulsed dye laser, glycolic acid peels, salicylic acid peels.

—Consider intralesional corticosteroids injections in treatment of individual acne nodules.

—Complementary/Alternative therapy: topical tea tree can be used, but study is limited.

—No specific dietary changes are supported by data; high glycemic index diet and skim milk may influence acne.

—Skin care advice:

- Use skin pH neutral or slightly acidic wash twice daily.
- Do not use oil-based or comedogenic skin care products, sunscreens, makeup.
- No picking or scratching lesions.

Comments

1. BP is effective in prevention of bacterial resistance.
2. Do not use topical abx as monotherapy because of risk of bacterial resistance.
3. Topical adapalene, tretinoin, and BP are safely used in preadolescent children.
4. Use systemic antibiotics for shortest duration and do not use as monotherapy without topicals.
5. Monitor LFTs, serum cholesterol and triglycerides, depression, and IBD while on isotretinoin. Females should be counseled on contraceptive methods.
6. Remember that OCP cannot be used in all patients.

Source

—Guidelines of care for the management of Acne Vulgaris. *J Am Acad Dermatol.* 2016;75(4): 945-973.

—www.nice.org.uk/guidance/ng198

ATOPIC DERMATITIS (AD)

Population

—Adults and children.

Organization

▶ AAD 2020

Recommendations

—Apply skin moisturizers after bathing with hypoallergenic neutral to low pH non-soap cleansers. No evidence for use of oils.

—Consider wet-wrap therapy with topical corticosteroids for moderate-to-severe AD during flares.

—Use twice-daily topical corticosteroids as first-line therapy.

—Consider topical calcineurin inhibitors (tacrolimus or pimecrolimus) for maintenance therapy.

—Consider bleach baths and intranasal mupirocin when signs of secondary bacterial infection.

—Do not use topical antihistamine therapy.

—Consider phototherapy for acute and chronic AD in both adults and children. NB-UVB is mostly used due to low-risk profile.

—Consider systemic immunomodulating agents for severe cases that are refractory to topical agents and phototherapy such as cyclosporine or methotrexate. Systemic steroids should be avoided except as bridge to another therapy.

—Do not use oral antibiotics unless there is clinical evidence of infection.
—Do not use skin prick tests or blood tests (eg, radioallergosorbent test) for the routine evaluation of atopic dermatitis.

Comment

1. Skin prick tests and RAST-type blood tests are useful to identify causes of allergic reactions, but not for diagnosing dermatitis or eczema. When testing for suspected allergies is indicated, patch testing with ingredients of products that come in contact with the patient's skin is recommended.

Sources

—AAD. *Atopic Dermatitis Clinical Guideline.* 2020. aad.org/clinical-quality/guidelines
—American Academy of Dermatology. *Choosing Wisely.* 2020.
—AAD. *Guidelines on Comorbidities Associated with Atopic Dermatitis.* 2022.

PRESSURE ULCERS

Population

—Adults at risk for pressure ulcers.

Organizations

▶ NICE 2014, ACP 2015

Recommendations

—Regularly document ulcer size.
—Debride any necrotic tissue if present with sharp debridement or autolytic debridement.
—Use hydrocolloid or foam dressings to reduce wound size.
—Provide nutritional supplementation for patients who are malnourished.
—Recommend a pressure-redistributing foam mattress.
—Consider electrical stimulation as adjunctive therapy to accelerate wound healing.
—Do not routinely use negative pressure wound therapy, electrotherapy, or hyperbaric oxygen therapy.
—Only use antibiotics for superimposed cellulitis or underlying osteomyelitis.

Comment

1. Moderate-quality evidence supports the addition of electrical stimulation to standard therapy to accelerate healing of Stage II–IV ulcers.

Sources

—http://www.guideline.gov/content.aspx?id=48026
—https://guidelines.gov/summaries/summary/49050

PSORIASIS, PLAQUE-TYPE

Population
—Adults.

Organization
▶ AAD 2009, AAD-NPF 2009, 2019

Recommendations
—Topical therapies are most effective for mild-to-moderate disease.
—Recommend emollients applied 1–3 times daily
—Use topical corticosteroids daily or BID as the cornerstone of therapy. Limit Class I (ie, high potency) topical steroids to 4 wk maximum.
—Topical agents that have proven efficacy when combined with topical corticosteroids:
  • Topical vitamin D analogues.
  • Topical tazarotene.
  • Topical salicylic acid.
—Reserve systemic therapies for severe, recalcitrant, or disabling psoriasis
  • Methotrexate (MTX):
    ○ Dose: 7.5–30 mg PO weekly (common 10–20 mg).
    ○ Monitor CBC and liver panel monthly (every 4 wk initially, while on higher doses and space to 8 wk for duration of treatment).
  • Cyclosporine:
    ○ Initial dose: 2.5–3 mg/kg divided BID (narrow therapeutic window).
    ○ Monitor for nephrotoxicity, HTN, and hypertrichosis.
  • Acitretin:
    ○ Dose: 10–50 mg PO daily.
    ○ Monitor: liver panel.
—Considerations for comorbidities:
  • Consider early and more frequent cardiovascular screening (obesity, HTN, HLD, DM, metabolic syndrome) in patients with psoriasis requiring systemic or phototherapy treatments, or psoriasis involving >10% of BSA.
  • Recommend screening for anxiety and depression in patients with psoriasis.
  • Recommend smoking cessation and limiting alcohol intake.
  • If a concern for comorbid IBD arises, refer the patient back to their PCP or to a gastroenterologist. Avoid IL-17 inhibitor therapy in patients with IBD.

Comments
1. Approximately 2% of population has psoriasis.
2. Eighty percent of patients with psoriasis have mild-to-moderate disease.

3. Topical steroid toxicity:
   a. Local: skin atrophy, telangiectasia, striae, purpura, or contact dermatitis.
   b. Hypothalamic–pituitary–adrenal axis may be suppressed with prolonged use of medium- to high-potency steroids.
4. MTX contraindications: pregnancy, breast-feeding, alcoholism, chronic liver disease, immunodeficiency syndromes, cytopenias, hypersensitivity reaction.
5. Cyclosporine contraindications: CA, renal impairment, uncontrolled HTN.
6. Acitretin contraindications: pregnancy, chronic liver, or renal disease.

Sources

—http://www.aad.org/File%20Library/Global%20navigation/Education%20and%20quality%20care/Guidelines-psoriasis-sec-3.pdf

—http://www.aad.org/File%20Library/Global%20navigation/Education%20and%20quality%20care/Guidelines-psoriasis-sec-4.pdf

—AAD-NPF. Joint AAD-NPF guidelines of care for the management and treatment of psoriasis with awareness and attention to comorbidities. *J Am Acad Dermatol.* 2019;90:1073-1113.

Appendices

33

ESTIMATE OF 10-Y CARDIAC RISK FOR MEN

ESTIMATE OF 10-Y CARDIAC RISK FOR MEN[a]

Age (y)		Points			
20–34		−9			
35–39		−4			
40–44		0			
45–49		3			
50–54		6			
55–59		8			
60–64		10			
65–69		11			
70–74		12			
75–79		13			
Total Cholesterol		**Points**			
	Age 20–39	Age 40–49	Age 50–59	Age 60–69	Age 70–79
<160	0	0	0	0	0
160–199	4	3	2	1	0
200–239	7	5	3	1	0
240–279	9	6	4	2	1
≥280	11	8	5	3	1
Nonsmoker	0	0	0	0	0
Smoker	8	5	3	1	1
High-Density Lipoprotein (mg/dL)		**Points**			
≥60		−1			
50–59		0			
40–49		1			
<40		2			

ESTIMATE OF 10-Y CARDIAC RISK FOR MEN[a] (*Continued*)

Systolic Blood Pressure (mmHg)		If Untreated		If Treated	
<120		0		0	
120–129		0		1	
130–139		1		2	
140–159		1		2	
≥160		2		3	
Point Total	**10-y Risk %**	**Point Total**	**10-y Risk %**		
<0	<1	9	5		
0	1	10	6		
1	1	11	8		
Age (y)		**Points**			
2	1	12	10		
3	1	13	12		
4	1	14	16		
5	2	15	20		
6	2	16	25		
7	3	≥17	≥30	**10-y Risk ____%**	
8	4				

[a]Framingham point scores.

Source: U.S. Department of Health and Human Services, Public Health Service, National Institutes of Health, National Heart, Lung, and Blood Institute. NIH Publication No. 01-3305, May 2001. https://www.nhlbi.nih.gov/files/docs/guidelines/atglance.pdf

ESTIMATE OF 10-Y CARDIAC RISK FOR WOMEN

ESTIMATE OF 10-Y CARDIAC RISK FOR WOMEN[a]

Age (y)		Points		
20–34		−7		
35–39		−3		
40–44		0		
45–49		3		
50–54		6		
55–59		8		
60–64		10		
65–69		12		
70–74		14		
75–79		16		
Total Cholesterol		**Points**		
	Age 20–39	**Age 40–49**	**Age 50–59**	**Age 60–69**	**Age 70–79**

Total Cholesterol	Age 20–39	Age 40–49	Age 50–59	Age 60–69	Age 70–79
<160	0	0	0	0	0
160–199	4	3	2	1	1
200–239	8	6	4	2	1
240–279	11	8	5	3	2
≥280	13	10	7	4	2
Nonsmoker	0	0	0	0	0
Smoker	9	7	4	2	1

High-Density Lipoprotein (mg/dL)		Points		
≥60		−1		
50–59		0		
40–49		1		
<40		2		

Systolic Blood Pressure (mmHg)		If Untreated		If Treated
<120		0		0
120–129		1		3
130–139		2		4

ESTIMATE OF 10-Y CARDIAC RISK FOR WOMEN[a]   *(Continued)*

140–159		3		5	
≥160		4		6	
Point Total	**10-y Risk %**	**Point Total**	**10-y Risk %**		
<9	<1	17	5		
9	1	18	6		
10	1	19	8		
11	1	20	11		
12	1	21	14		
13	2	22	17		
14	2	23	22		
15	3	24	27	**10-y Risk_____%**	
16	4	≥25	≥30		

[a]Framingham point scores.

Source: U.S. Department of Health and Human Services, Public Health Service, National Institutes of Health, National Heart, Lung, and Blood Institute. NIH Publication No. 01-3305, May 2001. https://www.nhlbi.nih.gov/files/docs/guidelines/atglance.pdf

95TH PERCENTILE OF BLOOD PRESSURE FOR BOYS

95TH PERCENTILE OF BLOOD PRESSURE FOR BOYS

Age (y)	Systolic Blood Pressure (mmHg) by Percentile of Height							Diastolic Blood Pressure (mmHg) by Percentile of Height						
	5%	10%	25%	50%	75%	90%	95%	5%	10%	25%	50%	75%	90%	95%
3	104	105	107	109	110	112	113	63	63	64	65	66	67	67
4	106	107	109	111	112	114	115	66	67	68	69	70	71	71
5	108	109	110	112	114	115	116	69	70	71	72	73	74	74
6	109	110	112	114	115	117	117	72	72	73	74	75	76	76
7	110	111	113	115	117	118	119	74	74	75	76	77	78	78
8	111	112	114	116	118	119	120	75	76	77	78	79	79	80
9	113	114	116	118	119	121	121	76	77	78	79	80	81	81
10	115	116	117	119	121	122	123	77	78	79	80	81	81	82
11	117	118	119	121	123	124	125	78	78	79	80	81	82	82
12	119	120	122	123	125	127	127	78	79	80	81	82	82	83
13	121	122	124	126	128	129	130	79	79	80	81	82	83	83
14	124	125	127	128	130	132	132	80	80	81	82	83	84	84
15	126	127	129	131	133	134	135	81	81	82	83	84	85	85
16	129	130	132	134	135	137	137	82	83	83	84	85	86	87
17	131	132	134	136	138	139	140	84	85	86	87	87	88	89

95TH PERCENTILE OF BLOOD PRESSURE FOR GIRLS

95TH PERCENTILE OF BLOOD PRESSURE FOR GIRLS

Age (y)	Systolic Blood Pressure (mmHg) by Percentile of Height							Diastolic Blood Pressure (mmHg) by Percentile of Height						
	5%	10%	25%	50%	75%	90%	95%	5%	10%	25%	50%	75%	90%	95%
3	104	104	105	107	108	109	110	65	66	66	67	68	68	69
4	105	106	107	108	110	111	112	68	68	69	70	71	71	72
5	107	107	108	110	111	112	113	70	71	71	72	73	73	74
6	108	109	110	111	113	114	115	72	72	73	74	74	75	76
7	110	111	112	113	115	116	116	73	74	74	75	76	76	77
8	112	112	114	115	116	118	118	75	75	76	76	77	78	78
9	114	114	115	117	118	119	120	76	76	76	77	78	79	79
10	116	116	117	119	120	121	122	77	77	77	78	79	80	80
11	118	118	119	121	122	123	124	78	78	78	79	80	81	81
12	119	120	121	123	124	125	126	79	79	79	80	81	82	82
13	121	121	123	124	126	127	128	80	80	80	81	82	83	83
14	123	123	125	126	127	129	129	81	81	81	82	83	84	84
15	124	125	126	127	129	130	131	82	82	82	83	84	85	85
16	125	126	127	128	130	131	132	82	82	83	84	85	85	86
17	125	126	127	129	130	131	132	82	83	83	84	85	85	86

Source: Blood Pressure Tables for Children and Adolescents from the *Fourth Report on the Diagnosis, Evaluation, and Treatment of High Blood Pressure in Children and Adolescents.* http://www.nhlbi.nih.gov/guidelines/hypertension/child_tbl.htm. Accessed June 3, 2008.

BODY MASS INDEX (BMI) CONVERSION TABLE

Height in inches (cm)	BMI 25 kg/m²	BMI 27 kg/m²	BMI 30 kg/m²
	Body weight in pounds (kg)		
58 (147.32)	119 (53.98)	129 (58.51)	143 (64.86)
59 (149.86)	124 (56.25)	133 (60.33)	148 (67.13)
60 (152.40)	128 (58.06)	138 (62.60)	153 (69.40)
61 (154.94)	132 (59.87)	143 (64.86)	158 (71.67)
62 (157.48)	136 (61.69)	147 (66.68)	164 (74.39)
63 (160.02)	141 (63.96)	152 (68.95)	169 (76.66)
64 (162.56)	145 (65.77)	157 (71.22)	174 (78.93)
65 (165.10)	150 (68.04)	162 (73.48)	180 (81.65)
66 (167.64)	155 (70.31)	167 (75.75)	186 (84.37)
67 (170.18)	159 (72.12)	172 (78.02)	191 (86.64)
68 (172.72)	164 (74.39)	177 (80.29)	197 (89.36)
69 (175.26)	169 (76.66)	182 (82.56)	203 (92.08)
70 (177.80)	174 (78.93)	188 (85.28)	207 (93.90)
71 (180.34)	179 (81.19)	193 (87.54)	215 (97.52)
72 (182.88)	184 (83.46)	199 (90.27)	221 (100.25)
73 (185.42)	189 (85.73)	204 (92.53)	227 (102.97)
74 (187.96)	194 (88.00)	210 (95.26)	233 (105.69)
75 (190.50)	200 (90.72)	216 (97.98)	240 (108.86)
76 (193.04)	205 (92.99)	221 (100.25)	246 (111.59)

Metric conversion formula = weight (kg)/ height (m²)	Nonmetric conversion formula = [weight (lb)/ height (in.²)] × 704.5
Example of BMI calculation: A person who weighs 78.93 kg and is 177 cm tall has a BMI of 25: weight (78.93 kg)/height (1.77 m²) = 25	Example of BMI calculation: A person who weighs 164 lb and is 68 in. (or 5′8″) tall has a BMI of 25: [weight (164 lb)/height (68 in.²)] × 704.5 = 25

BMI categories:
Underweight = <18.5
Normal weight = 18.5–24.9
Overweight = 25–29.9
Obesity = ≥30

Source: Adapted from NHLBI Obesity Guidelines in Adults. http://www.nhlbi.nih.gov/guidelines/obesity/bmi_tbl.htm. Accessed October 13, 2011. BMI online calculator. http://www.nhlbisupport.com/bmi/bmicalc.htm. Accessed October 13, 2011.

FUNCTIONAL ASSESSMENT SCREENING IN THE ELDERLY

FUNCTIONAL ASSESSMENT SCREENING IN THE ELDERLY

Target Area	Assessment Procedure	Abnormal Result	Suggested Intervention
Vision	Inquire about vision changes, Snellen chart testing.	Presence of vision changes; inability to read >20/40	Refer to ophthalmologist.
Hearing	Whisper a short, easily answered question such as "What is your name?" in each ear while the examiner's face is out of direct view. Use audioscope set at 40 dB; test using 1000 and 2000 Hz. Brief hearing loss screener.	Inability to answer question Inability to hear 1000 or 2000 Hz in both ears or inability to hear frequencies in either ear Brief hearing loss screen score ≥3	Examine auditory canals for cerumen and clean if necessary. Repeat test; if still abnormal in either ear, refer for audiometry and possible prosthesis.
Balance and gait	Observe the patient after instructing as follows: "Rise from your chair, walk 10 ft, return, and sit down." Check orthostatic blood pressure and heart rate.	Inability to complete task in 15 s	Performance-Oriented Mobility Assessment (POMA). Consider referral for physical therapy.
Continence of urine	Ask, "Do you ever lose your urine and get wet?" If yes, then ask, "Have you lost urine on at least 6 separate days?"	"Yes" to both questions	Ascertain frequency and amount. Search for remediable causes, including local irritations, polyuric states, and medications. Consider urologic referral.
Nutrition	Ask, "Without trying, have you lost 10 lb or more in the last 6 mo?" Weigh the patient. Measure height.	"Yes" or weight is below acceptable range for height	Do appropriate medical evaluation.
Mental status	Instruct as follows: "I am going to name three objects (pencil, truck, and book). I will ask you to repeat their names now and then again a few minutes from now."	Inability to recall all three objects after 1 min	Administer Folstein Mini-Mental State Examination. If score is <24, search for causes of cognitive impairment. Ascertain onset, duration, and fluctuation of overt symptoms. Review medications. Assess consciousness and affect. Do appropriate laboratory tests.

FUNCTIONAL ASSESSMENT SCREENING IN THE ELDERLY   (Continued)

Target Area	Assessment Procedure	Abnormal Result	Suggested Intervention
Depression	Ask, "Do you often feel sad or depressed?" or "How are your spirits?"	"Yes" or "Not very good, I guess"	Administer Geriatric Depression Scale or PHQ-9. If positive, check for antihypertensive, psychotropic, or other pertinent medications. Consider appropriate pharmacologic or psychiatric treatment.
ADL-IADL[a]	Ask, "Can you get out of bed yourself?" "Can you dress yourself?" "Can you make your own meals?" "Can you do your own shopping?"	"No" to any question	Corroborate responses with patient's appearance; question family members if accuracy is uncertain. Determine reasons for the inability (motivation compared with physical limitation). Institute appropriate medical, social, or environmental interventions.
Home environment	Ask, "Do you have trouble with stairs inside or outside of your home?" Ask about potential hazards inside the home with bathtubs, rugs, or lighting.	"Yes"	Evaluate home safety and institute appropriate countermeasures.
Social support	Ask, "Who would be able to help you in case of illness or emergency?"	—	List identified persons in the medical record. Become familiar with available resources for the elderly in the community.
Pain	Inquire about pain.	Presence of pain	Pain inventory.
Dentition	Oral examination.	Poor dentition	Dentistry referral.
Falls	Inquire about falls in past year and difficulty with walking or balance.	Presence of falls or gait/ balance problems	Falls evaluation.

[a]Activities of Daily Living–Instrumental Activities of Daily Living.
Source: Modified from Fleming KC, Evans JM, Weber DC, Chutka DS. Practical functional assessment of elderly persons: a primary-care approach. Mayo Clin Proc. 1995;70(9):890-910.

APPENDICES

GERIATRIC DEPRESSION SCALE

GERIATRIC DEPRESSION SCALE

Choose the best answer for how you felt over the past week

1. Are you basically satisfied with your life?	Yes/No
2. Have you dropped many of your activities and interests?	Yes/No
3. Do you feel that your life is empty?	Yes/No
4. Do you often get bored?	Yes/No
5. Are you hopeful about the future?	Yes/No
6. Are you bothered by thoughts you can't get out of your head?	Yes/No
7. Are you in good spirits most of the time?	Yes/No
8. Are you afraid that something bad is going to happen to you?	Yes/No
9. Do you feel happy most of the time?	Yes/No
10. Do you often feel helpless?	Yes/No
11. Do you often get restless and fidgety?	Yes/No
12. Do you prefer to stay at home, rather than going out and doing new things?	Yes/No
13. Do you frequently worry about the future?	Yes/No
14. Do you feel you have more problems with memory than most?	Yes/No
15. Do you think it is wonderful to be alive now?	Yes/No
16. Do you often feel downhearted and blue?	Yes/No
17. Do you feel pretty worthless the way you are now?	Yes/No
18. Do you worry a lot about the past?	Yes/No
19. Do you find life very exciting?	Yes/No
20. Is it hard for you to get started on new projects?	Yes/No
21. Do you feel full of energy?	Yes/No
22. Do you feel that your situation is hopeless?	Yes/No
23. Do you think that most people are better off than you are?	Yes/No
24. Do you frequently get upset over little things?	Yes/No
25. Do you frequently feel like crying?	Yes/No
26. Do you have trouble concentrating?	Yes/No
27. Do you enjoy getting up in the morning?	Yes/No
28. Do you prefer to avoid social gatherings?	Yes/No
29. Is it easy for you to make decisions?	Yes/No
30. Is your mind as clear as it used to be?	Yes/No

One point for each is response suggestive of depression. (Specifically "no" responses to questions 1, 5, 7, 9, 15, 19, 21, 27, 29, and 30, and "yes" responses to the remaining questions are suggestive of depression.)

A score of ≥15 yields a sensitivity of 80% and a specificity of 100%, as a screening test for geriatric depression. *Clin Gerontol*. 1982;1:37.

Source: Reproduced with permission from Yesavage JA, Brink TL, Rose TL, et al. Development and validation of a geriatric depression screening scale: a preliminary report. *J Psychiatr Res*. 1982-1983;17:37.

IMMUNIZATION SCHEDULE

CDC VACCINE SCHEDULES FOR CHILDREN AND ADOLESCENTS

Figure 1. Recommended immunization schedule for children and adolescents aged 18 y or younger—United States, 2021. (FOR THOSE WHO FALL BEHIND OR START LATE, SEE THE CATCH-UP SCHEDULE [FIGURE 2])

These recommendations must be read with the notes that follow. For those who fall behind or start late, provide catch-up vaccination at the earliest opportunity as indicated. To determine minimum intervals between doses, see the catch-up schedule (Figure 2). School entry and adolescent vaccine age groups are shaded in gray.

Vaccine	Birth	1 mo	2 mos	4 mos	6 mos	9 mos	12 mos	15 mos	18 mos	19–23 mos	2–3 yrs	4–6 yrs	7–10 yrs	11–12 yrs	13–15 yrs	16 yrs	17–18 yrs
Hepatitis B (HepB)	1st dose	←-- 2nd dose --→			←-- 3rd dose --→												
Rotavirus (RV): RV1 (2-dose series), RV5 (3-dose series)			1st dose	2nd dose	See Notes												
Diphtheria, tetanus, acellular pertussis (DTaP <7 yrs)			1st dose	2nd dose	3rd dose			←-- 4th dose --→				5th dose					
Haemophilus influenzae type b (Hib)			1st dose	2nd dose	See Notes		← 3rd or 4th dose, See Notes →										
Pneumococcal conjugate (PCV13)			1st dose	2nd dose	3rd dose		←-- 4th dose --→										
Inactivated poliovirus (IPV <18 yrs)			1st dose	2nd dose	←-- 3rd dose --→							4th dose					
Influenza (IIV)					Annual vaccination 1 or 2 doses								Annual vaccination 1 dose only				
or													or				
Influenza (LAIV4)											Annual vaccination 1 or 2 doses		Annual vaccination 1 dose only				
Measles, mumps, rubella (MMR)					See Notes		←-- 1st dose --→					2nd dose					
Varicella (VAR)							←-- 1st dose --→					2nd dose					
Hepatitis A (HepA)					See Notes		2-dose series, See Notes										
Tetanus, diphtheria, acellular pertussis (Tdap ≥7 yrs)														Tdap			
Human papillomavirus (HPV)													*	See Notes			
Meningococcal (MenACWY-D ≥9 mos, MenACWY-CRM ≥2 mos, MenACWY-TT ≥2years)			See Notes											1st dose		2nd dose	
Meningococcal B													See Notes				
Pneumococcal polysaccharide (PPSV23)											See Notes						

Range of recommended ages for all children | Range of recommended ages for catch-up immunization | Range of recommended ages for certain high-risk groups | Recommended based on shared clinical decision-making or *can be used in this age group | No recommendation/ not applicable

Source: https://www.cdc.gov/vaccines/schedules/hcp/imz/child-adolescent.html.

Figure 2. Catch-up immunization schedule for persons age 4 mo through 18 y who start late or who are more than 1 mo behind—United States, 2021.

The table below provides catch-up schedules and minimum intervals between doses for children whose vaccinations have been delayed. A vaccine series does not need to be restarted, regardless of the time that has elapsed between doses. Use the section appropriate for the child's age. **Always use this table in conjunction with Table 1 and the notes that follow.**

Vaccine	Minimum Age for Dose 1	Minimum Interval Between Doses			
		Dose 1 to Dose 2	Dose 2 to Dose 3	Dose 3 to Dose 4	Dose 4 to Dose 5
Children age 4 months through 6 years					
Hepatitis B	Birth	4 weeks	**8 weeks** *and* **at least 16 weeks after first dose.** Minimum age for the final dose is 24 weeks.		
Rotavirus	6 weeks Maximum age for first dose is 14 weeks, 6 days.	4 weeks	**4 weeks** Maximum age for final dose is 8 months, 0 days.		
Diphtheria, tetanus, and acellular pertussis	6 weeks	4 weeks	4 weeks	6 months	6 months
Haemophilus influenzae type b	6 weeks	**No further doses needed** if first dose was administered at age 15 months or older. **4 weeks** if first dose was administered before the 1st birthday. **8 weeks (as final dose)** if first dose was administered at age 12 through 14 months.	**No further doses needed** if previous dose was administered at age 15 months or older. **4 weeks** if current age is younger than 12 months *and* first dose was administered at younger than age 7 months *and* at least 1 previous dose was PRP-T (ActHib, Pentacel, Hiberix) or unknown. **8 weeks** *and* **age 12 through 59 months (as final dose)** if current age is younger than 12 months *and* first dose was administered at age 7 through 11 months; OR if current age is 12 through 59 months *and* first dose was administered before the 1st birthday *and* second dose was administered at younger than 15 months; OR if both doses were PRP-OMP (PedvaxHIB, Comvax) *and* were administered before the 1st birthday.	**8 weeks (as final dose)** This dose only necessary for children age 12 through 59 months who received 3 doses before the 1st birthday.	
Pneumococcal conjugate	6 weeks	**No further doses needed** for healthy children if first dose was administered at age 24 months or older. **4 weeks** if first dose was administered before the 1st birthday. **8 weeks (as final dose for healthy children)** if first dose was administered at the 1st birthday or after.	**No further doses needed** for healthy children if previous dose was administered at age 24 months or older. **4 weeks** if current age is younger than 12 months and previous dose was administered at <7 months old. **8 weeks (as final dose for healthy children)** if previous dose was administered between 7–11 months (wait until at least 12 months old); OR if current age is 12 months or older and at least 1 dose was administered before age 12 months.	**8 weeks (as final dose)** This dose only necessary for children age 12 through 59 months who received 3 doses before age 12 months or for children at high risk who received 3 doses at any age.	
Inactivated poliovirus	6 weeks	4 weeks	**4 weeks** if current age is <4 years. **6 months (as final dose)** if current age is 4 years or older.	**6 months (minimum age 4 years for final dose).**	
Measles, mumps, rubella	12 months	4 weeks			
Varicella	12 months	3 months			
Hepatitis A	12 months	6 months			
Meningococcal ACWY	2 months MenACWY-CRM 9 months MenACWY-D 2 years MenACWY-TT	8 weeks	See Notes	See Notes	
Children and adolescents age 7 through 18 years					
Meningococcal ACWY	Not applicable (N/A)	8 weeks			
Tetanus, diphtheria; tetanus, diphtheria, and acellular pertussis	7 years	4 weeks	**4 weeks** If first dose of DTaP/DT was administered before the 1st birthday. **6 months (as final dose)** If first dose of DTaP/DT or Tdap/Td was administered at or after the 1st birthday.	**6 months** if first dose of DTaP/DT was administered before the 1st birthday.	
Human papillomavirus	9 years	**Routine dosing intervals are recommended.**			
Hepatitis A	N/A	6 months			
Hepatitis B	N/A	4 weeks	**8 weeks** *and* **at least 16 weeks after first dose.**		
Inactivated poliovirus	N/A	4 weeks	**6 months** A fourth dose is not necessary if the third dose was administered at age 4 years or older and at least 6 months after the previous dose.	A fourth dose of IPV is indicated if all previous doses were administered at <4 years or if the third dose was administered <6 months after the second dose.	
Measles, mumps, rubella	N/A	4 weeks			
Varicella	N/A	**3 months** if younger than age 13 years. **4 weeks** if age 13 years or older.			

Source: https://www.cdc.gov/vaccines/schedules/hcp/imz/child-adolescent.html.

Figure 3. Vaccines that might be indicated for children and adolescents aged 18 y or younger based on medical indications.

VACCINE	Pregnancy	Immunocom-promised status (excluding HIV infection)	HIV infection CD4+ count[1]		Kidney failure, end-stage renal disease, or on hemodialysis	Heart disease or chronic lung disease	CSF leak or cochlear implant	Asplenia or persistent complement component deficiencies	Chronic liver disease	Diabetes
			<15% and total CD4 cell count of <200/mm³	≥15% and total CD4 cell count of ≥200/mm³						
Hepatitis B										
Rotavirus		SCID[2]								
Diphtheria, tetanus, and acellular pertussis (DTaP)										
Haemophilus influenzae type b										
Pneumococcal conjugate										
Inactivated poliovirus										
Influenza (IIV) or Influenza (LAIV4)						Asthma, wheezing: 2–4 yrs[3]				
Measles, mumps, rubella	*									
Varicella	*									
Hepatitis A										
Tetanus, diphtheria, and acellular pertussis (Tdap)										
Human papillomavirus	*									
Meningococcal ACWY										
Meningococcal B										
Pneumococcal polysaccharide										

Vaccination according to the routine schedule recommended

Recommended for persons with an additional risk factor for which the vaccine would be indicated

Vaccination is recommended, and additional doses may be necessary based on medical condition. See Notes.

Not recommended/contraindicated—vaccine should not be administered.
*Vaccinate after pregnancy.

Precaution—vaccine might be indicated if benefit of protection outweighs risk of adverse reaction

No recommendation/not applicable

1 For additional information regarding HIV laboratory parameters and use of live vaccines, see the *General Best Practice Guidelines for Immunization*, "Altered Immunocompetence," at www.cdc.gov/vaccines/hcp/acip-recs/general-recs/immunocompetence.html and Table 4-1 (footnote D) at www.cdc.gov/vaccines/hcp/acip-recs/general-recs/contraindications.html.
2 Severe Combined Immunodeficiency
3 LAIV4 contraindicated for children 2–4 years of age with asthma or wheezing during the preceding 12 months

Source: https://www.cdc.gov/vaccines/schedules/hcp/imz/child-adolescent.html.

Notes

Recommended Child and Adolescent Immunization Schedule for ages 18 years or younger, United States, 2021

For vaccination recommendations for persons ages 19 years or older, see the Recommended Adult Immunization Schedule, 2021.

Additional Information

COVID-19 Vaccination

ACIP recommends use of COVID-19 vaccines within the scope of the Emergency Use Authorization or Biologics License Application for the particular vaccine. Interim ACIP recommendations for the use of COVID-19 vaccines can be found at www.cdc.gov/vaccines/hcp/acip-recs/.

- Consult relevant ACIP statements for detailed recommendations at www.cdc.gov/vaccines/hcp/acip-recs/index.html.

- For information on contraindications and precautions for the use of a vaccine, consult the General Best Practice Guidelines for Immunization at www.cdc.gov/vaccines/hcp/acip-recs/general-recs/contraindications.html and relevant ACIP statements at www.cdc.gov/vaccines/hcp/acip-recs/index.html.

- For calculating intervals between doses, 4 weeks = 28 days. Intervals of ≥4 months are determined by calendar months.

- Within a number range (e.g., 12–18), a dash (–) should be read as "through".

- Vaccine doses administered ≤4 days before the minimum age or interval are considered valid. Doses of any vaccine administered ≥5 days earlier than the minimum age or minimum interval should not be counted as valid and should be repeated as age appropriate. **The repeat dose should be spaced after the invalid dose by the recommended minimum interval.** For further details, see Table 3-1, Recommended and minimum ages and intervals between vaccine doses, in General Best Practice Guidelines for Immunization at www.cdc.gov/vaccines/hcp/acip-recs/general-recs/timing.html.

- Information on travel vaccine requirements and recommendations is available at www.cdc.gov/travel/.

- For vaccination of persons with immunodeficiencies, see Table 8-1, Vaccination of persons with primary and secondary immunodeficiencies, in General Best Practice Guidelines for Immunization at www.cdc.gov/vaccines/hcp/acip-recs/general-recs/immunocompetence.html, and Immunization in Special Clinical Circumstances (In: Kimberlin DW, Brady MT, Jackson MA, Long SS, eds. Red Book: 2018 Report of the Committee on Infectious Diseases. 31st ed. Itasca, IL: American Academy of Pediatrics; 2018:67–111).

- For information about vaccination in the setting of a vaccine-preventable disease outbreak, contact your state or local health department.

- The National Vaccine Injury Compensation Program (VICP) is a no-fault alternative to the traditional legal system for resolving vaccine injury claims. All routine child and adolescent vaccines are covered by VICP except for pneumococcal polysaccharide vaccine (PPSV23). For more information, see www.hrsa.gov/vaccinecompensation/index.html.

Diphtheria, tetanus, and pertussis (DTaP) vaccination (minimum age: 6 weeks [4 years for Kinrix or Quadracel])

Routine vaccination

- 5-dose series at 2, 4, 6, 15–18 months, 4–6 years
  - **Prospectively:** Dose 4 may be administered as early as age 12 months if at least 6 months have elapsed since dose 3.
  - **Retrospectively:** A 4th dose that was inadvertently administered as early as age 12 months may be counted if at least 4 months have elapsed since dose 3.

Catch-up vaccination

- Dose 5 is not necessary if dose 4 was administered at age 4 years or older and at least 6 months after dose 3.
- For other catch-up guidance, see Table 2.

Special situations

- Wound management in children less than age 7 years with history of 3 or more doses of tetanus-toxoid-containing vaccine: For all wounds except clean and minor wounds, administer DTaP if more than 5 years since last dose of tetanus-toxoid-containing vaccine. For detailed information, see www.cdc.gov/mmwr/volumes/67/rr/rr6702a1.htm.

Haemophilus influenzae type b vaccination (minimum age: 6 weeks)

Routine vaccination

- **ActHIB, Hiberix, or Pentacel:** 4-dose series at 2, 4, 6, 12–15 months
- **PedvaxHIB:** 3-dose series at 2, 4, 12–15 months

Catch-up vaccination

- **Dose 1 at age 7–11 months:** Administer dose 2 at least 4 weeks later and dose 3 (final dose) at age 12–15 months or 8 weeks after dose 2 (whichever is later).
- **Dose 1 at age 12–14 months:** Administer dose 2 (final dose) at least 8 weeks after dose 1.
- **Dose 1 before age 12 months and dose 2 before age 15 months:** Administer dose 3 (final dose) 8 weeks after dose 2.
- **2 doses of PedvaxHIB before age 12 months:** Administer dose 3 (final dose) at 12–59 months and at least 8 weeks after dose 2.
- **1 dose administered at age 15 months or older:** No further doses needed.
- **Unvaccinated at age 15–59 months:** Administer 1 dose.
- **Previously unvaccinated children age 60 months or older who are not considered high risk:** Do not require catch-up vaccination.

For other catch-up guidance, see Table 2.

Special situations

- **Chemotherapy or radiation treatment:**
  - *12–59 months*
  - Unvaccinated or only 1 dose before age 12 months: 2 doses, 8 weeks apart
  - 2 or more doses before age 12 months: 1 dose at least 8 weeks after previous dose
  - *Doses administered within 14 days of starting therapy or during therapy should be repeated at least 3 months after therapy completion.*

- **Hematopoietic stem cell transplant (HSCT):**
  - 3-dose series 4 weeks apart starting 6 to 12 months after successful transplant, regardless of Hib vaccination history

- **Anatomic or functional asplenia (including sickle cell disease):**
  - *12–59 months*
  - Unvaccinated or only 1 dose before age 12 months: 2 doses, 8 weeks apart
  - 2 or more doses before age 12 months: 1 dose at least 8 weeks after previous dose
  - *Unvaccinated* persons age 5 years or older
  - 1 dose

- **Elective splenectomy:**
  - *Unvaccinated* persons age 15 months or older
  - 1 dose (preferably at least 14 days before procedure)

- **HIV infection:**
  - *12–59 months*
  - Unvaccinated or only 1 dose before age 12 months: 2 doses, 8 weeks apart
  - 2 or more doses before age 12 months: 1 dose at least 8 weeks after previous dose
  - *Unvaccinated* persons age 5–18 years
  - 1 dose

- **Immunoglobulin deficiency, early component complement deficiency:**
  - *12–59 months*
  - Unvaccinated or only 1 dose before age 12 months: 2 doses, 8 weeks apart
  - 2 or more doses before age 12 months: 1 dose at least 8 weeks after previous dose

*Unvaccinated = Less than routine series (through age 14 months) OR no doses (age 15 months or older)

Notes Recommended Child and Adolescent Immunization Schedule for ages 18 years or younger, United States, 2021

Hepatitis A vaccination
(minimum age: 12 months for routine vaccination)

Routine vaccination
- 2-dose series (minimum interval: 6 months) beginning at age 12 months

Catch-up vaccination
- Unvaccinated persons through age 18 years should complete a 2-dose series (minimum interval: 6 months).
- Persons who previously received 1 dose at age 12 months or older should receive dose 2 at least 6 months after dose 1.
- Adolescents age 18 years or older may receive the combined HepA and HepB vaccine, **Twinrix**, as a 3-dose series (0, 1, and 6 months) or 4-dose series (3 doses at 0, 7, and 21–30 days, followed by a booster dose at 12 months).

International travel
- Persons traveling to or working in countries with high or intermediate endemic hepatitis A (www.cdc.gov/travel/):
- **Infants age 6–11 months:** 1 dose before departure; revaccinate with 2 doses, separated by at least 6 months, between age 12–23 months.
- **Unvaccinated age 12 months or older:** Administer dose 1 as soon as travel is considered.

Hepatitis B vaccination
(minimum age: birth)

Birth dose (monovalent HepB vaccine only)
- **Mother is HBsAg-negative:** 1 dose within 24 hours of birth for **all** medically stable infants ≥2,000 grams. Infants <2,000 grams: Administer 1 dose at chronological age 1 month or hospital discharge (whichever is earlier and even if weight is still <2,000 grams).
- **Mother is HBsAg-positive:**
  - Administer **HepB vaccine** and **hepatitis B immune globulin (HBIG)** (in separate limbs) within 12 hours of birth, regardless of birth weight. For infants <2,000 grams, administer 3 additional doses of vaccine (total of 4 doses) beginning at age 1 month.
  - Test for HBsAg and anti-HBs at age 9–12 months. If HepB series is delayed, test 1–2 months after final dose.
- **Mother's HBsAg status is unknown:**
  - Administer **HepB vaccine** within 12 hours of birth, regardless of birth weight.
  - For infants <2,000 grams, administer **HBIG** in addition to HepB vaccine (in separate limbs) within 12 hours of birth. Administer 3 additional doses of vaccine (total of 4 doses) beginning at age 1 month.
  - Determine mother's HBsAg status as soon as possible. If mother is HBsAg-positive, administer **HBIG** to infants ≥2,000 grams as soon as possible, but no later than 7 days of age.

Routine series
- 3-dose series at 0, 1–2, 6–18 months (use monovalent HepB vaccine for doses administered before age 6 weeks)
- Infants who did not receive a birth dose should begin the series as soon as feasible (see Table 2).
- Administration of **4 doses** is permitted when a combination vaccine containing HepB is used after the birth dose.

- Minimum age for the final (3rd or 4th) dose: 24 weeks
- **Minimum intervals:** dose 1 to dose 2: 4 weeks / dose 2 to dose 3: 8 weeks / dose 1 to dose 3: 16 weeks (when 4 doses are administered, substitute "dose 4" for "dose 3" in these calculations)

Catch-up vaccination
- Unvaccinated persons should complete a 3-dose series at 0, 1–2, 6 months.
- Adolescents age 11–15 years may use an alternative 2-dose schedule with at least 4 months between doses (adult formulation **Recombivax HB** only).
- Adolescents age 18 years or older may receive a 2-dose series of HepB (**Heplisav-B**) at least 4 weeks apart.
- Adolescents age 18 years or older may receive the combined HepA and HepB vaccine, **Twinrix**, as a 3-dose series (0, 1, and 6 months) or 4-dose series (3 doses at 0, 7, and 21–30 days, followed by a booster dose at 12 months).
- For other catch-up guidance, see Table 2.

Special situations
- Revaccination is not generally recommended for persons with a normal immune status who were vaccinated as infants, children, adolescents, or adults.
- **Revaccination** may be recommended for certain populations, including:
  - **Infants born to HBsAg-positive mothers**
  - **Hemodialysis patients**
  - **Other immunocompromised persons**
- For detailed revaccination recommendations, see www.cdc.gov/vaccines/hcp/acip-recs/vacc-specific/hepb.html.

Human papillomavirus vaccination
(minimum age: 9 years)

Routine and catch-up vaccination
- HPV vaccination routinely recommended at **age 11–12 years** (can start at age 9 years) and catch-up HPV vaccination recommended for all persons through age 18 years if not adequately vaccinated
- 2- or 3-dose series depending on age at initial vaccination:
  - **Age 9–14 years at initial vaccination:** 2-dose series at 0, 6–12 months (minimum interval: 5 months; repeat dose if administered too soon)
  - **Age 15 years or older at initial vaccination:** 3-dose series at 0, 1–2 months, 6 months (minimum intervals: dose 1 to dose 2: 4 weeks / dose 2 to dose 3: 12 weeks / dose 1 to dose 3: 5 months; repeat dose if administered too soon)
- **Interrupted schedules:** If vaccination schedule is interrupted, the series does not need to be restarted.
- No additional dose recommended after completing series with recommended dosing intervals using any HPV vaccine.

Special situations
- **Immunocompromising conditions, including HIV infection:** 3-dose series as above
- **History of sexual abuse or assault:** Start at age 9 years.
- **Pregnancy:** HPV vaccination not recommended until after pregnancy; no intervention needed if vaccinated while pregnant; pregnancy testing not needed before vaccination

Influenza vaccination
(minimum age: 6 months [IIV], 2 years [LAIV4], 18 years [recombinant influenza vaccine, RIV4])

Routine vaccination
- Use any influenza vaccine appropriate for age and health status annually:
  - 2 doses, separated by at least 4 weeks, for **children age 6 months–8 years** who have received fewer than 2 influenza vaccine doses before July 1, 2020, or whose influenza vaccination history is unknown (administer dose 2 even if the child turns 9 between receipt of dose 1 and dose 2)
  - 1 dose for **children age 6 months–8 years** who have received at least 2 influenza vaccine doses before July 1, 2020
  - 1 dose for **all persons age 9 years or older**
- For the 2021–22 season, see the 2021–22 ACIP influenza vaccine recommendations.

Special situations
- **Egg allergy, hives only:** Any influenza vaccine appropriate for age and health status annually
- **Egg allergy with symptoms other than hives** (e.g., angioedema, respiratory distress, need for emergency medical services or epinephrine): Any influenza vaccine appropriate for age and health status annually. If using an influenza vaccine other than Flublok or Flucelvax, administer in a medical setting under supervision of health care provider who can recognize and manage severe allergic reactions.
- Severe allergic reactions to vaccines can occur even in the absence of a history of previous allergic reaction. All vaccination providers should be familiar with the office emergency plan and certified in cardiopulmonary resuscitation.
- A previous severe allergic reaction to influenza vaccine is a contraindication to future receipt of any influenza vaccine.
- **LAIV4 should not be used** in persons with the following conditions or situations:
  - History of severe allergic reaction to a previous dose of any influenza vaccine or to any vaccine component (excluding egg, see details above)
  - Receiving aspirin or salicylate-containing medications
  - Age 2–4 years with history of asthma or wheezing
  - Immunocompromised due to any cause (including medications and HIV infection)
  - Anatomic or functional asplenia
  - Close contacts or caregivers of severely immunosuppressed persons who require a protected environment
  - Pregnancy
  - Cochlear implant
  - Cerebrospinal fluid-oropharyngeal communication
  - Children less than age 2 years
  - Received influenza antiviral medications oseltamivir or zanamivir within the previous 48 hours, peramivir within the previous 5 days, or baloxavir within the previous 17 days

Notes Recommended Child and Adolescent Immunization Schedule for ages 18 years or younger, United States, 2021

Measles, mumps, and rubella vaccination
(minimum age: 12 months for routine vaccination)

Routine vaccination
- 2-dose series at 12–15 months, 4–6 years
- Dose 2 may be administered as early as 4 weeks after dose 1.

Catch-up vaccination
- Unvaccinated children and adolescents: 2-dose series at least 4 weeks apart
- The maximum age for use of MMRV is 12 years.

Special situations

International travel
- Infants age 6–11 months: 1 dose before departure; revaccinate with 2-dose series at age 12–15 months (12 months for children in high-risk areas) and dose 2 as early as 4 weeks later.
- Unvaccinated children age 12 months or older: 2-dose series at least 4 weeks apart before departure

Meningococcal serogroup A,C,W,Y vaccination
(minimum age: 2 months [MenACWY-CRM, Menveo], 9 months [MenACWY-D, Menactra], 2 years [MenACWY-TT, MenQuadfi])

Routine vaccination
- 2-dose series at 11–12 years, 16 years

Catch-up vaccination
- Age 13–15 years: 1 dose now and booster at age 16–18 years (minimum interval: 8 weeks)
- Age 16–18 years: 1 dose

Special situations

Anatomic or functional asplenia (including sickle cell disease), HIV infection, persistent complement component deficiency, complement inhibitor (e.g., eculizumab, ravulizumab) use:
- **Menveo**
  - Dose 1 at age 8 weeks: 4-dose series at 2, 4, 6, 12 months
  - Dose 1 at age 3–6 months: 3- or 4-dose series (dose 2 [and dose 3 if applicable] at least 8 weeks after previous dose until a dose is received at age 7 months or older, followed by an additional dose at least 12 weeks later and after age 12 months)
  - Dose 1 at age 7–23 months: 2-dose series (dose 2 at least 12 weeks after dose 1 and after age 12 months)
  - Dose 1 at age 24 months or older: 2-dose series at least 8 weeks apart
- **Menactra**
  - **Persistent complement component deficiency or complement inhibitor use:**
    - Age 9–23 months: 2-dose series at least 12 weeks apart
    - Age 24 months or older: 2-dose series at least 8 weeks apart
  - **Anatomic or functional asplenia, sickle cell disease, or HIV infection:**
    - Age 9–23 months: Not recommended
    - Age 24 months or older: 2-dose series at least 8 weeks apart
    - Menactra must be administered at least 4 weeks after completion of PCV13 series.

- **MenQuadfi**
  - Dose 1 at age 24 months or older: 2-dose series at least 8 weeks apart

Travel in countries with hyperendemic or epidemic meningococcal disease, including countries in the African meningitis belt or during the Hajj (www.cdc.gov/travel/):
- Children less than age 24 months:
  - **Menveo (age 2–23 months)**
    - Dose 1 at age 8 weeks: 4-dose series at 2, 4, 6, 12 months
    - Dose 1 at age 3–6 months: 3- or 4-dose series (dose 2 [and dose 3 if applicable] at least 8 weeks after previous dose until a dose is received at age 7 months or older, followed by an additional dose at least 12 weeks later and after age 12 months)
  - **Menactra (age 9–23 months)**
    - 2-dose series (dose 2 at least 12 weeks after dose 1; dose 2 may be administered as early as 8 weeks after dose 1 in travelers)
- Children age 2 years or older: 1 dose Menveo, Menactra, or MenQuadfi

First-year college students who live in residential housing (if not previously vaccinated at age 16 years or older) or military recruits:
- 1 dose Menveo, Menactra, or MenQuadfi

Adolescent vaccination of children who received MenACWY prior to age 10 years:
- **Children for whom boosters are recommended** because of an ongoing increased risk of meningococcal disease (e.g., those with complement deficiency, HIV, or asplenia): Follow the booster schedule for persons at increased risk.
- **Children for whom boosters are not recommended** (e.g., a healthy child who received a single dose for travel to a country where meningococcal disease is endemic): Administer MenACWY according to the recommended adolescent schedule with dose 1 at age 11–12 years and dose 2 at age 16 years.

Note: Menactra should be administered either before or at the same time as DTaP. For MenACWY **booster dose** recommendations for groups listed under "Special situations" and in an outbreak setting and additional meningococcal vaccination information, see www.cdc.gov/mmwr/volumes/69/rr/rr6909a1.htm.

Meningococcal serogroup B vaccination
(minimum age: 10 years [MenB-4C, Bexsero; MenB-FHbp, Trumenba])

Shared clinical decision-making
- **Adolescents not at increased risk** age 16–23 years (preferred age 16–18 years) based on shared clinical decision-making:
  - **Bexsero:** 2-dose series at least 1 month apart
  - **Trumenba:** 2-dose series at least 6 months apart; if dose 2 is administered earlier than 6 months, administer a 3rd dose at least 4 months after dose 2.

Special situations

Anatomic or functional asplenia (including sickle cell disease), persistent complement component deficiency, complement inhibitor (e.g., eculizumab, ravulizumab) use:
- **Bexsero:** 2-dose series at least 1 month apart
- **Trumenba:** 3-dose series at 0, 1–2, 6 months

Bexsero and Trumenba are not interchangeable; the same product should be used for all doses in a series.

For MenB **booster dose recommendations** for groups listed under "Special situations" and in an outbreak setting and additional meningococcal vaccination information, see www.cdc.gov/mmwr/volumes/69/rr/rr6909a1.htm.

Pneumococcal vaccination
(minimum age: 6 weeks [PCV13], 2 years [PPSV23])

Routine vaccination with PCV13
- 4-dose series at 2, 4, 6, 12–15 months

Catch-up vaccination with PCV13
- 1 dose for healthy children age 24–59 months with any incomplete* PCV13 series
- For other catch-up guidance, see Table 2.

Special situations

Underlying conditions below: When both PCV13 and PPSV23 are indicated, administer PCV13 first. PCV13 and PPSV23 should not be administered during same visit.

Chronic heart disease (particularly cyanotic congenital heart disease and cardiac failure); chronic lung disease (including asthma treated with high-dose, oral corticosteroids); diabetes mellitus:

Age 2–5 years
- Any incomplete* series with:
  - 3 PCV13 doses: 1 dose PCV13 (at least 8 weeks after any prior PCV13 dose)
  - Less than 3 PCV13 doses: 2 doses PCV13 (8 weeks after the most recent dose and administered 8 weeks apart)
- No history of PPSV23: 1 dose PPSV23 (at least 8 weeks after completing all recommended PCV13 doses)

Age 6–18 years
- No history of PPSV23: 1 dose PPSV23 (at least 8 weeks after completing all recommended PCV13 doses)

Cerebrospinal fluid leak, cochlear implant:

Age 2–5 years
- Any incomplete* series with:
  - 3 PCV13 doses: 1 dose PCV13 (at least 8 weeks after any prior PCV13 dose)
  - Less than 3 PCV13 doses: 2 doses PCV13 (8 weeks after the most recent dose and administered 8 weeks apart)
- No history of PPSV23: 1 dose PPSV23 (at least 8 weeks after any prior PCV13 dose)

Age 6–18 years
- No history of either PCV13 or PPSV23: 1 dose PCV13, 1 dose PPSV23 at least 8 weeks later
- Any PCV13 but no PPSV23: 1 dose PPSV23 at least 8 weeks after the most recent dose of PCV13
- PPSV23 but no PCV13: 1 dose PCV13 at least 8 weeks after the most recent dose of PPSV23

Notes Recommended Child and Adolescent Immunization Schedule for ages 18 years or younger, United States, 2021

Sickle cell disease and other hemoglobinopathies; anatomic or functional asplenia; congenital or acquired immunodeficiency; HIV infection; chronic renal failure; nephrotic syndrome; malignant neoplasms, leukemias, lymphomas, Hodgkin disease, and other diseases associated with treatment with immunosuppressive drugs or radiation therapy; solid organ transplantation; multiple myeloma:

Age 2–5 years
- Any incomplete* series with:
  - 3 PCV13 doses: 1 dose PCV13 (at least 8 weeks after any prior PCV13 dose)
  - Less than 3 PCV13 doses: 2 doses PCV13 (8 weeks after the most recent dose and administered 8 weeks apart)
- No history of PPSV23: 1 dose PPSV23 (at least 8 weeks after any prior PCV13 dose) and a 2nd dose of PPSV23 5 years later

Age 6–18 years
- No history of either PCV13 or PPSV23: 1 dose PCV13, 2 doses PPSV23 (dose 1 of PPSV23 administered 8 weeks after PCV13 and dose 2 of PPSV23 administered at least 5 years after dose 1 of PPSV23)
- Any PCV13 but no PPSV23: 2 doses PPSV23 (dose 1 of PPSV23 administered 8 weeks after the most recent dose of PCV13 and dose 2 of PPSV23 administered at least 5 years after dose 1 of PPSV23)
- PPSV23 but no PCV13: 1 dose PCV13 at least 8 weeks after the most recent PPSV23 dose and a 2nd dose of PPSV23 administered 5 years after dose 1 of PPSV23 and at least 8 weeks after a dose of PCV13

Chronic liver disease, alcoholism:

Age 6–18 years
- No history of PPSV23: 1 dose PPSV23 (at least 8 weeks after any prior PCV13 dose)

Incomplete series = Not having received all doses in either the recommended series or an age-appropriate catch-up series See Tables 8, 9, and 11 in the ACIP pneumococcal vaccine recommendations (www.cdc.gov/mmwr/pdf/rr/rr5911.pdf) for complete schedule details.

Poliovirus vaccination
(minimum age: 6 weeks)

Routine vaccination
- 4-dose series at ages 2, 4, 6–18 months, 4–6 years; administer the final dose on or after age 4 years and at least 6 months after the previous dose.
- 4 or more doses of IPV can be administered before age 4 years when a combination vaccine containing IPV is used. However, a dose is still recommended on or after age 4 years and at least 6 months after the previous dose.

Catch-up vaccination
- In the first 6 months of life, use minimum ages and intervals only for travel to a polio-endemic region or during an outbreak.
- IPV is not routinely recommended for U.S. residents age 18 years or older.

Series containing oral polio vaccine (OPV), either mixed OPV-IPV or OPV-only series:
- Total number of doses needed to complete the series is the same as that recommended for the U.S. IPV schedule. See www.cdc.gov/mmwr/volumes/66/wr/mm6601a6.htm?s_%20 cid=mm6601a6_w.
- Only trivalent OPV (tOPV) counts toward the U.S. vaccination requirements.
  - Doses of OPV administered before April 1, 2016, should be counted (unless specifically noted as administered during a campaign).
  - Doses of OPV administered on or after April 1, 2016, should not be counted.
- For guidance to assess doses documented as "OPV," see www.cdc.gov/mmwr/volumes/66/wr/mm6606a7.htm?s_ cid=mm6606a7_w.
- For other catch-up guidance, see Table 2.

Rotavirus vaccination
(minimum age: 6 weeks)

Routine vaccination
- **Rotarix:** 2-dose series at 2 and 4 months
- **RotaTeq:** 3-dose series at 2, 4, and 6 months
- If any dose in the series is either **RotaTeq** or unknown, default to 3-dose series.

Catch-up vaccination
- Do not start the series on or after age 15 weeks, 0 days.
- The maximum age for the final dose is 8 months, 0 days.
- For other catch-up guidance, see Table 2.

Tetanus, diphtheria, and pertussis (Tdap) vaccination
(minimum age: 11 years for routine vaccination, 7 years for catch-up vaccination)

Routine vaccination
- **Adolescents age 11–12 years:** 1 dose Tdap
- **Pregnancy:** 1 dose Tdap during each pregnancy, preferably in early part of gestational weeks 27–36
- Tdap may be administered regardless of the interval since the last tetanus- and diphtheria-toxoid-containing vaccine.

Catch-up vaccination
- **Adolescents age 13–18 years who have not received Tdap:** 1 dose Tdap, then Td or Tdap booster every 10 years
- **Persons age 7–18 years not fully vaccinated with DTaP:** 1 dose Tdap as part of the catch-up series (preferably the first dose); if additional doses are needed, use Td or Tdap.
- **Tdap administered at age 7–10 years:**
  - **Children age 7–9 years** who receive Tdap should receive the routine Tdap dose at age 11–12 years.
  - **Children age 10 years** who receive Tdap do not need the routine Tdap dose at age 11–12 years.
- **DTaP inadvertently administered on or after age 7 years:**
  - **Children age 7–9 years:** DTaP may count as part of catch-up series. Administer routine Tdap dose at age 11–12 years.
  - **Children age 10–18 years:** Count dose of DTaP as the adolescent Tdap booster.
- For catch-up guidance, see Table 2.

Special situations
- **Wound management in persons age 7 years or older** with history of 3 or more doses of tetanus-toxoid-containing vaccine: For clean and minor wounds, administer Tdap or Td if more than 10 years since last dose of tetanus-toxoid-containing vaccine; for all other wounds, administer Tdap or Td if more than 5 years since last dose of tetanus-toxoid-containing vaccine. Tdap is preferred for persons age 11 years or older who have not previously received Tdap or whose Tdap history is unknown. If a tetanus-toxoid-containing vaccine is indicated for a pregnant adolescent, use Tdap.
- For detailed information, see www.cdc.gov/mmwr/volumes/69/wr/mm6903a5.htm.

Fully vaccinated = 5 valid doses of DTaP OR 4 valid doses of DTaP if dose 4 was administered at age 4 years or older

Varicella vaccination
(minimum age: 12 months)

Routine vaccination
- 2-dose series at 12–15 months, 4–6 years
- Dose 2 may be administered as early as 3 months after dose 1 (a dose administered after a 4-week interval may be counted).

Catch-up vaccination
- Ensure persons age 7–18 years without evidence of immunity (see MMWR at www.cdc.gov/mmwr/pdf/rr/rr5604.pdf) have a 2-dose series:
  - **Age 7–12 years:** routine interval: 3 months (a dose administered after a 4-week interval may be counted)
  - **Age 13 years and older:** routine interval: 4–8 weeks (minimum interval: 4 weeks)
  - The maximum age for use of MMRV is 12 years.

Source: https://www.cdc.gov/vaccines/schedules/hcp/imz/child-adolescent.html.

CDC VACCINE SCHEDULES FOR ADULTS

Figure 4. Recommended immunization schedule for adults aged 19 y or older by age group, United States, 2021.

Vaccine	19–26 years	27–49 years	50–64 years	≥65 years
Influenza inactivated (IIV) or Influenza recombinant (RIV4)	1 dose annually			
Influenza live, attenuated (LAIV4)	1 dose annually			
Tetanus, diphtheria, pertussis (Tdap or Td)	1 dose Tdap each pregnancy; 1 dose Td/Tdap for wound management (see notes) 1 dose Tdap, then Td or Tdap booster every 10 years			
Measles, mumps, rubella (MMR)	1 or 2 doses depending on indication (if born in 1957 or later)			
Varicella (VAR)	2 doses (if born in 1980 or later)		2 doses	
Zoster recombinant (RZV)			2 doses	
Human papillomavirus (HPV)	2 or 3 doses depending on age at initial vaccination or condition	27 through 45 years		
Pneumococcal conjugate (PCV13)		1 dose		1 dose
Pneumococcal polysaccharide (PPSV23)	1 or 2 doses depending on indication			1 dose
Hepatitis A (HepA)	2 or 3 doses depending on vaccine			
Hepatitis B (HepB)	2 or 3 doses depending on vaccine			
Meningococcal A, C, W, Y (MenACWY)	1 or 2 doses depending on indication, see notes for booster recommendations			
Meningococcal B (MenB)	19 through 23 years	2 or 3 doses depending on vaccine and indication, see notes for booster recommendations		
Haemophilus influenzae type b (Hib)	1 or 3 doses depending on indication			

Recommended vaccination for adults who meet age requirement, lack documentation of vaccination, or lack evidence of past infection

Recommended vaccination for adults with an additional risk factor or another indication

Recommended vaccination based on shared clinical decision-making

No recommendation/ Not applicable

Vaccine	Pregnancy	Immuno-compromised (excluding HIV infection)	HIV infection CD4 count <200 mm³	HIV infection CD4 count ≥200 mm³	Asplenia, complement deficiencies	End-stage renal disease; or on hemodialysis	Heart or lung disease, alcoholism¹	Chronic liver disease	Diabetes	Health care personnel²	Men who have sex with men
HIV or RIV4 — or — LAIV4		Not Recommended				1 dose annually				— or — 1 dose annually	
Tdap or Td	1 dose Tdap each pregnancy				1 dose Tdap, then Td or Tdap booster every 10 years	Precaution					
MMR	Not Recommended*	Not Recommended			1 or 2 doses depending on indication						
VAR	Not Recommended*	Not Recommended			2 doses						
RZV					2 doses at age ≥50 years						
HPV	Not Recommended*	3 doses through age 26 years			2 or 3 doses through age 26 years depending on age at initial vaccination or condition						
PCV13					1 dose						
PPSV23					1, 2, or 3 doses depending on age and indication						
HepA					2 or 3 doses depending on vaccine						
HepB					2, 3, or 4 doses depending on vaccine or condition			<60 years / ≥60 years			
MenACWY		1 or 2 doses depending on indication, see notes for booster recommendations									
MenB	Precaution	2 or 3 doses depending on vaccine and indication, see notes for booster recommendations									
Hib		3 doses HSCT³ recipients only			1 dose						

Legend:
- Recommended vaccination for adults who meet age requirement, lack documentation of vaccination, or lack evidence of past infection
- Recommended vaccination for adults with an additional risk factor or another indication
- Precaution—vaccination might be indicated if benefit of protection outweighs risk of adverse reaction
- Recommended vaccination based on shared clinical decision-making
- Not recommended/ contraindicated—vaccine should not be administered. *Vaccinate after pregnancy.
- No recommendation/ Not applicable

1. Precaution for LAIV4 does not apply to alcoholism. 2. See notes for influenza; hepatitis B; measles, mumps, and rubella; and varicella vaccinations. 3. Hematopoietic stem cell transplant.

Source: https://www.cdc.gov/vaccines/schedules/hcp/imz/adult.html

Notes

Recommended Adult Immunization Schedule for ages 19 years or older, United States, 2021

For vaccine recommendations for persons 18 years of age or younger, see the Recommended Child/Adolescent Immunization Schedule.

Additional Information

COVID-19 Vaccination

ACIP recommends use of COVID-19 vaccines within the scope of the Emergency Use Authorization or Biologics License Application for the particular vaccine. Interim ACIP recommendations for the use of COVID-19 vaccines can be found at https://www.cdc.gov/vaccines/schedules/hcp/imz/child-adolescent.html

Haemophilus influenzae type b vaccination

Special situations

Anatomical or functional asplenia (including sickle cell disease): 1 dose if previously did not receive Hib; if elective splenectomy, 1 dose, preferably at least 14 days before splenectomy

Hematopoietic stem cell transplant (HSCT): 3-dose series 4 weeks apart starting 6–12 months after successful transplant, regardless of Hib vaccination history

Hepatitis A vaccination

Routine vaccination

Not at risk but want protection from hepatitis A (identification of risk factor not required): 2-dose series HepA (Havrix 6–12 months apart or Vaqta 6–18 months apart [minimum interval: 6 months]) or 3-dose series HepA-HepB (Twinrix at 0, 1, 6 months [minimum intervals: dose 1 to dose 2: 4 weeks / dose 2 to dose 3: 5 months])

Special situations

At risk for hepatitis A virus infection: 2-dose series HepA or 3-dose series HepA-HepB as above
- **Chronic liver disease** (e.g., persons with hepatitis B, hepatitis C, cirrhosis, fatty liver disease, alcoholic liver disease, autoimmune hepatitis, alanine aminotransferase [ALT] or aspartate aminotransferase [AST] level greater than twice the upper limit of normal)
- **HIV infection**
- **Men who have sex with men**
- **Injection or noninjection drug use**

- **Persons experiencing homelessness**
- **Work with hepatitis A virus** in research laboratory or with nonhuman primates with hepatitis A virus infection
- **Travel in countries with high or intermediate endemic hepatitis A** (HepA-HepB [Twinrix] may be administered on an accelerated schedule of 3 doses at 0, 7, and 21–30 days, followed by a booster dose at 12 months)
- **Close, personal contact with international adoptee** (e.g., household or regular babysitting) in first 60 days after arrival from country with high or intermediate endemic hepatitis A (administer dose 1 as soon as adoption is planned, at least 2 weeks before adoptee's arrival)
- **Pregnancy** if at risk for infection or severe outcome from infection during pregnancy
- **Settings for exposure, including** health care settings targeting services to injection or noninjection drug users or group homes and nonresidential day care facilities for developmentally disabled persons (individual risk factor screening not required)

Hepatitis B vaccination

Routine vaccination

Not at risk but want protection from hepatitis B (identification of risk factor not required): 2- or 3-dose series (2-dose series Heplisav-B at least 4 weeks apart [2-dose series HepB only applies when 2 doses of Heplisav-B are used at least 4 weeks apart] or 3-dose series Engerix-B or Recombivax HB at 0, 1, 6 months [minimum intervals: dose 1 to dose 2: 4 weeks / dose 2 to dose 3: 8 weeks / dose 1 to dose 3: 16 weeks]) or 3-dose series HepA-HepB (Twinrix at 0, 1, 6 months [minimum intervals: dose 1 to dose 2: 4 weeks / dose 2 to dose 3: 5 months])

Special situations

At risk for hepatitis B virus infection: 2-dose (Heplisav-B) or 3-dose (Engerix-B, Recombivax HB) series or 3-dose series HepA-HepB (Twinrix) as above
- **Chronic liver disease** (e.g., persons with hepatitis C, cirrhosis, fatty liver disease, alcoholic liver disease, autoimmune hepatitis, alanine aminotransferase [ALT] or aspartate aminotransferase [AST] level greater than twice upper limit of normal)
- **HIV infection**
- **Sexual exposure risk** (e.g., sex partners of hepatitis B surface antigen [HBsAg]-positive persons; sexually active persons not in mutually monogamous relationships; persons seeking evaluation or treatment for a sexually transmitted infection; men who have sex with men)

- **Current or recent injection drug use**
- **Percutaneous or mucosal risk for exposure to blood** (e.g., household contacts of HBsAg-positive persons; residents and staff of facilities for developmentally disabled persons; health care and public safety personnel with reasonably anticipated risk for exposure to blood or blood-contaminated body fluids; hemodialysis, peritoneal dialysis, home dialysis, and predialysis patients; persons with diabetes mellitus age younger than 60 years, shared clinical decision-making for persons age 60 years or older)
- **Incarcerated persons**
- **Travel in countries with high or intermediate endemic hepatitis B**
- **Pregnancy** if at risk for infection or severe outcome from infection during pregnancy (Heplisav-B not currently recommended due to lack of safety data in pregnant women)

Human papillomavirus vaccination

Routine vaccination

HPV vaccination recommended for all persons through age 26 years: 2- or 3-dose series depending on age at initial vaccination or condition:
- **Age 15 years or older at initial vaccination:** 3-dose series at 0, 1–2 months, 6 months (minimum intervals: dose 1 to dose 2: 4 weeks / dose 2 to dose 3: 12 weeks / dose 1 to dose 3: 5 months; repeat dose if administered too soon)
- **Age 9–14 years at initial vaccination and received 1 dose or 2 doses less than 5 months apart:** 1 additional dose
- **Age 9–14 years at initial vaccination and received 2 doses at least 5 months apart:** HPV vaccination series complete, no additional dose needed

Interrupted schedules: If vaccination schedule is interrupted, the series does not need to be restarted

No additional dose recommended after completing series with recommended dosing intervals using any HPV vaccine

Shared clinical decision-making

Some adults age 27–45 years: Based on shared clinical decision-making, 2- or 3-dose series as above

Special situations

Age ranges recommended above for routine and catch-up vaccination or shared clinical decision-making also apply in special situations

Notes   Recommended Adult Immunization Schedule, United States, 2021

- **Immunocompromising conditions, including HIV infection:** 3-dose series as above, regardless of age at initial vaccination
- **Pregnancy:** HPV vaccination not recommended until after pregnancy; no intervention needed if vaccinated while pregnant; pregnancy testing not needed before vaccination

Influenza vaccination

Routine vaccination

- **Persons age 6 months or older:** 1 dose any influenza vaccine appropriate for age and health status annually
- For additional guidance, see www.cdc.gov/flu/professionals/index.htm

Special situations

- **Egg allergy, hives only:** 1 dose any influenza vaccine appropriate for age and health status annually
- **Egg allergy—any symptom other than hives** (e.g., angioedema, respiratory distress): 1 dose any influenza vaccine appropriate for age and health status annually. If using an influenza vaccine other than RIV4 or ccIIV4, administer in medical setting under supervision of health care provider who can recognize and manage severe allergic reactions.
- Severe allergic reactions to any vaccine can occur even in the absence of a history of previous allergic reaction. Therefore, all vaccine providers should be familiar with the office emergency plan and certified in cardiopulmonary resuscitation.
- A previous severe allergic reaction to any influenza vaccine is a contraindication to future receipt of the vaccine.
- **LAIV4 should not be used** in persons with the following conditions or situations:
  - History of severe allergic reaction to any vaccine component (excluding egg) or to a previous dose of any influenza vaccine
  - Immunocompromised due to any cause (including medications and HIV infection)
  - Anatomic or functional asplenia
  - Close contacts or caregivers of severely immunosuppressed persons who require a protected environment
  - Pregnancy
  - Cranial CSF/oropharyngeal communications
  - Cochlear implant

- Received influenza antiviral medications oseltamivir or zanamivir within the previous 48 hours, peramivir within the previous 5 days, or baloxavir within the previous 17 days
  - Adults 50 years or older
- **History of Guillain-Barré syndrome within 6 weeks after previous dose of influenza vaccine:** Generally, should not be vaccinated unless vaccination benefits outweigh risks for those at higher risk for severe complications from influenza

Measles, mumps, and rubella vaccination

Routine vaccination

- **No evidence of immunity to measles, mumps, or rubella:** 1 dose
  - **Evidence of immunity:** Born before 1957 (health care personnel, see below), documentation of receipt of MMR vaccine, laboratory evidence of immunity or disease (diagnosis of disease without laboratory confirmation is not evidence of immunity)

Special situations

- **Pregnancy with no evidence of immunity to rubella:** MMR contraindicated during pregnancy; after pregnancy (before discharge from health care facility), 1 dose
- **Nonpregnant women of childbearing age with no evidence of immunity to rubella:** 1 dose
- **HIV infection with CD4 count ≥200 cells/mm³ for at least 6 months and no evidence of immunity to measles, mumps, or rubella:** 2-dose series at least 4 weeks apart; MMR contraindicated for HIV infection with CD4 count <200 cells/mm³
- **Severe immunocompromising conditions:** MMR contraindicated
- **Students in postsecondary educational institutions, international travelers, and household or close, personal contacts of immunocompromised persons with no evidence of immunity to measles, mumps, or rubella:** 2-dose series at least 4 weeks apart if previously did not receive any doses of MMR or 1 dose if previously received 1 dose MMR
- **Health care personnel:**
  - Born in 1957 or later with no evidence of immunity to measles, mumps, or rubella: 2-dose series at least 4 weeks apart for measles or mumps or at least 1 dose for rubella

- Born before 1957 with no evidence of immunity to measles, mumps, or rubella: Consider 2-dose series at least 4 weeks apart for measles or mumps or 1 dose for rubella

Meningococcal vaccination

Special situations for MenACWY

- **Anatomic or functional asplenia (including sickle cell disease), HIV infection, persistent complement component deficiency, complement inhibitor (e.g., eculizumab, ravulizumab) use:** 2-dose series MenACWY-D (Menactra, Menveo or MenQuadfi) at least 8 weeks apart and revaccinate every 5 years if risk remains
- **Travel in countries with hyperendemic or epidemic meningococcal disease, microbiologists routinely exposed to Neisseria meningitidis:** 1 dose MenACWY (Menactra, Menveo, or MenQuadfi) and revaccinate every 5 years if risk remains
- **First-year college students who live in residential housing (if not previously vaccinated at age 16 years or older) and military recruits:** 1 dose MenACWY (Menactra, Menveo, or MenQuadfi)
- For MenACWY booster dose recommendations for groups listed under "Special situations" and in an outbreak setting (e.g., in community or organizational settings and among men who have sex with men) and additional meningococcal vaccination information, see www.cdc.gov/mmwr/volumes/69/rr/rr6909a1.htm

Shared clinical decision-making for MenB

- **Adolescents and young adults age 16–23 years (age 16–18 years preferred) not at increased risk for meningococcal disease:** Based on shared clinical decision-making, 2-dose series MenB-4C (Bexsero) at least 1 month apart or 2-dose series MenB-FHbp (Trumenba) at 0, 6 months (if dose 2 was administered less than 6 months after dose 1, administer dose 3 at least 4 months after dose 2); MenB-4C and MenB-FHbp are not interchangeable (use same product for all doses in series)

Special situations for MenB

- **Anatomic or functional asplenia (including sickle cell disease), persistent complement component deficiency, complement inhibitor (e.g., eculizumab, ravulizumab) use, microbiologists routinely exposed to Neisseria meningitidis:** 2-dose primary series MenB-4C (Bexsero) at least one month apart or MenB-4C (Bexsero) at least 1 month apart or

Notes Recommended Adult Immunization Schedule, United States, 2021

- 3-dose primary series MenB-FHbp (Trumenba) at 0, 1–2, 6 months (if dose 2 was administered at least 6 months after dose 1, dose 3 not needed); MenB-4C and MenB-FHbp are not interchangeable (use same product for all doses in series); 1 dose MenB booster 1 year after primary series and revaccinate every 2–3 years if risk remains
- **Pregnancy:** Delay MenB until after pregnancy unless at increased risk and vaccination benefits outweigh potential risks
- For MenB **booster dose recommendations** for groups listed under "Special situations" and in an outbreak setting (e.g., in community or organizational settings and among men who have sex with men) and additional meningococcal vaccination information, see www.cdc.gov/ mmwr/volumes/69/rr/rr6909a1.htm

Source: https://www.cdc.gov/vaccines/schedules/hcp/imz/child-adolescent.html

Figure 5. Recommended immunization schedule for adults aged 19 years or older by medical condition and other indications, United States, 2021.

Pneumococcal vaccination

Routine vaccination
- **Age 65 years or older** (immunocompetent— see www.cdc.gov/mmwr/volumes/68/wr/mm6846a5. htm?s_cid=mm6846a5_w): 1 dose PPSV23
  - If PPSV23 was administered prior to age 65 years, administer 1 dose PPSV23 at least 5 years after previous dose

Shared clinical decision-making
- **Age 65 years or older** (immunocompetent): 1 dose PCV13 based on **shared clinical decision-making** if previously not administered.
  - PCV13 and PPSV23 should not be administered during the same visit
  - If both PCV13 and PPSV23 are to be administered, PCV13 should be administered first
  - PCV13 and PPSV23 should be administered at least 1 year apart

Special situations
(www.cdc.gov/mmwr/preview/mmwrhtml/mm6140a4.htm)
- **Age 19–64 years with chronic medical conditions** (chronic heart [excluding hypertension], lung, or liver disease, diabetes), alcoholism, or cigarette smoking: 1 dose PPSV23

- **Age 19 years or older with immunocompromising conditions** (congenital or acquired immunodeficiency [including B- and T-lymphocyte deficiency, complement deficiencies, phagocytic disorders, HIV infection], chronic renal failure, nephrotic syndrome, leukemia, lymphoma, Hodgkin disease, generalized malignancy, iatrogenic immunosuppression [e.g., drug or radiation therapy], solid organ transplant, multiple myeloma) or anatomical or functional asplenia (including sickle cell disease and other hemoglobinopathies): 1 dose PCV13 followed by 1 dose PPSV23 at least 8 weeks later, then another dose PPSV23 at least 5 years after previous PPSV23; at age 65 years or older, administer 1 dose PPSV23 at least 5 years after most recent PPSV23 (note: only 1 dose PPSV23 recommended at age 65 years or older)
- **Age 19 years or older with cerebrospinal fluid leak or cochlear implant:** 1 dose PCV13 followed by 1 dose PPSV23 at least 8 weeks later; at age 65 years or older, administer another dose PPSV23 at least 5 years after PPSV23 (note: only 1 dose PPSV23 recommended at age 65 years or older)

Tetanus, diphtheria, and pertussis vaccination

Routine vaccination
- **Previously did not receive Tdap at or after age 11 years:** 1 dose Tdap, then Td or Tdap every 10 years

Special situations
- **Previously did not receive primary vaccination series for tetanus, diphtheria, or pertussis:** At least 1 dose Tdap followed by 1 dose Td or Tdap at least 4 weeks after Tdap and another dose Td or Tdap 6–12 months after last Td or Tdap (Tdap can be substituted for any Td dose, but preferred as first dose), Td or Tdap every 10 years thereafter
- **Pregnancy:** 1 dose Tdap during each pregnancy, preferably in early part of gestational weeks 27–36
- **Wound management:** Persons with 3 or more doses of tetanus-toxoid-containing vaccine: For clean and minor wounds, administer Tdap or Td if more than 10 years since last dose of tetanus-toxoid-containing vaccine; for all other wounds, administer Tdap or Td if more than 5 years since last dose of tetanus-toxoid-containing vaccine. Tdap is preferred for persons who have not previously received Tdap or whose Tdap history is unknown. If a tetanus-toxoid-containing vaccine is indicated for a pregnant woman, use Tdap. For detailed information, see www.cdc.gov/mmwr/volumes/69/wr/mm6903a5.htm

Varicella vaccination

Routine vaccination
- **No evidence of immunity to varicella:** 2-dose series 4–8 weeks apart if previously did not receive varicella-containing vaccine (VAR or MMRV [measles-mumps-rubella-varicella vaccine] for children); if previously received 1 dose varicella-containing vaccine, 1 dose at least 4 weeks after first dose
  - Evidence of immunity: U.S.-born before 1980 (except for pregnant women and health care personnel [see below]), documentation of 2 doses varicella-containing vaccine at least 4 weeks apart, diagnosis or verification of history of varicella or herpes zoster by a health care provider, laboratory evidence of immunity or disease

Special situations
- **Pregnancy with no evidence of immunity to varicella:** VAR contraindicated during pregnancy; after pregnancy (before discharge from health care facility), 1 dose if previously received 1 dose varicella-containing vaccine or dose 1 of 2-dose series (dose 2: 4–8 weeks later) if previously did not receive any varicella-containing vaccine, regardless of whether U.S.-born before 1980
- **Health care personnel with no evidence of immunity to varicella:** 1 dose if previously received 1 dose varicella-containing vaccine; 2-dose series 4–8 weeks apart if previously did not receive any varicella-containing vaccine, regardless of whether U.S.-born before 1980
- **HIV infection with CD4 count ≥200 cells/mm³ with no evidence of immunity:** Vaccination may be considered (2 doses 3 months apart); VAR contraindicated for HIV infection with CD4 count <200 cells/mm³
- **Severe immunocompromising conditions:** VAR contraindicated

Zoster vaccination

Routine vaccination
- **Age 50 years or older:** 2-dose series RZV (Shingrix) 2–6 months apart (minimum interval: 4 weeks; repeat dose if administered too soon), regardless of previous herpes zoster or history of zoster vaccine live (ZVL, Zostavax) vaccination (administer RZV at least 2 months after ZVL)

Special situations
- **Pregnancy:** Consider delaying RZV until after pregnancy if RZV is otherwise indicated.
- **Severe immunocompromising conditions (including HIV infection with CD4 count <200 cells/mm³):** Recommended use of RZV under review

Source: https://www.cdc.gov/vaccines/schedules/hcp/imz/adult.html.

MODIFIED CHECKLIST FOR AUTISM IN TODDLERS, REVISED WITH FOLLOW-UP (M-CHAT-R/F)

MODIFIED CHECKLIST FOR AUTISM IN TODDLERS, REVISED WITH FOLLOW-UP (M-CHAT-R/F)	
Instructions: Please answer these questions about your child. Keep in mind how your child usually behaves. If you have seen your child do the behavior a few times, but he or she does not usually do it, then please answer no. Please circle YES or NO for every question. Thank you very much!	
1. If you point at something across the room, does your child look at it? (FOR EXAMPLE, if you point at a toy or an animal, does your child look at the toy or animal?)	YES or NO
2. Have you ever wondered if your child might be deaf?	YES or NO
3. Does your child play pretend or make-believe? (FOR EXAMPLE, pretend to drink from an empty cup, pretend to talk on a phone, or pretend to feed a doll or stuffed animal?)	YES or NO
4. Does your child like climbing on things? (FOR EXAMPLE, furniture, playground equipment, or stairs)	YES or NO

MODIFIED CHECKLIST FOR AUTISM IN TODDLERS, REVISED WITH FOLLOW-UP (M-CHAT-R/F)   (Continued)

5. Does your child make unusual finger movements near his or her eyes? (FOR EXAMPLE, does your child wiggle his or her fingers close to his or her eyes?)	YES or NO
6. Does your child point with one finger to ask for something or to get help? (FOR EXAMPLE, pointing to a snack or a toy that is out of reach)	YES or NO
7. Does your child point with one finger to show you something interesting? (FOR EXAMPLE, pointing to an airplane in the sky or a big truck in the road)	YES or NO
8. Is your child interested in other children? (FOR EXAMPLE, does your child watch other children, smile at them, or go to them?)	YES or NO
9. Does your child show you things by bringing them to you or holding them up for you to see—not to get help, but just to share? (FOR EXAMPLE, showing you a flower, a stuffed animal, or a toy truck)	YES or NO
10. Does your child respond when you call his or her name? (FOR EXAMPLE, does he or she look up, talk or babble, or stop what he or she is doing when you call his or her name?)	YES or NO
11. When you smile at your child, does he or she smile back at you?	YES or NO
12. Does your child get upset by everyday noises? (FOR EXAMPLE, does your child scream or cry to noise such as a vacuum cleaner or loud music?)	YES or NO
13. Does your child walk?	YES or NO
14. Does your child look you in the eye when you are talking to him or her, playing with him or her, or dressing him or her?	YES or NO
15. Does your child try to copy what you do? (FOR EXAMPLE, wave bye-bye, clap, or make a funny noise when you do)	YES or NO
16. If you turn your head to look at something, does your child look around to see what you are looking at?	YES or NO
17. Does your child try to get you to watch him or her? (FOR EXAMPLE, does your child look at you for praise, or say "look" or "watch me"?)	YES or NO
18. Does your child understand when you tell him or her to do something? (FOR EXAMPLE, if you don't point, can your child understand "put the book on the chair" or "bring me the blanket"?)	YES or NO
19. If something new happens, does your child look at your face to see how you feel about it? (FOR EXAMPLE, if he or she hears a strange or funny noise, or sees a new toy, will he or she look at your face?)	YES or NO
20. Does your child like movement activities? (FOR EXAMPLE, being swung or bounced on your knee)	YES or NO

Scoring: For all items except 2, 5, and 12, "NO" response indicates autism spectrum disorder risk.
Low-risk: 0–2; no further action required.
Medium-risk: 3–7; administer the follow-up (M-CHAT-R/F); if score remains ≥2, screening is positive.
High-risk: ≥8; refer immediately for diagnostic evaluation and early intervention.
Source: Reproduced with permission. © 2009 Diana Robins, Deborah Fein, & Marianne Barton. Follow-up questions and additional information can be found at www.mchatscreen.com.

SCREENING INSTRUMENTS: ALCOHOL ABUSE

SENSITIVITY AND SPECIFICITY OF SCREENING TESTS FOR PROBLEM DRINKING

Instrument Name	Screening Questions/Scoring	Threshold Score	Sensitivity/Specificity (%)	Source
CAGE[a]	See page 718	>1 >2[b] >3	77/58 53/81 29/92	*Am J Psychiatry.* 1974;131:1121 *J Gen Intern Med.* 1998;13:379
AUDIT	See page 718	>4 >5[b] >6	87/70 77/84 66/90	*BMJ.* 1997;314:420 *J Gen Intern Med.* 1998;13:379

[a]The CAGE may be less applicable to binge drinkers (eg, college students), the elderly, and minority populations.
[b]A CAGE score of 2 or an AUDIT score of 5 are generally accepted as "positive" screens.

SCREENING INSTRUMENTS: DEPRESSION

Instrument Name	Screening Questions/Scoring	Threshold Score	Source
Beck Depression Inventory (short form)	See page 584	0–4: None or minimal depression 5–7: Mild depression 8–15: Moderate depression >15: Severe depression	*Postgrad Med.* 1972;81
Geriatric Depression Scale	See page 564	≥15: Depression	*J Psychiatr Res.* 1983;17:37
PRIME-MD© (mood questions)	1. During the last month, have you often been bothered by feeling down, depressed, or hopeless? 2. During the last month, have you often been bothered by little interest or pleasure in doing things?	"Yes" to either question[a]	*JAMA.* 1994;272:1749 *J Gen Intern Med.* 1997;12:439

SCREENING INSTRUMENTS: DEPRESSION

| Patient Health Questionnaire (PHQ-9)© | http://www.pfizer.com/phq-9/ See page 721 | *Major depressive syndrome:* if answers to #1a or b and ≥5 of #1a–i are at least "More than half the days" (count #1i if present at all) *Other depressive syndrome:* if #1a or b and 2–4 of #1a–i are at least "More than half the days" (count #1i if present at all) 5–9: mild depression 10–14: moderate depression 15–19: moderately severe depression 20–27: severe depression | *JAMA.* 1999;282:1737 *J Gen Intern Med.* 2001;16:606 |

[a]Sensitivity 86%–96%; specificity 57%–75%.
Source: Pfizer Inc.

SCREENING INSTRUMENTS: DEPRESSION

PHQ-9 DEPRESSION SCREEN, ENGLISH

OVER THE PAST 2 WK, HOW OFTEN HAVE YOU BEEN BOTHERED BY ANY OF THE FOLLOWING PROBLEMS?

	Not at All	Several Days	>Half the Days	Nearly Every Day
a. Little interest or pleasure in doing things	0	1	2	3
b. Feeling down, depressed, or hopeless	0	1	2	3
c. Trouble falling or staying asleep, or sleeping too much	0	1	2	3
d. Feeling tired or having little energy	0	1	2	3

SCREENING INSTRUMENTS: DEPRESSION

e. Poor appetite or overeating	0	1	2	3
f. Feeling bad about yourself—or that you are a failure or that you have let yourself or your family down	0	1	2	3
g. Trouble concentrating on things, such as reading the newspaper or watching television	0	1	2	3
h. Moving or speaking so slowly that other people could have noticed? Or the opposite—being so fidgety or restless that you have been moving around a lot more than usual?	0	1	2	3
i. Thoughts that you would be better off dead or of hurting yourself in some way	0	1	2	3
For office coding: Total Score	— =	— +	— +	—

Major depressive syndrome: If ≥5 items present scored ≥2 and one of the items is depressed mood (b) or anhedonia (a). If item "i" is present, then this counts, even if score = 1.

Depressive screen positive: If at least one item ≥2 (or item "i" is ≥1).

Source: From Pfizer; Primary Care Evaluation of Mental Disorders Patient Health Questionnaire (PRIME-MD PHQ) by Dr. Robert L. et al. 1999.

SCREENING INSTRUMENTS: DEPRESSION

PHQ-9 DEPRESSION SCREEN, SPANISH

DURANTE LAS ÚLTIMAS 2 SEMANAS, ¿CON QUÉ FRECUENCIA LE HAN MOLESTADO LOS SIGUIENTES PROBLEMAS?

	Nunca	Varios dias	>La mitad de los dias	Casi todos los dias
a. Tener poco interés o placer en hacer las cosas	0	1	2	3
b. Sentirse desanimada, deprimida, o sin esperanza	0	1	2	3
c. Con problemas en dormirse o en mantenerse dormida, o en dormir demasiado	0	1	2	3
d. Sentirse cansada o tener poca energía	0	1	2	3
e. Tener poco apetito o comer en exceso	0	1	2	3
f. Sentir falta de amor propio—o qe sea un fracaso o que decepcionara a sí misma o a su familia	0	1	2	3
g. Tener dificultad para concentrarse en cosas tales como leer el periódico o mirar la televisión	0	1	2	3
h. Se mueve o habla tan lentamente que otra gente se podría dar cuenta—o de lo contrario, está tan agitada o inquieta que se mueve mucho más de lo acostumbrado	0	1	2	3
i. Se le han ocurrido pensamientos de que se haría daño de alguna manera	0	1	2	3
For office coding: Total Store	— =	— +	— +	—

Source: From Pfizer; Primary Care Evaluation of Mental Disorders Patient Health Questionnaire (PRIME-MD PHQ) by Dr. Robert L. et al. 1999.

SCREENING INSTRUMENTS: DEPRESSION

BECK DEPRESSION INVENTORY, SHORT FORM

Instructions: This is a questionnaire. On the questionnaire are groups of statements. Please read the entire group of statements in each category. Then pick out the one statement in that group that best describes the way you feel today, that is, right now! Circle the number beside the statement you have chosen. If several statements in the group seem to apply equally well, circle each one. Sum all numbers to calculate a score.

Be sure to read all the statements in each group before making your choice.

A. Sadness

3 I am so sad or unhappy that I can't stand it.
2 I am blue or sad all the time and I can't snap out of it.
1 I feel sad or blue.
0 I do not feel sad.

B. Pessimism

3 I feel that the future is hopeless and that things cannot improve.
2 I feel I have nothing to look forward to.
1 I feel discouraged about the future.
0 I am not particularly pessimistic or discouraged about the future.

C. Sense of failure

3 I feel I am a complete failure as a person (parent, husband, wife).
2 As I look back on my life, all I can see is a lot of failures.
1 I feel I have failed more than the average person.
0 I do not feel like a failure.

D. Dissatisfaction

3 I am dissatisfied with everything.
2 I don't get satisfaction out of anything anymore.
1 I don't enjoy things the way I used to.
0 I am not particularly dissatisfied.

E. Guilt

3 I feel as though I am very bad or worthless.
2 I feel quite guilty.
1 I feel bad or unworthy a good part of the time.
0 I don't feel particularly guilty.

F. Self-dislike

3 I hate myself.
2 I am disgusted with myself.
1 I am disappointed in myself.
0 I don't feel disappointed in myself.

G. Self-harm

3 I would kill myself if I had the chance.
2 I have definite plans about committing suicide.
1 I feel I would be better off dead.
0 I don't have any thoughts of harming myself.

SCREENING INSTRUMENTS: DEPRESSION (Continued)

H. Social withdrawal

3 I have lost all of my interest in other people and don't care about them at all.

2 I have lost most of my interest in other people and have little feeling for them.

1 I am less interested in other people than I used to be.

0 I have not lost interest in other people.

I. Indecisiveness

3 I can't make any decisions at all anymore.

2 I have great difficulty in making decisions.

1 I try to put off making decisions.

0 I make decisions about as well as ever.

J. Self-image change

3 I feel that I am ugly or repulsive looking.

2 I feel that there are permanent changes in my appearance and they make me look unattractive.

1 I am worried that I am looking old or unattractive.

0 I don't feel that I look worse than I used to.

K. Work difficulty

3 I can't do any work at all.

2 I have to push myself very hard to do anything.

1 It takes extra effort to get started at doing something.

0 I can work about as well as before.

L. Fatigability

3 I get too tired to do anything.

2 I get tired from doing anything.

1 I get tired more easily than I used to.

0 I don't get any more tired than usual.

M. Anorexia

3 I have no appetite at all anymore.

2 My appetite is much worse now.

1 My appetite is not as good as it used to be.

0 My appetite is no worse than usual.

Source: Reproduced with permission from Beck AT, Beck RW. Screening depressed patients in family practice: a rapid technic. *Postgrad Med.* 1972;52:81-85.

VULNERABLE SENIORS: PREVENTING ADVERSE DRUG EVENTS

For older adults, minimize exposure to potentially inappropriate medications. Below is a summary of the 2015 American Geriatric Society Beers Criteria to prevent adverse drug events in older patients.

SELECTED MEDICATIONS TO AVOID IN OLDER ADULTS

These medications carry risks specific to an older population and should be avoided except in specific situations.

Class of Medications	Reason to Avoid	Exceptions
First-Generation Antihistamines *(ie, diphenhydramine, hydroxyzine, promethazine, etc.)*	Clearance is reduced as age advances; risk of confusion and other anticholinergic effects	Diphenhydramine for acute allergic reaction may be appropriate
Antiparkinsonian agents *(ie, benztropine, trihexyphenidyl)*	More effective agents exist for Parkinson's disease	
Antispasmodics *(ie, atropine, belladonna alkaloids, dicyclomine, etc.)*	Risk of confusion and other anticholinergic effects	
Nitrofurantoin	Pulmonary, hepato-, and neurotoxicity with long-term use; safer alternatives exist for UTI ppx	
Alpha-1 blockers, peripheral *(ie, doxazosin, prazosin, terazosin)*	High risk of orthostatic hypotension	
Alpha blockers, central *(ie, clonidine, guanfacine, methyldopa)*	Risk of CNS effect, bradycardia, orthostatic hypotension	Clonidine may be appropriate in some cases as adjunctive agent in refractory HTN
Digoxin	AFib: More effective alternatives exist and mortality may increase	May be appropriate in some cases as adjunctive agent for refractory symptomatic atrial fibrillation or heart failure. If used, avoid doses >0.125 mg/d
	Heart failure: Benefit is arguable; mortality may increase	
Nifedipine	Risk of hypotension, myocardial ischemia	
Amiodarone	AFib: More toxicity than other agents	May be appropriate for rhythm control if LVH or significant heart failure
Antidepressants with anticholinergic profile *(ie, amitriptyline, nortriptyline, paroxetine)*	Sedating; orthostatic hypotension; anticholinergic effects including confusion	

VULNERABLE SENIORS: PREVENTING ADVERSE DRUG EVENTS

For older adults, minimize exposure to potentially inappropriate medications. Below is a summary of the 2015 American Geriatric Society Beers Criteria to prevent adverse drug events in older patients.

SELECTED MEDICATIONS TO AVOID IN OLDER ADULTS

Antipsychotics, first and second generation	Risk of CVA, cognitive decline	Schizophrenia, bipolar disorder
		Dementia/delirium: Only appropriate if nonpharmacologic options fail and patient threatens significant harm to self or others
Barbiturates (ie, phenobarbital, butalbital)	Risk of overdose at low dosages, dependence, escalating dose due to tolerance	
Benzodiazepines	Increased sensitivity with age, slower metabolism of longer-acting agents. Risk of cognitive impairment, falls, delirium	Seizure disorders, alcohol withdrawal, severe generalized anxiety, anesthesia
Nonbenzodiazepine hypnotics (ie, zolpidem, zaleplon, eszopiclone)	Similar to benzodiazepine risk; minimal improvement in sleep	
Androgens (ie, testosterone, methyltestosterone)	Cardiac problems; contraindicated in prostate cancer	Lab-verified symptomatic hypogonadism
Estrogen, +/− progestin	Risk of breast and endometrial cancer; no evidence for cardioprotection or cognitive protection in elderly	Vaginal estrogens safe/effective for vaginal dryness
Insulin on a sliding scale	Hypoglycemia risk; no outcome benefit in outpatient or inpatient settings	
Megestrol	Does not improve weight; higher risk of VTE and death	
Sulfonylureas of longer duration (ie, glyburide, chlorpropamide)	Severe prolonged hypoglycemia	
Metoclopramide	Extrapyramidal effects	Gastroparesis

VULNERABLE SENIORS: PREVENTING ADVERSE DRUG EVENTS

For older adults, minimize exposure to potentially inappropriate medications. Below is a summary of the 2015 American Geriatric Society Beers Criteria to prevent adverse drug events in older patients.

SELECTED MEDICATIONS TO AVOID IN OLDER ADULTS

Proton pump inhibitors	*Clostridium difficile* infection; osteopenia/osteoporosis	Short-courses (ie, <8 wk). May be appropriate to treat severe conditions such as erosive esophagitis, Barrett's esophagus, or for prevention in high-risk patients (ie, NSAID or corticosteroid use)
NSAIDs *(ie, high-dose aspirin, ibuprofen, naproxen, indomethacin, ketorolac, etc.)*	GI bleed or peptic ulcer disease. Some (ie, indomethacin, ketorolac) carry higher risk of AKI	Only use if alternative treatments are exhausted and patient can take PPI or misoprostol for gastroprotection (which reduces but does not eliminate risk)
Muscle relaxants *(ie, cyclobenzaprine, methocarbamol, carisoprodol)*	Anticholinergic effects, sedation, fracture risk; minimal efficacy	Urinary retention

Source: https://www.ncbi.nlm.nih.gov/pubmed/26446832

WHO INTEGRATED CARE FOR OLDER PEOPLE SCREENING TOOL

TABLE 1.

WHO ICOPE SCREENING TOOL

Priority conditions associated with declines in intrinsic capacity	Tests	Assess fully any domain with a checked circle
COGNITIVE DECLINE (Chapter 4)	1. Remember three words: flower, door, rice (for example)	
	2. Orientation in time and space: What is the full data today? Where are you now (home, clinic, etc.)?	◯ Wrong to either question or does not know
	3. Recalls the three words?	◯ Cannot recall all three words
LIMITED MOBILITY (Chapter 5)	Chair rise test: Rise from chair five times without using arms. Did the person complete five chair rises within 14 seconds?	◯ No
MALNUTRITION (Chapter 6)	1. Weight loss: Have you unintentionally lost more than 3 kg over the last three months?	◯ Yes
	2. Appetite loss: Have you experienced loss of appetite?	◯ Yes
VISUAL IMPAIRMENT (Chapter 7)	Do you have any problems with your eyes: difficulties in seeing far, reading, eye diseases or currently under medical treatment (eg diabetes, high blood pressure?	◯ Yes
HEARING LOSS (Chapter 8)	Hears whispers (whisper test) or Screening audiometry result is 35 dB or less or Passes automated app-based digits-in-noise test	◯ Fail
DEPRESSIVE SYMPTOMS (Chapter 9)	Over the past two weeks, have you been bothered by – feeling down, depressed or hopeless?	◯ Yes
	– little interest or pleasure in doing things?	◯ Yes

Source: Reproduced with permission from Integrated care for older people (ICOPE): Guidance for person-centred assessment and pathways in primary care. Geneva: World Health Organization; 2019 (WHO/FWC/ALC/19.1). Page 12.

WHO PAIN RELIEF LADDER

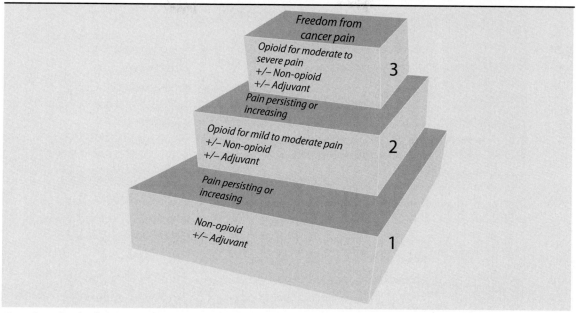

Source: Reproduced with permission of World Health Organization. https://www.who.int/cancer/palliative/painladder/en/

ORGANIZATIONS REFERENCED

PROFESSIONAL SOCIETIES AND GOVERNMENTAL AGENCIES

Abbreviation	Full Name	Internet Address
AACE	American Association of Clinical Endocrinologists	http://www.aace.com
AAD	American Academy of Dermatology	http://www.aad.org
AAFP	American Academy of Family Physicians	http://www.aafp.org
AAHPM	American Academy of Hospice and Palliative Medicine	http://www.aahpm.org
AAN	American Academy of Neurology	http://www.aan.com
AAO	American Academy of Ophthalmology	http://www.aao.org
AAO-HNS	American Academy of Otolaryngology—Head and Neck Surgery	http://www.entnet.org

PROFESSIONAL SOCIETIES AND GOVERNMENTAL AGENCIES   (*Continued*)

AAOS	American Academy of Orthopaedic Surgeons and American Association of Orthopaedic Surgeons	http://www.aaos.org
AAP	American Academy of Pediatrics	http://www.aap.org
ACC	American College of Cardiology	http://www.acc.org
ACCP	American College of Chest Physicians	http://www.chestnet.org
ACIP	Advisory Committee on Immunization Practices	http://www.cdc.gov/vaccines/acip/index.html
ACOG	American Congress of Obstetricians and Gynecologists	http://www.acog.com
ACP	American College of Physicians	http://www.acponline.org
ACR	American College of Radiology	http://www.acr.org
ACR	American College of Rheumatology	http://www.rheumatology.org
ACS	American Cancer Society	http://www.cancer.org
ACSM	American College of Sports Medicine	http://www.acsm.org
ADA	American Diabetes Association	http://www.diabetes.org
AGA	American Gastroenterological Association	http://www.gastro.org
AGS	American Geriatrics Society	http://www.americangeriatrics.org
AHA	American Heart Association	http://www.americanheart.org
ANA	American Nurses Association	http://www.nursingworld.org
AOA	American Optometric Association	http://www.aoa.org
ASA	American Stroke Association	http://www.strokeassociation.org
ASAM	American Society of Addiction Medicine	http://www.asam.org
ASCCP	American Society for Colposcopy and Cervical Pathology	http://www.asccp.org
ASCO	American Society of Clinical Oncology	http://www.asco.org
ASCRS	American Society of Colon and Rectal Surgeons	http://www.fascrs.org
ASGE	American Society for Gastrointestinal Endoscopy	http://asge.org
ASHA	American Speech-Language-Hearing Association	http://www.asha.org
ASN	American Society of Neuroimaging	http://www.asnweb.org
ATA	American Thyroid Association	http://www.thyroid.org
ATS	American Thoracic Society	http://www.thoracic.org

PROFESSIONAL SOCIETIES AND GOVERNMENTAL AGENCIES

AUA	American Urological Association	http://auanet.org
BASHH	British Association for Sexual Health and HIV	http://www.bashh.org
	Bright Futures	http://brightfutures.org
BGS	British Geriatrics Society	ihttp://www.bgs.org.uk/
BSAC	British Society for Antimicrobial Chemotherapy	http://www.bsac.org.uk
CDC	Centers for Disease Control and Prevention	http://www.cdc.gov
COG	Children's Oncology Group	http://www.childrensoncologygroup.org
CSVS	Canadian Society for Vascular Surgery	http://canadianvascular.ca
CTF	Canadian Task Force on Preventive Health Care	http://canadiantaskforce.ca
EASD	European Association for the Study of Diabetes	http://www.easd.org
EASL	European Association for the Study of the Liver	https://easl.eu
EAU	European Association of Urology	http://www.uroweb.org
ERS	European Respiratory Society	http://ersnet.org
ESC	European Society of Cardiology	http://www.escardio.org
ESH	European Society of Hypertension	http://www.eshonline.org
ARC	International Agency for Research on Cancer	http://screening.iarc.fr
ICSI	Institute for Clinical Systems Improvement	http://www.icsi.org
IDF	International Diabetes Federation	http://www.idf.org
KDIOG	Kidney Disease Improving Global Outcomes	https://kdigo.org
NAPNAP	National Association of Pediatric Nurse Practitioners	http://www.napnap.org
NCCN	National Comprehensive Cancer Network	http://www.nccn.org/cancer-guidelines.html
NCI	National Cancer Institute	http://www.cancer.gov/cancerinformation
NEI	National Eye Institute	http://www.nei.nih.gov
NGC	National Guideline Clearinghouse	http://www.guidelines.gov
NHLBI	National Heart, Lung, and Blood Institute	http://www.nhlbi.nih.gov
NIAAA	National Institute on Alcohol Abuse and Alcoholism	http://www.niaaa.nih.gov
NICE	National Institute for Health and Clinical Excellence	http://www.nice.org.uk

PROFESSIONAL SOCIETIES AND GOVERNMENTAL AGENCIES (*Continued*)		
NIDCR	National Institute of Dental and Craniofacial Research	http://www.nidr.nih.gov
NIHCDC	National Institutes of Health Consensus Development Program	http://www.consensus.nih.gov
NIP	National Immunization Program	http://www.cdc.gov/vaccines
NKF	National Kidney Foundation	http://www.kidney.org
NOF	National Osteoporosis Foundation	http://www.nof.org
NTSB	National Transportation Safety Board	http://www.ntsb.gov
SCF	Skin Cancer Foundation	http://www.skincancer.org
SGIM	Society of General Internal Medicine	http://www.sgim.org
SKI	Sloan-Kettering Institute	http://www.mskcc.org/mskcc/html/5804.cfm
SVU	Society for Vascular Ultrasound	http://www.svunet.org
UK-NHS	United Kingdom National Health Service	http://www.nhs.uk
USPSTF	United States Preventive Services Task Force	http://www.ahrq.gov/clinic/uspstfix.htm
WHO	World Health Organization	http://www.who.int/en

Index

Page references followed by "f" denote figures and "t" denote tables.